ACUTE RENAL FAILURE IN PRACTICE

ACUTE RENAL FAILURE IN PRACTICE

Paul Glynne

Andrew Allen

Charles Pusey

Imperial College of Science, Technology and Medicine
The Hammersmith Hospital
London

Imperial College Press

Published by

Imperial College Press
57 Shelton Street
Covent Garden
London WC2H 9HE

Distributed by

World Scientific Publishing Co. Pte. Ltd.
5 Toh Tuck Link, Singapore 596224
USA office: 27 Warren Street, Suite 401-402, Hackensack, NJ 07601
UK office: 57 Shelton Street, Covent Garden, London WC2H 9HE

British Library Cataloguing-in-Publication Data
A catalogue record for this book is available from the British Library.

ACUTE RENAL FAILURE IN PRACTICE

ISBN-13 978-1-86094-216-7
ISBN-10 1-86094-216-4
ISBN-13 978-1-86094-287-7 (pbk)
ISBN-10 1-86094-287-3 (pbk)

PREFACE

Acute renal failure is a relatively common medical emergency, and has been estimated to occur in up to 5% of hospital admissions. Since it may result from a wide range of disease processes, and may occur in many different clinical settings, it is likely to be encountered by physicians from all specialties. Patients will frequently require rapid and effective treatment, often before specialist help is available, so all physicians need a firm understanding of the principles of management. Although the metabolic consequences of acute renal failure are complex, and the provision of renal support is technically demanding, many aspects of the immediate management are straightforward and common to ARF resulting from different diseases. Treatment can be rewarding, because recovery of renal function is expected in the majority of patients who survive the acute illness.

The main aim of this volume is to review current practice in the treatment of acute renal failure, bearing in mind that this depends on a thorough understanding of disease mechanisms. The book therefore starts with consideration of normal renal physiology, and of the pathophysiology of acute renal failure. This is followed by a review of the general principles of diagnosis and management. The major causes of acute renal failure are then discussed individually; each of these chapters starts with a brief review of underlying disease mechanisms, which leads on to recommendations for treatment. There is a separate section with chapters on the development of acute renal failure in particular clinical settings, such as the Obstetric Unit or Intensive Care Unit. Each chapter is illustrated by clear tables and diagrams, and includes "practice points" which detail specific approaches in each clinical situation. There are useful appendices on prescribing and nutrition in acute renal failure.

Although sections on acute renal failure can be found in the large renal textbooks, this single volume provides an up-to-date and comprehensive guide to all aspects of acute renal failure in practice. We hope it will be a valuable tool for all clinicians, including those in training, who are involved in caring for these patients.

Paul Glynne
Andrew Allen
Charles Pusey
London, July 2002

ACKNOWLEDGEMENTS

We would like to thank all our colleagues who have helped us in the preparation of this book. These include Anjli Jagpal, Katy Glynne, Nick Price and Justin Green. Katie Darling prepared the illustrations used throughout the book.

LIST OF CONTRIBUTORS

Andrew R. Allen
Renal Section, Imperial College School of Medicine, Hammersmith Hospital, London

Richard Baker
Renal Unit, Hammersmith Hospital, London

Matthew A. Bailey
Centre For Nephrology, Royal Free & University College Medical School, London

Martin J.K. Blomley
Department of Imaging, Imperial College School of Medicine, Hammersmith Hospital, London

Stephen J. Brett
Intensive Care Unit, Hammersmith Hospital, London

Edwina Brown
Renal Unit, Charing Cross Hospital, London

Aine Burns
Renal Unit, The Royal Free Hospital, London

Giovambattista Capasso
Department of Nephrology, University of Naples, Naples, Italy

Afzal N. Chaudhry
Renal Section, Imperial College School of Medicine, Hammersmith Hospital, London

Peter Choi
Rheumatology Section, Imperial College School of Medicine, Hammersmith Hospital, London

Terry Cook
Department of Histopathology, Imperial College School of Medicine, Hammersmith Hospital, London

Jeremy Cordingley
Intensive Care Unit, Hammersmith Hospital, London

Susan M. Crail
Department of Renal Medicine, Basildon Hospital, Essex

Katie Darling
Department of Infectious Diseases, Imperial College School of Medicine, Hammersmith Hospital, London

Anthony Dorling
Renal Section, Imperial College School of Medicine, Hammersmith Hospital, London

Thomas J. Evans
Department of Infectious Diseases, Imperial College School of Medicine, Hammersmith Hospital, London

Richard Fielding
Renal Unit, Hammersmith Hospital, London

Luigi G. Forni
Department of Renal Medicine, St. Georges Hospital, London

Gill Gaskin
Renal Section, Imperial College School of Medicine, Hammersmith Hospital, London

Katy A. Glynne
Pharmacy Department, Hammersmith Hospital, London

Paul A. Glynne
Department of Infectious Diseases and Renal Section, Imperial College School of Medicine, Hammersmith Hospital, London

Lawrence Goldberg
Renal Unit, Sussex Royal County Hospital, Brighton

Megan Griffith
Renal Unit, Hammersmith Hospital, London

Christopher J. Harvey
Department of Imaging, Imperial College School of Medicine, Hammersmith Hospital, London

Rachel Hilton
Renal Unit, Guy's & St. Thomas' Hospitals, London

Steve Holt
Renal Unit, The Royal Free Hospital, London

Marie Kelly
Department of Nutrition and Dietetics, Hammersmith Hospital, London

Jeremy Levy
Renal Section, Imperial College School of Medicine, Hammersmith Hospital, London

Liz Lightstone
Renal Section, Imperial College School of Medicine, Hammersmith Hospital, London

Mark Little
Renal Unit, Hammersmith Hospital, London

Graham Lord
Department of Immunology and Renal Section, Imperial College School of Medicine, Hammersmith Hospital, London

Iain MacPhee
Department of Renal Medicine, St. Georges Hospital Medical School, London

Stephen H. Morgan
Department of Renal Medicine, South Essex Renal Services, Basildon Hospital, Essex

Nicholas M. Price
Department of Infectious Diseases, Imperial College School of Medicine, Hammersmith Hospital, London

Charles D. Pusey
Renal Section, Imperial College School of Medicine, Hammersmith Hospital, London

Peter D. Robins
Department of Imaging, Hammersmith Hospital, London

Michael G. Robson
Rheumatology Section, Imperial College School of Medicine, Hammersmith Hospital, London

Alan D. Salama
Renal Section, Imperial College School of Medicine, Hammersmith Hospital, London

David G. Shirley
Centre For Nephrology, Royal Free & University College Medical School, London

Lucy Smyth
Renal Section, Imperial College School of Medicine, Hammersmith Hospital, London

Paul E. Stevens
Renal Unit, Kent & Canterbury Hospital, Kent

Jo Thompson
Renal Unit, Hammersmith Hospital, London

Richard D. Thompson
BHF Cardiovascular Medicine Unit, Imperial College School of Medicine, Hammersmith Hospital, London

David Throssell
Sheffield Kidney Institute, Northern General Hospital, Sheffield

Raj Thuraisingham
Department of Nephrology, The Royal London Hospital, London

Robert J. Unwin
Centre For Nephrology, Royal Free & University College Medical School, London

Roger M.H. Walker
Institute of Urology and Nephrology, Royal Free & University College Medical School, London

Madhuri Warren
Department of Histopathology, Imperial College School of Medicine, Hammersmith Hospital, London

Anthony N. Warrens
Department of Immunology and Renal Section, Imperial College School of Medicine, Hammersmith Hospital, London

ABBREVIATIONS USED THROUGHOUT THE BOOK

AASV	ANCA-associated systemic vasculitis
Ab	antibody
ABG	arterial blood gas
ACE	angiotensin converting enzyme
ACEI	ACE inhibitor
ACT	activating clotting time
ADH	anti-diuretic hormone
AG	anion gap
AGE	advanced glycosylation end-product
AII	angiotensin II
AIN	acute ischaemic nephropathy
ANA	anti-nuclear antibody
ANCA	anti-neutrophil cytoplasmic antibodies
ANP	atrial natriuretic peptide
APTT	activated partial thromboplastin time
ARDS	acute respiratory distress syndrome
ARF	acute renal failure
ATIN	acute tubulointerstitial nephritis
ATIN	acute tubulointerstitial nephritis
ATN	acute tubular necrosis
BP	blood pressure
C-ANCA	cytoplasmic ANCA
CCU	coronary care unit
CO	cardiac output
CPAP	continuous positive airways pressure
CPK	creatine phosphokinase
CRP	C-reactive protein
CSF	cerebrospinal fluid
CVP	central venous pressure
CVVH	continuous venovenous haemofiltration
CVVHDF	continuous venovenous haemodiafiltration
DDAVP	1-deamino-8-d-arginine vasopressin
DIC	disseminated intravascular coagulation
DO_2	oxygen delivery
DTPA	diethylenetriaminepentacetic acid
ECG	electrocardiogram
ECV	effective circulating volume
ELISA	enzyme-linked immunosorbent assay
EM	electron microscopy
ESR	erythrocyte sedimentation rate
ET	endothelin
FBC	full blood count
FSGN	focal segmental glomerulonephritis
FSGS	focal segmental glomerulosclerosis
g	gram
GBM	glomerular basement membrane
GFR	glomerular filtration rate
GN	glomerulonephritis
h	hour
Hb	haemoglobin
HBV	hepatitis B virus
HCV	hepatitis C virus
HD	haemodialysis
HELLP	haemolysis, elevated liver enzymes and low platelets
HIV	human immunodeficiency virus
HLA	human leucocyte antigen

HRS	hepatorenal syndrome		PCT	proximal convoluted tubule
HUS	haemolytic uraemic syndrome		PD	peritoneal dialysis
ICAM	intercellular adhesion molecule		PEEP	positive end-expiratory pressure
ICU	intensive care unit		Pg/PG	prostaglandin
IF	immunofluorescence		PO_2	partial pressure of oxygen
IFNγ	interferon gamma		PR3	proteinase 3
Ig	immunoglobulin		PTH	parathyroid hormone
IGF	insulin-like growth factor		RAAS	renin-angiotensin-aldosterone
IH	immunohistochemistry			system
IL	interleukin		RBC	red blood cells
IV	intravenous		RBF	renal blood flow
JVP	jugular venous pressure		RPGN	rapidly progressive
L	litre			glomerulonephritis
LAP	left atrial pressure		RRT	renal replacement therapy
LDH	lactate dehydrogenase		SaO_2	oxygen saturation
LM	light microscopy		SC	sieving coefficient
LPS	lipopolysaccharide		SCD	sickle cell disease
MA	metabolic acidosis		SIRS	systemic inflammatory response
MAG3	mercaptoacetyltriglycerine			syndrome
MAHA	microangiopathic haemolytic		SLE	systemic lupus erythematosus
	anaemia		SNS	sympathetic nervous system
MAL	metabolic alkalosis		SRC	scleroderma renal crisis
MAP	mean arterial pressure		SvO_2	mixed venous oxygen saturation
MCGN	mesangiocapillary		SVR	systemic vascular resistance
	glomerulonephritis		TBM	tubular basement membrane
min	minute		TGFβ	transforming growth factor beta
MODS	multi-organ dysfunction syndrome		THP	Tamm-Horsfall glycoproteim
MPO	myeloperoxidase		TIN	tubulointerstitial nephritis
MSU	mid-stream specimen of urine		TLS	tumour lysis syndrome
NAE	Net acid excretion		TMP	transmembrane pressure
NFP	net filtration pressure		TNF	tumour necrosis factor
NO	nitric oxide		TTP	thrombotic thrombocytopaenic
NSAIDs	non-steroidal anti-inflammatory			purpura
	drugs		Tx	thromboxane
Osm	osmoles		UF	ultrafiltration
PA	pulmonary artery		UKM	urea kinetic modelling
PAF	platelet activating factor		US	ultrasound
P-ANCA	perinuclear ANCA		UTI	urinary tract infection
PaO_2	arterial oxygen tension		VO_2	oxygen consumption
PAOP	pulmonary artery occlusion		WBC	white blood cells
	pressure			

CONTENTS

SECTION 3. THE DISEASES

SECTION 4. SPECIALIST SCENARIOS

SECTION 1

FUNDAMENTALS OF RENAL PHYSIOLOGY

Chapter 1 _____

RENAL HAEMODYNAMICS AND GLOMERULAR FILTRATION
David Shirley, Giovambattista Capasso and Robert Unwin

The kidney has three homeostatic functions that can broadly be described as excretory, regulatory and hormonal. Excretory and regulatory functions are closely related: elimination of unwanted and potentially toxic products of tissue metabolism on the one hand; and the excretion or conservation of water and solutes, and thus the control of fluid and electrolyte balance and circulating volume, on the other. Several processes, beginning with the ultrafiltration of plasma and including the selective reabsorption and secretion of solutes and production of concentrated or dilute urine, achieve these functions. Here we discuss the first of these processes.

RENAL BLOOD FLOW

The normal renal blood flow is ~1200 mL/min, equivalent to ~25% of the resting cardiac output. Given that the kidneys make up <0.5% of the body weight, this clearly represents a massive blood flow. The magnitude of the blood supply is required not for the kidneys' metabolic needs but in order to maintain a high rate of glomerular filtration (ultrafiltration of blood plasma). A typical glomerular filtration rate is 120 mL/min (normal range 90–160 mL/min per 1.73 m^2); i.e. ~20% of the plasma perfusing the kidneys is normally filtered[1].

GLOMERULAR FILTRATION

The Filtration Barrier

Three layers separate the fluid in glomerular capillaries from that in Bowman's capsule (**Figure 1**). Plasma is forced through the *fenestrations* between glomerular endothelial cells (thereby excluding blood cells), then through the non-cellular *basement membrane* and the slits between the foot processes of the *podocytes* (glomerular epithelial cells) lining Bowman's capsule. As the plasma crosses the basement membrane and filtration slits, there is no hindrance to the passage of molecules with a diameter of <4 nm (<40 Å), while those with a diameter >8 nm are not filtered at all; between these figures there is graded filtration. Since most plasma constituents have a molecular diameter much less than 4 nm, while most plasma proteins are bigger than

---

[1]Assuming a normal haematocrit, the renal plasma flow is slightly greater than half the renal blood flow.

Figure 1. (A) Diagrammatic representation of the glomerular membranes; (B) Scanning electron micrograph of podocytes (P) as viewed from Bowman's space

The foot processes are wrapped around capillary loops. Taken, with permission, from Tisher CC and Madsen KM. Anatomy of the kidney; in The Kidney 4th ed., Brenner BM and Rector FC (eds.), Saunders, Philadelphia, 1991.

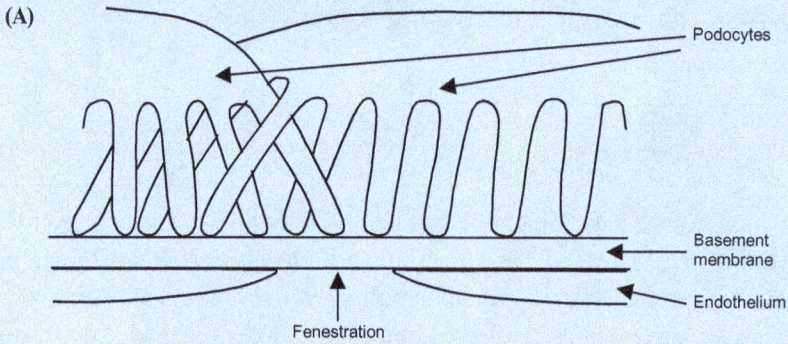

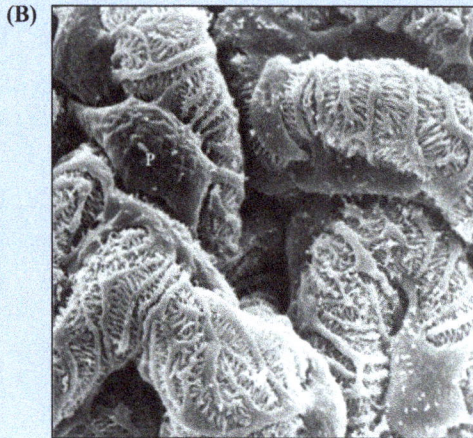

7 nm, the glomerular filtrate has a composition similar to plasma save for the virtual absence of protein (**Table 1**).

The glomerular barrier does not discriminate on the basis of size alone. A layer of *polyanionic glycoproteins* that covers the surface of the components of the filtration barrier repels large anions (i.e. proteins with a net negative charge like albumin) without significantly affecting small anions such as chloride or bicarbonate. Normal average urinary excretion of albumin in men and women is ~7 mg/24 h[2]; detection of albumin by dipstix has a threshold concentration of 100–200 mg/L. If the fixed negative charges on the filtration barrier are lost, as in some forms of glomerular disease (e.g. minimal change nephropathy), the filterability of albumin increases significantly from its normal value of <0.1%, causing significant proteinuria. Some plasma

---

[2]Up to 18 mg/24 h in men and 32 mg/24 h in women.

Table 1. Relationship between molecular diameter and filtration across glomerular membranes		
Substance	**Molecular diameter (nm)**	**Filterability* (%)**
Sodium	~0.4 (hydrated)	100
Chloride	~0.6 (hydrated)	100
Glucose	0.72	100
β_2 microglobulin	3.2	100
Myoglobin	3.9	75
Bence-Jones protein	5.5	10
Haemoglobin	6.5	3
Albumin	7.2	<0.1
γ-globulin	11.1	0

*100% filterability indicates that the substance is freely filtered, i.e. its concentration in Bowman's space equals that in plasma.

proteins, e.g. β_2 microglobulin (molecular diameter ~3.2 nm), are small enough to be filtered even under normal circumstances. Haemoglobin (molecular diameter ~6.5 nm), even if released into plasma, becomes bound to haptoglobin and very little is filtered. However, myoglobin (molecular diameter ~3.9 nm), if released into plasma due to muscle damage (see **Chapter 12**), undergoes major filtration (**Table 1**).

Pressures Responsible for Glomerular Filtration

Ultimately, the glomerular filtrate is forced across the glomerular membranes by the hydrostatic pressure in the glomerular capillaries (P_{GC}). This pressure is sufficient to overcome the opposing two pressures: the hydrostatic pressure in Bowman's capsule (P_{BC}) and the colloid osmotic (oncotic) pressure in the glomerular capillaries (π_{GC}) (**Figure 2**). The driving force for filtration is known as the *net filtration pressure* (NFP). The colloid osmotic pressure in Bowman's capsule is negligible, owing to the virtual exclusion of proteins from the filtrate.

The rate of filtration (GFR) is determined by the product of NFP and the ultrafiltration coefficient (K_f), the latter being a composite of the surface area available for filtration (which is large) and the hydraulic conductance of the glomerular membranes (which is high).

Although direct measurements of P_{GC} and P_{BC} are unavailable in humans, extrapolation from animal studies allows the following estimates of the pressures at the start (*afferent* end) of the glomerular capillary bed:

$$P_{GC} \sim 50 \text{ mmHg}$$
$$P_{BC} \sim 15 \text{ mmHg}$$
$$\pi_{GC} \sim 25 \text{ mmHg}$$

Therefore, NFP ~10 mmHg.

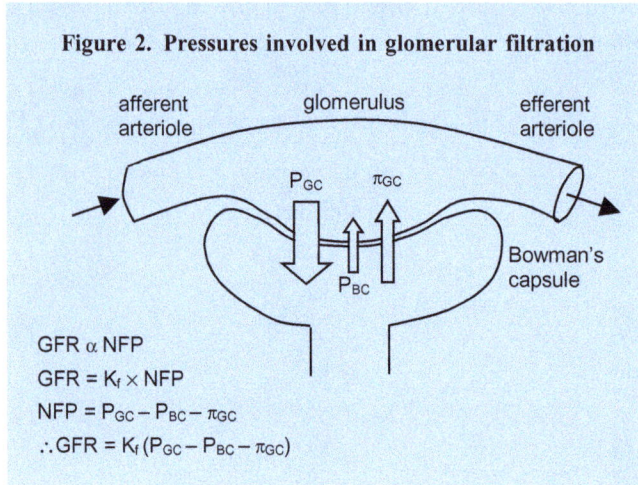

Figure 2. Pressures involved in glomerular filtration

afferent arteriole   glomerulus   efferent arteriole

P_{GC} π_{GC}

P_{BC}

Bowman's capsule

$GFR \; \alpha \; NFP$

$GFR = K_f \times NFP$

$NFP = P_{GC} - P_{BC} - \pi_{GC}$

$\therefore GFR = K_f (P_{GC} - P_{BC} - \pi_{GC})$

Owing to the low resistance of the glomerular capillaries, P_{GC} does not decrease appreciably along the capillary bed. However, as (protein-free) fluid is filtered, the protein concentration of unfiltered plasma remaining in the glomerular capillary increases, thereby raising π_{GC} and reducing NFP. In some species, *filtration equilibrium* is achieved, whereby NFP = 0, before the end of the capillary bed (*efferent* end). In humans, it is thought that this situation is rarely, if ever, attained; nevertheless, NFP clearly decreases as the glomerular capillaries are traversed. If renal blood flow increases, the percentage of plasma filtered per unit length of capillary will decrease; therefore, π_{GC} will rise less rapidly and NFP will fall more slowly. Thus the mean NFP along the capillary will be increased, resulting in a raised GFR. In this way, GFR is linked to renal blood flow. Although the average value for NFP is probably <10 mmHg, ~180 litres of glomerular filtrate are formed each 24 h. This points to the extraordinarily high K_f of glomerular capillaries.

AUTOREGULATION OF RENAL BLOOD FLOW AND GFR

Given the low resting value for NFP, even small changes in any of the filtration pressures can have profound effects on GFR. Nevertheless, under normal circumstances, despite fluctuations in arterial pressure that would be expected to influence P_{GC}, GFR changes very little. This is due to the phenomenon of *autoregulation* whereby, over a mean arterial pressure (MAP) range of ~80–180 mmHg[3], the renal vascular resistance automatically changes as the blood pressure changes (**Figure 3**). The change in resistance occurs in the *afferent* arterioles, which has the important consequence that not only is renal blood flow autoregulated but so is GFR, since only a small proportion of the change in MAP is transmitted to the glomerular capillaries, i.e. P_{GC} changes only marginally (**Figure 4**). Without autoregulation, relatively small fluctuations in MAP would cause major changes in P_{GC} and GFR, and in excretion rates.

---

[3]MAP is calculated as 1/3 systolic BP +2/3 diastolic BP; BP limits for autoregulation are approximately 90/70 and 260/140 mmHg.

Figure 3. Renal autoregulation

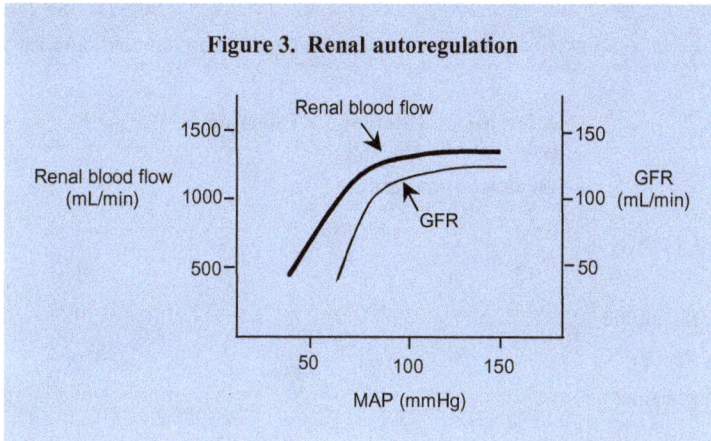

Figure 4. Autoregulation of glomerular filtration rate

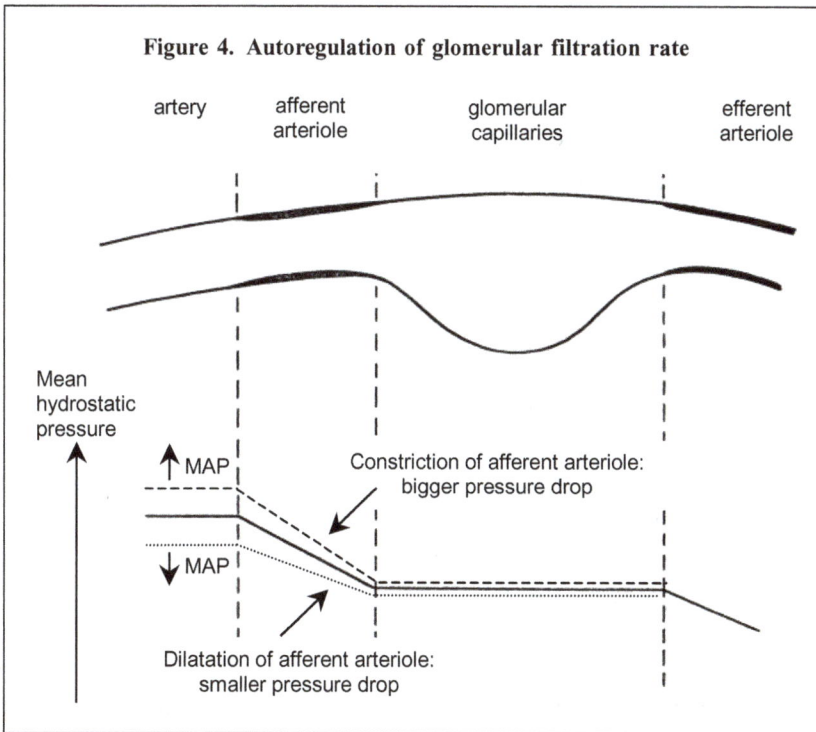

   The intrarenal mechanism underlying autoregulation is not fully understood. It is probably in part a *myogenic* mechanism whereby the smooth muscle of the afferent arteriolar wall intrinsically responds to being stretched (due to a rise in MAP) by contracting, thereby increasing the vascular resistance. The other possible contributory factor is *tubulo-glomerular feedback*, a negative feedback mechanism whereby an initial increase in GFR (resulting from a raised MAP) leads to an increased delivery of NaCl in the tubular fluid arriving at the *macula densa* region of the nephron (last part of the thick ascending limb of the loop of Henle), which, by some unknown mechanism involving angiotensin II and other vasoconstrictors (such as adenosine and ATP), triggers vasoconstriction of the adjacent afferent arteriole.

Table 2. Effects of vasoactive agents on glomerular haemodynamics

	Afferent arteriole resistance	Efferent arteriole resistance	Effect on NFP	K_f	Effect on GFR
Renal Sympathetic Nerves	↑	↑	↓	↓	↓
Angiotensin II	↑	↑↑	→ or ↑	↓	↓
Epinephrine/Norepinephrine	↑	↑	→ or ↑	?	→ or ↓
Atrial Natriuretic Peptide	↓	→	↑	→ or ↑	↑
Vasodilator Prostaglandins	↓	↓	↑	↓	→
Thromboxanes	↑	↑	→	↓	↓
Adenosine	↑	→	↓	→	↓
Endothelin-1	↑	↑↑	→ or ↑	↓	↓
Nitric Oxide	↓	↓	?	↑(?)	?
Dopamine	↓	↓	?	?	↑

N.B. The arrows represent directional changes seen when the agent is applied in high dose in isolation. The actual changes that occur will be influenced greatly by both dosage and experimental setting.

Factors Affecting Renal Blood Flow and GFR

Outside the autoregulatory range, e.g. in circulatory shock, renal blood flow and GFR change with blood pressure. Even within the autoregulatory range, blood pressure does have some influence on renal haemodynamics (**Figure 3**). Furthermore, a number of *extrinsic* factors can override the *intrinsic* influence of autoregulation. These extrinsic factors can affect renal blood flow and P_{GC} by altering the resistance of afferent and/or efferent arterioles; or they can change K_f by inducing *mesangial cell* contraction or relaxation, thereby altering the glomerular surface area available for filtration (**Table 2**).

Afferent arteriolar constriction will reduce renal blood flow and reduce P_{GC}, causing a reduction in GFR.

Efferent arteriolar constriction will reduce renal blood flow but increase P_{GC}; these changes act in opposite directions with respect to GFR and the net effect on GFR is minimal.

A reduction in K_f will reduce GFR.

Any given vasoactive agent may have a spectrum of effects (on afferent/efferent arteriolar tone or K_f), making the net effect on GFR difficult to predict. Thus, angiotensin II, a major regulator of glomerular function, causes constriction of both afferent *and* efferent[4] arterioles, as well as reducing K_f. The overall outcome for GFR depends on the relative magnitudes of these actions, which vary in different pathophysiological conditions.

---

[4]The efferent arteriole is particularly sensitive to angiotensin II, which is why blockade of its action can precipitate ARF in the setting of renal hypoperfusion.

A period of renal hypoperfusion, systemic or local, underlies most cases of ARF. Therefore, an obvious therapeutic target is to reverse afferent arteriolar vasoconstriction, and/or mesangial cell contraction, but without significantly reducing efferent arteriolar tone. This selective approach is not easy to achieve in practice, although various experimental studies have reported beneficial effects of antagonists of endothelin and adenosine, and of nitric oxide donors. However, due to the varying aetiology and underlying complexity of even haemodynamic ARF, it is apparent that no single agent will be fully protective.

For further reading please refer to the end of Chapter 2.

Chapter 2 _____

RENAL TUBULAR FUNCTION
David Shirley, Giovambattista Capasso, Matthew Bailey and Robert Unwin

Of the 180 litres of water filtered at the glomeruli per day, the tubules usually reabsorb ~99%, leaving only 1–2 litres to be excreted. Reabsorption on this scale also applies to filtered sodium, chloride, bicarbonate, calcium and magnesium, while net potassium excretion is usually equivalent to ~15% of the filtered load (although most urinary potassium is not derived from the glomerular filtrate). Here we give a brief overview of events in the major subdivisions of the nephron, followed by an account of the renal handling of specific solutes. Finally, the mechanisms of action of important classes of diuretics are discussed.

PROXIMAL CONVOLUTED TUBULE

The main function of the proximal convoluted tubule (PCT), which makes up the first two thirds of the proximal tubule, is the reabsorption of the bulk of the glomerular filtrate, although some secretion also occurs (**Table 1**). The PCT reabsorbs approximately 50% of the filtered sodium and water, reabsorption at this site being isosmotic (i.e. no significant osmotic gradient is established). Considerably more than 50% of filtered bicarbonate is reabsorbed, while reabsorption of chloride and potassium lags slightly behind that of sodium.

Table 1. Principal functions of the proximal convoluted tubule

Reabsorption	Secretion
~50% of filtered Na^+	Organic anions, e.g. bile salts, penicillin, salicylate, furosemide, chlorothiazide
~50% of filtered H_2O	Organic cations, e.g. creatinine, atropine, cimetidine, amiloride
~45% of filtered K^+	H^+
~45% of filtered Cl^-	NH_4^+
Most filtered HCO_3^-	
Most filtered phosphate	
Most filtered urate	
All filtered glucose	
All filtered amino acids	

Figure 1. Sodium reabsorption in the proximal convoluted tubule

The figure represents a proximal tubular epithelial cell. There is an apical (luminal) and basolateral (interstitial) surface. In this and subsequent diagrams, closed circles represent pumps requiring a direct energy source (hydrolysis of ATP), i.e. primary active transport, while open circles represent co-transporters or counter-transporters (secondary active transport). The stoichiometry of linked solute fluxes is not shown.

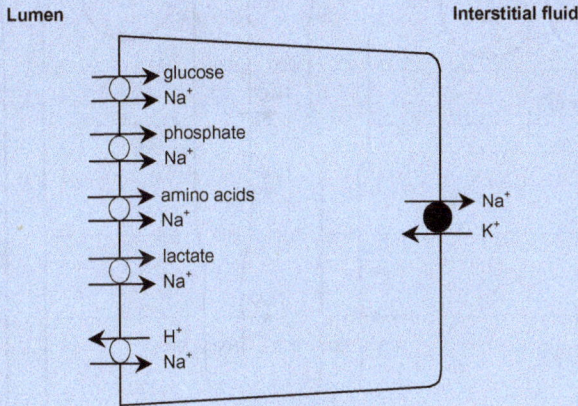

Secretory transport mechanisms exist for organic anions and cations. These are important with respect to the renal elimination of many drugs; they also ensure that diuretics which require access to the luminal membrane are effective. Some diuretics, e.g. furosemide, are protein-bound and are therefore not filtered to any appreciable extent.

Virtually all transport in the PCT appears to be linked, directly or indirectly, to sodium reabsorption. Throughout the nephron, transcellular sodium reabsorption occurs by passive entry into the cell at the *luminal* membrane and active extrusion across the *basolateral* membrane via the ubiquitous Na^+/K^+-ATPase ("sodium pump"); only the mode of passive entry of sodium at the luminal membrane differs from segment to segment. In the PCT, sodium entry uses a series of carriers, each of which co-transports a second solute (**Figure 1**). The energy from the "downhill" movement of sodium is used to move the second solute "uphill"; this is known as secondary active transport. There are separate carriers for H^+ (counter-transport), glucose, phosphate and each class of amino acid (co-transport).

LOOP OF HENLE

The loop of Henle is usually defined as that segment of the nephron between the PCT and the distal tubule. As such, it includes the final third of the proximal tubule — the proximal straight tubule (*pars recta*) — as well as the thin descending and (in deep nephrons only) ascending limbs and the thick ascending limb (TALH). As a whole, this heterogeneous nephron segment reabsorbs considerable amounts of solute (e.g. sodium reabsorption is ~40% of the filtered load) and water (~30% of the filtered load).

The water reabsorption occurs (by osmosis) in two regions: (i) the *pars recta*, where it is assumed to follow solute reabsorption isosmotically; and (ii) the thin descending limb, where it

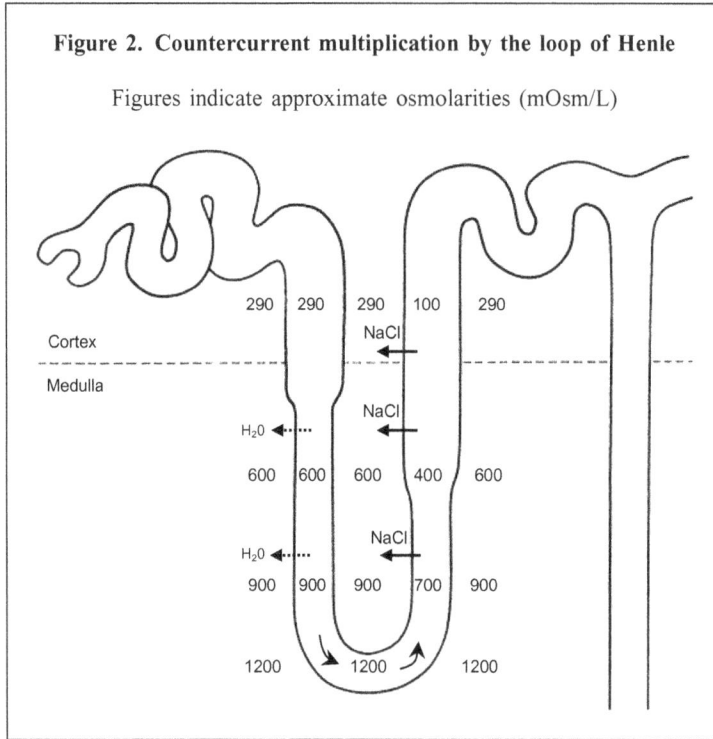

Figure 2. Countercurrent multiplication by the loop of Henle

Figures indicate approximate osmolarities (mOsm/L)

is drawn into the *hypertonic medullary interstitium*, thereby rendering the fluid remaining within the descending limb hypertonic.

The ascending limb of Henle is almost completely impermeable to water, but significant quantities of sodium, chloride, potassium, calcium and magnesium are reabsorbed; thus the fluid in the ascending limb becomes progressively diluted.

The solute reabsorption in the water-impermeable ascending limb, combined with osmotic equilibration in the descending limb and counter-current flow of tubular fluid in the descending and ascending limbs, generates a progressive osmotic gradient in the medullary interstitium, which in humans reaches ~1200 mOsm/L in the deepest region (**Figure 2**). The energy source for this process (*countercurrent multiplication*) is the active transport of sodium in the TALH. Na^+ ions enter the cell on a carrier that also transports K^+ and Cl^- ions (the $Na^+/K^+/2Cl^-$ co-transporter) and are pumped across the basolateral membrane by the Na^+/K^+-ATPase (**Figure 3**). The transport processes in the TALH result in a lumen-positive transepithelial potential difference (PD) that drives the reabsorption of additional cations (including ~50% of the Na^+ reabsorbed along the TALH) through the cation-selective paracellular pathway. Recently, in the basolateral membrane of the TALH, a calcium-sensing receptor has been found that inhibits ion transport when activated by hypercalcaemia.

The reabsorption of sodium along the *thin ascending limb* is believed to be passive, using simple diffusion. This can occur as a consequence of the high urea concentration in the inner medullary interstitium (see below), which helps to draw water out of the *thin descending limb* and thereby raises the sodium concentration of the fluid delivered to the tip of the loop and entering the thin ascending limb.

Figure 3. Sodium chloride transport in the thick ascending limb of the loop of Henle

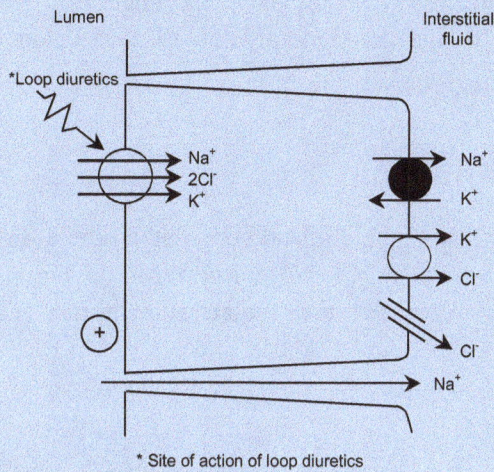

* Site of action of loop diuretics

Figure 4. Countercurrent exchange in the vasa recta

Figures indicate approximate osmolarities (mOsm/L)

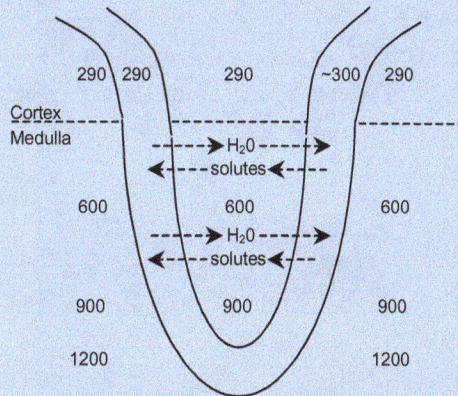

As a consequence of the actions of the loop of Henle, the following are achieved:

- Reabsorption of large proportions of the filtered solutes and water.
- Establishment of a hypertonic interstitium in the medulla, which can be utilised to produce a concentrated urine in the collecting ducts (see below).
- Delivery of *hypotonic* fluid to the distal tubule, which allows the production of a dilute urine when required (see below).

The medullary blood supply does not dissipate the cortico-medullary osmotic gradient because of the special arrangement of the deep nephron post-glomerular capillaries known as *vasa recta* (**Figure 4**). These capillaries form vascular bundles intermingling with, and mirroring, the corresponding loops of Henle. Their descending and ascending limbs passively "exchange" fluid and solutes (between limbs and with the interstitium) and so there is minimal disturbance to the medullary osmotic gradient — *countercurrent* exchange. However, these exchange processes do not occur instantaneously, and consequently the vasa recta do remove some solute from the medulla.

EARLY DISTAL TUBULE

The main event in the early distal tubule (distal convoluted tubule) is the reabsorption of sodium and chloride as NaCl. This uses a Na^+/Cl^- co-transporter in the luminal membrane, coupled with Na^+ extrusion via the Na^+/K^+-ATPase on the basolateral membrane (**Figure 5**). This segment also actively reabsorbs calcium (see later).

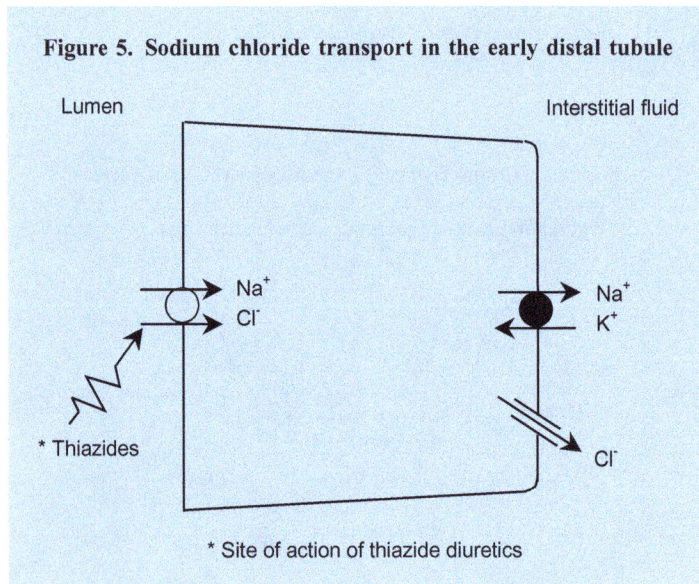

Figure 5. Sodium chloride transport in the early distal tubule

Lumen

Interstitial fluid

Na^+
Cl^-

Na^+
K^+

* Thiazides

Cl^-

* Site of action of thiazide diuretics

LATE DISTAL TUBULE AND CORTICAL COLLECTING DUCT

Two types of cells make up the late distal tubule and cortical collecting duct: *principal* cells (the majority cell type), which reabsorb sodium and water and secrete potassium (**Figure 6**); and *intercalated* cells, which secrete either H^+ or HCO_3^- ions (see later section).

Luminal sodium entry into principal cells is by simple diffusion through Na^+ channels; basolateral exit is via the Na^+/K^+-ATPase. Potassium secretion occurs because the luminal membrane of these cells contains K^+ channels through which K^+ ions enter the lumen. This potassium secretion is the major determinant of potassium excretion.

The hormone *vasopressin*, secreted from the neurohypophysis when osmoreceptors in the hypothalamus detect a rise in plasma osmolarity, binds to receptors on the basolateral membrane of principal cells and causes increased insertion of water channels (*aquaporins*) in the luminal

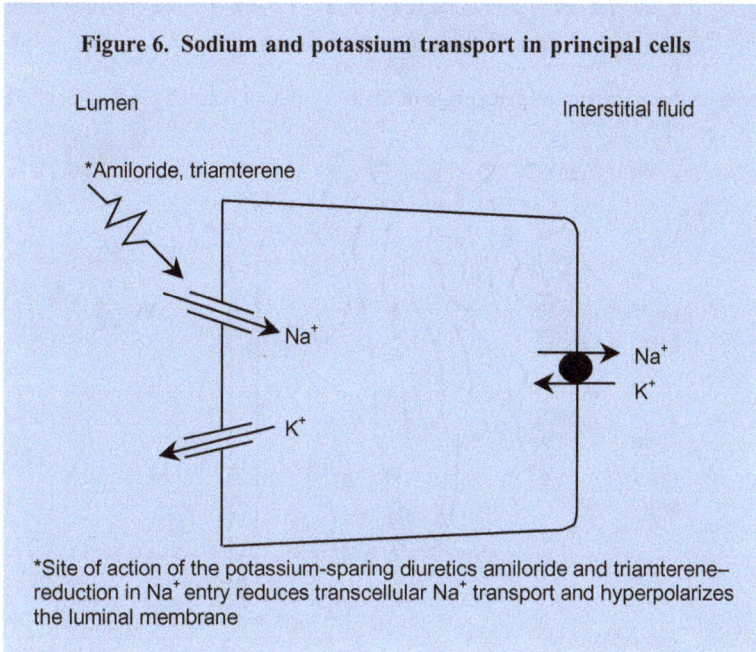

Figure 6. Sodium and potassium transport in principal cells

Lumen

Interstitial fluid

*Amiloride, triamterene

Na$^+$

Na$^+$

K$^+$

K$^+$

*Site of action of the potassium-sparing diuretics amiloride and triamterene–
reduction in Na$^+$ entry reduces transcellular Na$^+$ transport and hyperpolarizes
the luminal membrane

membrane. Maximal stimulation by vasopressin allows the fluid within the late distal tubule and cortical collecting duct to come into osmotic equilibrium with the surrounding interstitial fluid (which is itself isotonic). This causes the reabsorption of approximately 2/3 of the water arriving at the distal tubule.

MEDULLARY COLLECTING DUCT

This is a heterogeneous segment whose function is not as well defined as that of the cortical collecting duct. It consists of modified principal cells and probably some intercalated cells. Active reabsorption of sodium occurs, but potassium secretion is absent. Vasopressin increases the osmotic water permeability of the entire medullary collecting duct (just as in the cortical collecting duct) and thereby allows the final urine osmolarity to reach that of the deepest part of the medullary interstitium (~1200 mOsm/L). In the absence of vasopressin, the hypotonic fluid delivered from the loop of Henle remains hypotonic; indeed, because of continuing solute (principally sodium) reabsorption in the virtual absence of water reabsorption, the final urine osmolarity can be as low as 50 mOsm/L.

RENAL HANDLING OF SPECIFIC SOLUTES

SODIUM

Using mechanisms outlined above, most sodium reabsorption (~90%) occurs in the PCT and loop of Henle, while a further 5% is reabsorbed in the early distal tubule (**Figure 7**). Therefore, approximately 5% of the filtered load normally reaches the late distal tubule, and it is in the

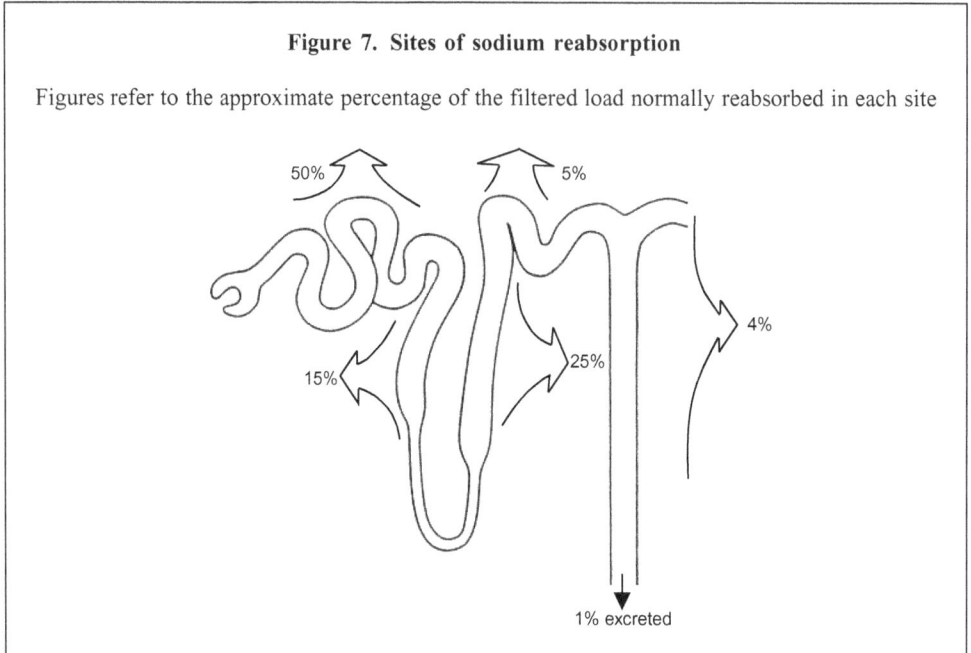

Figure 7. Sites of sodium reabsorption

Figures refer to the approximate percentage of the filtered load normally reabsorbed in each site

late distal tubule and collecting duct that the day-to-day control of sodium excretion occurs. However, in more extreme circumstances, other nephron segments contribute to altered sodium excretion.

Control of Sodium Excretion

- *Angiotensin II*, which is generated systemically when the effective circulating volume is reduced (**Figure 8**) and which may also be produced within the tubular lumen, stimulates sodium reabsorption along the proximal tubule. This effect is complemented by an action of the *sympathetic nerves* that innervate the proximal tubule.
- *Dopamine*, which is synthesised locally, inhibits Na^+/K^+-ATPase and sodium reabsorption in the proximal tubule and further downstream (see later).
- *Aldosterone* stimulates sodium reabsorption by increasing the activity (and, in the longer term, number) of basolateral Na^+/K^+-ATPase units of the principal cells in the late distal tubule/ cortical collecting duct and also by increasing the activity of luminal Na^+ channels (see **Figure 6**). Aldosterone is secreted from the *zona glomerulosa* of the adrenal cortex. The main stimulus to its release is angiotensin II. Other (patho-) physiological stimuli for aldosterone secretion are:

  — decreased plasma Na^+ concentration
  — increased plasma K^+ concentration (a more potent stimulus than Na^+)

- *Atrial natriuretic peptide* (ANP), released from the atria in response to volume overload and consequent atrial stretch, increases sodium excretion by inhibiting sodium reabsorption in the medullary collecting duct. ANP also indirectly increases sodium excretion by inhibiting the release of renin and aldosterone.

Figure 8. Factors affecting aldosterone secretion

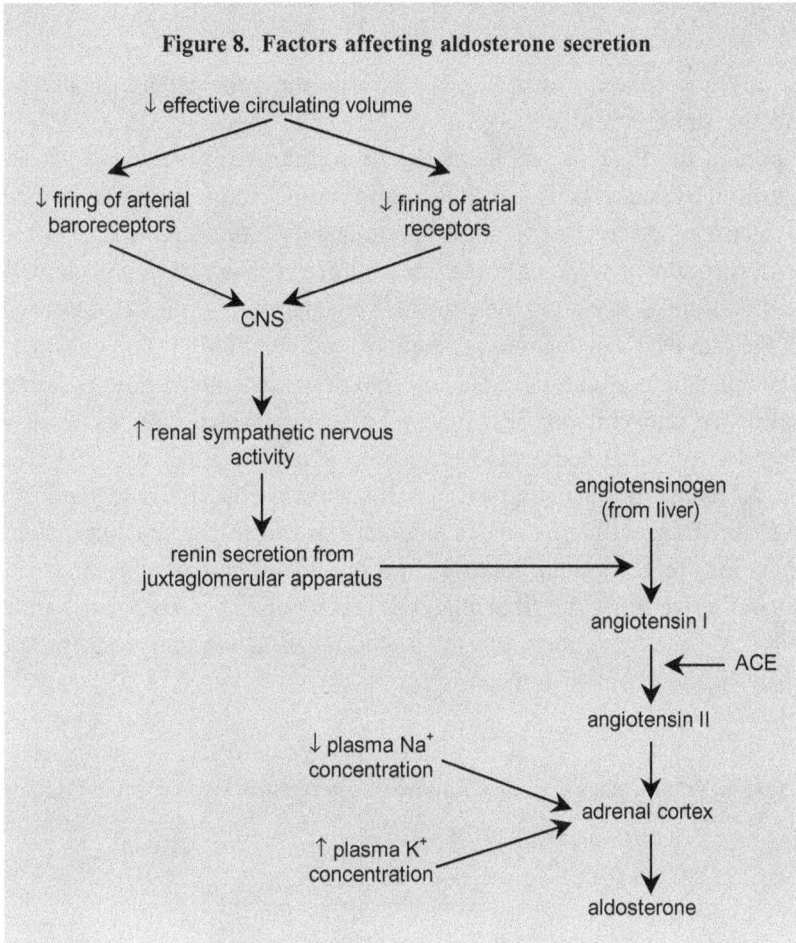

Practice Point 1

Urinary sodium concentration is commonly measured in an attempt to distinguish potentially reversible pre-renal failure from established and intrinsic renal failure. It is generally stated than a urine sodium concentration of <10 mmol/L indicates enhanced tubular sodium reabsorption in the setting of reduced renal perfusion and GFR, and therefore pre-renal failure; whereas a sodium concentration of >20 mmol/L suggests impaired tubular function and intrinsic renal damage. However, a more reliable and equally simple measurement on a spot urine sample is to estimate the fractional excretion of sodium from the ratio of urine sodium:plasma sodium divided by urine creatinine:plasma creatinine, thus:

$$([U_{Na}]/[P_{Na}])/([U_{Cr}]/[P_{Cr}])$$

This fraction (which can be applied to any solute in urine) when multiplied by 100 gives the percent fractional excretion of sodium. A value of >1% indicates tubular dysfunction.

CHLORIDE

In general, chloride reabsorption is linked to, and follows the same pattern as, sodium reabsorption and is subject to the same controls.

In the early part of the PCT (S_1 segment), some sodium reabsorption is associated with co-transport of neutral substances such as glucose and amino acids. In consequence, this sodium reabsorption is electrogenic, creating a small lumen-negative transepithelial PD (~-2 mV). This PD drives the reabsorption of some chloride paracellularly. However, chloride reabsorption lags behind that of sodium (and water), and the chloride concentration within the tubular fluid therefore rises slightly. In the late PCT (S_2 segment), the raised tubular fluid/plasma chloride concentration ratio leads to some paracellular chloride reabsorption down its concentration gradient; this in turn causes a reversal of the transepithelial PD (to $\sim+2$ mV, lumen-positive), which drives the further (passive) reabsorption of some sodium.

Not all chloride reabsorption in the PCT is by simple diffusion and paracellular. Some is secondary active and transcellular, using a counter-transporter in the luminal membrane that deposits organic anions (e.g. formate, oxalate) into the lumen and acts in concert with a luminal Na^+/H^+ exchanger (**Figure 9**). In the final analysis, this secondary active transport depends on the basolateral Na^+/K^+-ATPase, which maintains a low intracellular sodium concentration that in turn drives the luminal Na^+/H^+ counter-transporter.

Figure 9. Transcellular chloride reabsorption in the proximal convoluted tubule

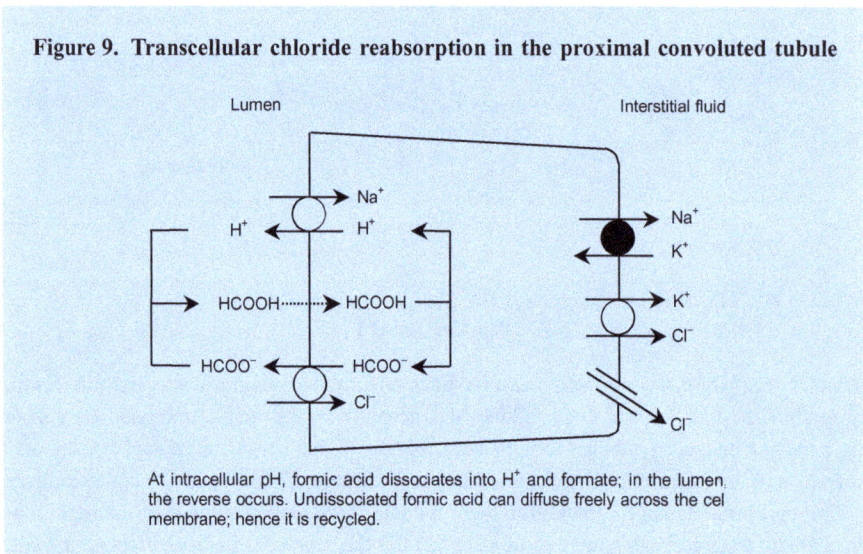

At intracellular pH, formic acid dissociates into H^+ and formate; in the lumen, the reverse occurs. Undissociated formic acid can diffuse freely across the cell membrane; hence it is recycled.

The mechanism of chloride reabsorption in the *pars recta* is unknown. Nor is it known whether chloride (or sodium) reabsorption occurs in the thin descending limb. In the thin ascending limb, chloride reabsorption is thought to be passive, by simple diffusion (as for sodium), while in the TALH chloride reabsorption is secondary active, entering the cell on the $Na^+/K^+/Cl^-$ co-transporter and leaving via Cl^- channels and possibly a K^+/Cl^- co-transporter (see **Figure 3**). In the early distal tubule, chloride uses the luminal Na^+/Cl^- co-transporter (see **Figure 5**), and in the more distal nephron segments it is believed to be reabsorbed paracellularly (despite this being a "tight" epithelium), driven by a large lumen-negative PD created by active sodium reabsorption.

POTASSIUM

Renal potassium transport is summarised in **Figure 10**. Much of the filtered potassium is reabsorbed in the PCT. In the early segment (S_1), there is little potassium reabsorption and the tubular fluid potassium concentration therefore rises slightly. In the main part of the PCT (S_2), there is a small lumen-positive transepithelial PD (see above); the combination of a small concentration gradient and the electrical gradient may be sufficient to drive significant quantities of potassium reabsorption paracellularly by simple diffusion. The remainder is probably by solvent drag, whereby reabsorbed fluid entrains any solute whose permeance exceeds zero (**Figure 11**). There is little evidence for active potassium reabsorption in the PCT.

In the thin descending limb, potassium enters the lumen by passive diffusion from the medullary interstitium. However, in the ascending limb it is reabsorbed to a major extent. In the TALH, potassium enters the cells on the $Na^+/K^+/2Cl^-$ co-transporter, but much of it recycles across the luminal membrane through K^+ channels. On the basolateral membrane, potassium enters the cell on the Na^+/K^+-ATPase and leaves again via K^+ channels or a K^+/Cl^- co-transporter. It is likely that the main route of net potassium reabsorption in the TALH is paracellular, driven by the lumen-positive PD (**Figure 12**).

As a consequence of net potassium reabsorption in the proximal tubule and loop of Henle, ~10% of filtered potassium normally arrives at the distal tubule. This figure varies little, regardless of potassium balance. Therefore, the large variations in potassium excretion that can be achieved result from variations in potassium handling in the distal nephron. Potassium is normally secreted

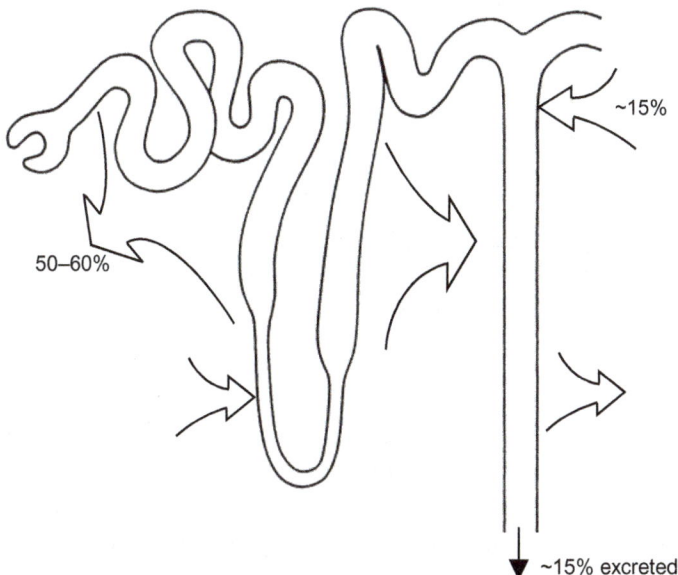

Figure 10. Normal renal potassium handling

Where figures are not given, this is because quantitative information is unavailable.

The extent of secretion in the late distal tubule/cortical collecting duct varies enormously.

~15%

50–60%

~15% excreted

Figure 11. Potassium reabsorption in the proximal convoluted tubule (S_2 segment)

Lumen

Interstitial fluid

K⁺

(+)

Diffusion down
electrochemical gradient

H_2O/K^+

Solvent drag: entrained
in reabsorbed water

Figure 12. Potassium transport in the thick ascending limb of the loop of Henle

Lumen

Interstitial fluid

Na⁺
2Cl⁻
K⁺

K⁺

Na⁺
K⁺

K⁺

K⁺
Cl⁻

K⁺

(+)

K⁺

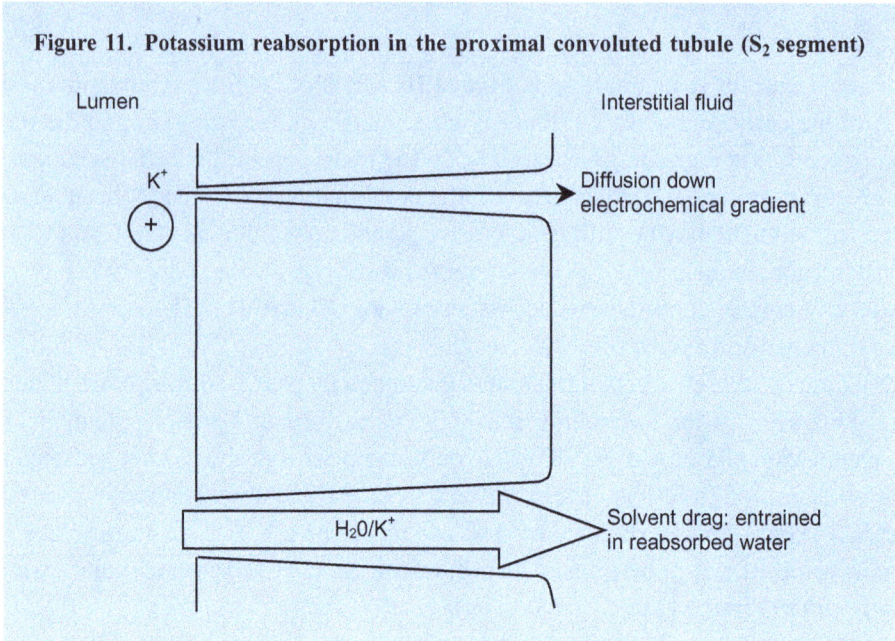

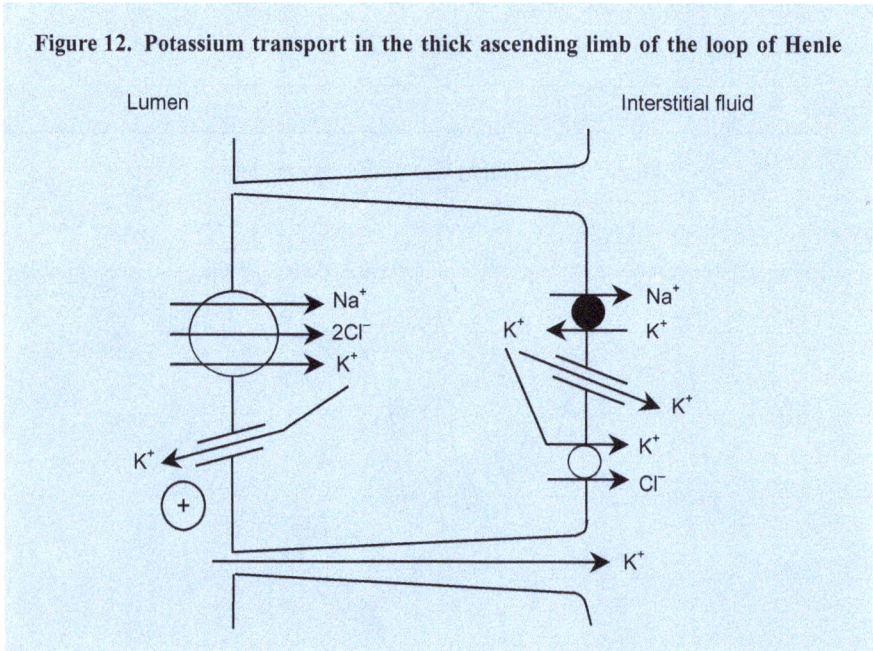

by the principal cells in the late distal tubule and cortical collecting duct (see **Figure 6**), and this secretion masks potassium reabsorption by the intercalated cells. During potassium loading or in renal insufficiency, net potassium secretion by functioning principal cells is greatly increased; in potassium depletion it can be reduced to zero, so that net potassium reabsorption becomes evident. The final nephron segment (medullary collecting duct) is thought to reabsorb potassium under most circumstances, which contributes to the high potassium concentration in the medullary interstitium.

Factors Affecting Potassium Secretion and Excretion

- *Aldosterone*, as well as stimulating sodium reabsorption by principal cells, also stimulates potassium secretion. It does this partly by stimulating the basolateral Na^+/K^+ pump and partly by increasing luminal sodium entry, which in turn depolarises the luminal membrane and increases the electrochemical gradient for potassium exit into the lumen. Aldosterone may also increase the activity of the luminal K^+ channels.
- *An increase in plasma potassium*, by increasing net entry of potassium at the basolateral membrane, increases the driving force for luminal potassium exit.
- *Increased tubular fluid flow rate* through the distal nephron (e.g. during diuretic treatment) stimulates potassium secretion and can lead to hypokalaemia. This results from enhancement of the driving force for potassium secretion across the luminal membrane; the high flow rate, by quickly flushing secreted potassium downstream, maintains a high concentration gradient for further potassium secretion.
- *Acid-base imbalances* have profound effects on potassium secretion. Alkalosis increases the activity of luminal K^+ channels, thereby increasing potassium secretion and inducing hypokalaemia, while acute acidosis has the opposite effect. In *chronic* acidosis, however, potassium excretion is not reduced. This is because chronic acidosis inhibits proximal tubular reabsorption, which leads to an increase in tubular fluid flow rate through the distal nephron, which itself stimulates potassium secretion.

Practice Point 2

Hyperkalaemia is the most life-threatening electrolyte disturbance in ARF: there may be loss of nephrons, reduced GFR and tubular fluid flow rate, and acute acidosis, all of which contribute to potassium retention by reducing distal potassium secretion. Correction, which is only temporary in the absence of normal renal function, depends on the extra-renal control of potassium distribution inside and outside cells. Correcting acidosis with sodium bicarbonate, giving insulin plus glucose and administering β-agonists, all move K^+ into cells. In addition, the aldosterone-sensitive colon, which secretes potassium like the late distal tubule, can be used to promote potassium loss by giving ion exchange resins as enemas (see also **Chapter 8.3**).

BICARBONATE

1. Bicarbonate Reabsorption

Under normal circumstances, practically all filtered bicarbonate is reabsorbed, the bulk of it in the proximal tubule, the remainder in the TALH and collecting duct (**Figure 13**). The mechanism of reabsorption is indirect, whereby H^+ and HCO_3^- ions are generated in tubular cells (with the aid of carbonic anhydrase), and the H^+ ions are secreted into the lumen while the HCO_3^- ions

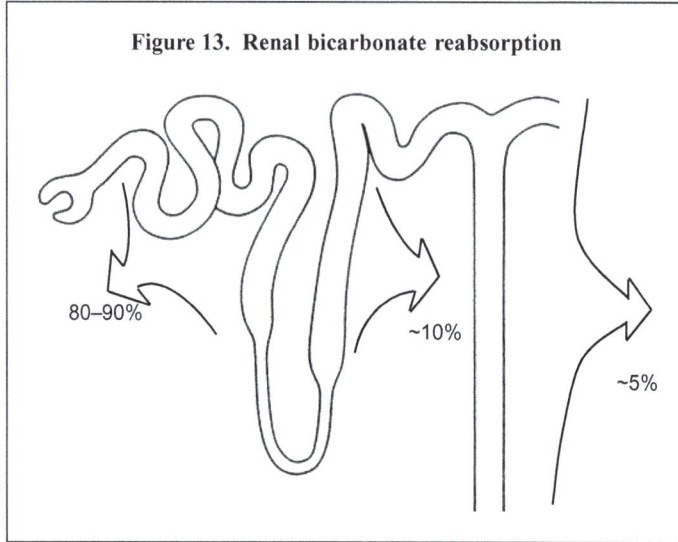

Figure 13. Renal bicarbonate reabsorption

80–90%

~10%

~5%

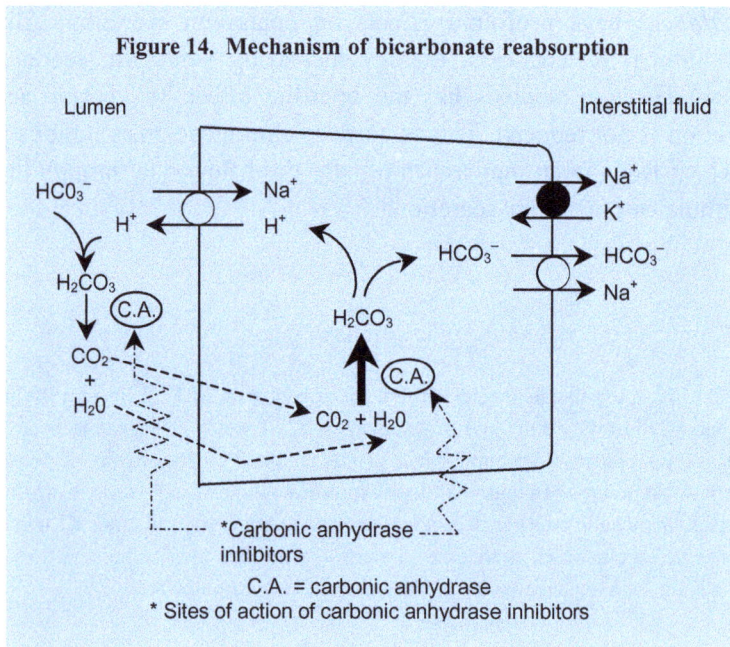

Figure 14. Mechanism of bicarbonate reabsorption

Lumen

Interstitial fluid

HCO_3^-

H^+ → Na^+

H^+

H_2CO_3

C.A.

CO_2 + H_2O

Na^+

K^+

HCO_3^- → HCO_3^-

H_2CO_3

C.A.

CO_2 + H_2O

Na^+

*Carbonic anhydrase inhibitors

C.A. = carbonic anhydrase
* Sites of action of carbonic anhydrase inhibitors

enter the plasma (**Figure 14**). In the proximal tubule and TALH, most of the H^+ secretion is via a Na^+/H^+ counter-transporter in the luminal membrane, although there is also some primary active H^+ secretion by an H^+-ATPase. The secreted H^+ ions react with filtered HCO_3^- ions to form H_2CO_3, which is rapidly converted to CO_2 and H_2O by carbonic anhydrase present along the luminal membrane; the CO_2 and H_2O diffuse into the cell. The net outcome is that a filtered HCO_3^- ion is removed while another one replaces it in plasma.

2. Addition of "New" Bicarbonate to Plasma

The vast majority of H$^+$ ions generated within tubular cells are used in the way described above to *reclaim* filtered bicarbonate (>4,000 mmol/day). However, under normal circumstances, when metabolism of food produces an excess of acid in the body (~50 mmol/day), it is necessary to add "new" (extra) bicarbonate to the plasma to replace the bicarbonate and other buffer anions that have been used to buffer this acid load. This is achieved by continuing to generate H$^+$ and HCO$_3^-$ within tubular cells, over and above those needed to effect HCO$_3^-$ reabsorption. The extra HCO$_3^-$ ions (~50 mmol/day) enter the plasma so that the bicarbonate content of the blood in the renal vein slightly exceeds that in the renal artery. The fate of the H$^+$ ions produced simultaneously is a little more complicated. The simplest thing would be to secrete them directly into the tubular lumen and excrete them in the urine. However, the excretion of ~50 mmol of free H$^+$ ions per day in the urine would lower urine pH to ~1, a feat the kidneys cannot achieve (minimum urine pH ~4.5). These extra H$^+$ ions are therefore dealt with by two alternative mechanisms:

(i) *Excretion of titratable acid*

Some of the extra H$^+$ ions are secreted into the lumen, where they can react with buffer anions in the tubular fluid (principally filtered HPO$_4^{2-}$); any buffer remaining unreabsorbed will rid the body of unwanted acid (**Figure 15**). The total amount of H$^+$ lost in the urine in this way can be determined by back-titrating the urine with a strong base (e.g. NaOH) until the urine pH is raised to 7.4 (i.e. that of arterial plasma); hence the term "titratable acid". It usually amounts to ~20 mmol/day. Approximately half the titratable acid production occurs in the proximal tubule, where tubular fluid pH falls to ~6.8 (equal to the pK of the HPO$_4^{2-}$/H$_2$PO$_4^-$ buffer system). The remainder occurs in the collecting duct, where H$^+$ ions can be secreted against a much higher concentration gradient and consequently, as indicated above, urine pH can fall to ~4.5.

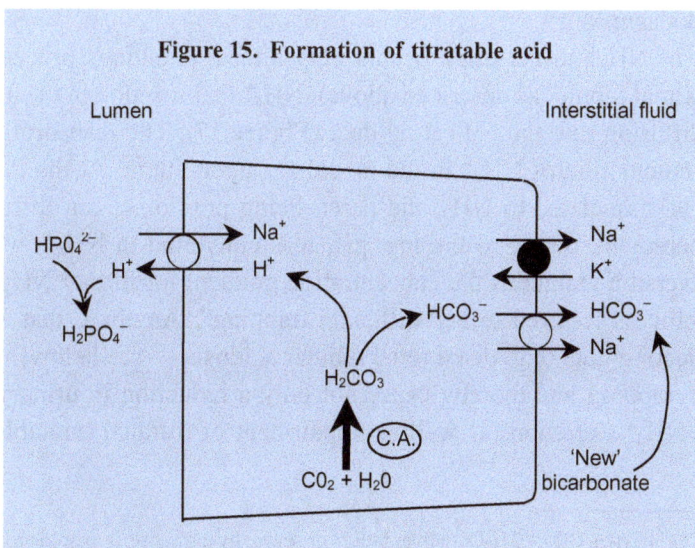

Figure 15. Formation of titratable acid

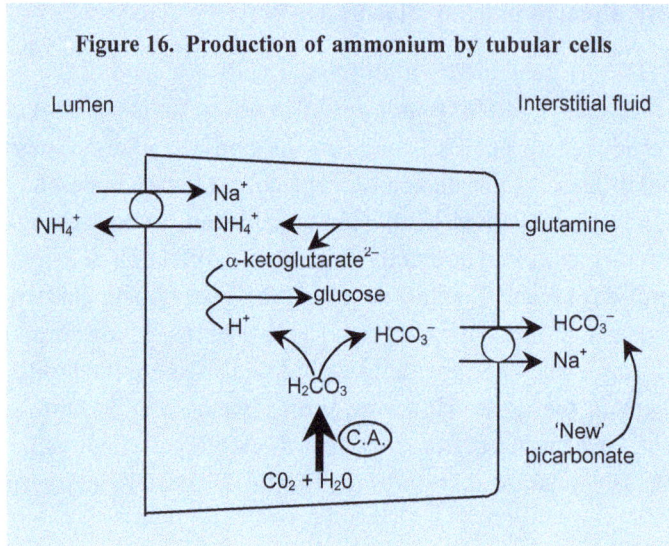

Figure 16. Production of ammonium by tubular cells

(ii) *Excretion of ammonium*

The proximal tubular cells are capable of taking up the amino acid glutamine and deaminating it to form ammonium ions and α-ketoglutarate. The ammonium ions are secreted into the tubular lumen (substituting for H^+ on the Na^+/H^+ counter-transporter) and are eventually excreted, while the α-ketoglutarate is converted, through a series of reactions that consume H^+, to glucose. The H^+ ions are generated in the usual way (from CO_2 and H_2O) and the HCO_3^- ions formed simultaneously are added to plasma (**Figure 16**). It is important that the NH_4^+ produced from glutamine enters the tubular fluid and *not* the plasma; otherwise it would be taken to the liver with bicarbonate, and converted to urea and CO_2, effectively neutralising the bicarbonate[1]. The NH_4^+ system for the generation of "new" bicarbonate is adaptable: the activity of the glutaminase enzyme that deaminates glutamine is enhanced during acidosis (including intracellular acidosis, as in chronic hypokalaemia).

The elimination of NH_4^+ in the urine occurs only after a circuitous process involving NH_4^+ secretion in the proximal tubule (as described above), NH_4^+ reabsorption in the TALH, and, finally, NH_3 secretion by diffusion into the collecting duct (**Figure 17**). The reabsorption of NH_4^+ in the TALH results in accumulation of NH_4^+ in the medullary interstitium. At the interstitial fluid pH, some of the NH_4^+ is dissociated to NH_3; the latter, being non-ionic, can diffuse freely into the collecting duct, whereupon, owing to the low pH, it is converted to NH_4^+, which is trapped in the lumen. The conversion maintains the concentration gradient for further NH_3 diffusion into the collecting duct, a process referred to as "diffusion trapping". Anything that interferes with H^+ secretion in the collecting duct (e.g. distal renal tubular acidosis — see below) would be expected to reduce diffusion trapping and thereby cause not only a reduction in urinary acidification but also a reduction in NH_4^+ excretion (as well as impairment of residual titratable acid formation).

---

[1] $2NH_4^+ + 2HCO_3^- \rightarrow CO(NH_2)_2 + CO_2 + 3H_2O$. In liver failure or severe liver disease, impaired production of urea reduces the consumption of bicarbonate and causes metabolic alkalosis.

Practice Point 3

In patients with distal renal tubular acidosis, titratable acid excretion is reduced, but NH_4^+ excretion is not impaired in all cases. In patients with so-called "incomplete" distal renal tubular acidosis, NH_4^+ excretion is normal and this may be why their plasma bicarbonate concentration remains within the normal range. If they develop nephrocalcinosis and renal stones (a frequent complication), progressive renal damage will reduce NH_4^+ excretion and contribute to worsening acidosis.

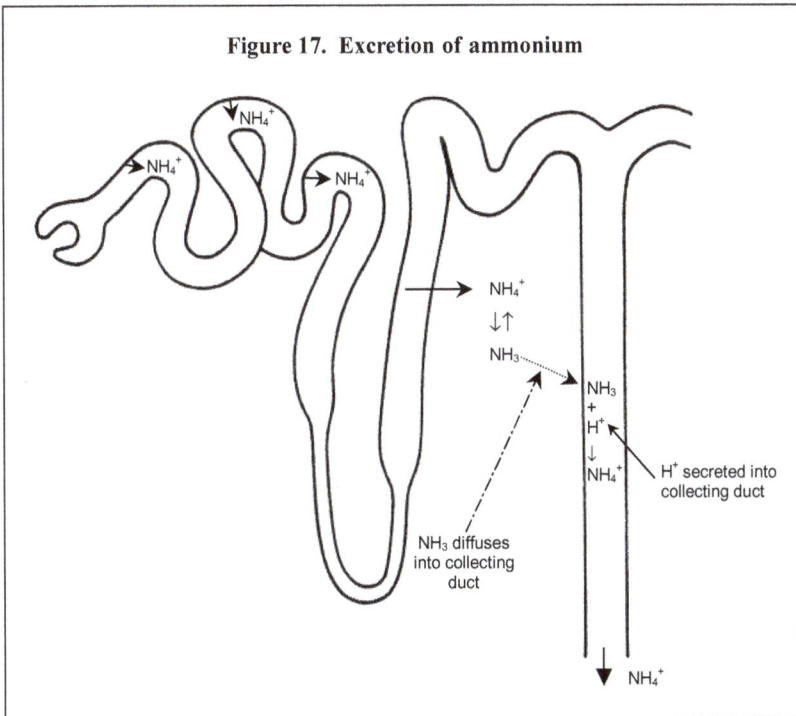

Figure 17. Excretion of ammonium

Intercalated Cells

Intercalated cells, present in the late distal tubule and collecting duct, are of at least two types, α- and β-cells; evidence for further types is evolving. The α-intercalated cells secrete H^+ into the lumen using H^+-ATPase and/or H^+/K^+-ATPase, while the β-intercalated cells secrete HCO_3^- ions, via a luminal HCO_3^-/Cl^- counter-transporter. Generally, the activity of α-cells predominates, but during variations in acid-base balance, either cell type can adapt appropriately.

Regulation of Renal Bicarbonate Handling

• *Respiratory acid-base disorders*

An increase in arterial pCO_2 (caused by respiratory acidosis — CO_2 retention) stimulates the generation of H^+ and HCO_3^- within tubular cells (see **Figure 14**) and thereby increases HCO_3^-

reabsorption and addition of new HCO_3^- to plasma. NH_4^+ generation is also increased in response to respiratory acidosis, which adds to the generation of new bicarbonate. The importance of the renal adaptation to respiratory acidosis is underlined by the fact that in severe acidaemia (pH < 7.2) the survival rate is poorer in those patients who also have renal failure. A decrease in arterial pCO_2 (e.g. during hyperventilation) reduces H^+ and HCO_3^- generation and results in insufficient H^+ secretion to reclaim all the filtered HCO_3^-; consequently, some HCO_3^- is lost in the urine and the plasma HCO_3^- concentration falls. These responses, which bring about appropriate adjustments of plasma HCO_3^- to correct systemic pH[2], constitute the renal compensation for respiratory acid-base disorders.

- *Metabolic acid-base disorders (of non-renal origin)*

Changes in systemic pH are reflected by changes in renal intracellular pH and consequently affect H^+ secretion directly. In addition, over a period of days, NH_4^+ generation is modified appropriately (see above) and insertion of H^+-ATPase and H^+/K^+-ATPase into the luminal membrane of intercalated cells may be affected (increased insertion in acidosis and retrieval in alkalosis).

- *Aldosterone*

Aldosterone stimulates H^+ secretion in the late distal tubule and collecting duct, partly through a direct effect on α-intercalated cells and partly through stimulation of sodium reabsorption by principal cells; the latter process increases the lumen-negative transepithelial PD and thereby favours proton secretion.

- *Extracellular volume fluctuations*

Changes in extracellular volume affect renal bicarbonate handling as a result of altered sodium reabsorption. For example, extracellular volume contraction enhances proximal tubular sodium reabsorption at least partly by increasing the activity of the Na^+/H^+ exchanger, thereby increasing HCO_3^- reabsorption. In addition, the associated rise in plasma aldosterone concentration itself stimulates H^+ secretion in the late distal tubule and collecting duct (see above).

- *Hypokalaemia*

Hypokalaemia, by causing a compensatory exit of potassium ions across the basolateral membrane of renal cells, induces the reciprocal movement of H^+ into cells. The raised intracellular H^+ concentration leads to increased H^+ secretion and HCO_3^- reabsorption, causing a metabolic alkalosis. Another contributory factor may be stimulation (or increased insertion) of the luminal H^+/K^+-ATPase in α-intercalated cells. Recent evidence suggests that increased insertion of luminal H^+-ATPase might also be involved. Moreover, hypokalaemia increases NH_4^+ generation and excretion, which also promotes HCO_3^- addition to plasma. Hyperkalaemia has the opposite effect.

---

[2]pH ∝ $[HCO_3^-]/pCO_2$

URATE

At physiological pH, the end product of purine metabolism, uric acid, is ionised to urate. Renal urate transport is restricted to the proximal tubule; it is both reabsorbed and secreted at this site. In some species secretion predominates, but in humans it is minor: the net result is that approximately 10% of the filtered load is usually excreted.

Urate is taken up in the proximal tubular cells by an anion exchanger in the luminal membrane. A number of intracellular anions can occupy the exchanger; metabolic disorders can affect the availability of these anions and thereby influence the reabsorption of urate. Urate ions leave the cells across both luminal and basolateral membranes by voltage-dependent diffusion. Urate reabsorption is increased by volume depletion (and, together with urea, a raised plasma urate can be a useful clue). Low-dose aspirin reduces urate excretion, while high-dose aspirin increases it.

UREA

Usually 30–50% of filtered urea is excreted, the final figure being a consequence of both reabsorption and secretion in various nephron segments. In the PCT, urea is reabsorbed passively down a concentration gradient created by water reabsorption; urea reabsorption lags slightly behind that of water. In the final segment of the pars recta (S_3), which is located in the outer medulla, urea is secreted; it is also secreted in the thin descending and ascending limbs, probably by simple passive diffusion down a concentration gradient. The wall of the TALH has a low permeability to urea, and throughout the distal tubule and most of the collecting duct the urea permeability is even less. In contrast, in the very deepest region of the medullary collecting duct the walls are very permeable to urea. When the hormone vasopressin is present and water is reabsorbed from the late distal tubule and collecting duct, the urea remaining in the lumen becomes concentrated. When this high concentration of urea reaches the terminal collecting duct, it is reabsorbed into the inner medullary interstitium and contributes to the high osmolarity in this region. The mechanism of reabsorption in the medullary terminal collecting duct is facilitated diffusion (i.e. carrier mediated, but passive), using specific transporters[3].

Vasopressin increases urea reabsorption in the terminal collecting duct in two ways:

- It increases water reabsorption in the collecting duct, thereby raising the intraluminal urea concentration.
- It directly increases the number of urea transporters.

CREATININE

The rate of excretion of creatinine, which is derived from the metabolism of muscle creatine, is usually similar to the rate of its filtration. Consequently, the clearance of creatinine is routinely used as an estimate of GFR. However, although creatinine is not reabsorbed by any nephron segment, it is secreted to some extent by the proximal tubular organic cation secretory system

---

[3]Recently, three Na^+-dependent urea transporters have been characterised.

(see **Table 1**); thus, the amount in the urine exceeds that in the filtrate. In healthy individuals, the proportion of creatinine secreted (in relation to the amount filtered) is minor and varies little; however, if the plasma creatinine concentration rises (as in renal failure), this proportion increases and the clearance of creatinine can then grossly overestimate the true GFR.

Practice Point 4

In volume depletion states, with accompanying GFR reduction, there is often a greater increase in plasma urea concentration than in plasma creatinine concentration. When detected, this is a useful pointer to the need for rehydration. The disproportionate rise in plasma urea occurs because the fractional reabsorption of urea increases in the PCT (as part of the proximal tubular response to volume depletion) and in the terminal collecting duct (as a consequence of enhanced fractional water reabsorption throughout the collecting duct). In contrast, proximal tubular creatinine secretion tends to increase as GFR falls (see above).

CALCIUM

Since ~40% of total plasma calcium is bound to protein, only the remaining 60% is freely filtered. Of this, ~98% is usually reabsorbed. The reabsorptive sites are shown in **Figure 18**. Reabsorption is by a combination of transcellular (active) and paracellular (passive) routes (**Figure 19**). Throughout the nephron, calcium entry into the cell from the lumen occurs through channels down a large

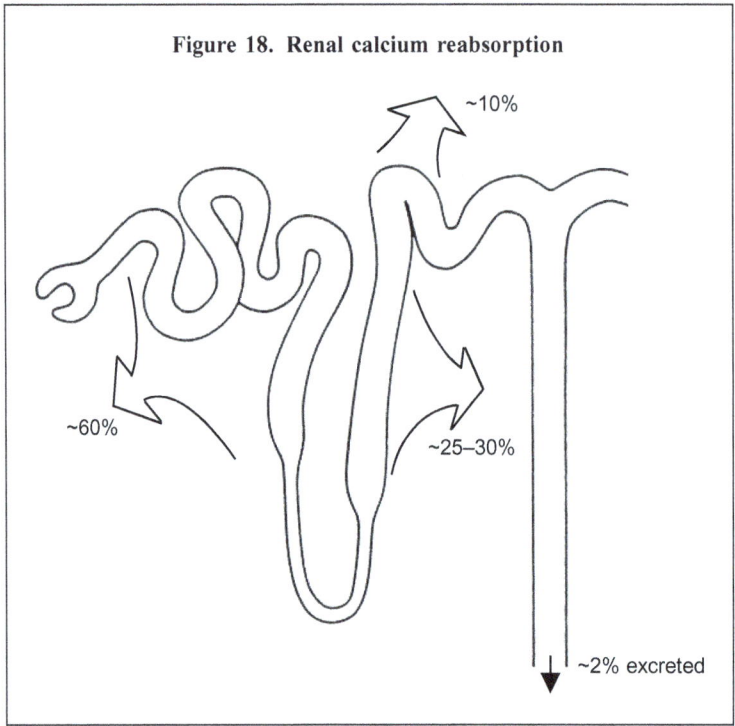

Figure 18. Renal calcium reabsorption

~10%

~60%

~25–30%

~2% excreted

Figure 19. Mechanisms of calcium reabsorption

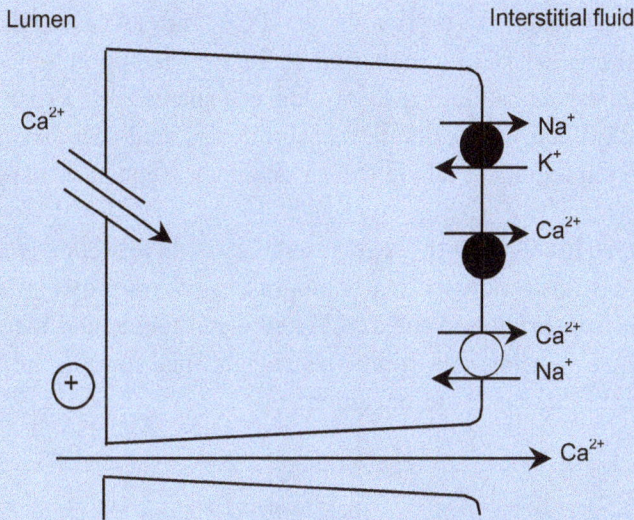

Voltage-driven paracellular Ca^{2+} reabsorption occurs only in the S$_2$ segment of the PCT and in the TALH

electrochemical gradient; exit across the basolateral membrane is uphill and is either primary active (Ca^{2+}-ATPase) or secondary active (Na$^+$/Ca^{2+} exchange).

Most reabsorption is in the S$_2$ segment of the PCT, where a combination of the lumen-positive transepithelial PD (see earlier under Chloride) and a tubular fluid: plasma concentration ratio >1 drives passive paracellular reabsorption; solvent drag may also be involved. In addition, some transcellular reabsorption takes place. The mechanisms of calcium reabsorption in the TALH are thought to be similar to those in the PCT (except that no solvent drag is possible, owing to the absence of water reabsorption). The larger transepithelial PD in the TALH ensures a high proportion of passive paracellular transport. If the PD is reduced, e.g. during treatment with loop diuretics, paracellular reabsorption is reduced and hypercalciuria ensues. In the distal tubule, a "tight" epithelium, calcium reabsorption is exclusively transcellular.

High affinity Ca^{2+}-binding proteins, such as calbindin, facilitate the entry step for Ca^{2+}. These proteins act as cytosolic buffers and maintain a low intracellular Ca^{2+} concentration and thus a favourable gradient for Ca^{2+} entry. Cyclosporin inhibits calbindin expression, which might explain the *hypercalciuria* sometimes seen in patients on this drug. Thiazide diuretics, which inhibit NaCl reabsorption in the early distal tubule (see later), *enhance* calcium reabsorption in this segment, resulting in *hypocalciuria*. There are two likely reasons for this:

- By blocking NaCl entry into early distal tubular cells, thiazides reduce intracellular sodium and thereby enhance basolateral Na$^+$/Ca^{2+} exchange.
- By blocking NaCl entry into early distal tubular cells, thiazides also reduce intracellular chloride. This causes hyperpolarisation of the cells, thereby increasing the driving force for calcium entry through luminal calcium channels.

Factors Affecting Calcium Excretion

- Because of the partial dependence of calcium reabsorption on Na^+/Ca^{2+} exchange and the transepithelial PD, calcium reabsorption in the PCT and TALH tends to parallel sodium transport in these segments; factors inhibiting sodium reabsorption, e.g. extracellular volume expansion, will also reduce calcium reabsorption and increase its excretion.
- A second important influence on calcium reabsorption is acid-base balance; acidosis inhibits calcium reabsorption in the distal tubule (by an unknown mechanism) and therefore increases calcium excretion[4].
- The principal hormone involved in the regulation of calcium excretion is *parathyroid hormone* (PTH). Although PTH has a non-specific inhibitory effect on proximal tubular reabsorption, it enhances calcium reabsorption in the TALH and distal tubule and thereby reduces calcium excretion. Curiously, *calcitonin* also stimulates calcium reabsorption in the TALH and distal tubule[5]. The effects of *calcitriol* are uncertain.

Practice Point 5

The action of loop diuretics on calcium reabsorption in the TALH (as described above) is the basis of their use in severe acute hypercalcaemia to increase calcium excretion.

PHOSPHATE

Inorganic phosphate (P_i) is present in plasma as HPO_4^{2-} and $H_2PO_4^-$. Approximately 10% of the filtered P_i is usually excreted. Quantitatively, the most significant reabsorptive site is the proximal tubule, where ~80% of filtered P_i is reabsorbed by secondary active transport involving carriers in both luminal and basolateral membranes. Up to 10% of filtered P_i is reabsorbed beyond the loop of Henle by unknown mechanisms.

Factors Affecting Phosphate Excretion

- Because P_i reabsorption is almost exclusively proximal, any factor influencing proximal tubular reabsorption (e.g. extracellular volume status) will affect P_i excretion.
- Proximal P_i reabsorption is influenced by dietary phosphate; increased intake stimulates (and decreased intake inhibits) the luminal Na^+/P_i co-transporters.

---

[4]A change in the concentration of free, and therefore filterable, calcium may also be important in acidosis and alkalosis, causing an increase and decrease, respectively.

[5]In view of this anticalciuric action of calcitonin, it may seem puzzling that it is used to treat malignant hypercalcaemia; however, in this setting, what is important therapeutically is its inhibitory effect on bone osteoclast activity.

- Acid-base status is an important factor, acidosis being associated with reduced P_i reabsorption.
- Hormonal control is by PTH, which inhibits P_i reabsorption by reducing the number of luminal co-transporters. PTH is therefore a major factor increasing P_i excretion.

MAGNESIUM

Approximately 70% of plasma magnesium is ultrafilterable, of which ~97% is usually reabsorbed **(Figure 20)**. Uniquely, the major reabsorptive site is the TALH, with only moderate reabsorption in the proximal tubule. Although the reabsorptive mechanisms are not fully understood, it is believed that passive paracellular transport predominates; certainly there is strong evidence that magnesium reabsorption in the TALH is driven largely by the transepithelial PD.

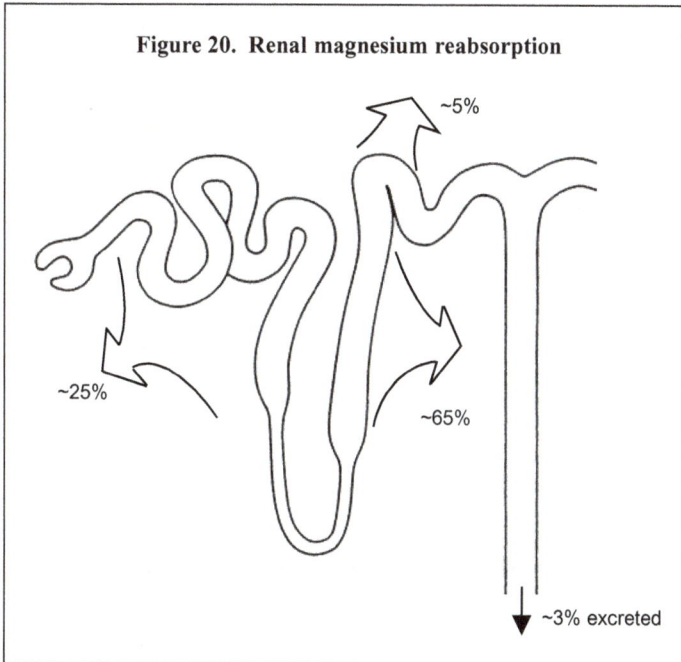

Figure 20. Renal magnesium reabsorption

~5%

~25%

~65%

~3% excreted

Factors Affecting Magnesium Excretion

It is likely that most quantitatively significant changes in magnesium excretion result largely from altered magnesium reabsorption in the TALH, which in turn is dependent on the size of the reabsorptive driving force. Factors involved include:

- loop diuretics: $\downarrow$ Mg^{2+} reabsorption
- increased/decreased dietary magnesium: $\downarrow/\uparrow$ Mg^{2+} reabsorption
- extracellular volume expansion/contraction: $\downarrow/\uparrow$ Mg^{2+} reabsorption
- acidosis/alkalosis: $\downarrow/\uparrow$ Mg^{2+} reabsorption
- hypercalcaemia/hypocalcaemia: $\downarrow/\uparrow$ Mg^{2+} reabsorption
- PTH: $\uparrow$ Mg^{2+} reabsorption

Practice Point 6

The magnesium loss induced by loop diuretics can (through unknown mechanisms) prevent correction of hypokalaemia by potassium supplements; alcoholics are particularly susceptible to this problem. Amiloride has the advantage that it is both potassium- and magnesium-sparing, which indicates that some magnesium reabsorption must be transcellular and also must occur beyond the loop of Henle. However, the importance of the paracellular route for magnesium reabsorption along the TALH has been confirmed recently in patients with a familial form of magnesium-wasting nephropathy. In this syndrome, a mutation in a renal tight junction (paracellular) protein called paracellin-1 (a channel-like protein) has been found.

DIURETICS

Strictly speaking, the term "diuretic" embraces any substance that increases urine flow rate. However, by convention, diuretics are generally regarded as agents that inhibit sodium and water reabsorption in one or more nephron segments. The classes of diuretic still in use are:

- osmotic diuretics
- carbonic anhydrase inhibitors
- loop diuretics
- thiazide diuretics
- potassium-sparing diuretics.

Their sites of action along the nephron are indicated in **Figure 21**.

Osmotic Diuretics

Any substance that is poorly reabsorbed in the proximal tubule will cause retention of fluid and sodium within the nephron and, if present in sufficient amount, will act as an osmotic diuretic. The best-known example is mannitol.

As indicated earlier, reabsorption in the proximal tubules is isosmotic. When administered, mannitol contributes to the total osmolarity of the filtrate and, since it is not reabsorbed, its presence reduces water reabsorption in the proximal tubule. The concentration of sodium in the isosmotic reabsorbate will exceed that in plasma (because, unlike plasma, the reabsorbate contains no mannitol), and consequently the sodium concentration of the fluid remaining in the tubule falls until a limiting concentration gradient is established, against which no further sodium can be reabsorbed. In this way, the delivery of sodium and water to the end of the proximal tubule is increased.

Normally, any increase in sodium delivery from the proximal tubules would be largely offset by enhanced reabsorption in the loop of Henle. In this instance, however, the reabsorptive capacity of the loop is impaired. This is because NaCl reabsorption in the TALH is concentration dependent, i.e. it can proceed only until a limiting NaCl concentration is achieved. Therefore, if the NaCl concentration of the fluid entering the TALH is already lowered (as when mannitol is present), the amount reabsorbed in the TALH will be reduced.

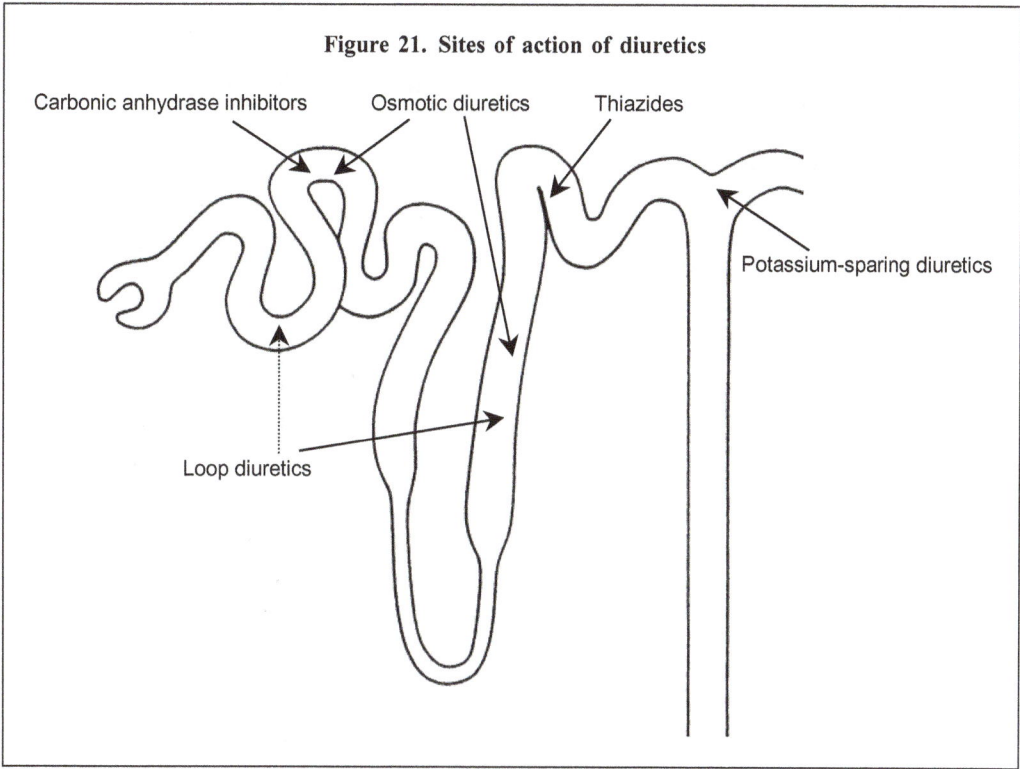

Figure 21. Sites of action of diuretics

The diuretic effect of mannitol is increased by a further factor; for reasons that are not yet clear, mannitol increases the renal medullary blood flow, which in turn tends to cause some "washout" of the medullary hypertonicity (see earlier). This reduces water reabsorption in the thin descending limb of Henle and also limits the ability to concentrate the urine in the collecting duct.

Practice Point 7

Both urea and glucose (as in heavy glycosuria) can act as osmotic diuretics. This action of urea may contribute to the polyuric phase of recovery from ARF (acute tubular necrosis) and the polyuria seen in some patients following renal transplantation. A danger of administering an osmotic diuretic like mannitol (which must be given intravenously) to a patient with a low and fixed GFR, or impaired cardiac function, is sudden expansion of the intravascular volume and circulatory overload, leading to acute pulmonary oedema. This occurs because fluid is drawn in osmotically from the extravascular (interstitial) space and cannot be rapidly filtered and excreted.

Carbonic Anhydrase Inhibitors

Isoforms of the enzyme carbonic anhydrase are present in all those regions of the nephron where H^+ secretion occurs: proximal tubule, TALH and the intercalated cells of the distal nephron. However, since the vast bulk of H^+ secretion occurs in the proximal tubule, this is the principal site of action of carbonic anhydrase inhibitors (e.g. acetazolamide, methazolamide). By interfering with the action of the enzyme, these agents: (i) inhibit the generation of H^+ ions within the cells, thereby limiting the supply of H^+ for Na^+/H^+ exchange; and (ii) inhibit the dehydration of H_2CO_3 (to CO_2 and H_2O) in the lumen, thereby increasing the luminal H^+ concentration and preventing further H^+ secretion (see **Figure 14**). Not only do these actions inhibit sodium bicarbonate reabsorption in the proximal tubule (where sodium bicarbonate reabsorption normally accounts for ~1/3 of all sodium reabsorption), they also reduce sodium chloride reabsorption. The latter effect arises from the fact that the preferential reabsorption of HCO_3^- in the early PCT normally raises the intratubular Cl^- concentration, which facilitates passive Cl^- reabsorption in the late PCT.

Despite disrupting a significant proportion of proximal reabsorption, the overall effect of carbonic anhydrase inhibitors on sodium and water excretion is relatively minor. This is a consequence of the compensatory action of the TALH and (to a lesser extent) distal tubule, which increase their sodium reabsorptive rates in response to the increased delivery.

Practice Point 8

The diuretic effect of oral acetazolamide used to treat glaucoma is sometimes over-looked; it can cause significant hypokalaemia (see later). Since carbonic anhydrase inhibitors require adequate filtered HCO_3^- for their diuretic action, this effect is blunted in the presence of metabolic acidosis and to that extent is self-limiting due to urinary losses of HCO_3^-.

Loop Diuretics

Agents that inhibit sodium reabsorption in the TALH (furosemide, bumetanide, torasemide, ethacrynic acid) are the most potent diuretics available. This is principally because ~25% of filtered sodium is normally reabsorbed in the TALH, while the ability of the downstream nephron segments to reabsorb the extra delivered load of sodium is limited.

Loop diuretics block the $Na^+/K^+/2Cl^-$ co-transporter by competing with Cl^- ions for occupation of the second Cl^- binding site on the transporter protein. In consequence, transport of sodium into the cell is lowered, thereby reducing its extrusion across the basolateral membrane (see **Figure 3**). Blockade of the $Na^+/K^+/2Cl^-$ co-transporter also prevents entry of Cl^- and K^+ into the cell; therefore, K^+ recycling across the luminal membrane and Cl^- exit across the basolateral membrane are inhibited. As a result, the transepithelial PD is reduced or abolished. Therefore, in addition to their inhibitory effects on net NaCl reabsorption, loop diuretics also promote the excretion of those cations normally reabsorbed in the TALH by passive paracellular transport (K^+, Ca^{2+}, Mg^{2+}).

Since, in the final analysis, countercurrent multiplication is dependent on NaCl reabsorption in the TALH (see earlier), loop diuretics cause major disruption of the medullary osmotic gradient, resulting in:

- reduced water reabsorption in the thin descending limb.
- an inability to concentrate the urine in the collecting duct.

The net effect is the excretion of large volumes of virtually isotonic urine.

In addition to their primary action in the TALH, there is good evidence that, at the doses usually employed, loop diuretics have some inhibitory effect on proximal tubular reabsorption (possibly through inhibition of carbonic anhydrase). Clearly, any such action could not be buffered by enhanced reabsorption in the loop and would therefore augment loop diuretic potency. This is the principle behind combining diuretics with different sites of action to treat "refractory" oedema.

Loop diuretics in acute renal failure

There is some evidence that loop diuretics may prevent the development of ARF. This could result in part from a renal vasodilator effect and in part from the flushing out of intraluminal debris. A third factor might be that, by reducing the metabolic needs of TALH cells, the potential for ischaemic injury in this sensitive nephron site is lessened.

Thiazide Diuretics

Thiazide diuretics (e.g. chlorothiazide, hydrochlorothiazide, chlortalidone, bendroflumethiazide) inhibit the NaCl co-transporter in the early distal tubule and therefore block NaCl reabsorption at this site (see **Figure 5**). Because the extent of sodium reabsorption in the early distal tubule is usually only of the order of 5% of the filtered load, thiazide diuretics are only moderately natriuretic. Some thiazides (notably chlortalidone and chlorothiazide) have significant carbonic anhydrase inhibitory activity and therefore have a subsidiary inhibitory effect on proximal tubular reabsorption. The anticalciuric effect of thiazides has been described in an earlier section.

Potassium-Sparing Diuretics

As explained earlier, all diuretics that act proximally to the late distal tubule/cortical collecting duct (i.e. all those dealt with so far) will increase the delivery of sodium and fluid to the potassium secretory site and therefore will enhance potassium secretion and excretion. In an attempt to prevent the hypokalaemia that would otherwise ensue, potassium-sparing diuretics are frequently co-prescribed. These are of two types: those that act directly on luminal Na^+ channels of principal cells (amiloride, triamterene) and those that act indirectly by antagonising the action of aldosterone (spironolactone). The net effect of the two types is similar: a mild natriuresis (only 2–3% of filtered sodium is normally reabsorbed in this segment) and, more importantly, inhibition of potassium secretion.

Blockade of luminal Na^+ channels prevents sodium entry into principal cells (see **Figure 6**). This reduces potassium secretion in two ways:

- The reduction in intracellular sodium lowers the rate of sodium extrusion by the basolateral Na^+/K^+-ATPase, which in turn lowers the rate of entry of potassium into the cell and thus reduces intracellular potassium.

- The electrical profile across the luminal membrane is altered. Na^+ entry from the lumen normally depolarises the luminal membrane (i.e. makes the cell interior less negative with respect to the lumen), which increases the electrochemical gradient favouring potassium secretion. Blockade of the Na^+ channels will hyperpolarise the luminal membrane, which will *reduce* (usually to zero) the electrochemical gradient favouring potassium secretion.

Dopamine

Dopamine is an endogenous catecholamine that in certain circumstances is administered clinically as a diuretic. It is synthesised by proximal tubular cells (its production being increased during volume expansion) and appears to act not only in the proximal tubule but also in the TALH and the cortical collecting duct to inhibit basolateral Na^+/K^+-ATPase activity, which in turn leads to reduced entry of sodium from the lumen. It is not known whether the effects downstream from the proximal tubule result from dopamine being carried in the tubular fluid. Two broad types of dopamine receptor have been classified: DA_1 and DA_2 (although several subtypes have now been described). The renal actions of dopamine appear to be mediated largely by DA_1 receptors, which activate adenylate cyclase, leading to raised levels of intracellular cAMP.

When administered, dopamine and dopamine agonists (e.g. dopexamine, fenoldopam) cause renal vasodilatation (and $\uparrow$ GFR) as well as inhibition of tubular sodium reabsorption. Although some authorities believe that dopamine helps prevent ARF in some patients (owing largely to its ability to increase renal blood flow), the evidence is inconclusive. More promising are reports that dopamine might help in *recovery* from ARF, although the timing of its administration may be critical.

FURTHER READING

Aronson PS, Giebisch G (1997) Mechanisms of chloride transport in the proximal tubule. *American Journal of Physiology*; 273: F179–F192

Giebisch G (1998) Renal potassium transport: Mechanisms and regulation. *American Journal of Physiology*; 274: F817–F833

Ichikawa I, Harris RC (1991) Angiotensin actions in the kidney: Renewed insight into the old hormone. *Kidney International*; 40: 583–596

Schnermann JB, Sayegh SI (eds.) (1998) Kidney physiology. Philadelphia: Lippincott-Raven

Seldin D, Giebisch G (eds.) (1997) Diuretic agents. San Diego: Academic Press

(This list covers both **Chapters 1** and **2**)

SECTION 2

ACUTE RENAL FAILURE — COMMON PRINCIPLES

Chapter 3 _____

THE AETIOLOGY OF ACUTE RENAL FAILURE
Andrew Allen

DEFINITION

Acute renal failure (ARF) can be defined as a rapid loss of glomerular filtration and tubular function, leading to abnormal water, electrolyte and solute balance. This occurs over hours to days (distinguishing it from chronic renal failure), although ARF can be superimposed upon a background of chronic renal impairment, so-called acute-on-chronic renal failure. The diagnosis of ARF is often first made upon noting rises in plasma urea and creatinine concentrations; clinically overt sequelae such as pulmonary oedema and hypertension tend to occur only once ARF is fully established. ARF is most commonly related to renal ischaemia, and this often occurs as part of a multi-system disorder, such as septic shock or severe trauma. It is important to recognise developing ARF quickly, since it may be reversible if appropriate treatment is instituted rapidly, and established ARF brings with it the burdens of increased morbidity, mortality, hospital stay and cost.

In the majority of patients, ARF is associated with oliguria, defined as urine production of <400 mL/day. Anuria (<100 mL/day) is also common. Some patients however (20–40%), develop non-oliguric ARF (e.g. following administration of radiocontrast media), and this is associated with a better prognosis, i.e. a lower likelihood of requiring dialysis. For this reason, conversion of oliguric to non-oliguric renal failure is regarded as a valuable goal in the therapy of ARF.

EPIDEMIOLOGY

It is difficult to ascertain an accurate figure for the population incidence of ARF, since definitions of ARF can vary from a plasma creatinine of >150 μmol/L to the temporary requirement for dialysis. Nevertheless, population studies relying upon laboratory databases to identify patients with elevated urea/creatinine, have suggested values for ARF incidence of 80–140 per million population (pmp) per year. 50–70 pmp/year will require dialysis. Most strikingly, the incidence rises dramatically with increasing age: for those below 50 years of age the figure is 17 pmp/year, whereas for those between 80 and 89 it is 949 pmp/year. In such community-based studies, prostatic disease is the commonest cause of renal failure, although much of this may represent progressive chronic renal impairment rather than true ARF.

With regard to ARF in hospital, a large prospective American series examining over 2200 consecutive medical and surgical admissions found that some degree of ARF developed in ~5%. Dialysis was required in around 0.5% of all patients. Studies of particular subgroups of patients, such as those undergoing aortic aneurysm surgery, will typically provide much higher estimates of ARF incidence. The majority of cases of ARF in hospital are due to acute tubular necrosis.

Prior to 1960 or so, post-surgical and obstetric cases of ARF were very common, comprising the majority of patients. Improvements in post-operative and obstetric care have increased the percentage of "medical" patients contributing to ARF series. This phenomenon also reflects a diminishing reluctance to refer and treat elderly patients with ARF from a variety of medical reasons. Indeed, the mean age of referred patients seen at a major British renal unit increased from 41 years in the 1950s to 61 years in the 1980s. There are also geographic factors which influence both the incidence and aetiology of ARF. In India, for example, copper sulphate (widely used in agriculture and tanning) is a common cause of ARF due to direct nephrotoxicity and haemoglobinuria. In Africa, herbal medicines containing toxins, together with infections, contribute to many cases of ARF.

The mortality of ARF due to military trauma fell from 90% to 5% following the advent of dialysis in the 1950s. Unfortunately, this success has not been mirrored in the civilian population, for whom ARF is associated with a 50–60% mortality rate which has changed little over the last 20–30 years. It is felt that this reflects the increasingly sick nature of patients taken on for temporary renal replacement therapy, and that changes in ARF management are unlikely to change the overall mortality very much. Patients with isolated ARF, i.e. single-system failure, have a very good prognosis; but as increasing numbers of organ systems fail, mortality rises swiftly (see **Chapter 28**). In current practice, patients may die with renal failure, but they seldom die from it.

AETIOLOGY

ARF has many potential causes, which often conflate within a given individual, making it unclear as to which, if any, is the dominant aetiologic factor. Broadly (and helpfully), the causes of ARF can be divided into 3 groups to help clarify the diagnostic process. These are:

- **Pre-renal** — implying failure of the "circulation" (through loss of volume and/or pressure) to provide the kidney with sufficient plasma flow to maintain steady-state blood chemistry and fluid balance.
- **Renal** — Intrinsic renal disease causing loss of glomerular filtration — this can be through glomerular disease (**Chapter 16**), tubulointerstitial disease (**Chapter 18**) or vascular disease, e.g. thrombotic microangiopathy (**Chapter 15**).
- **Post-renal** — due to obstruction of the renal tract which can be anywhere from renal pelvis to urethra (see **Chapter 23**).

Pre-Renal Failure

Following the definition(s) of ARF given above, the commonest cause of a rapid loss of glomerular filtration is a reduction in renal perfusion, below the level at which homeostatic mechanisms can compensate. Thus oliguria and a rise in serum creatinine will ensue, although restoration of renal perfusion (typically by restoring intravascular volume) will often lead to rapid return of normal urine flow and correction of the electrolyte/metabolite disturbances. This reversible form of renal

Table 1. Major causes of pre-renal failure/azotaemia	
Hypovolaemia	**Renal hypoperfusion**
Haemorrhage	Renal artery thrombosis
Burns	Bilateral renal artery stenosis (especially if ACEI given)
3rd-spacing (pancreatitis, crush injury, intestinal obstruction)	NSAIDs (especially in elderly, hypovolaemic patient)
GI losses (enteric fistulae/tube drainage, diarrhoea, vomiting)	Abdominal aortic aneurysm affecting renal vessels
Renal losses (glycosuria, post-obstructive diuresis, diuretics)	
Hypotension	**Oedematous states**
Shock (cardiogenic or septic)	Congestive cardiac failure
Over-aggressive therapy of hypertension	Hepatic cirrhosis (including hepatorenal syndrome)
	Minimal change glomerulonephritis with ARF

decompensation is called pre-renal failure. In the US, the term pre-renal azotaemia is often used, which is appealing since there is no suggestion of renal failure, simply insufficient renal perfusion and glomerular filtration to permit maintenance of normal, steady-state electrolyte/metabolite concentrations. Common causes of pre-renal azotaemia are listed in **Table 1** and are segmented according to reduction in either (effective) blood volume or pressure.

"Intrinsic" Renal Failure

As described above, intrinsic ARF can be divided into three groups — tubular, glomerular and vascular. The former is by far the commonest, since it lies on a continuum with pre-renal ARF and is associated with the same broad set of causes. If renal hypoperfusion is prolonged, then ischaemic damage to the kidney will occur, which typically manifests as acute tubular necrosis (ATN). The widespread use of drugs, such as NSAIDs and ACE inhibitors (ACEI), which modulate intra-renal blood flow adversely, has probably had a major part to play in increasing the frequency of ATN in clinical practice. ATN can also be secondary to direct tubule epithelial cell toxicity from agents as varied as aminoglycoside antibiotics and snake venom (**Table 2**). The histopathology of ATN is discussed in **Chapter 7**, and is characterised by flattening of proximal convoluted tubule cell microvilli, tubule epithelial cell flattening, and obstruction of the tubule lumen by shed epithelial cells and precipitating proteins. Mitosis of epithelial cells may be seen, particularly in the recovery phase of ATN, as cells regenerate.

Given that the kidney receives approximately 20% of cardiac output, it is at first rather puzzling that the same organ is particularly susceptible to ischaemic insults which most other organs readily tolerate. The answer to this lies in the subtleties of the kidney's circulatory arrangements. The normal kidney has a very low oxygen extraction ratio, and its vessels are arranged such that oxygenated blood perfuses the parenchyma starting at the outer cortex. All arterioles and capillaries supplying the deeper, medullary tubules are post-glomerular, and are arranged in countercurrent parallel loops, akin to the loops of Henle. These vasa rectae allow

Table 2. Major causes of acute tubular necrosis	
Post-ischaemic	**Toxin-related**
As above under pre-renal failure	Drugs, e.g. aminoglycosides, cisplatin, amphotericin B
	Radiocontrast agents (particularly in volume-depleted patients)
	Haem pigments, e.g. rhabdomyolysis, myoglobinuria
	Snake venom
	Heavy metals, e.g. lead, mercury

oxygen to perfuse freely across their walls, and their countercurrent arrangement means that the cortex is relatively well oxygenated, whereas the normal medulla is relatively hypoxic. This process is comparable to the high medullary osmolality generated by the loops of Henle (see **Chapter 2**). The metabolic demands of tubule epithelial cells are also substantial, given their dependence upon the basolateral membrane Na^+/K^+-ATPase for normal tubule function. As a consequence of their high ATP demands in a region of relative hypoxia, tubule epithelial cells are prone to injury following renal ischaemia. Experimental studies in rats have suggested that the thick ascending limb of the loop of Henle and the S_3 segment of the proximal tubule are particularly susceptible to hypoxic damage. Intense intra-renal vasoconstriction may also occur after relatively minor insults, to compound the tendency towards ischaemic injury. The pathophysiology of ischaemic acute tubule injury is discussed further in **Chapters 8** and **19**.

Acute tubulointerstitial nephritis (ATIN) is another major cause of "tubular" intrinsic ARF, and is described in detail in **Chapter 18**. One overlap disorder is crystalluria, such as that of hyperoxaluria, which can cause intense tubulointerstitial inflammation as well as tubular obstruction (see below).

Glomerular causes of ARF are principally those forms of glomerulonephritis (GN) associated with the clinical syndrome of rapidly progressive GN (RPGN), as discussed in detail in **Chapter 16**. Special mention should perhaps be made of the clinical syndrome of ARF with the otherwise benign glomerular lesion of minimal change nephropathy. Although poorly understood, the presence of ARF in minimal change nephropathy at presentation is well described in adults, and usually attributed to a combination of relative hypovolaemia (perhaps related to over-zealous diuresis), reduced filtration surface area (through foot process fusion) and, perhaps, renal parenchymal oedema. The prognosis is usually good, and function improves rapidly as oedema resolves. A key differential of this syndrome is minimal change nephropathy plus associated TIN, as occasionally seen with certain NSAIDs (especially fenoprofen).

Vascular causes of ARF are relatively uncommon, but very important since they typically demand immediate therapy to avoid permanent loss of function or life. Large vessel obstruction can be through aortic dissection with occlusion of the renal vessels, or from arterial embolism or venous thrombosis. Renal vein thrombosis is an important differential in nephrotic patients who experience sudden deterioration in renal function, usually associated with loin pain and haematuria. Microvascular occlusion is also important, typically from a thrombotic angiopathy,

Table 3. Common causes of renal tract obstruction causing acute renal failure	
Site of obstruction	**Disorder**
Renal pelvis	Calculus
	Sloughed papilla
Ureter	Carcinoma
	Calculus
	Blood clot
	Pregnancy
	Surgical error (ligation)
	Retroperitoneal disorder, e.g. carcinomatous infiltration, idiopathic fibrosis, lymphoma
Bladder (neck)	Bladder carcinoma
	Prostatic enlargement (benign or malignant)
	Acutely neurogenic bladder
Urethra	Stricture/stenosis

such as those associated with pre-eclampsia, haemolytic uraemic syndrome, thrombotic thrombocytopaenic purpura, scleroderma or malignant hypertension.

Post-Renal Failure

Obstruction of the urinary tract is a common cause of renal failure, particularly in the community, where prostatic disease causes much (chronic) renal impairment. Acute renal failure from urinary obstruction is less common, but still important to diagnose accurately since urgent intervention is usually mandated. The major causes are given in **Table 3**.

INVESTIGATION

The relevant investigations to pinpoint the exact aetiology of ARF are detailed in **Chapters 4–7**. A standard clinical approach to the patient with (acute) renal failure has been outlined well by Firth, and comprises the following steps:

1. Establish whether ARF is truly acute — typically by measuring renal size. CRF is associated with two small, shrunken (often scarred) kidneys, whereas true ARF is associated with normal or large kidneys.
2. Exclude urinary obstruction — most conveniently by renal ultrasonography. Rarely there can occur obstructive ARF with non-dilated renal calyces, most frequently with renal tract malignancy. If suspicion of "non-dilated" obstruction exists, serial ultrasound scans can be performed, or a CT scan, which delineates renal anatomy more accurately than ultrasonography. A dynamic test can, alternatively, be performed, such as a nuclear medicine scan (MAG3 renogram — see **Chapter 6**). In the final instance, retrograde ureteropyelograms can be carried out under general anaesthesia.

3. Exclude intrinsic ARF from glomerular, tubulointerstitial or vascular disease as a cause of renal failure. If present, the medical history is usually suggestive of multi-systemic disease, and physical examination can be informative (skin rashes of systemic vasculitis can be easily missed). Urine microscopy to identify the classic "active" sediment of acute GN should always be performed in cases of ARF.

4. Has acute vascular occlusion occurred? The clinical setting is typically suggestive of such an event, and renal vascular Doppler studies are usually adequate to support the diagnosis, although angiography may be required.

The vast majority of remaining cases will be secondary to pre-renal disease or ATN, for which the clinical approach is similar in the first instance, i.e. optimisation of fluid balance and systemic haemodynamics with a peripheral role for pharmacologic intervention such as diuretics and dopamine. Of note, absolute anuria is suggestive of renal tract obstruction, renal cortical necrosis or necrotising GN.

TREATMENT

Prevention of ARF should be a key principle for all physicians managing vulnerable patients, which category includes all elderly patients, all those with pre-existing renal impairment, and all with multisystem disease. Simple principles of maintaining normal fluid balance and avoiding nephrotoxins (particularly drugs) wherever possible should guide all medical interventions.

If ARF develops, however, its treatment falls into two categories — life-saving emergency measures for ARF, irrespective of cause, and subsequent specific therapies targeted at the individual aetiology.

The possible life-threatening consequences of ARF are:

1. Hyperkalaemia with ventricular arrhythmia.
2. Profound metabolic acidosis with disturbance of cardiac rhythm and contractility.
3. Fluid overload and pulmonary oedema.
4. Severe uraemia with uraemic coma or pericarditis.

The emergent treatment of each of these dangerous complications is described in detail in **Chapter 8**.

Specific therapies for the various forms of ARF vary according to aetiology, but a common principle is to optimise fluid balance and systemic haemodynamics. These simple manoeuvres may be sufficient, in cases of pre-renal ARF or non-oliguric ATN, to reverse renal failure and, in the case of ATN, obviate the need for renal replacement. Fluid replacement can be carried out according to clinical examination in the emergency setting, but central venous pressure monitoring is often used to guide this key aspect of management. Details of invasive monitoring are provided in **Chapter 5**.

The patient with ARF is at major risk of sepsis, through both relative immunosuppression and the intensive instrumentation (particularly indwelling dialysis catheters) needed for management of such patients. Close attention to all vascular lines is mandated, with removal necessary if evidence of infection is detected. Nutrition is also important, with aggressive nutritional supplementation necessary in many patients, particularly those with intense protein catabolism (see **Appendix B**).

Many experimental therapies have been found effective in various animal models of ARF, but their translation into clinical practice has proven remarkably difficult. Synthetic atrial natriuretic peptide (ANP) was one of the leading candidates to emerge from pre-clinical studies, but a pivotal clinical trial in over 500 critically ill patients with ATN proved very disappointing. Only small effects were evident after 24 h of intravenous ANP analogue infusion (anaritide) in a prospectively defined subgroup of oliguric patients, with slightly higher dialysis-free survival in the treated group. Further trials of ANP have proven similarly disappointing, and hope has transferred to a variety of growth factors, such as insulin-like growth factor (IGF), which have generated slightly more encouraging early-stage clinical data (see **Chapter 8**). Further data are eagerly awaited.

OUTCOME

Unsurprisingly, there is no simple predictor of outcome for a disorder as diverse as ARF. Generally, non-oliguric ARF carries a better prognosis than oligoanuria, particularly for ATN, presumably reflecting the lesser severity of renal injury in the former cases. This simple observation underpins much of the effort made to "convert" oliguric to non-oliguric ATN using pharmacotherapy (loop diuretics, mannitol and dopamine). Controlled trial data in support of this approach are notably lacking. For patients who develop established oligo-anuric ATN, recovery classically follows a biphasic pattern with initial polyuria followed by normal restoration of urine flow. This can occur at any point between 1–2 weeks or 2–3 months following acute injury, although even later recovery is well described. The polyuric phase is ascribed to partial recovery of the kidney, with improved glomerular filtration but impaired tubular function, such that urinary concentration is defective and large quantities of dilute urine are produced. The particular importance of the polyuric recovery phase of ATN is that, if it goes unrecognised, volume depletion may develop and renal injury recur. Treatment usually comprises intravenous fluid replacement with a combination of normal saline and 5% dextrose (in a 1:2–3 ratio), since the urinary sodium concentration is around 50–70 mmol/L. In clinical practice, polyuric ATN is most typically seen in renal transplant recipients in whom the transplanted kidney developed ATN during its cold ischaemic period. Hypokalaemia can also develop in such patients, and replacement can be guided by measurement of urinary potassium losses.

FURTHER READING

Conger J (1998) Prophylaxis and treatment of acute renal failure by vasoactive agents: The facts and the myths. *Kidney International*; 53(Suppl. 64): S23

Feest TG, Round A, Hamad S (1993) Incidence of severe acute renal failure in adults: Results of a community-based study. *British Medical Journal*; 306: 481

Firth JD (1997) The clinical approach to the patient with acute renal failure. In: Winnearls C, Cameron JS, Ledingham D, Ritz E and Davison AM (eds.). *Oxford Textbook of Clinical Nephrology* (2nd Edition). Oxford: Oxford University Press; pp. 1557–1582

Firth JD (1998) Medical treatment of acute tubular necrosis. *Quarterly Journal of Medicine*; 91: 321

Hou SH, Bushinsky DA, Wish JB, *et al.* (1983) Hospital-acquired renal insufficiency: A prospective study. *American Journal of Medicine*; 74: 243

Klahr S, Miller SB (1998) Acute oliguria. *The New England Journal of Medicine*; 338: 671

Chapter 4 _____

CLINICAL APPROACH AND LABORATORY INVESTIGATION

4.1 History and examination (pages 47–50)
4.2 Urine output and urinalysis (pages 51–64)
4.3 Haematological investigations (pages 65–67)
4.4 Biochemical investigations (pages 67–70)
4.5 Immunological investigations (pages 71–75)

This chapter describes the clinical assessment of patients with acute renal failure (ARF). The diverse aetiology of ARF often necessitates the use of a range of laboratory, physiological and radiological investigations to aid the clinician in determining diagnoses and guiding therapy. **Table 1** provides a useful check-list of important investigations for patients presenting with ARF of undetermined aetiology.

Table 1. The acute renal failure investigations "check-list"

The relevant book chapters which describe each test in more detail are shown in parentheses.

HISTORY AND EXAMINATION (Chapter 4.1)

URINE (Chapter 4.2)
Dipstick
Microscopy, culture
24 h collection for creatinine clearance & protein excretion
Bence Jones protein
Urinary electrolytes/osmolality

HAEMATOLOGY (Chapter 4.3)
All patients
Full blood count & ESR
Coagulation (INR, APTT)
Hb electrophoresis (in appropriate ethnic groups)
When indicated by results of the above
Blood film, reticulocyte count
Direct Coomb's test
Lactate dehydrogenase, haptoglobin
Fibrinogen, thrombin time, fibrin degradation products
Lupus anticoagulant (and anti-cardiolipin antibodies)

BIOCHEMISTRY (Chapter 4.4)
Urea, creatinine and electrolytes
Albumin, calcium, phosphate
C-reactive protein
Glucose and HbA1C
Liver function tests
Creatine kinase

IMMUNOLOGY (Chapter 4.5)
Immunoglobulins
Serum protein electrophoresis
C3, C4, CH50, anti-C1q Ab
ANA, anti-dsDNA Ab, ENA
Rheumatoid factor & other autoantibodies
Cryoglobulins
ANCA
Anti-GBM antibodies

PHYSIOLOGICAL INVESTIGATION (Chapter 5)
Blood pressure
Electrocardiogram
Arterial blood gases
Pulse oximetry

IMAGING (Chapter 6)
X-ray (CXR, KUB)
Renal tract ultrasound/Doppler studies

MICROBIOLOGY/VIROLOGY (Chapter 20)
Urine culture
Blood cultures
ASOT
Hepatitis serology
HIV
Cytomegalovirus

4.1 HISTORY AND EXAMINATION
Katie Darling

Thorough history-taking and clinical examination form an essential part of the assessment of all patients with ARF. The aims of this clinical assessment are to elucidate the underlying cause of ARF and to identify life threatening complications.

THE HISTORY

Symptoms

Sub-dividing causes of ARF into pre-renal, renal and post-renal (see **Chapter 3**) helps to direct patient questioning. ARF can present with a wide range of symptoms, some which are common to all causes of ARF, and others which reflect more specific aetiologies. **Figure 1** provides an overview of many of the symptoms associated with ARF; where relevant, the reader is referred to the appropriate chapter for more detail.

Past Medical History

- Previous urea and electrolyte results (acute or chronic renal failure?)
- Previous health checks (for insurance/employment)
- Systemic conditions (e.g. diabetes, hypertension, ischaemic heart disease, jaundice)
- Previous urinary symptoms (pyelonephritis, urinary tract infection)
- Recent procedures/instrumentation (surgery, angiography, other radiological procedures)
- Known immunosuppression (transplant patients, HIV, lymphoproliferative disorders).

Drug History

ARF caused by toxins and drugs is discussed in **Chapter 11**. The drug history should include non-prescribed medication such as over-the-counter formulations (notably NSAIDs) and herbal remedies such as Chinese medicines and slimming treatments.

Family History

- Ethnic origin (inherited disorders of metabolism)
- Hereditary causes of renal impairment (polycystic kidney disease, hereditary nephritis)
- Diabetes, ischaemic heart disease, rheumatic disease etc.

Figure 1. Symptoms associated with acute renal failure

The relevant chapters within the book are shown in parentheses

Fever
Infection (19, 20)
Rhabdomyolysis (12)
Vasculitis (16)

Constitutional Symptoms
Nausea & vomiting
Thirst
Diarrhoea

General Malaise

Dyspnoea
Fluid overload (8.2)
Anaemia
Acid-base disturbance (8.4)

Haemoptysis
Vasculitis (16)

Abdominal Pain
Hantaan virus (20)
Leptospirosis (20)

Testicular Pain
Polyarteritis nodosa (16)

Muscular Pain
Rhabdomyolysis

Arthralgia
Vasculitis
Connective tissue diseases (17)

Peripheral oedema
Fluid overload
Nephrotic syndrome

Numbness and weakness
Neuropathy
e.g. diabetes, uraemia,
vasculitis, cryoglobulins

Altered conscious level
Liver failure
Uraemia
Cerebral SLE/ vasculitis

Red eyes, epistaxes, sinusitis
Vasculitis (16)

Hearing / vestibular disturbance
Aminoglycosides (11)
Vasculitis (16)

Pruritis + jaundice
Uraemia (8.6)
Liver disease (25)

Rash
Vasculitis (16)
SLE, cryoglobulins (17)
Cholesterol emboli (13)

Palpitations
Electrolyte imbalance

Orthopnoea
Cardiac Failure (8.2)

Renal Tract Pain (23)

Colic
Calculus
Sloughed papilla
Blood clot

Loin pain
Pyelonephritis
Interstitial rephritis

Urinary Symptoms (4.2)
Volume & appearance
Frequency
Prostatism
Infection

Dysuria, suprapubic pain
Retention
Infection

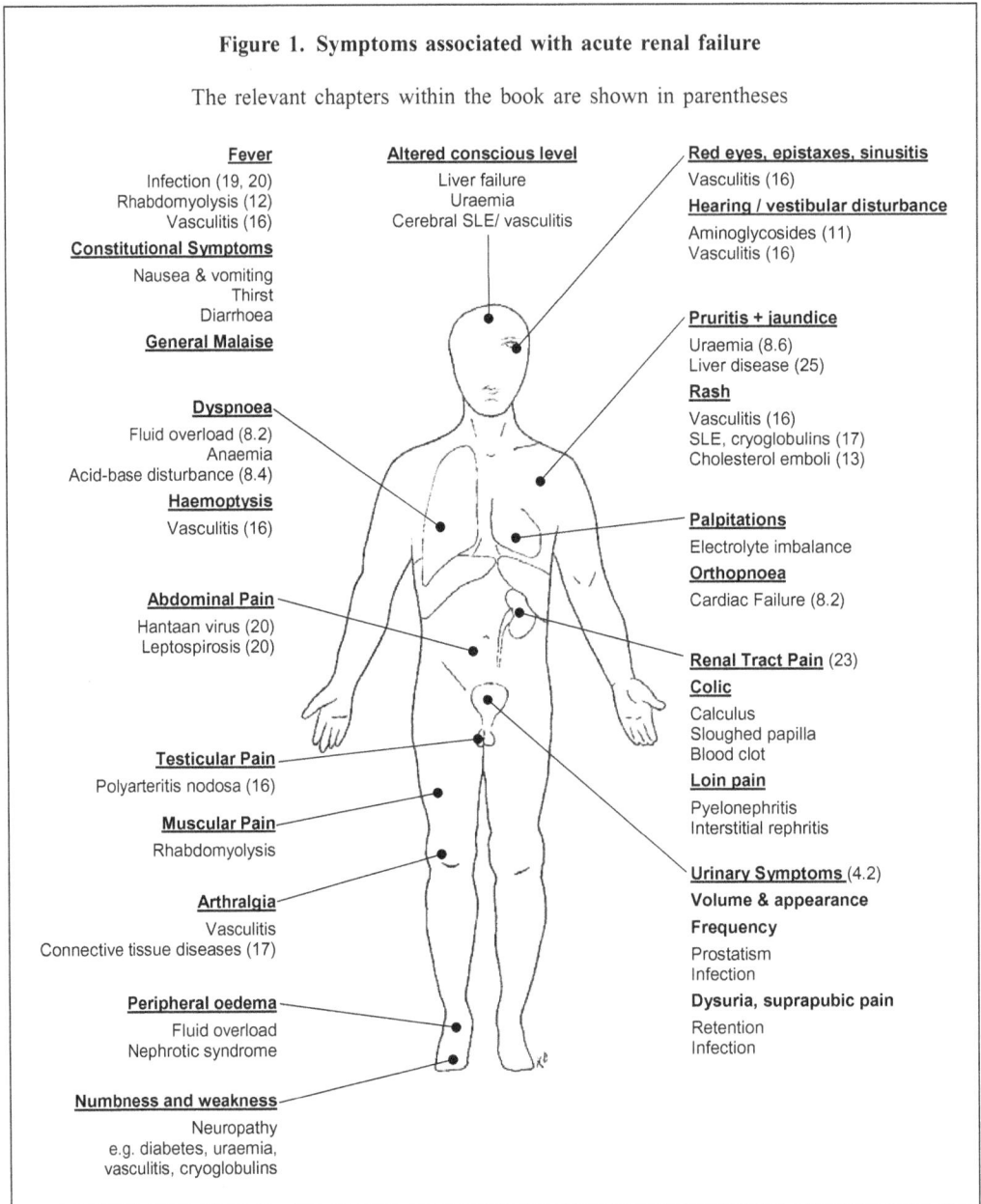

Social History

- Smoking (malignancy)
- Occupation (e.g. exposure to β-naphthaline dyes in chemical/rubber industries — bladder neoplasia)
- Foreign travel (e.g. malaria, schistosomiasis)
- Exposure to waterways or sewage systems (leptospirosis)
- Exposure to rodents in rural areas or disused building sites in endemic areas (Hantaan virus).

CLINICAL EXAMINATION

Initial Clinical Assessment

ARF is a potentially life-threatening condition and a rapid assessment should always be made of the patient's vital signs, level of consciousness and intravascular volume status.

1. *Vital signs*
   Airway, Breathing, Circulation (see **Chapter 5**)

2. *Level of consciousness*
   Glasgow Coma Scale[1]

3. *Assessment of intravascular volume status*
   Degree of hydration is assessed clinically by:

   - Examination of mucous membranes and skin turgor.

     Skin turgor is best measured by twisting the skin over the anterior chest wall or over the forehead as other areas, notably over the backs of the hands, have reduced turgor with advancing age.

   - Measuring heart rate, lying and standing blood pressure (postural hypotension in dehydration).

     In the absence of autonomic neuropathy or cardiac conduction anomaly, any drop in pressure should be accompanied by an increase in heart rate.

   - Assessing jugular venous pressure (JVP) with the patient reclining at 45°.

     Normal JVP is between 0–3 cm above the sternal angle, which corresponds to a right atrial pressure of approximately 8 cm H_2O. If the JVP is difficult to visualise, *gentle* pressure over the liver to increase venous return can be helpful (the hepatojugular reflex).

   - Examining the patient's peripheries.

     Check for capillary return by gentle pressure over the nail bed. A useful technique in a sick patient unable to lie comfortably at 45° is to examine the venous filling over the back of the hand with the arm held at rest beside the body and then when elevated. In fluid overload, venous filling persists on elevation of the outstretched hand to above the level of the right atrium.

   - Recording daily weights in conjunction with fluid balance charts and clinical examination.

---

[1]**Glasgow Coma Scale**

Best verbal response		Best motor response		Eye opening	
Orientated speech	5	Obeys verbal commands	6	Spontaneous	4
Confused speech	4	Localises painful stimuli	5	To speech	3
Inappropriate words	3	Withdraws to pain	4	To painful stimuli	2
Incomprehensible sounds	2	Flexion to pain	3	No response	1
No response	1	Extension to pain	2		
		No response	1		

Further Clinical Examination

Figure 2 highlights important clinical signs associated with a wide range of causes of ARF.

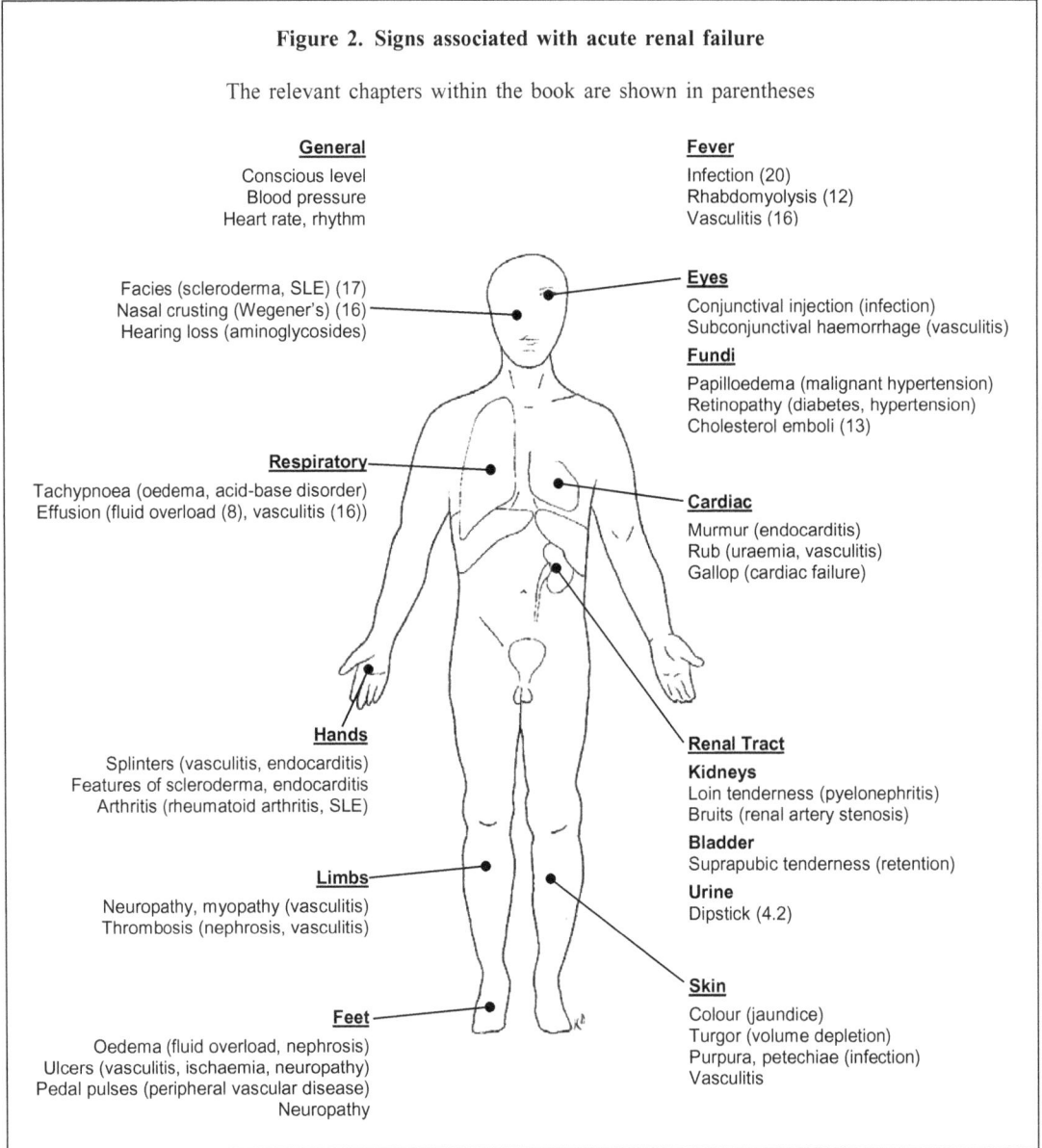

Figure 2. Signs associated with acute renal failure

The relevant chapters within the book are shown in parentheses

General
Conscious level
Blood pressure
Heart rate, rhythm

Fever
Infection (20)
Rhabdomyolysis (12)
Vasculitis (16)

Facies (scleroderma, SLE) (17)
Nasal crusting (Wegener's) (16)
Hearing loss (aminoglycosides)

Eyes
Conjunctival injection (infection)
Subconjunctival haemorrhage (vasculitis)

Fundi
Papilloedema (malignant hypertension)
Retinopathy (diabetes, hypertension)
Cholesterol emboli (13)

Respiratory
Tachypnoea (oedema, acid-base disorder)
Effusion (fluid overload (8), vasculitis (16))

Cardiac
Murmur (endocarditis)
Rub (uraemia, vasculitis)
Gallop (cardiac failure)

Hands
Splinters (vasculitis, endocarditis)
Features of scleroderma, endocarditis
Arthritis (rheumatoid arthritis, SLE)

Renal Tract
Kidneys
Loin tenderness (pyelonephritis)
Bruits (renal artery stenosis)

Bladder
Suprapubic tenderness (retention)
Urine
Dipstick (4.2)

Limbs
Neuropathy, myopathy (vasculitis)
Thrombosis (nephrosis, vasculitis)

Skin
Colour (jaundice)
Turgor (volume depletion)
Purpura, petechiae (infection)
Vasculitis

Feet
Oedema (fluid overload, nephrosis)
Ulcers (vasculitis, ischaemia, neuropathy)
Pedal pulses (peripheral vascular disease)
Neuropathy

4.2 URINE OUTPUT AND URINALYSIS

Iain MacPhee

Urine should be examined in all cases of ARF. The study of the composition of urine and its contents yields much useful information about both the function of the kidney and about pathological processes at specific regions throughout the renal tract. Examination of urine remains a simple process that can be performed quickly, and contributes significantly to the diagnosis of ARF. Up to 50% of patients with ARF present with early oliguria. Indeed, oliguria may be the first and only sign of underlying renal pathology, as other clinical and biochemical features often take 2–3 days to develop. It follows that there is often oligo-anuria at a time when examination of the urine is likely to yield the most important diagnostic information. It is therefore important to obtain a sample of any urine passed as rapidly as possible, for prompt and thorough examination.

URINE VOLUME

Normal 24 h urine output is extremely variable (approximately 800–2500 mL) and primarily reflects water intake. Urine output is modulated by changes in the plasma concentration of a number of neuroendocrine factors, including anti-diuretic hormone (vasopressin), mineralocorticoids and atrial natriuretic peptide (ANP), in response to changes in blood pressure, blood volume and osmolality (see **Chapter 2**). An arbitrary figure of 400–500 mL/24 h is considered to be the lower end of the normal range, which translates approximately to 30 mL/h. The volume of urine produced in ARF can vary from oligo-anuria to extreme polyuria (see **Chapters 3** and **8**). In patients with ARF a urinary catheter is usually passed to exclude obstruction distal to the bladder, and allows accurate measurement of hourly urine output. Measurement of hourly urine volumes is useful in monitoring the initial response to fluid resuscitation until the patient is adequately fluid filled and haemodynamics have been optimised. Once this state is reached, hourly urine volumes are less useful in guiding treatment and increased urine flow should not be regarded as a primary treatment goal. When patients are established to be oligo-anuric, the urinary catheter should be removed after 24 h to reduce the risk of infection. In apparent anuria, bilateral ureteric obstruction should be considered as well as the possibility of a blocked or incorrectly placed catheter. Careful charting of urine volume is essential throughout the course of ARF, in particular to guide appropriate fluid replacement during the polyuric phase of recovery. Unless the patient is incontinent this should be possible without urinary catheterisation. In practice, weighing the patient daily probably gives a more accurate assessment of fluid status than measurement of the urine volume.

URINE EXAMINATION

Appearance

A mid-stream specimen of urine (MSU) should be examined within 60 min of collection. Much can be gleaned simply by inspecting the urine. A number of pathologies, drugs and ingested pigments change the colour of urine as summarised in Table 2.

Table 2. Urine colour			
COLOUR	**POSSIBLE EXPLANATION**		
	Pathology	Drugs	Artefact
Colourless	diabetes mellitus diabetes insipidus		dilute urine
Red	haematuria	rifampicin	anthrocyanin (pigment in beetroot and blackberries)
	haemoglobinuria myoglobinuria acute intermittent porphyria	doxorubicin phenytoin phenolphthalein (in alkaline urine) phenazopyridine	red food dyes
Red-brown	urobilinogen bilirubin	codanthrusate nitrofurantoin primaquine chloroquine metronidazole imipenem-cilastatin	
Brown-black	acidified haemoglobin/myoglobin alkaptonuria melanin (in melanoma)	senna cascara levodopa	rhubarb
Yellow		riboflavin quinacrine	normal
Amber		pyridium sulphasalazine	concentrated urine
Green	biliverdin *Pseudomonas* bacteriuria	methylene blue amitriptyline triamterene	
Milky white	Pyuria, chyluria		

Yellow urine

Urochromes give urine its normal yellow colour which is more intense when concentrated.

Red urine

Red is the most commonly seen change in urine colour. Following urine centrifugation, if the colour is in the urinary sediment it is due to erythrocytes; if the colour is in the supernatant and is dipstick positive for blood then myoglobinuria, haemoglobinuria or lysed erythrocytes (erythrocytes in hypo-osmolar dilute urine tend to be lysed completely) are responsible for the colour change. Myoglobinuria and haemoglobinuria are discussed further in **Chapter 12**.

As little as 1 mL of blood in 1 L of urine produces a bright red colour and very small amounts of blood produce a "smoky" colour. Visible blood clots in urine indicate bleeding distal to the renal tubule. Less common causes of red urine include acute intermittent porphyria, where urine left to stand for several hours turns pink due to the presence of large amounts of urinary porphobilinogen. This process can be accelerated by the addition of Ehrlich's aldehyde solution. On ingestion of beetroot, urine turns red in individuals with increased intestinal absorption of the pigment anthrocyanin (approximately 14% of the population).

Cloudy urine

Urine may appear cloudy due to pyuria, bacteriuria, chyluria or the deposition of amorphous phosphate in alkaline urine which can be a normal finding.

Smell

Tasting of urine has thankfully been dropped from clinical practice but it is impossible to avoid the aroma of urine when handling samples. Infected urine has a characteristic pungent smell and the presence of ketones gives a sweet fruity smell.

URINE MICROSCOPY

Urine microscopy is mandatory in the investigation of ARF and all renal units admitting patients with ARF should be equipped with a microscope and centrifuge.

Microscopy can reveal the presence of:

* Cells
* Casts
* Crystals
* Organisms.

In non-specialist units, a satisfactory urine microscopy service is provided by the Microbiology Department, in terms of microbiological diagnosis and the counting of erythrocytes and white blood cells. Ideally, microscopy should be performed by the clinician who probably has more experience and greater interest in detecting and describing urinary casts and crystals.

Urine should be examined both unspun and after centrifugation at 2000–3000 rpm for 5–10 min, preferably using a phase contrast microscope, although a conventional bright-field microscope will suffice. If using a conventional microscope, methylene blue can be added to the urine to add definition. After centrifugation, the supernatant is poured off and the sediment resuspended using a Pasteur pipette. A single drop of urine is placed on a glass slide under a cover slip. The slide should first be examined at low power (magnification x100) and then at high power (magnification x400).

Cells

Erythrocytes

Normal erythrocytes appear as discs 6–8 μm in diameter but may develop a crenated appearance on standing in concentrated urine (**Figure 3A**). The normal erythrocyte excretion rate in urine is less than 10^5/h. However, in the immediate clinical setting it is impractical to use methods to quantify accurately the concentration of cells in urine and it is acceptable to count the number of cells per high-power field in the urinary sediment. There is some discrepancy between studies as to the number of erythrocytes that are found in normal urine by this method, with estimates ranging from 2–10 per high power field (equivalent to 1000–5000 erythrocytes/mL). Conventionally, a figure of 2 is taken as the upper limit of normal. This corresponds to the threshold of detection of dipsticks for haemoglobin. The presence of greater than 20% dysmorphic erythrocytes or acanthocytes (ring forms with vesicle-shaped protrusions) suggests glomerular disease, although the finding is not specific (**Figure 3B**). Sickled erythrocytes may be found with sickle cell disease. Other common causes of erythrocytes in urine are urinary tract infection, malignancy, stones and polycystic kidney disease. Urothelial trauma following catheterisation or as a result of self-mutilation are possible causes of erythrocytes arising from the lower urinary tract. Menstruation may result in contamination of the urine with erythrocytes.

White blood cells

The normal excretion rate for white blood cells (WBC) is less than 5×10^5/h. On spun urine, greater than 4 WBC per high power field is considered to be abnormal. Without staining it is difficult to differentiate between the types of WBC, but neutrophils occur most commonly.

- **Neutrophil polymorphs** (pus cells) appear granular with multi-lobed nuclei and are about twice the size of erythrocytes at 10–12 μm in diameter (**Figure 3C**). Their presence suggests inflammation in the urinary tract due to infection, glomerulonephritis, acute tubulo-interstitial nephritis or stones.
- **Lymphocytes**, which are closer in size to erythrocytes at 7–8 μm in diameter, are found in sterile pyuria due to renal tuberculosis or chronic tubulo-interstitial diseases such as sarcoidosis.
- **Eosinophils** in urine suggest a diagnosis of acute tubulo-interstitial nephritis, especially when drug-induced, but can also be seen with urinary tract infection and cholesterol embolism. Hansel's or Wright's stains allow the detection of eosinophils, but their use is beyond most ward side-rooms.

Epithelial cells

Epithelial cells from anywhere in the urinary tract from the renal tubule to the urethra can enter urine. They vary in size from 13–50 μm in diameter. The presence of squamous urothelial cells is a normal finding of no significance (**Figure 3D**). Renal tubule epithelial cells containing absorbed lipids suggest a diagnosis of nephrotic syndrome.

Figure 3. Cells found on urine microscopy

(A) Normal erythrocytes. Note that they may have a crenated appearance (lower panel), often the result of urine with a high osmolality. (B) Dysmorphic erythrocytes. (C) White blood cells: neutrophil polymorphs with granular-appearance and multi-lobed nuclei. (D) Squamous (i) and transitional (ii) epithelial cells. Photographs (A) and (D) reproduced with permission from: Ruthanne Hyduke, M.A., University of Iowa from Virtual Hospital® (www.vh.org), copyright University of Iowa, (B) with permission from Hans Kohler, MD and (C) Frances Andrus BA. (B) and (C) were both reproduced from Post, TW, Rose BD. Urinalysis in the diagnosis of renal disease. In: UpToDate, Rose, BD (Ed), UpToDate, Wellesley, MA, 2000. Copyright 2000, UpToDate, Inc (www.uptodate.com).

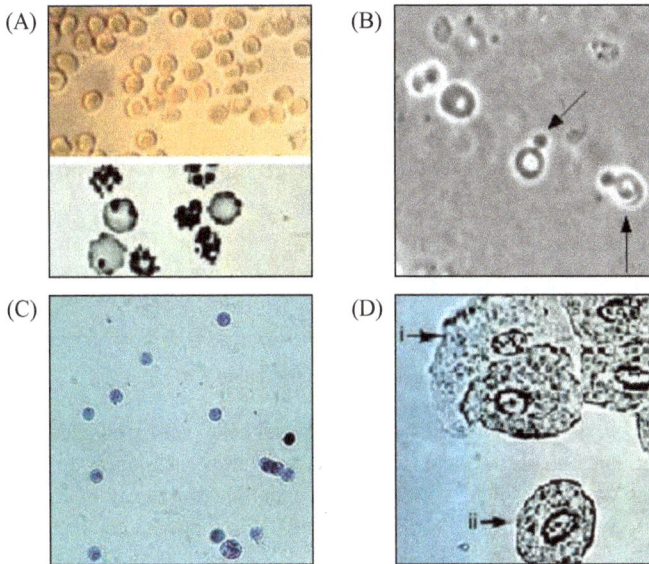

Malignant cells

Identification of malignant cells should be performed by cytologists.

Urinary Casts

When cellular debris and the Tamm-Horsfall mucoprotein are deposited in the lumen of distal tubules and collecting ducts, the mass sometimes coalesces and breaks off as a cylindrical "cast", with subsequent passage into urine. In normal spun urine one cast may be found in 10–20 low power fields. There are several different forms of cast which provide a clue as to the underlying pathology.

Red cell casts

Red cell casts (**Figure 4A**) are virtually diagnostic of glomerulonephritis or vasculitis, but are present in only 25–30% of patients with glomerulonephritis. The term "active urinary sediment" is often used when red cell casts are present in association with haematuria.

White cell casts

The presence of white cell casts **(Figure 4B)** indicates inflammation of the renal parenchyma and occurs in acute tubulo-interstitial nephritis, pyelonephritis and in some cases of glomerular disease.

Epithelial casts

Casts composed of renal tubule epithelial cells **(Figure 4C)** are often found in ATN, but can occasionally be seen with hyperbilirubinaemia.

Granular casts

Granular casts **(Figure 4D)** represent degenerating cellular casts of all types, which over time become finely granular and then waxy. They therefore suggest pathology but are a non-specific finding. The presence of waxy casts, which take a long time to form, is suggestive of a low urine flow-rate and they are usually only seen with advanced renal failure.

Figure 4. Urinary casts

(A) Red cell, (B) white cell, (C) epithelial cell (note that the epithelial cells are larger than the white blood cell (arrowed)), (D) granular. Photographs (A) and (D) reproduced with permission from: Ruthanne Hyduke, M.A., University of Iowa from Virtual Hospital® (www.vh.org), copyright University of Iowa and (B) and (C) with permission from Frances Andrus BA from Post, TW, Rose BD. Urinalysis in the diagnosis of renal disease. In: UpToDate, Rose, BD (Ed), UpToDate, Wellesley, MA, 2000. Copyright 2000, UpToDate, Inc (www.uptodate.com).

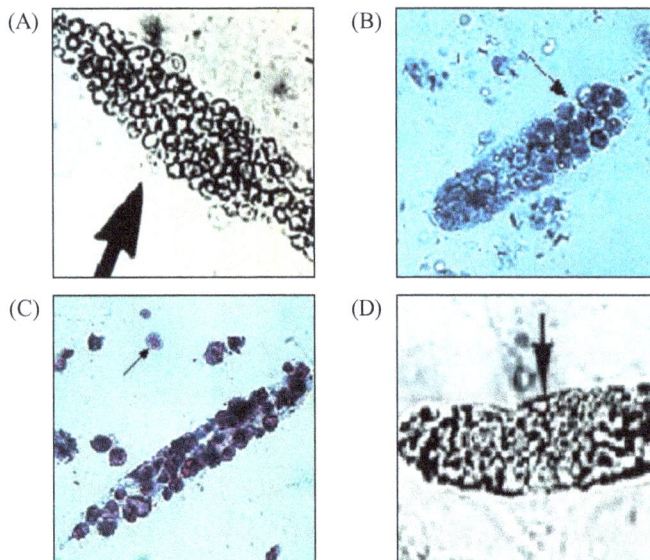

Fatty casts

Fatty casts may be seen in patients with proteinuria, especially if nephrotic. Under polarised light the fat droplets have a "Maltese cross" appearance. Isolated oval fat bodies may also be present.

Hyaline casts

These are composed of Tamm-Horsfall protein alone and are of no clinical significance. They are present in small numbers in normal urine, especially when concentrated or after vigorous exercise.

Urinary Crystals

Most urinary crystals form because the solubility product of the minerals concerned is reduced by concentration, acidity, or cooling of urine and do not indicate pathology. Refrigeration causes the precipitation of phosphates and urate. Occasionally, oxalate, urate and phosphate crystals are found in normal urine. The finding of crystals is usually of little significance except in patients with renal stones, where the type of crystal may indicate the underlying metabolic defect.

Oxalate crystals

The formation of oxalate crystals is pH-independent. Usually, calcium oxalate monohydrate crystals are dumb-bell-shaped and calcium oxalate dihydrate crystals are bipyramidal (**Figure 5A**), but needle-shaped forms are seen occasionally. The presence of oxalate crystals is usually of little clinical significance but does occur in ARF due to ethylene glycol poisoning. A high urinary oxalate concentration resulting in crystal formation is often found in malabsorption states or primary hyperoxaluria.

Urate crystals

Urate crystals only form in acid urine. The pleomorphic rhombic plates or rosettes are yellow or reddish brown. Urate crystals are found in acute urate nephropathy, most commonly associated with the tumour lysis syndrome.

Phosphate crystals

Phosphate crystals form only in alkaline urine, usually in association with urease-producing organisms. Magnesium ammonium phosphate (triple phosphate or struvite) crystals are rectangular and have been described as being shaped like coffin lids (**Figure 5B**).

Cystine crystals

Hexagonal cystine crystals (**Figure 5C**) are diagnostic of the autosomal recessive condition cystinuria, and are seen at initial urine microscopy in 25% of cases.

Figure 5. Urinary crystals

(A) Dumb-bell shaped calcium oxalate monohydrate crystal (arrowed) and bipyramidal calcium oxalate dihydrate crystals, (B) rectangular phosphate crystal, (C) hexagonal cystine crystals. Photograph (A) reproduced with permission from Frances Andrus BA from Post, TW, Rose BD. Urinalysis in the diagnosis of renal disease. In: UpToDate, Rose, BD (Ed), UpToDate, Wellesley, MA, 2000. Copyright 2000, UpToDate, Inc (www.uptodate.com) and (B) and (C) reproduced with permission from: Ruthanne Hyduke, M.A., University of Iowa from Virtual Hospital® (www.vh.org), copyright University of Iowa.

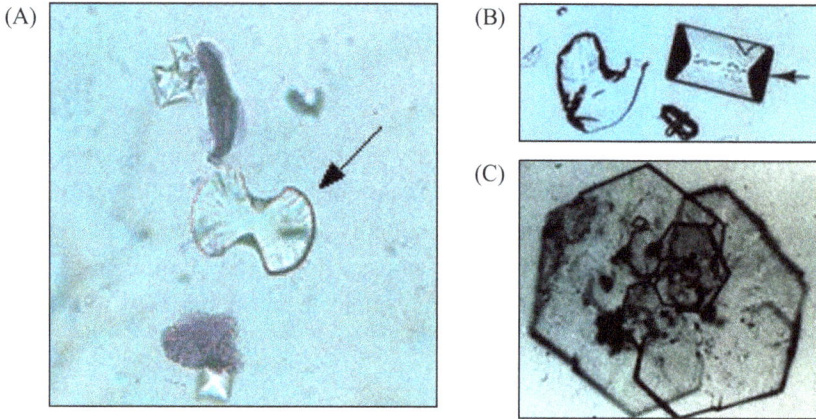

Others

Needle-shaped sulphonamide crystals may be present in sulphonamide toxicity and calcium carbonate-apatite crystals can form in the presence of urease-producing organisms. Microliths or small stones may be seen.

Organisms

It is usual to see some bacteria in spun urine (up to 20 per high-power field) but the finding of bacteria in unspun urine is significant. Unless there is pyuria there is unlikely to be significant urinary infection. Yeasts, *Trichomonas vaginalis* or *Schistosoma haematobium* ova may also be seen. Characterisation of organisms should be performed by the microbiology laboratory.

URINALYSIS USING DIPSTICKS

Urine dipsticks are chemically impregnated plastic strips that measure the presence of a number of substances in urine in a semi-quantitative manner. It should be ensured that the dipsticks have not passed their expiry date and that they are read at the time interval specified on the bottle.

Blood

The dipstick test for blood is based on the peroxidase activity of haemoglobin and myoglobin. Intact erythrocytes lyse on the matrix forming green spots while free haemoglobin or myoglobin produce a diffuse green colour. Dipsticks are capable of detecting the equivalent of 2–3 erythrocytes per high-power field in spun urine (equivalent to approximately 1000 cells/mL) with sensitivity of 97%. A distinction should be made between dipstick-positive haematuria and microscopic haematuria. If the dipstick test is positive with no erythrocytes on urine microscopy, this is suggestive of myoglobinuria, haemoglobinuria due to intravascular haemolysis, or complete lysis of the erythrocytes in urine, as discussed above. A false negative reading may be obtained in the presence of large concentrations of ascorbic acid and false positive results can occur in the presence of oxidising agents such as povidone iodine. False positive results for haematuria with dipsticks are common and false negative results are uncommon.

Albumin

The test is based on binding of negatively charged proteins especially albumin. Therefore positively charged proteins, such as immunoglobulins and Bence-Jones protein, are not detected. Albumin concentrations above 250 mg/L are detectable.

Calibration is on a semiquantitative scale, e.g.:

+	0.3 g/L
++	1 g/L
+++	5 g/L

False positive results may be found in alkaline urine and in the presence of iodinated radiocontrast. Testing should be delayed until 24 h after the administration of contrast. The sensitivity of dipsticks for detection of proteinuria is 32–46% with specificity of 97–100%. It should be noted that in the context of significant haematuria, plasma leads to dipstick-positive proteinuria. Microalbuminuria is best detected by radioimmunoassay (see below), but dipsticks are available.

Glucose

Glycosuria occurs when the plasma glucose concentration exceeds the renal threshold for glucose excretion, which is usually approximately 10 mmol/L. This may be due to hyperglycaemia, or with normal plasma glucose concentrations in normal pregnancy and in renal tubular disorders that lower the renal threshold, such as the Fanconi syndrome and acute tubular necrosis. Large quantities of ketones or ascorbic acid interfere with the colour-change reaction.

pH

Normal urine is acid with pH between 4.5 and 7.8. Urease-producing organisms such as *Proteus mirabilis* raise urinary pH and a very high pH (>8.0) nearly always indicates urinary tract infection. In the presence of systemic acidosis urine pH should be 5.3 or less. If not then a diagnosis of renal tubular acidosis should be suspected.

Ketones

The ketones aceto-acetate, acetone and beta-hydroxybutyrate are present in urine in diabetic ketoacidosis, starvation ketosis and alcoholic ketosis. Only aceto-acetate and acetone are detected by dipsticks, which may give a misleading result. Substances in urine containing sulphydryl groups, such as levodopa metabolites and captopril, may give a false positive result.

Specific Gravity

Specific gravity is the ratio of the weight of a fluid to the weight of an equal volume of water and is used as a surrogate for measurement of urine osmolality. Water has a specific gravity of 1.0; the presence of solutes increases the specific gravity depending on the weight of the solutes. In normal urine, where the main solutes are urea, sodium, chloride, potassium, ammonium and phosphate ions, each 30–35 mOsm/kg rise in osmolality raises the specific gravity by 0.001. Therefore a specific gravity of 1.010 represents a urine osmolality of 300–350 mOsm/kg. Normal urine specific gravity varies from 1.002–1.030. Larger solutes such as glucose and radiological contrast give a disproportionate increase in specific gravity.

Specific gravity can be directly measured using a hydrometer but this is rarely done in practice. Dipsticks measure specific gravity by an indirect method that depends on the displacement of hydrogen ions bound to a polyanionic polymer by competing cations in urine, resulting in a pH-dependent colour change. Readings are falsely high when urine pH is less than 6.0 and falsely low when urine pH is greater than 7.0. Albumin, glucose and urea are not reflected in this measurement. In general, if it is important to determine the concentration of urine, a directly measured osmolality should be used.

Diagnosis of Urinary Infection using Dipsticks

- *Leucocytes*

This test is based on the detection of neutrophil esterases. High concentrations of glucose, albumin, ascorbic acid, tetracycline or cephalexin may inhibit the reaction. Nitrofurantoin and rifampicin in urine interfere with interpretation because the change in urine colour interferes with visual interpretation of the test strip.

- *Nitrite*

Urinary Gram-negative bacteria convert nitrate to nitrite. A positive nitrite test suggests the presence of greater than 10^5 Gram negative organisms per mL of urine. A negative test is found with several urinary pathogens including *Streptococcus faecalis*, *Neisseria gonorrhoeae*, some Pseudomonas species and *Mycobacterium tuberculosis*. There are several causes of false negative results. Conversion from nitrate to nitrite can take up to 4 h so inadequate bladder retention time or urinary catheterisation may allow insufficient time for the reaction. Nitrites break down with prolonged storage of urine. High concentrations of ascorbic acid in the urine and high urine concentration interfere with the reaction on the test-strip. Prolonged exposure of urine to light results in conversion of nitrate to nitrite giving a false positive result.

In using leucocyte esterase and nitrite dipsticks together in the diagnosis of suspected urinary tract infection, sensitivity is 95% with specificity 75%. The positive predictive value for a suspected diagnosis of urinary infection is 30–40% with a negative predictive value of 99%.

URINE CULTURE

A MSU should be collected. The first sample in the morning is the most sensitive as the urine is more concentrated and bacteria will have had the opportunity to multiply in the bladder. If a sample cannot be examined immediately, bacteria will survive without multiplying if stored overnight at 4°C but leucocytes will be altered. If urine cannot be refrigerated within 2 h, then storage bottles containing preservative such as 1.8% boric acid should be used. Conventionally a growth of greater than 10^5 colonies/mL of urine is considered to represent significant urinary infection. If tuberculosis is suspected, urine from the first void of the day, on 3 separate days, should be sent for culture (early morning urine, EMU).

URINE BIOCHEMISTRY

Urinary sodium excretion varies with dietary salt intake with a normal range of 40–220 mmol/day, but can be used as an indicator of renal tubule function. In volume-depleted states and in heart failure, salt and water are retained as a homeostatic mechanism to increase intravascular volume, resulting in low urine sodium concentration (usually less than 20 mmol/L) with a high osmolality (usually in excess of 500 mOsm/kg) — so-called "pre-renal" renal failure. In ATN this mechanism is disrupted, primarily due to medullary ischaemia, with loss of response to anti-diuretic hormone. Urinary sodium concentration is usually greater than 40 mmol/L with osmolality similar to that of plasma (less than 350 mOsm/kg).

Urinary sodium excretion can also be expressed as the fractional excretion of sodium (FENa) which relates sodium excretion to creatinine excretion and can be calculated by the equation:

$$\text{FENa} = \text{sodium clearance/creatinine clearance}$$

$$= \frac{[Na]_{urine} \times \text{Urine vol/unit time}}{[Na]_{plasma}} \div \frac{[creatinine]_{urine} \times \text{Urine vol/unit time}}{[creatinine]_{plasma}}$$

$$= \frac{[Na]_{urine}(mmol/L) \times [creatinine]_{plasma}(\mu mol/L)}{[Na]_{plasma}(mmol/L) \times [creatinine]_{urine}(\mu mol/L)} \times 100$$

Typically, in volume-depleted states the fractional excretion of sodium is less than 1% and in acute tubular necrosis (ATN) greater than 2%. Clearly these values can be altered by diuretic treatment (diuretics will increase urine sodium) and measurement should be made prior to commencing diuretic treatment if possible. These urinary biochemical parameters are shown in **Table 3**.

The importance of distinguishing ATN from pre-renal renal failure based on these measurements is probably over-emphasised. In practice there is little value in making this distinction as the clinical management of these problems is essentially the same: adequate fluid resuscitation with caution not to fluid-overload.

Table 3. Diagnosis of pre-renal renal failure on urine biochemistry

	Pre-renal renal failure	ATN
Urine Na	<20 mmol/L	>40 mmol/L
Urine osmolality	>500 mOsm/L	<350 mOsm/L
Fractional excretion of sodium (FENa)	<1%	>2%

Low urine sodium concentrations may also be seen with radio-contrast nephropathy, haemoglobinuria and vasculitis, in the absence of hypovolaemia, and in patients with ATN who have an ongoing pre-renal pathology such as the hepato-renal syndrome or cardiac failure. A very low urinary sodium (<10 mmol/L) can be helpful in confirming a diagnosis of hepato-renal syndrome. In myoglobinuric ARF, FENa is often <1% reflecting tubule obstruction rather than necrosis (see **Chapter 12**).

In polyuric states, including the diuretic phase of ARF, measurement of urinary sodium and potassium can be used to guide appropriate electrolyte replacement. Measurement of potassium in an unidentified yellow body fluid can be helpful in differentiating between urine, which should have a high potassium concentration (typically >10 mmol/L), and serous fluid which should have the same potassium concentration as plasma. Normal urinary potassium excretion is 25–125 mmol/day.

Protein

The gold-standard for quantification of proteinuria is a 24 h urine collection, but any accurately timed collection is adequate. Urine should be collected into a bottle containing preservative such as "Thymol". Normal 24 h urinary protein excretion is less than 150 mg, composed mostly of proteins with molecular weight less than 25 kDa such as β2-microglobulin, immunoglobulin light chains and retinol binding protein, with albumin excretion less than 30 mg. Fever, exercise, heart failure, seizures and poor glycaemic control can all transiently elevate urinary albumin excretion. Urinary protein excretion is arbitrarily defined as microalbuminuria when albumin excretion is 30–300 mg/day and as proteinuria at greater albumin excretion rates. Microalbuminuria is a marker for early diabetic nephropathy and for vascular disease in non-diabetics. A diagnosis of microalbuminuria requires at least 3 separate samples because of variability in daily albumin excretion.

An estimate of 24 h urinary protein excretion can be made by calculating the albumin/creatinine ratio for a spot sample of urine using the formula:

$$24\,\text{h urinary protein} \, (g/1.73\,m^2\,\text{body surface area}) \approx \frac{\text{urine protein}\,(mg/L)\times 0.088}{\text{urine creatinine}\,(mmol/L)}$$

This formula will underestimate protein excretion in individuals with proportionately higher urinary creatinine concentration due to a large muscle mass, and overestimate it in cachectic patients with a low muscle mass (the same caveat as applies to using serum creatinine to estimate GFR).

Proteinuria can be further defined by electrophoresis to determine the molecular weight of proteins present. This is of particular value in the detection of Bence-Jones proteins. Otherwise further characterisation of the proteins present is of little value in the diagnosis of ARF.

Creatinine Clearance

Urinary creatinine clearance (CrCl) using 24 h urine collections in bottles containing preservative such as "Thymol" can be used as a marker of GFR. CrCl is calculated from the following equation:

$$\text{Creatinine clearance (mL/min)} = \frac{\text{Urinary creatinine concentration (µmol/L)} \times \text{urine volume (mL)}}{\text{Plasma creatinine (µmol/L)} \times 1440}$$

This technique has been criticised as being inaccurate, largely due to incomplete or poorly timed urine collections. It has been suggested that using the modified Cockcroft-Gault calculation based on serum creatinine concentration and weight is more accurate (see **Appendix A**). In practice, in ARF where the serum creatinine concentration is elevated outside the normal range more complicated measurements of GFR add little to management.

Osmolality

Urine osmolality is measured by the degree of depression of the freezing point of a liquid by solutes (so any contribution of volatile alcohols to osmolality is not detected). Alteration of urine osmolality, with a wide normal range of 50–1400 mOsm/kg, in response to anti-diuretic hormone, plays a central role in the tight regulation of plasma osmolality to around 285 mOsm/kg. It is more important that the urine osmolality is appropriate to the patient's salt and water status than the absolute value. Concentrating or acidifying defects suggest tubular disease.

Stone Substrates

In patients with renal stones it is important to measure urinary calcium, urate, oxalate, cystine and citrate. Normal values are given in **Appendix C**.

URINARY FINDINGS IN ACUTE RENAL FAILURE

Urinalysis does not usually allow a precise diagnosis but the pattern of findings narrows the differential diagnosis to allow rational planning of further investigation. In particular, the urinary findings often dictate whether or not renal biopsy is indicated. The typical urinary findings for the main causes of ARF are summarised in **Table 4**.

Table 4. Urine abnormalities in acute renal failure

Diagnosis	Urine appearance	Microscopy	Dip-stick testing[2]	Chemistry
Acute tubular necrosis	normal	epithelial cell casts	normal	Urinary Na$^+$ >40 mmol/L
Rapidly progressive glomerulonephritis/vasculitis	turbid/red	normal & dysmorphic RBCs red cell casts, epithelial cell casts	+ve blood +ve protein	Albuminuria
Acute tubulointerstitial nephritis	normal	white cell casts epithelial cell casts neutrophils & eosinophils "Sometimes RBCs namely red cell casts" to this list?	may be normal or +ve protein sometimes +ve blood	
Renovascular disease	normal	unremarkable	usually normal occasionally +ve protein	
Myeloma	normal	unremarkable	+ve protein but may be −ve (Bence-Jones protein not detected)	Bence-Jones proteins
Rhabdomyolysis	brown	unremarkable or tubular cell casts	+ve blood	Myoglobin
Contrast nephropathy	normal	unremarkable	possible false +ve protein	
Acute pyelonephritis	turbid	erythrocytes, white cells bacteria, white cell casts	+ve blood, +ve protein +ve leucocyte esterase, +ve nitrite	High urinary pH
Haemolytic uraemic syndrome	normal	occasionally erythrocytes and red cell casts	occasionally +ve protein	
Accelerated hypertension	turbid/red	normal and dysmorphic erythrocytes	+ve blood, +ve protein	
Cholesterol embolisation	normal	eosinophils	normal	
Acute urate nephropathy	normal	urate crystals	normal	
Obstructive nephropathy	normal	normal	normal	

[2] +ve = positive, −ve = negative.

4.3 HAEMATOLOGICAL INVESTIGATIONS
Lawrence Goldberg

Many diseases which cause ARF are associated with derangements in haematological test results. Knowledge of the significance of these haematological abnormalities can often provide valuable clues as to the cause of ARF.

HAEMOGLOBIN

It is a commonly held assumption that when a patient presents with renal failure, a normal haemoglobin (Hb) indicates ARF, whilst anaemia is indicative of chronic renal failure. There are however many exceptions to this "rule". The possible causes of anaemia in ARF are listed in **Table 5**. A normal Hb may be found in patients with end stage renal failure if they are haemoconcentrated as part of their acute illness, or in patients with underlying adult polycystic kidney disease, where the Hb is typically maintained.

WHITE CELL COUNT AND DIFFERENTIAL

Leucopaenia. A low total white cell count (WCC), whilst being a normal variant in patients of African descent, may indicate severe sepsis or active SLE. If a low WCC is associated with a pancytopaenia, this may represent marrow infiltration, e.g. multiple myeloma with acute myeloma cast nephropathy (see **Chapter 22**), lymphoma with renal infiltration (see **Chapter 21**), prostatic carcinoma with bilateral ureteric or urethral obstruction (see **Chapter 23**).

Neutrophilia whilst suggestive of sepsis, is also found in acute ANCA-associated vasculitic illnesses.

Eosinophilia would suggest a drug-induced interstitial nephritis or Churg-Strauss syndrome.

PLATELETS AND BLEEDING TIME

Thrombocytopaenia in ARF is seen with disseminated intravascular coagulation (DIC), thrombotic microangiopathies, SLE, the anti-phospholipid syndrome and marrow infiltration with malignancy.

Thrombocytosis is commonly seen in systemic vasculitis, other non-lupoid inflammatory diseases and malignancy.

Abnormal platelet function is very common in ARF, causing prolongation of the bleeding time (see **Chapter 8.6**). The aetiology of abnormal platelet function is unclear; it is known that as yet unspecified molecules accumulate in ARF and interfere with fibrinogen binding to platelet glycoprotein IIb-IIIa. In addition, increased nitric oxide production from platelets and the vascular endothelium during uraemia prolongs the bleeding time.

Table 5. Potential causes of anaemia in patients with acute renal failure

Process causing anaemia	Specific conditions
Intra-vascular haemolysis	Thrombotic microangiopathies — see **Chapter 15**
	Disseminated intra-vascular coagulation (severe sepsis, haemorrhagic viral infections, placental abruption/amniotic fluid embolus)
	Bacterial toxins (e.g. *Clostridium perfringens*)
	Falciparum malaria ("black water fever") — see **Chapter 20**
	Poisoning (arsine, chlorates)
	Paroxysmal nocturnal haemoglobinuria
Extra-vascular haemolysis	Auto-immune haemolytic anaemia:
	Warm type (SLE, lymphomas [with renal infiltration])
	Cold type (Mycoplasma infection ["cold haemagglutinins"], paroxysmal cold haemoglobinuria, lymphoma)
Haemorrhage	Traumatic
	Gastro-intestinal
	Pulmonary (as part of pulmonary-renal syndromes) — see **Chapter 16**
	– Wegener's granulomatosis
	– Microscopic polyangiitis
	– Goodpasture's disease
	– Henoch-Schönlein purpura
	– Type II cryoglobulinaemia
Chronic inflammatory disease causing ARF	Sarcoidosis
	Wegener's granulomatosis
	Polyarteritis nodosa

The bleeding time can be shortened prior to invasive procedures by:

- Administration of 1-deamino-8-D-arginine vasopressin (DDAVP) 0.3 µg/kg as an intravenous infusion, which stimulates the release of factor VIII and von Willebrand factor (Factor VIII-related antigen) from the endothelium. Further details are given in **Chapter 8.6**.
- Blood transfusion if the patient is anaemic, as this tends to increase platelet-endothelial contact in the vasculature.

COAGULATION

An increased INR and prolonged activated partial thromboplastin time (APTT) together are highly suggestive of DIC, and can be confirmed by finding elevated levels of fibrin degradation products, reduced fibrinogen and often red cell fragments on the blood film (though the latter is less marked than in the thrombotic microangiopathies).

An increased INR alone may indicate acute liver failure with associated ARF, whether due to acute viral hepatitis, paracetamol overdose or other cause, or severe chronic liver disease with ensuing hepato-renal syndrome (see **Chapter 25**).

The anti-phospholipid syndrome can cause ARF through either large vessel (aortic, renal artery or renal vein) thrombosis, or renal microvascular thrombosis (often in association with lupus nephritis). This is diagnosed by the presence of either the lupus anticoagulant and/or anti-cardiolipin antibodies. The presence of the lupus anticoagulant usually causes an isolated increase in the APTT (or the prothrombin time, depending on the reagents used by individual laboratories). This is not reversed by 1:1 dilution with normal control plasma.

ERYTHROCYTE SEDIMENTATION RATE

The ESR is completely unreliable as an inflammatory marker in ARF, as it is usually elevated, often markedly so, even in the absence of an inflammatory response. C-reactive protein levels are not influenced by renal failure *per se*.

DIAGNOSIS OF THROMBOTIC MICROANGIOPATHIES

The thrombotic microangiopathies (TMA) are a group of conditions characterised by intra-vascular haemolysis, which cause ARF by intra-renal microvascular thrombosis. These disorders and their haematological features are described in **Chapter 15**. The cardinal feature of TMA is the presence of red blood cell fragments (schistocytes) on a blood film, caused by red cell disruption as they pass through narrowed small vessels lined by diseased endothelium.

4.4 BIOCHEMICAL INVESTIGATIONS
Lawrence Goldberg

The biochemistry laboratory provides invaluable help, not only with the diagnosis of ARF, but also in the establishment of its cause. ARF indicates a rapid reduction in the glomerular filtration rate (GFR), which is evidenced by a rapid rise in the plasma creatinine concentration, which may or may not be associated with oliguria.

Interpretation of Plasma Creatinine in Acute Renal Failure

It must be remembered that significant renal impairment may exist before the plasma creatinine concentration rises above the "normal" range, as the relationship between plasma creatinine and CrCl is not linear but hyperbolic (see **Figure 6**). Therefore whilst a halving of the GFR from 60 mL/min to 30 mL/min may double the plasma creatinine, a reduction from 120 mL/min to

Figure 6. Relationship of plasma creatinine to glomerular filtration rate (creatinine clearance)

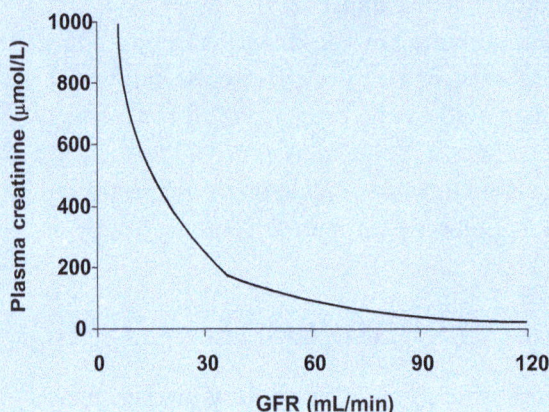

60 mL/min may only result in a minor elevation of plasma creatinine. In practical terms, this means that a rise in plasma creatinine from 90 to 120 µmol/L can indicate a marked reduction in GFR Therefore, the development of ARF may be diagnosed early if this relationship is understood.

In addition, the interpretation of an individual's plasma creatinine is dependent on the patient's size, sex and age (as per the Cockcroft-Gault equation for CrCl — see **Appendix A**). A plasma creatinine of 120 µmol/L in a 40 year old man weighing 80 kg equates to a CrCl of 84.6 mL/min, whilst the same plasma creatinine of 120 µmol/L in an 80 year old woman weighing 45 kg equates to a CrCl of 24.2 mL/min.

ACUTE OR CHRONIC RENAL FAILURE?

It is vital to establish, whenever possible, that the detection of renal impairment in a patient when first seen represents an acute deterioration and is not simply the presentation of previously asymptomatic chronic renal failure. If previous renal impairment is not apparent from the clinical history, it may be possible to obtain previous creatinine measurements from the general practitioner, or from current, referring or other hospitals' records or laboratories; every effort should be made to obtain such data.

Patients may however develop acute renal deterioration on a background of chronic renal dysfunction, either due to an exacerbation of an underlying renal disease (such as SLE, vasculitis, interstitial nephritis), or due to unrelated renal insults (e.g. hypovolaemia, sepsis, nephrotoxins).

Biochemical Indicators of Acute or Chronic Renal Failure

There is no reliable way to differentiate acute from chronic renal failure on the initial biochemical screen (in the absence of knowledge of previous renal function). However certain biochemical features may suggest one or the other.

Urea and creatinine

Patients with a slow onset of renal failure (chronic) have had time potentially to adapt to the consequent biochemical and osmotic derangement. Therefore patients with very high plasma urea (>50 mmol/L) or creatinine (>1000 μmol/L) levels, who do not appear acutely unwell, are more likely to have slowly progressive or chronic renal failure.

Potassium

This feature does not distinguish between acute and chronic renal disease, but high plasma levels (>6.0 mmol/L) are better tolerated when deterioration of renal function has been gradual (see **Chapter 8.3**).

Calcium and phosphate

Chronic renal disease is associated with reduced activity of the enzyme 1-α hydroxylase, which results in a reduction of the metabolically active 1,25 di-OH vitamin D. Untreated patients are therefore usually hypocalcaemic. The presence of a normal or high serum calcium is therefore likely to indicate ARF (with the caveat that hypercalcaemia-inducing diseases which affect the kidney such as sarcoidosis and multiple myeloma may have a slow, "chronic" evolution — see **Chapter 8.5**).

PRE-RENAL, RENAL OR POST-RENAL ACUTE RENAL FAILURE?

ARF can be due to pre-renal, intra-renal or post-renal causes (see **Chapter 3**). Whilst plasma and urine biochemistry are usually unhelpful in determining an obstructive cause, these can help to distinguish pre-renal from renal causes, especially ATN.

Plasma Urea and Creatinine

Renal hypoperfusion due to any cause of hypotension (e.g. dehydration, haemorrhage, sepsis, cardiac failure) often results in a disproportionate increase in the plasma urea:creatinine ratio, as urea is re-absorbed passively along with sodium and water (unlike creatinine which is not re-absorbable).

However, such a **raised** urea:creatinine ratio may also be produced by a high protein diet, increased catabolism (surgery, infection, trauma), gastrointestinal bleeding, corticosteroid therapy and tetracyclines. Alternatively, it can result from a reduction in the plasma creatinine concentration due to reduced body muscle mass. **The urea:creatinine ratio must therefore be interpreted with caution.**

Importantly, myoglobinuric ARF is associated with a **low** urea:creatinine ratio. In rhabdomyolysis, creatine released as a result of muscle cell lysis leads to a disproportionately high serum creatinine concentration (see **Chapter 12**). Note that a **low** urea:creatinine ratio also results from suppressed urea synthesis, due to malnutrition (reduced protein intake) or liver disease (reduced amino acid catabolism), or from increased urea elimination (elevated GFR, e.g. pregnancy). In addition, certain drugs increase serum creatinine levels by reducing tubular secretion of creatinine, e.g. cimetidine, trimethoprim, amiloride and spironolactone.

Biochemical Testing of the Urine

The main purpose of measuring urine biochemistry is for the diagnosis of pre-renal ARF. As a result of renal hypoperfusion, the kidneys respond by re-absorbing sodium from the glomerular filtrate, which draws water and to some extent urea with it. As a result, the urinary concentration of sodium falls to very low levels, associated with a low fractional excretion of sodium. Due to excessive concentration of the urine, the urinary osmolality rises. Urine biochemistry is discussed in detail in **Chapter 4.2**.

BIOCHEMICAL TESTS TO ESTABLISH CAUSE OF ARF

The biochemical tests that help establish the cause of ARF and which should be performed at the time the patient presents, together with the diseases commonly causing such abnormalities, are shown in **Table 6**.

Table 6. Biochemical tests which help establish the cause of acute renal failure	
Biochemical test	**Possible cause of renal failure if abnormal**
Calcium	If high: hypercalcaemia itself (whatever the cause) myeloma cast nephropathy sarcoidosis with interstitial nephritis renal tract outflow obstruction due to tumour (e.g. prostate, bladder) If low: acute pancreatitis rhabdomyolysis (pre-existing chronic renal failure)
CK (creatine kinase)	Rhabdomyolysis
Amylase	Acute pancreatitis
Liver function tests	Acute hepatic failure Septicaemia Haemolysis
LDH	Intravascular haemolysis (e.g. haemolytic uraemic syndrome) Tissue necrosis (e.g. classical polyarteritis nodosa, bowel infarction)
Acid-base assessment	Metabolic acidosis usual in ARF (see **Chapter 8.4**)
Urine and blood screen for toxins	Paracetamol, polyethylene glycol or methanol poisoning (see **Chapter 11**)
Serum protein and urine electrophoresis	Myeloma cast nephropathy (see **Chapter 22**)

4.5 IMMUNOLOGICAL INVESTIGATIONS
Megan Griffith

Immunological investigations play a key role in the diagnosis of ARF, and should be considered even in the absence of stigmata of systemic disease. This section describes the immunological investigations that are often undertaken as part of the work-up of the patient with ARF (summarised in **Table 7**). For a more detailed discussion of the associated diseases the reader is referred to the appropriate chapters in the book.

Table 7. Immunological investigations in acute renal failure	
Investigation	**Comments**
Serum electrophoresis	Monoclonal band in myeloma Light Chain Deposition Disease Amyloidosis
Immunoglobulins	Immune paresis in myeloma Raised IgA in IgA disease Polyclonal increase in SLE, chronic infections, e.g. infective endocarditis
Complement	SLE C3↓ C4↓ Infective endocarditis C3↓ C4↓ Post streptococcal glomerulonephritis C3↓ C4↓ Essential mixed cryoglobulinaemia C4↓ C3 normal Mesangiocapillary glomerulonephritis type II C3↓ C4 normal
ANCA	C-ANCA positive in Wegener's granulomatosis C-ANCA or P-ANCA positive in microscopic polyangiitis
Anti-GBM	Goodpasture's disease
ANA/anti-dsDNA/anti-C1q	SLE

IMMUNOGLOBULINS AND ELECTROPHORESIS

Serum IgG, IgA and IgM should be measured along with serum electrophoresis. Myeloma can present with ARF due to a variety of causes including cast nephropathy and ATN (see **Chapter 22**). Electrophoresis of urine should also be performed, even in the absence of serum abnormalities, as free light chains are excreted in urine but may not be apparent on serum electrophoresis (myelomas and low-grade plasma cell dyscrasias will otherwise be missed). Measurement of serum immunoglobulin is useful for quantifying monoclonal gammopathies and identifying an associated immune paresis. A non-specific hypergammaglobulinaemia is seen in other diseases such as SLE, bacterial endocarditis and other chronic infections. IgA nephropathy is a rare cause of ARF, and serum IgA is elevated in 35 to 50% of cases.

AUTOANTIBODIES

ANTINUCLEAR ANTIBODIES

Antinuclear antibodies (ANA) were first discovered in the 1940s using the LE test. Most laboratories now use Hep2 cells (human epithelial tumour cell line) which contain large nucleoli. ANA binding to these cells are detected via immunofluorescence (IF). ANA are highly sensitive for some autoimmune diseases including SLE, scleroderma, mixed connective tissue disease and Sjogren's syndrome, and are often positive in others including polymyositis, pauciarticular juvenile chronic arthritis and rheumatoid arthritis. Therefore they are a good screening test for autoimmune disease. They are not however specific for autoimmune disease and can be found in infections such as infective endocarditis and tuberculosis, and in some lymphoproliferative disorders. False positive ANA are also seen, particularly in women and the elderly, usually in low titre. Different patterns of ANA staining occur depending on the nucleolar antigens recognised by the ANA. However these staining patterns are difficult to interpret and have been superseded by more specific tests such as ELISA and immunoblotting for individual antigens. Certain specificities of ANA are associated with particular autoimmune diseases (**Table 8**). Hence the presence of ANA in high titre should raise suspicions of an autoimmune cause of ARF and is an important screening test. However, it is relatively non-specific and if positive should be investigated in more detail to determine its significance.

Table 8. ANA specificities and their associations with auto-immune disease

Type of ANA	Disease association
Anti Ro/SSA & La/SSB antibodies	Sjogren's syndrome Subacute cutaneous LE Neonatal LE
Anti-Scl-70 antibodies	Scleroderma
Anti-centromere antibodies	CREST variant of scleroderma (limited scleroderma)
Anti-U1-RNP	Mixed connective tissue disease
Anti-RNA polymerase I and II	Renal involvement in scleroderma

ANTI-DOUBLE STRANDED DNA ANTIBODIES

Anti-double stranded DNA (dsDNA) antibodies are highly specific for SLE. They are therefore useful for diagnosis, although less sensitive than ANA. Anti-dsDNA antibodies can be detected by immunoprecipitation (Farr assay), indirect IF following binding to a DNA rich unicellular flagellate (Crithidia luciliae assay) or ELISAs with differing sensitivity and specificity. High titres of anti-dsDNA antibodies have been shown to correlate with active lupus nephritis and can also be used to follow disease activity.

ANTI-C1Q ANTIBODIES

Anti-C1q antibodies are found in patients with SLE and mesangiocapillary glomerulonephritis, and recent reports suggest they may be present in IgA nephropathy. The highest titres of anti-C1q antibodies are found in active lupus nephritis, and rising levels in an individual patient may predict renal relapse. The positive predictive value of anti-C1q in lupus nephritis has been reported as only 50%, but the negative predictive value is much higher (96–100%) and hence they are a useful marker for renal disease. There are however pitfalls in the measurement of anti-C1q antibodies, as immune complexes with and without dsDNA can cause false positive results — this can usually be prevented by altering the ionic strength of the incubation media in solid phase assays.

ANTI-NEUTROPHIL CYTOPLASMIC ANTIBODIES (ANCA)

ANCA were first described in 1982 and subsequently found to be associated with both Wegener's granulomatosis and microscopic polyangiitis. ANCA are detected by indirect IF following binding to ethanol fixed human neutrophils. There are two main patterns of ANCA, cytoplasmic (C) and perinuclear (P), as defined by their IF appearances (**Figure 7**). Both C-ANCA and P-ANCA bind to neutrophil granule enzymes. The main target antigen of C-ANCA is proteinase 3 (PR3). P-ANCA have a wider range of antigenic specificities, but in systemic vasculitis are usually specific for myeloperoxidase (MPO). Most patients with Wegener's granulomatosis have proteinase 3 specific ANCA, patients with Churg Strauss syndrome often have anti-myeloperoxidase specific ANCA, and patients with microscopic polyangiitis may have either. The specificity of ANCA can be determined by MPO and PR3 specific ELISA. ANCA have also been detected in patients with diseases other than primary systemic vasculitis, such as inflammatory bowel disease, primary sclerosing cholangitis and rheumatoid arthritis, but the specificity in these patients is usually for different neutrophil granule enzymes such as lactoferrin and cathepsin G. Therefore, a positive

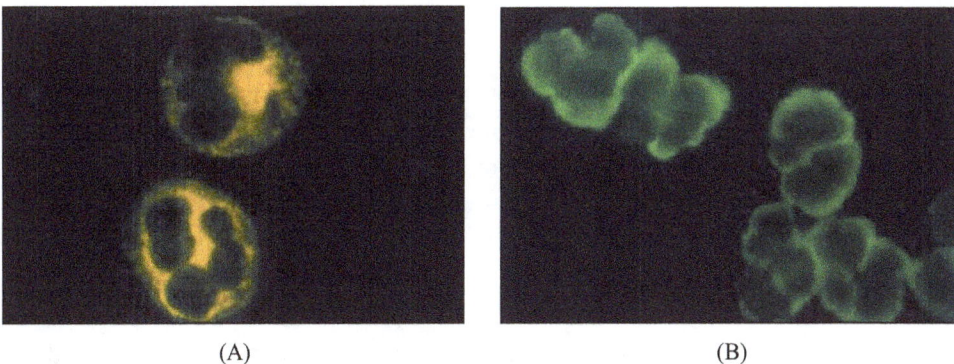

Figure 7. ANCA immunofluorescence

(A) cytoplasmic staining pattern, C-ANCA; (B) perinuclear staining pattern, P-ANCA

(A)   (B)

ANCA result should always be interpreted in conjunction with the antigen specificity by ELISA, as this greatly increases the diagnostic specificity. The specificity of the combination of C-ANCA and anti-PR3 or P-ANCA and anti-MPO for primary systemic vasculitis has been measured as 99%. ANCA have been found not only to correlate with the pattern of disease but also with disease activity. Levels generally fall after treatment and subsequent rises often precede clinical relapse; hence they are also useful for monitoring treatment. However, a small sub-group of patients remains persistently ANCA positive even in remission.

ANTI-GLOMERULAR BASEMENT MEMBRANE ANTIBODIES

Circulating anti-glomerular basement membrane (anti-GBM) antibodies are specific for the α3 chain of type IV collagen and are pathognomonic of Goodpasture's disease. They can now be detected by radio-immunoassay or ELISA in most major hospital laboratories. Although these assays are usually both sensitive and specific, if there is any doubt the result can be confirmed by Western blotting. Detection of linear staining of glomerular basement membrane by direct IF of the renal biopsy is still the most sensitive method of detection. Antibodies have not been found in normal controls or relatives. ANCA can also be detected in 10–20% of patients with Goodpasture's disease, while anti-GBM antibodies may be detected in 2% of ANCA positive patients. Patients who have both antibodies tend to respond to treatment in a manner more typical of vasculitis; this has therapeutic implications particularly for those presenting with dialysis dependent renal failure and in monitoring patients for relapse. This is discussed in more detail in **Chapter 16**.

COMPLEMENT

The most widespread assays for complement are immunoassays for C3, C4 and a functional assay for the total haemolytic complement (CH50). The CH50 measures the ability of the serum to lyse sheep erythrocytes coated with rabbit antibody. This requires all components of the classical and terminal pathways and hence is a good screen for complement pathway abnormalities. C3, C4 and factor B can also be used to screen for abnormalities in the classical and alternative pathways, and in serial measurement to monitor certain diseases such as SLE. Measurement of the proteolytic fragments of C3, C5, C2 and factor B can also be measured and are more sensitive markers of *in vivo* complement activation, as they are not affected by the acute phase response. Care must be taken with serum samples as several of the complement proteins are heat labile and the serum should be assayed the same day or stored frozen to prevent false positive results.

Disorders with high levels of circulating immune complexes, such as SLE, post streptococcal glomerulonephritis and mixed cryoglobulinaemia are associated with hypocomplementaemia. Hypocomplementaemia is also common in mesangiocapillary glomerulonephritis (MCGN). In type 1 MCGN there is mainly classical pathway activation presumably secondary to circulating immune complexes. In type 2 MCGN massive alternative pathway activation is seen due to persistent catabolism of C3. This is due to an IgG antibody, C3 nephritic factor, which binds to C3 convertase (C3bBb) preventing its inactivation and thus resulting in accelerated activation of C3. Occasionally a different nephritic factor can also result in complement activation in type

1 MCGN. Inherited deficiencies of complement can also predispose to certain diseases, the most common being C1q deficiency which results in SLE and occasionally isolated mesangiocapillary glomerulonephritis. Abnormalities of factor H are associated with familial haemolytic uraemic syndrome.

CRYOGLOBULINS

Cryoglobulins are immunoglobulins which reversibly precipitate in the cold. They should be considered as the cause for ARF especially in patients presenting with a rash, arthralgia, peripheral neuropathy or abnormal liver function tests, and in those patients known to have a lymphoproliferative disorder or hepatitis C. The patient's blood sample needs to be placed immediately in a thermos flask containing water warmed to 37°C and transported to the laboratory for immediate testing. There are three types of cryoglobulinaemia. In type I, the cryoglobulin is a single monoclonal antibody and is found in patients with myeloma, Waldenstrom's macroglobulinaemia and MGUS (monoclonal gammopathy of unknown significance). In types II and III the cryoprecipitants are mixed, containing polyclonal IgG which binds to another immunoglobulin that acts as a rheumatoid factor, i.e. has IgG binding properties. In type II the rheumatoid factor is usually subclass IgM and is monoclonal, whereas in type III it is polyclonal. Severe glomerulonephritis is more common in type II cryoglobulinaemia.

FURTHER READING

History and Examination

Davison AM, Cameron JS, Grunfeld J-P, Kerr DNS, Ritz E, Winearls CG (eds.) (1998) *Oxford Textbook of Clinical Nephrology* (2nd Edition). Oxford: Oxford University Press

Urine and Urinalysis

Froom P, Ribak J, Benbassat J (1984) Significance of microhaematuria in young adults. *British Medical Journal*; 288: 20–22

Kiel DP, Moskowitz MA (1987) The urinalysis: A critical appraisal. *Medical Clinics of North America*; 71: 607–624

Klatt EC (1999) Tutorial on Urinalysis on University of Utah Pathology Web site. http://medstat.med.utah.edu/WebPath/TUTORIAL/URINE/URINE.html

Wright WT (1959) Cell counts in urine. *Archives of Internal Medicine*; 103: 76–78

Immunological Investigations

Cameron JS, Turner DR, Heaton J, *et al.* (1983) Idiopathic mesangiocapillary glomerulonephritis. Comparison of types I and II in children and adults and long term prognosis. *American Journal of Medicine*; 74: 175–192

Hagen EC, Daha MR, Hermans J, *et al.* (1998) Diagnostic value of standardised assays for anti-neutrophil cytoplasmic antibodies in idiopathic systemic vasculitis. EC/BCR project for ANCA Assay Standardisation. *Kidney International*; 53(3): 796–798

Hahn BH (1998) Antibodies to DNA. *The New England Journal of Medicine*; 338: 1359–1368

Pusey CD, Gaskin G (1997) Disease associations with anti-neutrophil cytoplasmic antibodies. In: Gross WL (ed.). ANCA-associated vasculitides: Immunological and clinical aspects. New York: Plenum Press; pp. 145–155

Savage COS, Winearls CG, Jones S, *et al.* (1987) Prospective study of radioimmunoassay for antibodies directed against neutrophil cytoplasm in the diagnosis of systemic vasculitis. *Lancet*; 1: 1389–1393

Tervaert J, Van de Woude FJ, Fauci AS, *et al.* (1989) Association between active Wegener's granulomatosis and anticytoplasmic antibodies. *Archives of Internal Medicine*; 149: 2461–2465

Chapter 5 _____

PHYSIOLOGICAL INVESTIGATION
Lui Forni

INTRODUCTION

The patient with acute renal failure (ARF) presents complex management problems. Whilst *clinical* investigation involving the pathology and radiology departments is awaited, *physiological* investigation and assessment of the patient can provide invaluable data. This may not only provide key information as to the aetiology of ARF but may also guide appropriate initial therapy. With the ever increasing array of invasive techniques available it is sometimes all too easy to neglect the basic clinical examination as well as the information accrued from relatively straightforward monitoring. Some of the techniques described were once the sole bastion of the intensive care unit (ICU) but with the advent of the high dependency unit (HDU) these procedures are now readily available. Indeed, several renal units have practised intensive physiological monitoring for some time. It is not the remit of this book to provide an in-depth description of the techniques available in the intensivists armoury — for these the reader is directed elsewhere. Rather this chapter outlines methods available which **supplement** the current clinical skills practised by nephrologists.

MONITORING: BASIC PRINCIPLES

Regardless of the type of monitoring systems available the following principles should be adhered to:

- Regular clinical examination should never be neglected.
- Simple physical signs may yield as much information as data displayed on state of the art monitors.
- Changes in the monitored variable must be promptly identified, correctly interpreted and an effective therapy should be available and administered without delay.
- Where conflict between clinical assessment and monitoring occur, the monitor should be presumed to be wrong until all sources of error have been eliminated.
- Changes and trends are more important than any single absolute number.

ECG MONITORING

There is frequently an increased risk of cardiac arrythmias in patients with ARF, most commonly as a result of severe electrolyte imbalance (see **Chapter 8**). Standard ECG monitoring consists of single lead monitoring which records heart rate and aids in the rapid diagnosis of rhythm change. The main components for effective ECG monitoring include: a reliable ECG display, the ability to detect arrhythmias and available facilities for correcting the arrythmia disturbance. In the UK, usual practice is three lead monitoring with lead II, the standard limb lead, being the norm. Lead II is obtained by attaching the negative electrode to the right arm and the positive electrode to the left leg. To eliminate or reduce electrical interference in the ECG when using lead II for monitoring, a third, electrically neutral ground electrode is attached, often to the left upper chest, although this can be attached anywhere. In coronary care units (CCU) the practice tends to five lead placement where further information can be gathered from the chest leads.

ECG monitoring is indicated in patients presenting with ARF who have the following:

- Severe electrolyte/acid-base disturbance.
- Severe hypoxaemia.
- Shock.
- Potential arrhythmogenic drug toxicity or initiation of arrhythmogenic drugs.
- Documented cardiac history (e.g. recent myocardial infarction).
- Documented arrhythmia.
- Concurrent acute coronary syndrome or myocardial infarction.

BLOOD PRESSURE MONITORING

Non-Invasive Blood Pressure Monitoring

Blood pressure can be measured manually with a sphygmomanometer or with a digital device such as a Dynamap® monitor. Manual measurement is recommended in the case of hyper- or hypo-tension. A cuff of suitable size must be used; blood pressure will be overestimated if the cuff is too small. Ideally, the cuff width should be at least 40% of arm circumference with a bladder length at least 80% of arm circumference. There is less error if the cuff is too wide than if too narrow, so it is advisable to use a wide cuff bladder (15 cm) for adults unless the patient is very thin.

Blood pressure should be measured with the patient lying and standing to check for postural hypotension. In the absence of autonomic neuropathy or cardiac conduction anomaly, any drop in pressure should be accompanied by an increased heart rate.

The maintenance of an adequate circulation is essential and vigilant measurement of the blood pressure is paramount. Although the standard sphygmomanometer is more than adequate, the repeated measurement of blood pressure led to the development of automated non-invasive devices. These tend to overestimate at low arterial pressures and underestimate at higher pressures. They most accurately record the mean arterial blood pressure (MAP) calculated from:

$$MAP = 1/3 \text{ systolic BP} + 2/3 \text{ diastolic BP}$$

Over the normotensive range the 95% confidence limits are ±15 mmHg. The most important determinant of measurement accuracy is cuff size (see above). Other limitations of non-invasive systems include erroneous results with arrhythmias such as atrial fibrillation, ulnar nerve injury, limb oedema and problems with infusions.

Invasive Blood Pressure Monitoring

The development of single use systems coupled with the availability of computerised bedside monitors has allowed convenient and accurate invasive arterial blood pressure to be obtained. Clearly this remains an ICU/HDU technique but it does have several advantages. Firstly, it allows accurate and continuous assessment of arterial pressures. Secondly, repeated blood sampling can be performed for blood gas analysis and monitoring of electrolytes, which is of direct relevance to the patient in ARF. Indeed, the morbidity associated with five or more arterial punctures is greater than that with arterial cannulation.

The basic equipment needed for monitoring blood pressure is *the plumbing system* and *the monitoring system*. Detailed descriptions of such systems are available elsewhere, but of most importance is that the system must be zeroed correctly. This involves opening of the appropriate zeroing stopcock to atmosphere and aligning the fluid-air interface point at zero. This is conventionally taken as the mid-axillary line. The position of the transducer relative to the mid-axillary line will change and so this should be verified frequently. Invasive arterial monitoring may also overestimate systolic pressure through a phenomenon known as systolic overshoot which can be overcome by increasing the damping in the system. The most convenient method is the use of smaller gauge tubing although this does detract from the sensitivity. Complications of intraarterial monitoring include ischaemia distal to the cannula, exsanguination and infection — hence the need for regular inspection of the arterial puncture site.

PULSE OXIMETRY

Hypoxaemia may complicate ARF in a variety of settings, the most common of which is volume overload. The degree of a patient's oxygenation is difficult to assess by physical examination alone, being affected by skin perfusion, skin pigmentation and the haemoglobin concentration. Clinically apparent cyanosis does not develop until the deoxyhaemoglobin level has risen to some 5 g/dL which corresponds to an arterial oxygen saturation (SaO_2) of approximately 67%. Arterial blood gas analysis was for many years the accepted method of detecting hypoxemia but this often does not provide immediate or continuous data. The non-invasive nature of pulse oximetry together with its relative affordability has lead to almost universal adoption of this technique for the assessment of arterial oxygen saturation and has been referred to, in some quarters, as the fifth vital sign.

Basic Principles of Pulse Oximetry

A full description of the mathematics and physics involved in pulse oximetry is beyond the scope of this text; however, a brief outline enables the limitations of the technique to be understood. The principal behind pulse oximetry is that haemoglobin changes colour depending on its arterial oxygen saturation. Deoxyhaemoglobin absorbs light principally in the red band of the spectrum (600–750 nm). Oxyhaemoglobin absorbs in the infrared (850–1000 nm) as well as all wavelengths below about 630 nm (visible spectrum) **apart** from the red region (hence its colour!). By applying the Beer-Lambert law the concentrations of both deoxy and oxyhaemoglobin can then be derived. It is relatively easy to see how this can be applied to the laboratory situation, whereas the application of this spectrophotometric principle to a non-invasive device, where tissue is of varying thickness and blood flows in a pulsatile manner, is considerably more difficult. Modern pulse oximeters address these factors through the use of two wavelengths of light and complex microprocessors. Absorbance at the determined wavelengths is used to estimate saturation, which is derived from the ratio of oxyhaemoglobin to the sum of oxyhaemoglobin plus deoxyhaemoglobin according to:

$$SaO_2 \ (\%) = (OxyHb/(OxyHb + DeOxyHb)) \times 100$$

Pulse oximeter probes consist of a photodetector and two light-emitting diodes which commonly emit light at 660 nm and 940 nm. The detector and emitters are positioned facing each other through the interposed tissue. The photodiodes are triggered on and off several hundred times per second, so that light absorption by oxyhaemoglobin and deoxyhaemoglobin is recorded during pulsatile and non-pulsatile flow. Absorption during pulsatile flow relates to the arterial blood plus background tissue and venous blood, whereas absorption during non-pulsatile flow is due to the background tissue and venous blood alone. Absorption at the two wavelengths during pulsatile flow is divided by absorption during non-pulsatile flow, and these ratios are fed into an algorithm in the microprocessor to yield a saturation value. The displayed value is an average based on the previous three to six seconds. Rather surprisingly, the microprocessors of pulse oximeters are calibrated using reference tables compiled by exposing healthy volunteers to decreasing FiO_2 to yield SaO_2 ranging from 75 to 100%. Although manufacturers claim that reported values between 70 and 100% are accurate to within $\pm2\%$ of the true value, in practice the cut-off for acceptable accuracy is felt by many clinicians to be 80%.

Pulse Oximetry in Practice

Pulse oximetry is indicated in any clinical setting where hypoxaemia may occur; this includes initial investigation of the patient, as well as procedures which may affect oxygenation such as the placing of a central venous catheter or the first treatment with dialysis. Pulse oximetry offers the advantage of providing data on haemoglobin saturation rather than the PaO_2. SaO_2 reflects the 98% of arterial oxygen content that is normally carried by haemoglobin, while the PaO_2 directly measures only the small amount of oxygen that is dissolved in plasma. Although the dissolved and haemoglobin-bound oxygen pools are in equilibrium, and PaO_2 is commonly used to estimate arterial oxyhaemoglobin saturation, changes in pH, temperature, and 2,3-diphosphoglycerate concentration alter the PaO_2–SaO_2 relationship and may result in misleading calculations of oxyhaemoglobin saturation. What should also be borne in mind is that pulse oximetry tells us that the haemoglobin is loaded with oxygen and that the lungs must be reasonably well perfused, with underlying adequate gas exchange. Pulse oximetry provides little information with regard to oxygen delivery. In the *healthy* patient arterial oxygen saturation should be at least 96% and stable. If the readings are consistently below this the cause of the respiratory failure should be investigated. The derived oxygen saturation may also be used in the calculation of total blood oxygen content as well as oxygen delivery (see below). Sudden falls in SaO_2 may be caused by a variety of conditions including pneumothorax, a fall in cardiac output, thick secretions blocking the proximal bronchial tree or, indeed, error.

Limitations of Pulse Oximetry

While pulse oximetry is a convenient way of measuring arterial oxygenation, it does not assess ventilation or underlying oxygen delivery. Therefore, its use should be supplemented with arterial blood gas analysis when hypoventilation may be a concern. In addition, because it does not measure PaO_2, over-reliance on pulse oximetry may delay detection of clinically significant hypoxemia. A large decrease in PaO_2 will not produce a significant fall in SaO_2 until the steeper portion of the oxygen haemoglobin dissociation curve is encountered at a PaO_2 of approximately 60 to 70 mmHg. Also pulse oximetry results are signal-averaged over several seconds and may not detect a hypoxemic event until well after it has occurred. This is of most significance when the device is being used for monitoring during intubation. Interpretation of pulse oximetry readings should also consider other factors which may influence the results (**Table 1**). Carboxyhaemoglobin absorbs approximately the same amount of 660 nm light as does oxyhaemoglobin which results in an inaccurate summation of oxyhaemoglobin and carboxyhaemoglobin. Therefore, in cases of carbon monoxide poisoning, a falsely reassuring pulse oximetry reading may mask life-threatening arterial desaturation. Methaemoglobin absorbs at both 660 and 940 nm and similar errors can be made. If carboxyhaemoglobinemia is suspected, co-oximetry is required to accurately measure oxyhaemoglobin. Co-oximeters, which use four rather than two wavelengths of light, detect oxyhaemoglobin, deoxyhaemoglobin, carboxyhaemoglobin, and methaemoglobin, but require a sample of arterial whole blood. If a saturation reading is in doubt, a quick quality assurance test can be done by putting the probe on your own finger!

Table 1. Conditions where pulse oximetry may be unreliable

Anaemia	Excessive patient movement
Low cardiac output states	Motion artefact
Methaemoglobin	Poor peripheral perfusion
Carboxyhaemoglobin	High ambient light levels
Abnormal haemoglobins	Electromagnetic radiation (e.g. MRI)

CENTRAL VENOUS PRESSURE MONITORING

The use of central venous catheters is openly advocated in most treatment algorithms for the management of ARF. Their use is not only limited to that of monitoring, and the applications of central venous catheters lines are growing. Both the techniques and materials involved in this procedure have evolved; the catheter through needle technique has given way to the guide-wire technique, and multi-lumen devices have largely replaced single lumen catheters. This area continues to develop, with much current research related to catheter materials and methods to prevent long-term complications.

Indications for Central Venous Pressure Monitoring

The major indications for central venous catheter insertion are outlined in **Table 2**. Volume resuscitation alone is not an indication for central venous access. Because resistance to flow is related to both the length and diameter of a catheter, short, large-bore peripheral intravenous lines are better suited for rapid volume resuscitation. For example, a 2.5 inch, 16-gauge catheter used to cannulate a peripheral vein has twice the maximal flow rate as an 8-inch central venous catheter of identical bore. The use of central venous catheters with regard to physiological monitoring includes the monitoring of the central venous pressure (CVP) and the use of the pulmonary artery catheter. The two most common sites of central access employed for physiological monitoring are the internal jugular and subclavian veins. The internal jugular vein has several advantages, including a lower risk of pneumothorax, ease of compressibility of the vessel in the event of bleeding, and the straight path from the right internal jugular to the superior vena cava, which facilitates the passage of catheters to the heart. However, landmarks may be difficult to appreciate in obese or oedematous patients, patient comfort and ease of dressing is less than with a subclavian approach, and the site is easily infected if a tracheostomy is present. This will be covered in more depth in **Chapter 9.6**.

Table 2. Indications for central venous catheterisation
Haemodynamic monitoring
Administration of parenteral nutrition
Infusion of drugs likely to induce phlebitis when administered through a peripheral vein
Lack of peripheral venous access
Temporary trans-venous cardiac pacing
Haemodialysis or continuous renal replacement therapies

Central Venous Pressure Monitoring: Basic Principles

Assessment of the CVP occupies a critical position in the diagnosis of the patient with ARF. The CVP gives an indication of the state of the distension of the venous collecting system and the relative efficiency of the heart in dealing with this. The CVP is directly proportional to the venous return which is regulated by the blood volume as well as the capacitance of the venous system. Therefore the CVP provides a guide to the filling of the right ventricle (RV) in that it reflects right ventricular end diastolic pressure. Right ventricular preload, however, is determined by end diastolic volume (not pressure) and therefore an isolated reading of the CVP may be of limited value without some knowledge of cardiac function. However, it does provide a means of recognising changes in the venous system before the development of clinical signs. What cannot be over stated is that the CVP is not directly proportional to the blood volume, although continuous measurement of the CVP with respect to volume expansion or contraction may provide a useful guide to fluid therapy. For example, in severe hypovolaemia the right atrial pressure may be sustained by peripheral venoconstriction and fluid resuscitation may initially produce little or no change in the CVP. As with the monitoring of other pressures within the circulation, the measurement must be relative to some fixed point. Several landmarks are used and it is essential that this is known before any treatment is started. The sternal angle has several advantages in that it is convenient, and does not have the uncertainties associated with monitoring if the patient cannot lie flat. The CVP measured from here has a normal range of −5 to +3 cm of water which, although not an SI unit, is the unit used on general wards and where the pressure is not directly transduced.

Before discussing the use of the CVP in the investigation of a patient with ARF, a word of caution. In many patients who present with ARF, the jugular venous pressure can be seen and the intravascular volume can be readily assessed through clinical examination. In such cases, any additional benefit from the insertion of a central venous catheter may not outweigh the risks associated with it. The slavish adherence to rigid protocols rather than to sensible analysis of the clinical situation is to be avoided. With this in mind, in certain cases the data obtained from the insertion of a CVP line can provide information that cannot be obtained clinically.

Use of Central Venous Pressure Monitoring

The role of CVP monitoring in the face of ARF depends, to some degree, on the aetiology. The causes of ARF are discussed elsewhere, but in general the state of the circulation will dictate the clinician's response as well as the degree of invasive procedures undertaken. Initial clinical management must include some assessment of the circulation. Where there is circulatory collapse and oligo/anuria, CVP measurement will provide useful information (see **Chapters 8 and 10**). In certain cases the intravascular volume status can be difficult to ascertain and CVP measurements may avoid potentially dangerous therapeutic manoeuvres. Although the limitations of isolated CVP readings have been outlined above, when coupled with simple clinical examination they provide a useful guide to a systematic approach to the patient with circulatory insufficiency.

Practice Point 1 provides simple guidelines with which the patient with ARF can be initially assessed. These guidelines give some help as to the aetiology of circulatory collapse in a patient with low systemic blood pressure and oliguria. In many cases the CVP can be used as a guide to right ventricular filling, with the caveats stated above. Where the CVP is low but systemic circulation is adequate, implying volume depletion, the administration of colloid (50–250 mL over 10–15 min) and observing the effect on CVP is a reasonable response. If the CVP does not rise by more than 4 cm, further volume loading may be required. If the CVP rises by more than 6 cm, fluid loading is probably maximal. In most patients, adequate right ventricular filling reflects adequate left ventricular filling, providing the patient has normal heart and lungs, in that the relationship between right and left sided pressures is consistent. Where this is not the case, such as in impaired right ventricular function or in underlying lung disease, the next manoeuvre may be the insertion of a pulmonary artery catheter.

Practice Point 1. Flow diagram for the initial assessment of the CVP

Adapted from RD Bradley & DF Treacher (1997)

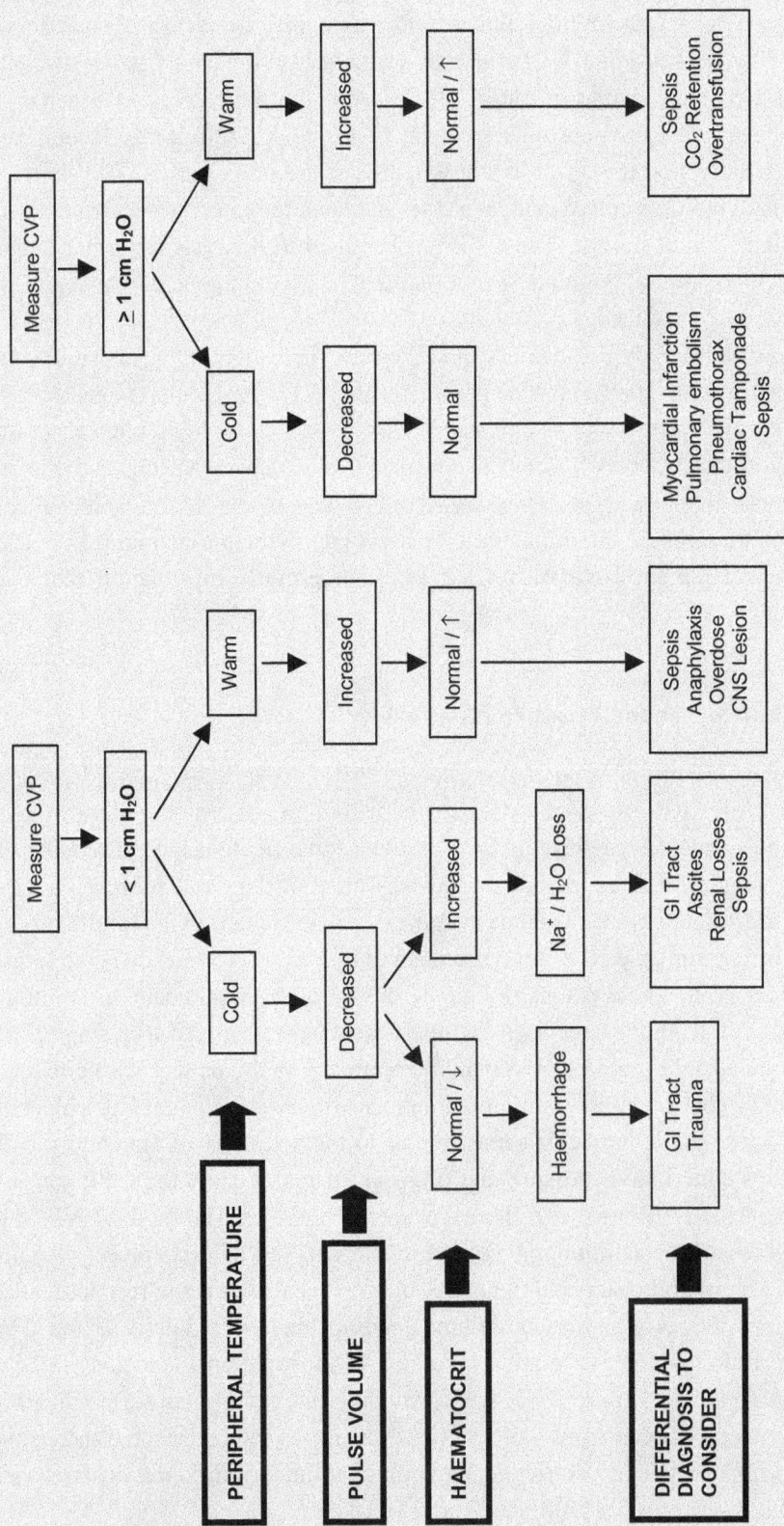

PULMONARY ARTERY CATHETERISATION

Placement of a pulmonary artery catheter allows the clinician to measure intravascular pressures in the right atrium (RA), right ventricle (RV), and pulmonary artery (PA). Left atrial pressure (LAP) can also be assessed **indirectly** from the PA occlusion pressure (also called pulmonary capillary wedge pressure) and samples of blood can be obtained from the PA. Furthermore, various haemodynamic parameters can be assessed including the cardiac output (CO) and the vascular resistance in both the systemic and pulmonary vascular beds.

Pulmonary Artery Catheter Insertion

The choice of insertion site depends on the individual patient. The left subclavian and the right internal jugular approaches probably permit easiest passage of the catheter into the PA, although the femoral approach is also used (**Figure 1**). Most modern catheters have an inflatable balloon which facilitates the passage of the catheter and simplifies the estimation of the LAP. The balloon is inflated when the tip of the catheter enters the RA. Continuous pressure monitoring during the procedure, after correct zeroing and calibration, allows correct positioning of the catheter without fluoroscopic control, although fluoroscopy may be necessary in more difficult insertions — including patients with marked right atrial or ventricular dilatation or severe tricuspid regurgitation. Most commercially available catheters are marked at 10 cm intervals, which may help when advancing the catheter, given that anatomic and corresponding haemodynamic changes occur at approximately 10 cm intervals, the so-called "rule of 10's" (**Table 3**). If the catheter must be withdrawn, the balloon **must** first be deflated.

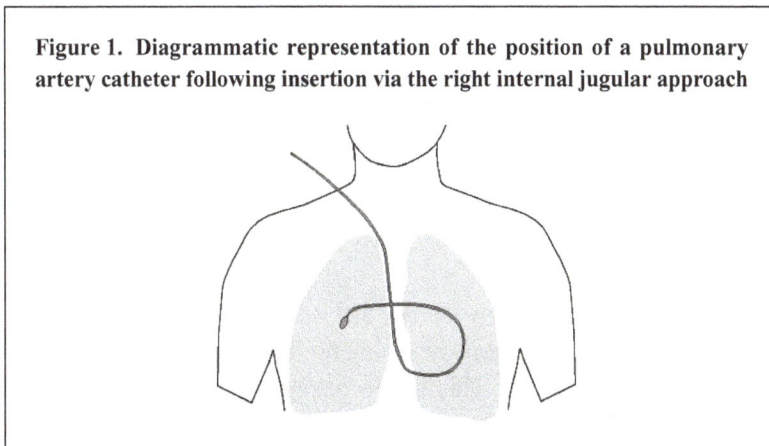

Figure 1. Diagrammatic representation of the position of a pulmonary artery catheter following insertion via the right internal jugular approach

Figure 2 outlines the characteristic pressure tracings observed as the catheter is advanced. On entering the RV from the RA, the pressure tracing changes in keeping with the higher pressures generated in the RV. This is the location with the greatest risk of arrhythmias, and advancement into the PA should proceed without delay. Arrival in the PA is accompanied by a further change in the morphology of the pressure tracing (**Figure 2**). The characteristic dicrotic notch should

Table 3. Guide for pulmonary artery catheter insertion sites

Insertion site	RA (cm)	RV (cm)	PA (cm)
Internal jugular	15–20	30	40
Subclavian	15–20	30	40
Femoral	30	40	50

Approximate distances from the insertion site to the chambers listed, in cm.

Figure 2. Diagrammatic representation of the pressure waveforms expected by location of the pulmonary artery catheter tip

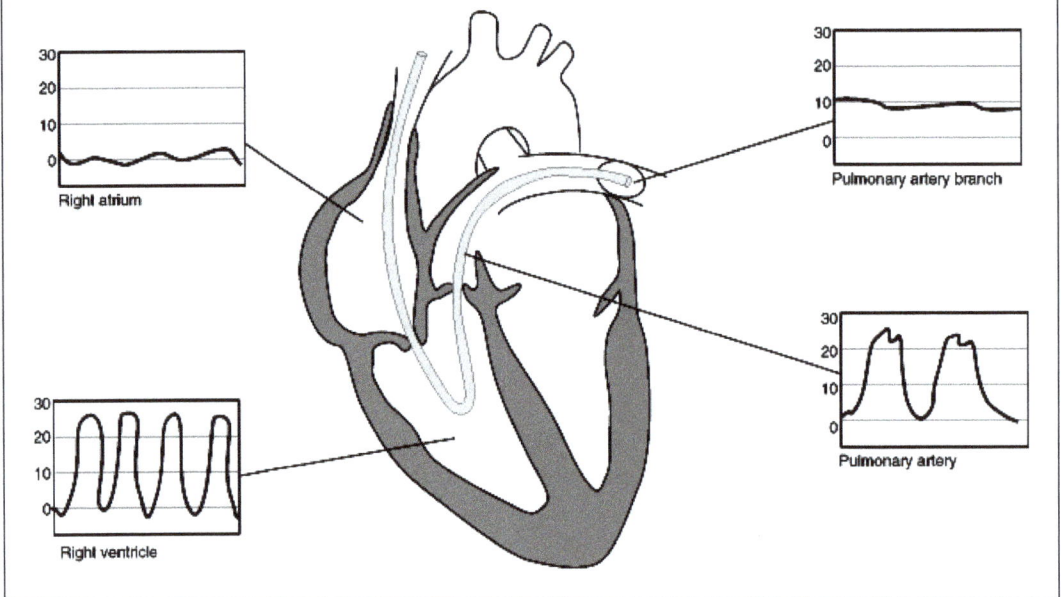

appear and the diastolic pressure will rise above that seen in the RV. From the PA, the catheter should be advanced (with the balloon still inflated) until a fall in the systolic pressure is noted compared with the pressure in the PA. This is the pulmonary artery occlusion pressure (wedge pressure). On balloon deflation the PA tracing should reappear. If the wedge tracing persists, the catheter should be withdrawn until the PA tracing is seen. The catheter must be positioned in the PA such that the wedge position is achieved after 75 to 100% of the full inflation volume of the balloon. If the wedge position occurs on minimal balloon filling, the catheter tip is positioned too distally and further inflation risks rupture of the PA. Alternatively, if too much balloon volume is required to reach wedge position (i.e. more than the full inflation volume), the catheter is too proximal and may slip back into the RV, with the associated risk of arrhythmias and intracardiac damage.

The accuracy of the occlusion pressure also depends on the position of the catheter tip within the lung. If the pressure in the surrounding alveoli exceeds the capillary pressure, the pressure recorded at the catheter tip will reflect alveolar pressure and not the LAP. The pulmonary artery occlusion pressure is only an accurate estimation of the LAP when the pulmonary capillary pressure exceeds the mean alveolar pressure. This occurs in the most dependent area of the lung, referred to as West's zone III, and ideally the catheter should be positioned below the level of the left atrium. The position can be verified by aspirating blood from the distal port of the catheter following occlusion of the PA. After removal of the dead space the arterial saturation in this sample should be greater than that in arterial blood. Other features of a correctly positioned catheter include an occlusion pressure less than the diastolic PA pressure, as well as a normal atrial curve and atrioventricular waves seen on the pressure trace. Therefore a chest X-ray should be obtained to confirm the position of the catheter tip, which should be no more than 3 to 5 cm from the midline, and daily chest X-rays are also recommended to monitor for catheter movement.

Indications for Pulmonary Artery Catheter Insertion

Despite the common use of PA catheters in ICU, there is no conclusive evidence that their deployment has led to decreased mortality, and the technique has undergone somewhat of an onslaught in the medical press of late. However, in many patients they can provide unexpected information which may change therapy. Also, blame cannot be apportioned to the PA catheter if the data obtained is misinterpreted or used incorrectly. The major indications for PA catheterisation include:

- Volume assessment/fluid management where there is impaired RV and/or LV function.
- Assessment of left atrial filling pressures.
- Evaluation of pulmonary hypertension.
- Diagnosis of intracardiac shunt.
- Cardiac output measurement.
- Mixed venous saturation measurement.

This list is by no means exhaustive. The best indicator for PA catheter placement is if a specific question regarding the patient's circulation cannot be answered either clinically or through less invasive measures, and if that the answer would change the management of the patient. More specific recommendations for PA catheterisation were published in a 1998 American College of Cardiology consensus statement.

Complications of Pulmonary Artery Catheter Insertion

Clearly, insertion of a PA catheter carries the same risks as the insertion of any central venous catheter. In addition, the PA catheter has specific risks given its course through the heart.
  These include:

- *Atrial and ventricular arrhythmias*

These are mostly self-limiting. Sustained ventricular arrhythmias occur in 0–3% of patients. Right bundle branch block develops in approximately 5% of catheter insertions, placing patients with pre-existing left bundle branch block at risk for complete heart block, although this is extremely rare. Thus catheter insertion should not be undertaken in such patients without the ability to institute immediate cardiac pacing.

• *Knotting of the catheter*

This can generally be avoided if the individual passing the catheter is careful not to exceed the expected distance from the insertion point to the RV or PA. When knotting occurs, the catheter can usually be removed transvenously.

• *Trauma related*

This includes perforation of the myocardium as well as PA rupture. Pulmonary infarction and thromboembolic events may also occur. The most feared complication is PA rupture which carries a mortality in excess of 30%. This complication is often due to balloon inflation of a distally placed catheter. Certain individuals are at particular risk for this complication, including patients with pulmonary hypertension and mitral valve disease.

Cardiac Output Estimation

The PA catheter facilitates measurement of CO through several methods, the most common of which is the thermodilution technique. More recent catheter designs incorporate continuous oximetric monitoring of PA SaO_2 through fibreoptic reflectance spectrophotometry, which enables continuous CO estimation. Continuous thermodilution catheters are also available and correlate reasonably well with bolus thermodilution methods. The thermodilution method uses a bolus of cold 0.9% saline or 5% dextrose injected through the proximal port of the PA catheter which mixes with blood in the RV. This mixing lowers the temperature of the blood which is then detected by a distal thermistor port. The thermistor records the temperature change and electronically displays a temperature versus time plot. The area under this curve is inversely proportional to the flow rate in the PA and, assuming there is no intracardiac shunt, this flow rate equals cardiac output. This technique has been well validated, although important sources of error do exist.

These include:

• *Tricuspid regurgitation*

This leads to an attenuated peak and a prolonged washout phase of the temperature versus time plot through reflux of the injectate back into the vena cava. The net effect is an underestimation of CO.

• *Intracardiac shunts*

Right-to-left and left-to-right intracardiac shunts can produce falsely elevated CO estimations. Right-to-left intracardiac shunts result in the injectate passing into the left heart which lowers the peak of the temperature versus time plot and overestimates CO. Left-to-right shunting results in increased right heart volume and relative dilution of the injectate, producing a falsely elevated estimate of CO. However, at best, the error involved in CO measurement is of the order of 10%.

Estimation of the CO can also be determined by other methods such as the oesophageal doppler. However, this technique is the reserve of the sedated patient and as such is not discussed further here.

Interpretation of Pulmonary Artery Catheter Measurements

The principal use of PA catheters is haemodynamic monitoring. **Table 4** outlines the pressures measured using the PA catheter and expected normal values. In the patient with circulatory collapse this may aid in diagnosis, but also may be of benefit when evaluating the effect of therapy. In the patient with multi-organ failure, ARF is associated, in part, with the degree of circulatory collapse — hence investigation of these patients is tailored to the underlying cause of circulatory disturbance. Where ARF is found together with poor myocardial performance (an increasingly prevalent scenario), the PA catheter is useful in determining the LAP and degree of left ventricular filling. However, left ventricular compliance may also invalidate the observed PA occlusion pressure and further measures such as echocardiography should be considered. The most efficient way of increasing the CO is through optimisation of the preload; this is covered in **Chapter 28**.

Table 4. Normal pressures measured by pulmonary artery catheter			
Site	cm H$_2$0	mmHg	kPa
Right atrium (mean)	1–10	1–7	0.13–0.93
Right ventricle (systolic)	20–33	15–25	2.0–3.3
Right ventricle (diastolic)	0–11	0–8	0–1.1
Pulmonary artery systolic	20–33	15–25	2.0–3.3
Pulmonary artery diastolic	11–20	8–15	1.1–2.0
Pulmonary artery mean	13–26	10–20	1.3–2.6
Pulmonary artery occlusion pressure	8–20	6–15	0.8–2.0

MIXED VENOUS OXYGEN SATURATION MONITORING

Advocates of mixed venous oxygen saturation (SvO$_2$) measurement suggest that it is probably the best single indicator of the adequacy of whole body oxygen transport. However, in keeping with other forms of monitoring, there is little supportive evidence. The principle behind SvO$_2$ measurement is that it reflects the balance between supply and demand with respect to tissue oxygen tension. Clearly it does not reflect the status of individual tissues. Sampling from the RV ensures adequate mixing and therefore gives a general appreciation of oxygen delivery. The most common indication for the use of SvO$_2$ monitoring is cardiovascular failure with hypotension or unexplained metabolic acidosis.

In brief, the normal SvO_2 is 75%. This falls if oxygen demand increases or oxygen delivery falls. When SvO_2 falls as low as 30%, delivery is insufficient to meet tissue oxygen demands. In terms of management of the patient with a low SvO_2, initial aims must be to increase the CO initially through intravascular fluid optimisation. If SvO_2 remains low, the blood pressure will determine whether after load reduction or the introduction of inotropes will increase CO. The measurement of SvO_2 does not have a pivotal role in the management of ARF but can provide useful information in the setting of multi-organ failure.

ARTERIAL BLOOD GAS ANALYSIS

Contemporary arterial blood gas analysers measure arterial **pH**, **PaO₂** and **PaCO₂**. In addition, other calculated variables are also given including the **standard bicarbonate** and the **base excess or deficit**:

Standard bicarbonate was introduced to try and provide an estimate of the metabolic component of the acid base disturbance in isolation. It represents what the plasma bicarbonate *would* be if the $PaCO_2$ was normal (40 mmHg, 5.33 kPa).

Base deficit represents the concentration of alkali in mmol/l needed to restore one litre of the patient's blood to normal pH at a $PaCO_2$ of 5.33 kPa.

However, both these variables are calculated from *in vitro* data and ignore the fact that the buffering capacity of blood *in vivo* is considerably different, given the contribution from intracellular and interstitial buffers which are in equilibrium with the blood. The base excess is also confusing in that standard compensatory mechanisms may be mistaken for an underlying pathology. For example, the patient with chronic respiratory insufficiency will have a raised base excess through renal retention of bicarbonate; this should not be interpreted as an underlying metabolic alkalosis as well as the known respiratory acidosis.

The arterial blood gas also quantifies the arterial oxygen concentration (PaO_2) at a given inspired oxygen concentration. A $PaO_2 < 10.6$ kPa (80 mmHg) defines hypoxaemia although in practice clinically significant hypoxaemia is present if the $PaO_2 < 8$ kPa (60 mmHg). The degree of hypoxaemia can be estimated from the relationship between the fractional inspired concentration of oxygen (FiO_2) and the PaO_2. This is of use clinically in assessing ventilation. For an increase in FiO_2 of 10% (0.1) there is an increase in the inspired oxygen tension by 10% [i.e. 10 kPa (75 mmHg) at sea level] and an increase in PaO_2 by approximately 6.7 kPa (50 mmHg). Therefore the predicted PaO_2 at a given FiO_2 can be easily calculated. If the calculated value is higher than that measured it can be assumed that the patient would be hypoxaemic when inspiring room air.

Interpretation of Arterial Blood Gas Results

1. *Assessment of the PaCO₂ and pH*

This is described in detail in **Chapter 8.4**.

2. *Assessment of arterial oxygenation*

After assessment of the $PaCO_2$ and pH values, the question of arterial oxygenation should be addressed. This involves three variables:

- PaO_2.
- Oxyhaemoglobin saturation.
- Haemoglobin concentration.

As well as a predictable relationship with the FiO_2 the arterial oxygen tension (PaO_2) has a predictable relationship with the SaO_2, assuming a normal haemoglobin affinity for oxygen. The efficiency of oxygenation may be calculated from the alveolar-arterial oxygen gradient which is derived from subtraction of the arterial oxygen tension from the calculated alveolar oxygen tension. The alveolar oxygen concentration may be calculated from the alveolar gas equation:

$$PAO_2 = (FiO_2 \times [Patm - PH_2O]) - (PaCO_2 \div R)$$

where:

- PAO_2 = alveolar oxygen tension (mmHg)
- FiO_2 = fractional inspired oxygen concentration
- Patm = atmospheric pressure (mmHg)
- PH_2O = partial pressure of water (47 mmHg at 37°C)
- R = respiratory quotient (approximately 0.8 at steady state).

This is a simplification of the actual derived relationship and the result may deviate up to 10 mmHg when $FiO_2 = 1.0$. Also, the values used in the equation may not be precisely known, particularly the FiO_2 (unless on room air) and the value of the respiratory quotient. The alveolar–arterial oxygen gradient also known as the A-a gradient, is obtained through subtracting the measured arterial oxygen tension from the calculated alveolar tension. This may be estimated from:

$$\text{A-a gradient} = 2.5 + 0.21 \times \text{age in years}$$

The normal A-a gradient varies with age and ranges from 7 to 14 mmHg when breathing room air. With higher inspired oxygen concentrations, the A-a gradient also increases. Other simple indices of oxygenation include the ratio of arterial oxygen tension to calculate alveolar oxygen tension:

$$PaO_2 \div PAO_2$$

This is commonly employed on the ICU and approximates the change in PaO_2 which will occur when the FiO_2 is varied, the lower limit of normal being 0.77–0.82. Also the ratio of arterial oxygen tension to FiO_2 may be used to determine clinically significant problems with gas exchange:

$$PaO_2 \div FiO_2$$

The normal value is 300–500. A value of <250 indicates significant gas exchange derangement. The main causes of hypoxaemia are shown in **Table 5**.

Table 5. Causes of hypoxaemia
Hypoventilation
Drug overdose
CNS lesions involving the respiratory centre
Disorders of neural conduction
Respiratory muscular weakness
Diseases of the chest wall
Ventilation-perfusion mismatch
Obstructive lung disease
Pulmonary vascular disease
Lung parenchymal diseases
Right-to-left shunts
Diffusion impairment
Fibrotic lung disease
Reduced inspired oxygen

Oxygen Delivery

Delivery of oxygen to the tissues is determined by both the arterial oxygen content and the CO:

$$DO_2 = CO \times CaO_2$$

$$\therefore DO_2 = CO \times [(Hb \times SaO_2 \times 1.34) + (PaO_2 \times 0.003)]$$

where DO_2 = oxygen delivery (mL O_2/min); CO = cardiac output (L/min); CaO_2 = arterial oxygen content (mL O_2/100 mL blood). Clearly, the oxygen content of the blood will be governed by the concentration and affinity state of haemoglobin. Reduced CO states will lead to reduced DO_2 which may result in cellular hypoxia and ensuing lactic acidosis.

However, the mechanisms behind this are complex and tissue hypoxia may occur despite adequate DO_2. This has lead to the development of so called "goal oriented" haemodynamic therapy in high-risk surgical patients as well as the critically ill in whom DO_2 is augmented to above normal values. This is a controversial area which will not be discussed further.

FURTHER READING

Bradley RD (1977) *Studies in Heart Failure*. London: Edward Arnold

Bradley RD, Treacher DF (1996) Intensive care medicine. *Oxford Textbook of Medicine*. Oxford University Press; 2563–2588

Levine RL, Fromm Jr RE (eds.) (1995) *Critical Care Monitoring*. Mosby-Year Book Inc. St Louis, Missouri, USA

Oh TE (ed.) (1997) *Intensive Care Manual*. 4th Edition. Butterworth Heinemann Press

Singer M, Webb A (eds.) (1997) *Oxford Handbook of Critical Care*. Oxford: Oxford University Press

Webb AR, Shapiro MJ, Singer M, Suter PM (eds.) (1999) *Oxford Textbook of Critical Care*. Oxford Medical Press

Chapter 6 _____

IMAGING IN ACUTE RENAL FAILURE
Christopher Harvey, Peter Robins and Martin Blomley

Imaging and the discipline of uroradiology are central to the diagnosis and management of ARF. Uroradiology encompasses the various imaging and interventional techniques involving the urogenital tract. The renal tract may be imaged by ultrasound (US), intravenous urography (IVU), radionuclide scans, computed tomography (CT), magnetic resonance imaging (MRI) and angiography. The imaging technique of choice should be based on diagnostic yield, radiation burden, cost and possible complications. One of the most important roles of imaging in the context of ARF is to confirm or exclude obstruction as this is a potentially reversible cause of loss of renal function. This chapter will discuss the role of the imaging modalities in the investigation and management of ARF and the acutely failing renal transplant.

IMAGING MODALITIES

ULTRASONOGRAPHY

Ultrasound has replaced IVU as the modality of choice for the initial investigation of ARF and is often able to provide sufficient diagnostic information to make further imaging unnecessary. Ultrasound has the advantage of producing real time two dimensional images whilst being non-invasive, quick, portable (for intensive care patients) and inexpensive, without using ionising radiation. Real time US imaging allows renal biopsy and guides interventions such as nephrostomy placement. The normal renal outline appears smooth with an echogenic (bright) central renal sinus [made up of the pelvicalyceal system (PC), vessels and fat]. The renal cortex is of slightly less echogenicity than the adjacent liver and spleen, and the medullary pyramids are identified as triangular areas of lower echogenicity than the cortex (**Figure 1**). The ureters are not usually visualised.

Intrinsic parenchymal renal disease, such as the glomerulonephritides, are commonly associated with an increased renal cortical echogenicity, although this is a non-specific finding and is unhelpful in the differential diagnosis of the cause. In the context of ARF, normal or enlarged kidneys shown by US may warrant a renal biopsy depending on other clinical features.

Doppler ultrasound can be used to assess vessel patency, direction of flow and degree of stenosis, e.g. renal artery stenosis. The technique is based on the principle that when incident sound waves are reflected from a moving structure, the frequency is shifted by

Figure 1. Normal longitudinal ultrasound scan of the right kidney (inferior to the liver) showing renal cortex (arrowhead), echogenic central renal sinus (broken arrow) and pyramids (small straight arrows)

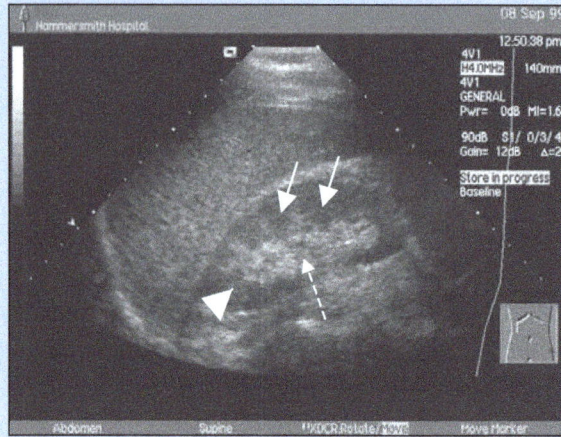

Figure 2. Doppler ultrasound study of a normal kidney

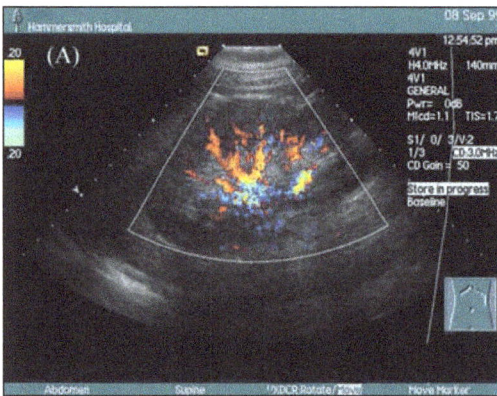

(A) Colour Doppler with red indicating flow towards the transducer.

(B) Colour and Spectral Doppler with the Spectral Doppler cursor positioned over an artery and vein. The arterial trace is seen above the baseline (indicating flow towards the transducer) and the venous trace below.

(C) Power Doppler demonstrating peripheral cortical flow.

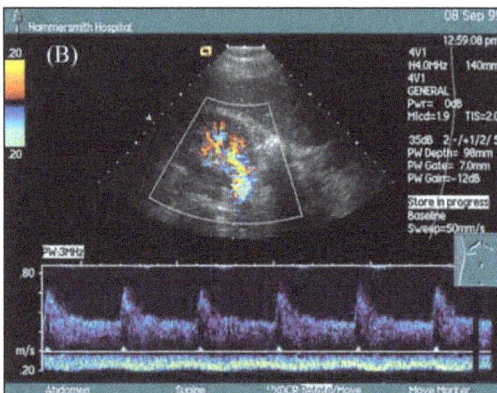

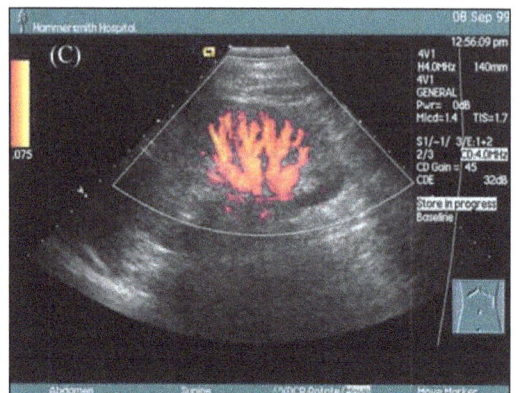

an amount proportional to the velocity of the reflector (e.g. red blood cell), and this can be quantified and displayed as a spectral Doppler or a colour overlay (colour Doppler) (**Figure 2A**). Flow towards the transducer is conventionally red and away blue. Spectral Doppler interrogation of a vessel gives a time dependent velocity profile useful in assessing vascular stenoses (**Figure 2B**). Power Doppler shows the intensity of the Doppler shift as a colour display; directional and flow information is lost but sensitivity may be increased (**Figure 2C**).

Imaging modalities vary in the amount of anatomical and functional information they provide. US and CT provide anatomical detail but little functional information. Radionuclide studies offer more functional information than either IVU, US or CT, but poorer anatomical detail. In addition, the likely diagnostic information obtained must be balanced against the amount of ionising radiation the patient is exposed to when using CT, radionuclides and IVU.

NUCLEAR MEDICINE

The dynamic renogram is most commonly used in the assessment of ARF, while the static renal scan is occasionally helpful. The dynamic renogram is used to diagnose or exclude obstruction. Dynamic renography uses radiolabelled tracers that are rapidly excreted by the kidneys and their arrival, uptake and elimination can be imaged using a gamma camera. The tracers are technetium-99m labelled diethylenetriaminepentacetic acid (Tc-99m DTPA) or mercaptoacetyltriglycerine (Tc-99m MAG3). DTPA is filtered at the glomerulus whereas MAG3 is also secreted by the proximal tubules. For most clinical purposes these two agents are interchangeable with normal renal function, however with increasing renal impairment MAG3 is superior because of a higher extraction efficiency.

The patient is injected with the radionuclide and imaging is performed over a 20 min period. Furosemide can be used to increase urine flow through the kidney and may be administered 5 min prior to the study (T minus 5 protocol) or more commonly 15–20 min into the study and imaging continued for a further 20 min (T plus 20 protocol). The computer generated time-activity curves are used to assess overall renal function and quantify differential perfusion, excretion and relative renal function. The normal renogram has three phases: vascular or perfusion phase (initial sharp rise), cortical uptake or functional phase (slower rise), and finally the excretory or clearance phase (fall of activity) (**Figures 3A** and **3B**). Captopril renography (Captopril 25 mg orally 1 h prior to the scan) may be used to assess renal artery stenosis, where there is a relative decrease in function on the affected side compared to a baseline study. This helps to determine the significance of the stenosis and may give prognostic information with regards to outcome following intervention. It has a limited role in the assessment of ARF compared to its use in evaluation of the hypertensive patient.

The static renal scan uses technetium-99m dimercaptosuccinic acid (Tc-99m DMSA), which binds to proximal convoluted tubules. The kidneys are imaged 2–4 h post injection when approximately 40–50% of the tracer remains bound in the kidneys. It is mainly used to identify areas of renal cortical scarring associated with pyelonephritis in childhood reflux nephropathy.

Figure 3. Dynamic renogram of a normal kidney

(A) Normal dynamic renogram images from which the time-activity data is obtained. Perfusion as well as excretion and drainage can be assessed; (B) Normal dynamic renogram demonstrating the three phases of the time-activity curve; 1st phase — perfusion (30–60 s), 2nd phase — cortical uptake (1–3 min) and 3rd phase — excretion and clearance of collecting system

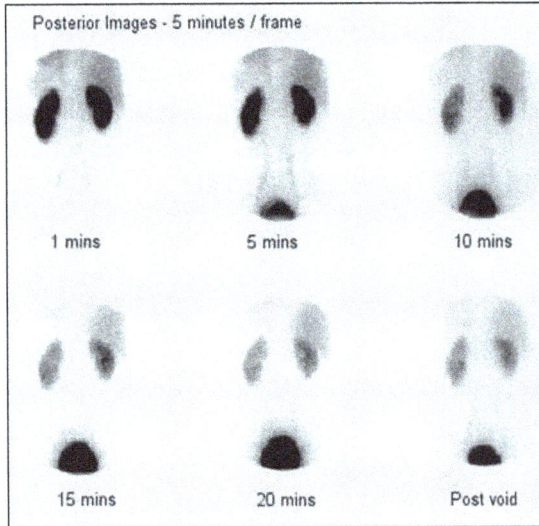

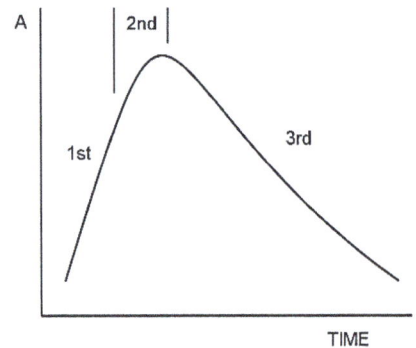

(A)   (B)

INTRAVENOUS UROGRAPHY (IVU)

Ultrasound has largely superseded IVU in the investigation of ARF. The principle of the IVU is dependent on the filtration and excretion of an iodinated contrast medium, thus producing excellent anatomical information as well as some indication of function. In a normal IVU, following contrast medium administration a "nephrogram" is seen coinciding with the highest concentration of contrast in the nephrons. Subsequently a pyelogram is obtained representing urinary opacification of the PC system. In renal impairment it may be difficult to perform a diagnostic IVU, requiring higher doses of contrast medium.

COMPUTED TOMOGRAPHY (CT)

CT has the advantage of excellent anatomical demonstration in addition to some functional information on renal perfusion and filtration. Using fast modern spiral CT the kidney can be imaged initially in the parenchymal nephrogram phase followed by the pyelogram phase (analogous to the IVU) (**Figure 4**). Spiral CT angiography demonstrates the renal vasculature, useful in renal artery stenosis, and showing the relationship of renal arteries to aortic aneurysms. CT can also be used to distinguish stones from transitional cell carcinomas when a PC filling defect is seen on IVU or US.

Figure 4. Spiral CT of a normal kidney

(A) Unenhanced image; (B) Nephrogram phase with cortical enhancement (white arrow). The scan was performed during the arterial phase, note the aortic enhancement (black arrow); (C) Pyelogram phase with contrast medium (white arrow) seen in the renal collecting systems

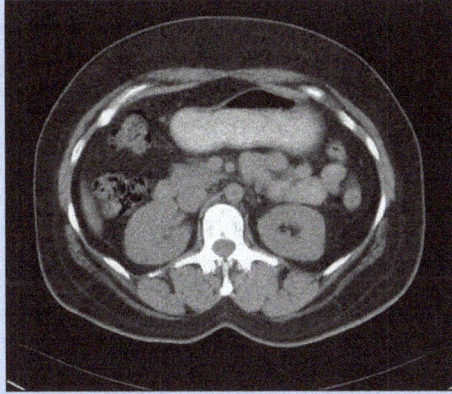

(A)

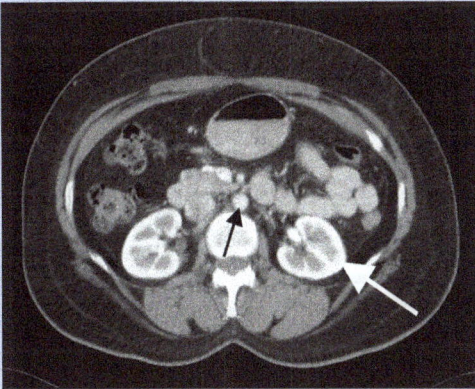

(B)

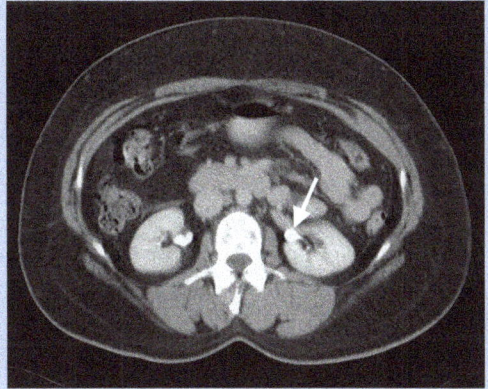

(C)

MAGNETIC RESONANCE IMAGING (MRI)

MRI is based on the fact that protons spin and have an associated magnetic field. When an external radiofrequency pulse is delivered the protons resonate (energy is transferred to the protons). When the pulse is switched off the acquired magnetization decays and the time decay curve is characteristic of tissue types and thus pathological processes. MRI has the advantage of not using ionising radiation but is expensive. Currently MR is mainly used as an alternative to CT. Many new applications are emerging including angiography (MRA) and urographic imaging (MRU), with interventional MR now a reality.

ANGIOGRAPHY

The use of renal angiography has declined since the introduction of CT and ultrasound. It is usually performed using digital subtraction equipment where the image is subtracted from the background. It is still performed, in many centres, on live renal transplant donors to document the number and pattern of renal arteries as well as normality of the other kidney. Management of stenoses can be by angioplasty (balloon dilatation) or endovascular stenting (**Figure 5**) which is attracting considerable interest. Venography can be performed to demonstrate renal venous patency.

Figure 5. Transplant kidney renal artery stenosis

(A) Iliac angiogram shows a complex stenosis (arrow) of an end to end anastomosis between the renal and iliac arteries; (B) Angiogram following placement of a metallic Wallstent across the stenosis showing an excellent result

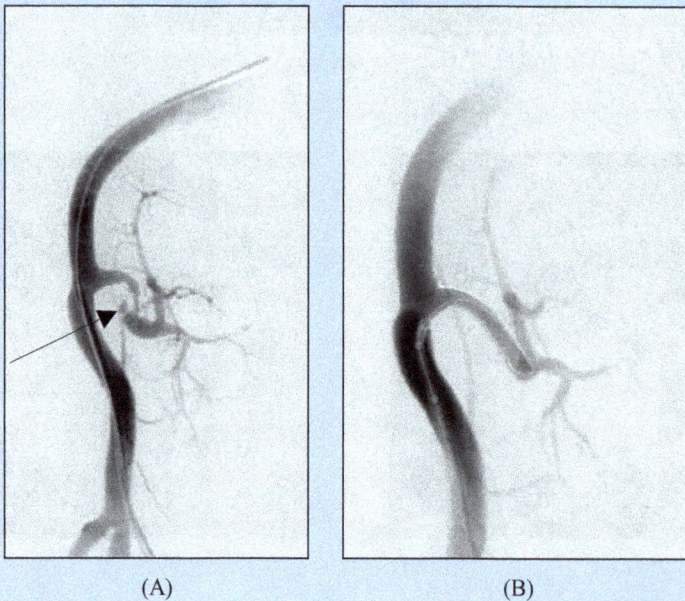

(A)   (B)

CONTRAST AGENT NEPHROTOXICITY

The iodinated contrast agents used for IVU, angiography and CT are potentially nephrotoxic, and this needs to be borne in mind when requesting imaging studies. Important risk factors include pre-existing renal insufficiency, diabetes mellitus, dehydration, myeloma, old age and the use of large doses of contrast. Although transient decreases in renal blood flow and glomerular filtration rate (GFR) are commonly seen (approximately 10% of patients with renal impairment show a reversible rise in serum creatinine), these are only clinically significant in a small proportion (2% of patients with raised creatinine levels) using modern non-ionic contrast agents. Other considerations are that contrast agents carry a significant osmolar load and that potential interactions may occur with biguanides producing lactic acidosis. Currently it is recommended that metformin should be stopped for 48 h after the use of iodinated contrast agents and the serum creatinine checked prior to recommencement.

RENAL TRACT OBSTRUCTION

Diagnosis

The two most important aims of imaging in ARF are to demonstrate or exclude obstruction and to measure renal size. Ultrasound can accurately measure renal size, without the magnification effects associated with an IVU. The normal adult renal length, measured by ultrasound, is 9–12 cm. Renal size and parenchymal cortical thickness can be used to give an indication of whether the aetiology is acute or acute on chronic renal failure. Ultrasound is the modality of choice in the initial investigation of obstruction and often demonstrates the cause. US is able to demonstrate calculi (**Figure 6**), tumours of the renal pelvis, bladder, prostate and pelvis as well as retroperitoneal pathologies. Ultrasound is a very sensitive detector of PC dilatation, the hallmark of obstruction. False negatives occur due to the absence of PC dilatation (e.g. in early obstruction and dehydrated states). Conversely, if the policy that PC dilatation equates with obstruction is adopted, a false positive rate of up to 20% can be expected as there are several causes of non-obstructive PC dilatation (**Table 1**). The commonest of these causes is a "baggy" renal pelvis (i.e. a slightly dilated non-obstructed pelvis) which can be easily diagnosed by US, IVU or CT as there is no calyceal dilatation or functional evidence of obstruction. Furthermore, the degree of PC dilatation does not equate with the level of obstruction: the duration and degree of obstruction being more important factors. Colour Doppler ultrasound is useful in demonstrating the bilateral ureteric "jets" of urine into the bladder, the presence of which exclude obstruction proximal to

Figure 6. Longitudinal ultrasound scan of an obstructed hydronephrotic kidney secondary to a calculus (note the characteristic posterior acoustic shadowing) in the proximal ureter

Measurement cursors have been placed on the calculus

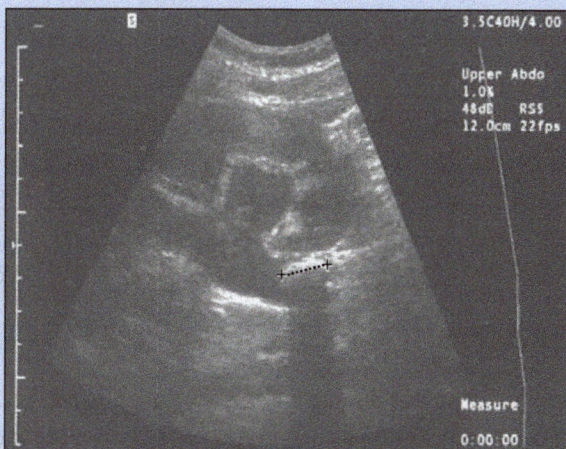

Table 1. Causes of pelvicalyceal dilatation without obstruction

Cause	Examples
Normal variants	"baggy" renal pelvis secondary to a full bladder congenital megacalyces
Dilated PC system from pre-existing renal disease	post-obstructive dilatation or infection
Non-obstructed dilated calyces	reflux nephropathy papillary necrosis pregnancy
Increased urine flow	overhydration, diuresis due to medications

Table 2. Ultrasonography cannot exclude obstruction in the following situations

Clinical situation	Reason/Examples
Technical problems	When the kidneys are difficult to identify: • small irregular kidneys with increased parenchymal echogenicity • obese patients
Cystic disease	A dilated pelvicalyceal system is difficult to visualise in: • polycystic kidney disease • multiple simple cortical cysts • parapelvic cysts
Calculus disease	Large stones filling and distending the pelvicalyceal system
Failure of dilatation of an obstructed system	In severe parenchymal disease (e.g. acute tubular necrosis) Infiltrative processes (e.g. retroperitoneal fibrosis) Early in acute obstruction

the ureterovesical junction. Ultrasound may be unable to exclude obstruction in some situations (**Table 2**). Under these circumstances further investigation is necessary. This may involve antegrade pyelography as part of a nephrostomy, radionuclide studies, high-dose urography or CT. An algorithm for the radiological management of suspected ARF is given in the **Practice Point** at the end of the chapter.

HIGH-DOSE UROGRAPHY

This technique is of value when renal impairment is mild and can provide better anatomical information about the calyces then either ultrasound or CT. It is especially useful in excluding obstruction in polycystic and multicystic kidneys. IVU provides functional information as well as anatomical detail about the degree, level and cause of obstruction. The presence of renal impairment necessitates increasing the contrast medium dose to 600 mg I/kg (double that of a routine IVU) to obtain diagnostic urinary opacification. A preliminary control film is important as this may show renal tract calculi. Tomography may be useful precisely to localise renal stones.

In the presence of acute obstruction an increasingly dense nephrogram may be seen due to hyperconcentration of contrast medium as it slowly progresses down the tubules. Other urographic features that may be present in acute obstruction are:

- renal enlargement
- delayed pyelogram
- opacification of a dilated collecting system and ureter
- pyelosinus extravasation of contrast medium.

The pyelogram appears after a variable delay depending on the degree of obstruction. Additional films can be obtained to demonstrate the level of obstruction. There are no definite rules regarding the timing of these films. In general if a pyelogram is seen not present by 15 min after contrast administration the next film should not be obtained until at least 2 h later ("rule of eights"). Obstruction is excluded if contrast is seen within a non-dilated collecting system within 30 min. In unilateral distal ureteric obstruction a standing column of contrast from the kidney to the site of holdup may be seen. A standing column may be seen in normal subjects so it is important to obtain a postmicturition film to distinguish true obstruction from ureteric stasis secondary to a full bladder.

Extravasation of contrast is seen in up to 25% of cases of acute obstruction and is due to a raised PC system pressure (**Figure 7**). It is due to rupture of the collecting system at its weakest point, the calyceal fornix, where the calyx attaches to the papilla. Contrast then enters the renal

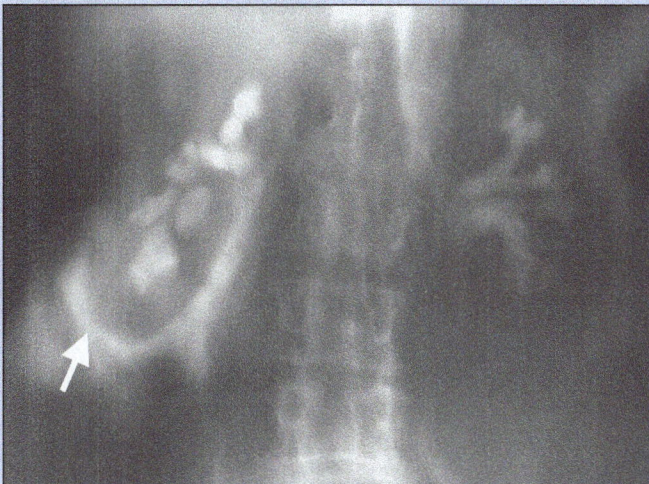

Figure 7. Extravasation of contrast medium during urography in an acutely obstructed right kidney. Note the contrast medium tracking into the subcapsular region outlining the kidney (arrow). Spontaneous resolution occurred once the obstructing calculus had been removed

sinus, the space around the PC system, and may extend inferiorly to outline the ureter. Less commonly contrast may track into lymphatics, subcapsular region, perinephric space or into the venous system (intravasation). Usually extravasation is a benign process with spontaneous resolution unless the urine is infected. A perinephric collection (urinoma) may form in unrelieved obstruction. This may become infected or cause an inflammatory response. Management consists of drainage of the urinoma and correction of the obstruction.

COMPUTED TOMOGRAPHY

In the further investigation of obstruction, or when US is unable to exclude obstruction (**Table 2**), CT is indicated. CT demonstrates retroperitoneal and pelvic anatomy in great detail (**Figure 8**). Unenhanced CT is also able to identify a proportion of the US false positives by demonstrating absence of intrarenal collecting system dilatation, but gives a less accurate measure of renal size compared to US. Recently spiral CT has been shown to rival and in some cases surpass IVU, the traditional gold standard, in the assessment of acute renal colic. It is a sensitive way of demonstrating calculi, especially radiolucent stones, not revealed by IVU. CT has the advantage of providing more anatomical information and is quicker than an IVU. CT is able to show retroperitoneal fibrosis, lymphadenopathy and pelvic tumours. CT can also demonstrate parenchymal thinning, indicative of chronic obstruction in cases of acute on chronic renal failure.

Figure 8. Abdominal CT showing a hydronephrotic right kidney with a dilated pelvicalyceal (PC) system (thick white arrow). The left kidney is normal demonstrating the pyelogram phase with contrast seen in a non-dilated PC system. Malignant lymphadenopathy is seen around the calcified aorta (straight arrow)

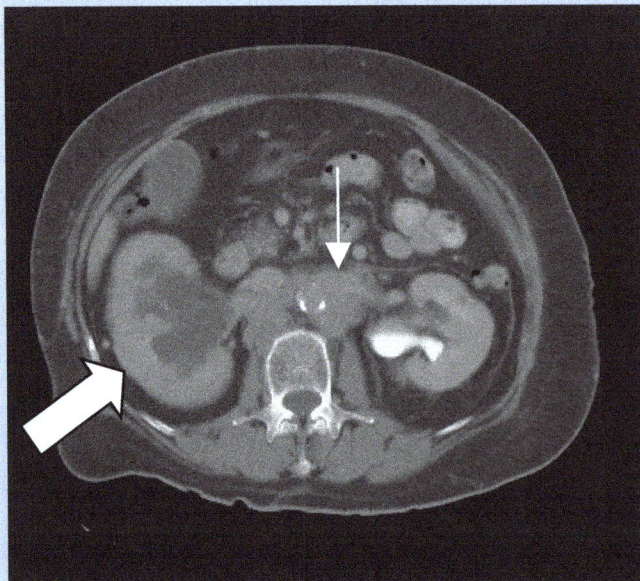

RADIONUCLIDE SCANS

Renography gives useful information on the presence or absence of obstruction, relative renal function and assessment of renovascular compromise. It is also used to assess renal transplant perfusion, function and drainage. The patient should always be well hydrated and diuretic stress can be used to augment functional information with respect to drainage. In obstruction there is a delay in the cortical uptake phase of the curve and a rise in whole kidney activity in the excretory phase. The vascular phase of the renal curve remains normal in the early stage of obstruction, but deteriorates with severe or long-standing obstruction. Where a dilated collecting system is present, furosemide (20 mg IV or an increased dose in renal failure) given intravenously at 15–20 min post tracer injection allows the amount of washout to be calculated (**Figure 9**).

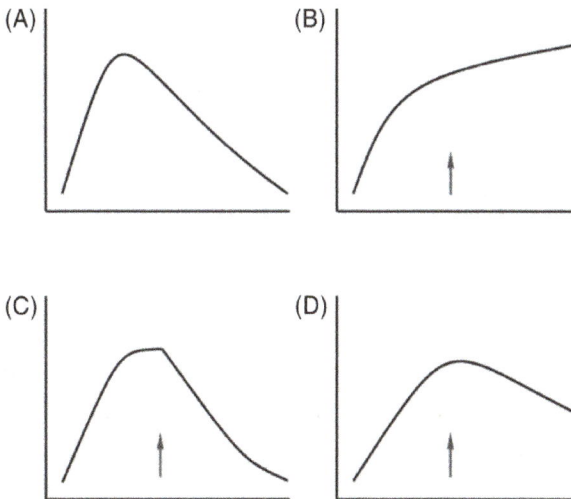

Figure 9. Dynamic renogram curves with time (horizontal axis) versus activity (vertical axis) in normal (A), obstructed (B) and dilated non-obstructed systems (C), showing the effect of furosemide at 20 min (arrows). An indeterminate curve (D) may result when clearance occurs slower than expected despite furosemide, but this may be due to other causes than obstruction

A furosemide half-clearance time (time for 50% decrease in renal activity after diuretic) of less than 10 min is considered normal, while greater than 20 min indicates obstruction. This is particularly useful in confirmation of suspected pelvi-ureteric junction (PUJ) obstruction. A half-clearance time between 10 and 20 min should be considered indeterminate as this may be due to other causes such as reduced urine production in renal failure or dehydration, rather than true obstruction. In the hydronephrotic kidney, the dilated pelvi-calyceal system is often seen as a photopenic defect early that slowly fills in over time (**Figure 10**).

Figure 10. **Obstructed left kidney with hydronephrosis causing central photopaenia on the early images, which progressively fills in, and retention of activity in the dilated collecting system which does not clear with furosemide**

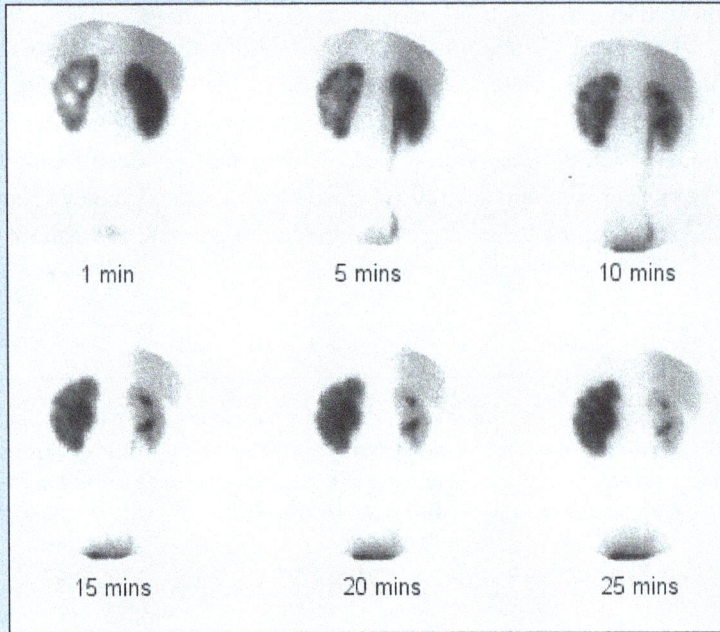

1 min   5 mins   10 mins

15 mins   20 mins   25 mins

INVASIVE TECHNIQUES

Antegrade Pyelography

As with all invasive procedures, clotting and platelets levels should be checked beforehand. Under US or fluoroscopic guidance the collecting system is punctured percutaneously. A guidewire is then inserted, over which a catheter is introduced. Films are taken of the upper tract and ureter as contrast is injected. Antegrade pyelography may be performed as a prelude to nephrostomy, to identify the level of obstruction (e.g. when IVU has failed to do so) and to obtain urine for bacteriological and cytological investigation. Antegrade pyelography is usually able to distinguish intraluminal from mural and extrinsic ureteric obstruction. Further evaluation with CT may be necessary to reach a diagnosis when the level of obstruction is identified.

Retrograde Pyelography

This technique is rarely used now because of improvements in other imaging modalities. It is most useful in the investigation of haematuria (in suspected transitional cell carcinoma which is seen as filling defects) and when there is a contraindication to contrast medium. Following cystoscopic retrograde insertion of ureteric catheters, contrast is introduced to opacify the ureters and upper tracts.

MANAGEMENT OF OBSTRUCTION

Nephrostomy

Nephrostomy is indicated in obstruction in the presence of a pyonephrosis, severe loin pain and in order to preserve renal function. It may be performed using fluoroscopic or US guidance, allowing a pigtail catheter to be inserted. Nephrostomy forms the initial part of a number of procedures. It may be converted to double J stents when long-term drainage is necessary. Percutaneous nephrolithotomy (PCNL) may be performed to extract calculi from the renal pelvis. This is done by dilating the nephrostomy track thus allowing direct endoscopic inspection. Small calculi may be removed intact and larger stones may be broken up using ultrasonic probes. Any residual stones may be fragmented by extracorporeal shock wave lithotripsy (ESWL).

Technique of Nephrostomy

Nephrostomy may be performed using fluoroscopic or real-time US guidance, allowing a pigtail catheter to be inserted. Intravenous contrast may be used to aid fluoroscopic localisation. The Seldinger technique is the most commonly used approach, employing a sheathed needle and guidewire. A calyx is punctured and the track is dilated to allow the insertion of typically a 7 French pigtail catheter. Urine samples are sent for culture and cytology. Complications include septicaemia, which should be covered by prophylactic antibiotics, haemorrhage and arteriovenous fistula formation (incidence 0.5%). Haematuria is usually mild and lasts for 12–24 hours.

ROLE OF IMAGING IN THE ACUTELY FAILING RENAL TRANSPLANT

The causes of dysfunction of a renal transplant are multiple (**Table 3**). Close liaison with the imaging department is extremely important in the early post-transplantation period to assess function and for the prompt diagnosis and management of complications (see also **Chapter 24**).

Table 3. Complications of renal transplantation

1. Rejection	Acute
	Chronic
2. Urological	Obstruction
	Reflux
	Perinephric collections — lymphocoele, urinoma, haematoma, abscess
3. Vascular	Renal artery thrombosis/stenosis
	Renal vein thrombosis
	Arteriovenous fistula
4. Acute tubular necrosis	
5. Cyclosporin toxicity	

Acute Tubular Necrosis (ATN) and Acute Rejection

ATN is the commonest cause of ARF following transplantation. The differentiation of ATN from acute rejection in the early post-transplant period is difficult. Scintigraphy remains the best means of distinguishing between the two. In ATN, renography shows a normal perfusion phase, uptake consisting of blood pool only, and no excretory phase (**Figure 11**), whereas rejection is characterised by a decrease in perfusion and function. Follow up scans in ATN demonstrate progressive recovery.

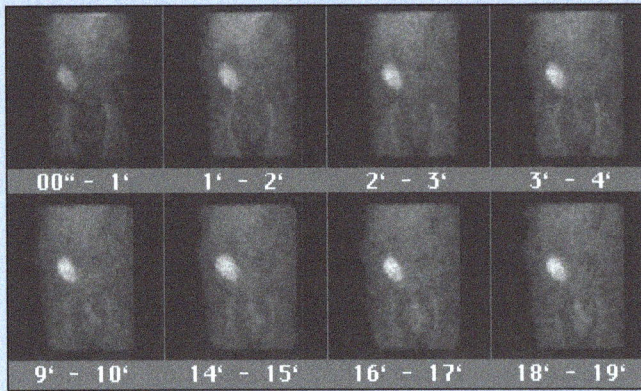

Figure 11. ATN in early post-operative transplant kidney, which has normal perfusion, but delayed uptake and excretion with reduced clearance

There are no specific sonographic features, with renal enlargement, pyramidal swelling and a decrease in the renal sinus echogenicity occurring in both conditions. Indeed normal US appearances may be present. The value of US lies the fact that serial scans can be compared with a baseline. Spectral Doppler was formerly widely used to diagnose acute rejection since the reduced diastolic flow in the intrarenal arteries can be expressed as a reduced Pulsatility Index or an elevated Resistive Index[1] (RI). A ratio of greater than 0.7 was taken as abnormal. However, it has since been shown that similar findings occur in ATN and any other cause of renal swelling, e.g. obstruction. Renal biopsy is therefore necessary to make a diagnosis and is performed under US guidance. Cyclosporin toxicity has no specific imaging features.

Obstruction

As previously discussed, US is a very sensitive means of detecting dilatation of the collecting system. There are numerous causes of obstruction of a renal transplant. In the early postoperative period, mild hydronephrosis may occur due to oedema at the ureteroneocystostomy and this usually resolves spontaneously (**Figure 12**). Stricture at this site may occur later as a result of rejection or vascular insufficiency. The commonest cause of obstruction is ureteric stricture, with other causes including perinephric collections, calculus, clot and fistulae. Functional PC dilatation

---

[1]RI = peak systolic flow velocity-minimal diastolic flow velocity/peak systolic flow velocity.

Figure 12. Acutely obstructed transplant kidney

(A) A longitudinal ultrasound shows gross pelvicalyceal dilatation (thick black arrow) and submucosal oedema (thin black arrows); (B) Antegrade pyelogram demonstrates a tight stricture at the neoureterovesical junction (thick black arrow). Some contrast is seen in the bladder (thin black arrow)

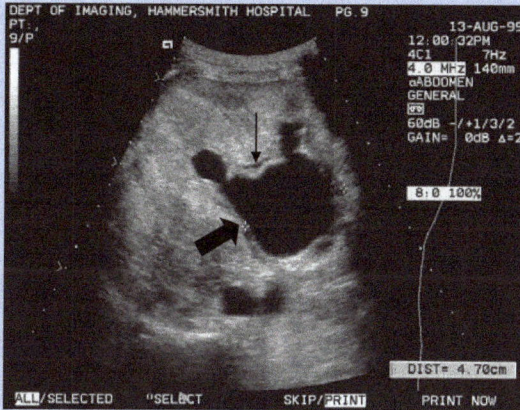
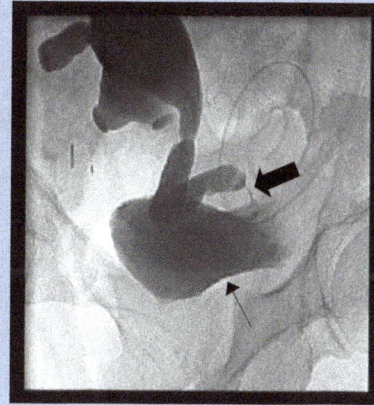

(A)   (B)

due to bladder distension needs to be excluded. US and radionuclide studies are the best modalities for diagnosing obstruction in transplants, with an anatomical level and cause optimally shown by IVU (when renal impairment is mild) or antegrade pyelography. The renogram in obstruction shows reduced perfusion with respect to ATN, with progressive accumulation of tracer due to delayed transit, which does not wash out with furosemide, as described before.

Management consists of nephrostomy and correction of the cause. Ureteric stents and angioplasty are employed in ureteric stricture.

Perinephric Collections

US is the modality of choice in the diagnosis of perinephric collections (**Figure 13**). Fluid collections are seen in up to 50% of transplants and their clinical significance is that they may cause obstruction or indicate a urinary leak. The most common cause is lymphocoeles which usually occur 1–3 weeks post-transplant. They tend to be larger than abscesses or urinomas and are usually related to the inferior pole. Sonographically they may be septated.

Urinomas result from leaks from the renal pelvis, bladder or ureteroneocystostomy. They occur near the lower pole or bladder. The renogram may demonstrate leakage of urinary activity on delayed images. Nonspecific hepatobiliary excretion of MAG3 into bowel may obscure leaked urinary activity on delayed images, but this does not occur with DTPA. Their suspected diagnosis should prompt either antegrade pyelography or urography.

Abscesses usually occur about 5 weeks post-transplant. A haematoma is less common and its site variable.

US cannot differentiate between the various fluid collections, but internal echoes, debris and a capsule point to infection or haemorrhage as likely aetiologies. The collections can be aspirated or drained under US or CT guidance.

Figure 13. Perinephric collection adjacent to the upper pole of a transplant kidney

(A) Ultrasound shows a perinephric infected haematoma (black arrow) containing echogenic contents which was drained percutaneously. Transplant kidney (white arrow); (B) CT demonstrates the perinephric collection (curved arrows) adjacent to the transplant (arrow) and extending between loops of small bowel

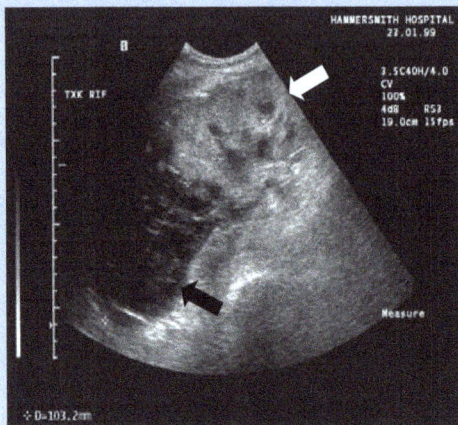 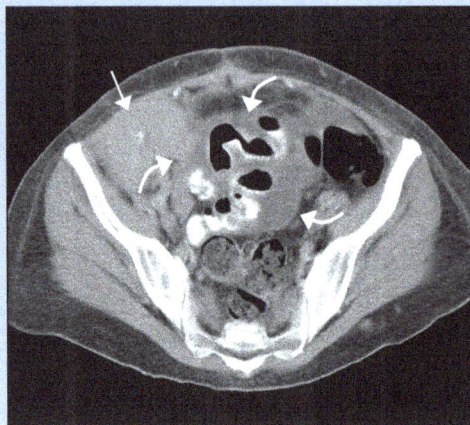

(A)   (B)

Vascular Complications

Renal artery occlusion presents with acute anuria and the diagnosis may be confirmed by Doppler US, renography (**Figure 14**) or angiography.

Renal artery stenosis occurs at the anastomotic site as a late complication. Whilst angiography remains the definitive test, Doppler US has a high detection accuracy. Angioplasty or stenting can be performed as part of the angiographic procedure.

Renal vein thrombosis is best evaluated with Doppler US but can also be diagnosed by angiography. Doppler interrogation may show absence of normal renal venous signal,

Figure 14. Acute lower pole segmental infarct complicating a renal transplant kidney in the right iliac fossa

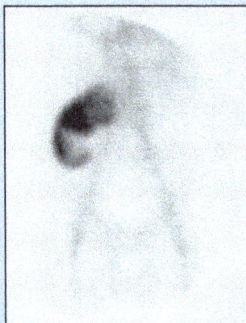

and the renal arterial waveforms may show sharp systolic peaks with diastolic reversal of flow.

Arteriovenous fistulae may result from renal biopsy and can be detected using Colour Doppler (**Figure 15**). Doppler features include pulsatile venous flow and increased velocity with low resistance flow in the feeding artery.

Figure 15. Renal transplant arteriovenous (AV) fistula

(A) Doppler ultrasound shows a lower pole AV fistula (arrow) and its feeding vessel; (B) Spectral Doppler of the transplant vein shows arterialisation of the venous trace

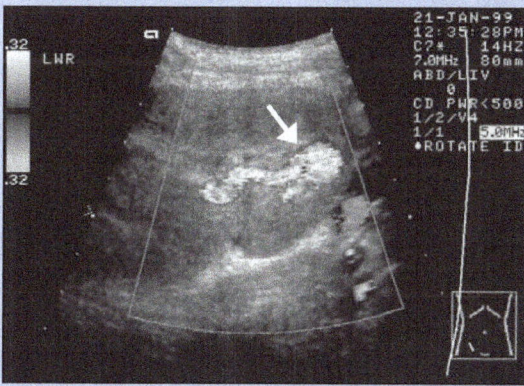
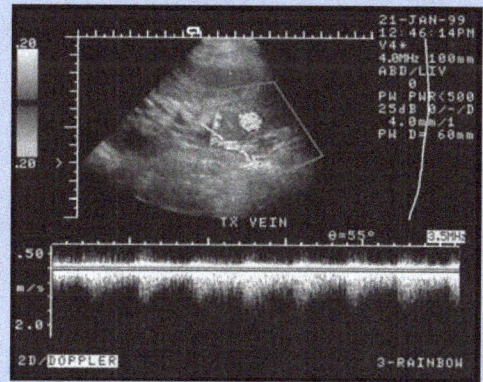

(A)   (B)

Figure 16. Post biopsy arteriovenous (AV) fistula of a transplant kidney

(A) A selective renal angiogram demonstrates an AV fistula (thick black arrow) with characteristic early venous opacification (arrowheads); (B) Angiogram following successful embolisation with platinum microcoils (arrow). There is complete occlusion of the fistula with preservation of the normal arterial branches to the lower pole

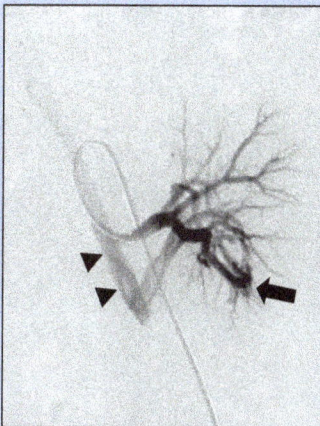
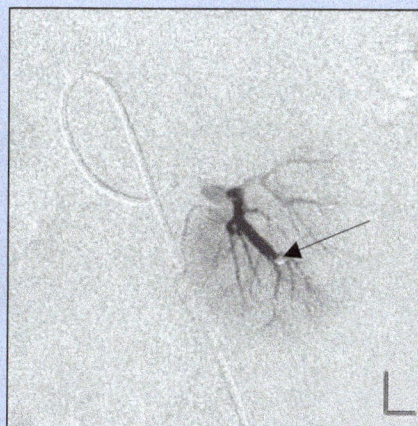

(A)   (B)

Angiography is required to localise the fistula (**Figure 16**) or aneurysm (**Figure 17**) as a prelude to embolisation. Highly-selective embolisation may be performed using modern co-axial catheters, sparing as much normal tissue as possible.

Haemorrhage may occur secondary to biopsy, nephrostomy or other percutaneous procedures. Haemorrhage usually occurs into the collecting system, causing obstruction (**Figure 18**) but may be perinephric. The treatment of choice is embolisation since surgical options are limited.

Figure 17. Transplant pseudoaneurysm secondary to biopsy

(A) A selective renal angiogram shows a 3 cm pseudoaneurysm (arrow) arising from a lower pole branch artery; (B) Post-embolisation angiogram shows successful occlusion of the pseudoaneurysm but with accompanying sacrifice of the lower pole artery. Note the platinum microcoils (arrow)

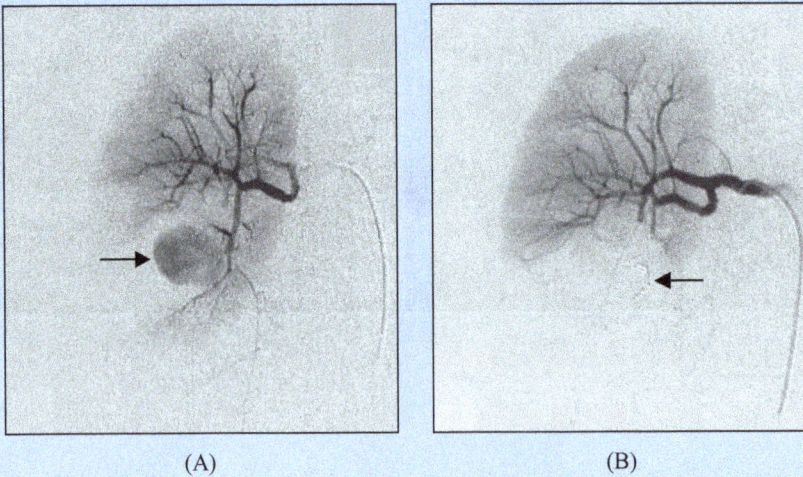

(A)   (B)

Figure 18. Ultrasound shows post biopsy haematoma (arrows) in the collecting system causing obstruction of a transplant kidney

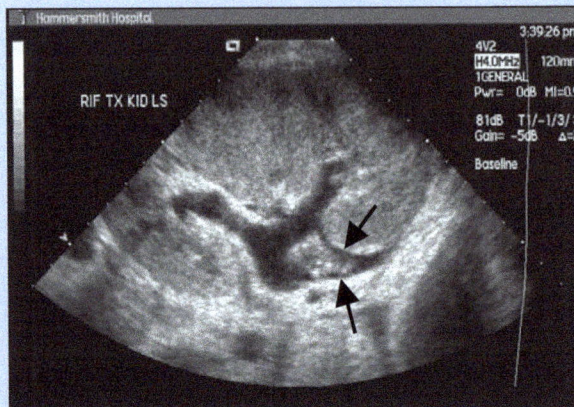

Practice Point. Algorithm for the radiological management of suspected ARF[2]

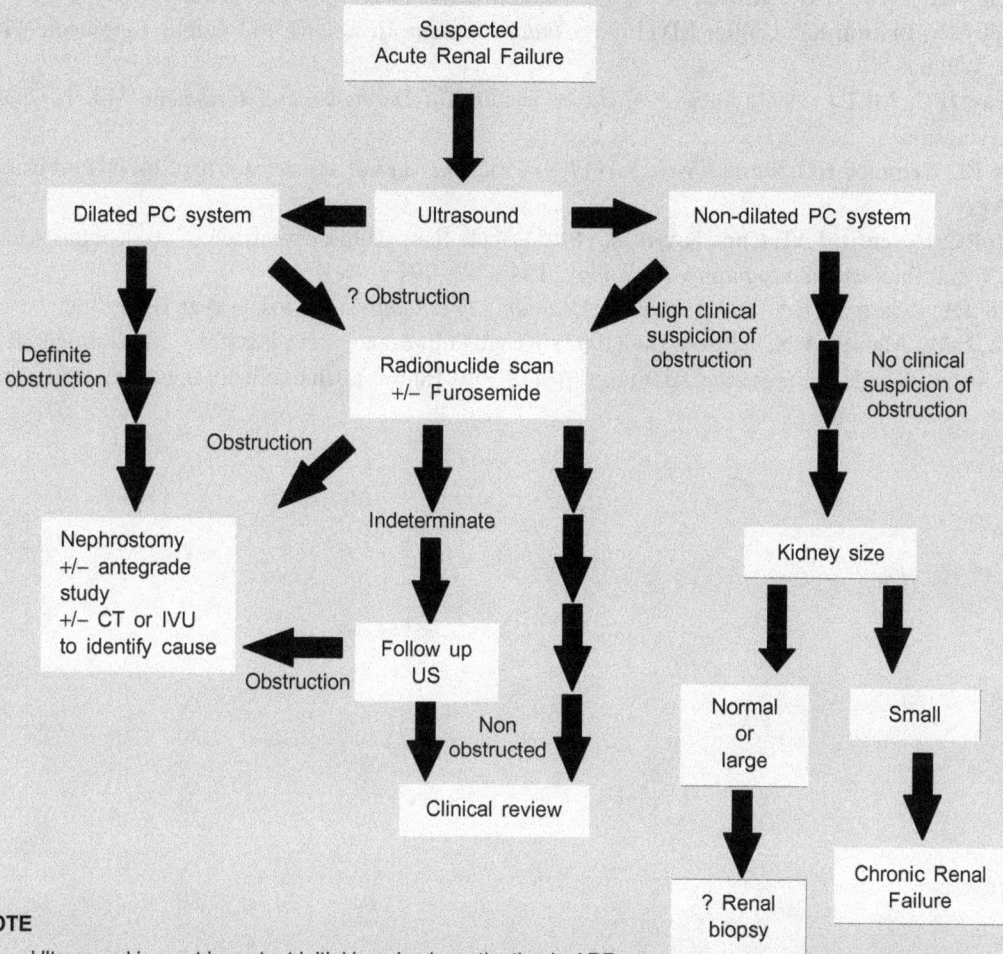

```
                        ┌──────────────────┐
                        │    Suspected     │
                        │ Acute Renal Failure │
                        └──────────────────┘
                                  │
                                  ▼
┌──────────────────┐     ┌──────────────┐     ┌────────────────────┐
│ Dilated PC system │ ◀── │  Ultrasound  │ ──▶ │ Non-dilated PC system │
└──────────────────┘     └──────────────┘     └────────────────────┘
```

- Dilated PC system
  - Definite obstruction
  - ? Obstruction
- Ultrasound
- Non-dilated PC system
  - High clinical suspicion of obstruction
  - No clinical suspicion of obstruction

Radionuclide scan +/− Furosemide

Obstruction

Nephrostomy +/− antegrade study +/− CT or IVU to identify cause

Indeterminate

Follow up US

Obstruction

Non obstructed

Clinical review

Kidney size

Normal or large

Small

? Renal biopsy

Chronic Renal Failure

NOTE

- Ultrasound is most important initial imaging investigation in ARF
- The most important role of imaging in the context of ARF is to confirm or exclude obstruction
- Radionuclide studies impart functional information whereas radiological techniques mainly give anatomical and structural detail
- MAG3 is better than DTPA in ARF
- DTPA may be better than MAG3 for delayed images of urinomas due to late non-specific gut activity with the latter
- **Beware:**   Divided renal function measurements are unreliable in acute obstruction

   Reduced renal function may result in an indeterminate study for obstruction

---

[2]Abbreviations: US, ultrasound, PC, pelvicalyceal, IVU, intravenous urogram, CT, computed tomography.

FURTHER READING

Cattell WR, Webb JAW, Hillson A (1989) *Clinical Renal Imaging*. London: John Wiley

Maisey MN, Britton KE, Collier BD (1998) *Clinical Nuclear Medicine* (3rd Edition). Lippincott Williams & Wilkins

Murray IPC, Ell PJ (1994) *Nuclear Medicine in Clinical Diagnosis and Treatment*. Vol. 1. Churchill-Livingstone

Sharp PF, Gemmell HG, Smith FW (eds.) (1989) *Practical Nuclear Medicine*. Chap. 14. Oxford University Press

Smith RC, Rosenfield AT, Choe KA, *et al.* (1995) Acute flank pain: Comparison of non-contrast-enhanced CT and intravenous urography. *Radiology*; 194: 789–794

Thrall JH, Zeissman HA (1995) *Nuclear Medicine: The Requisites*. Mosby-Year Book, Inc.

Webb JAW, Maisey MN, Allison DJ (1997) Renal failure and transplantation. In: Grainger RG and Allison DJ (eds.). *Diagnostic Radiology*. Vol. 2 (3rd Edition). Churchill-Livingstone; 1491–1511

Chapter 7 _____

RENAL BIOPSY IN ACUTE RENAL FAILURE
Madhuri Warren, Mark Little and Terry Cook

INDICATIONS FOR RENAL BIOPSY

Renal biopsy should be considered when clinical and laboratory investigations are insufficient to identify disease aetiology, to assess prognosis, and to guide therapy in patients presenting with acute renal failure (ARF) and normal kidney size. Renal biopsy is usually performed percutaneously with a spring-loaded needle and is associated with a small but real risk of complications. Therefore, before proceeding to biopsy, it is imperative to consider carefully the usefulness of information obtainable from histological examination of renal tissue, particularly since data available from non-invasive investigations are ever increasing.

"Pre-renal" and "post-renal" causes of ARF can usually be diagnosed clinically and with appropriate imaging (see **Chapter 3**); they should be excluded assiduously before considering renal biopsy. Equally, the finding of shrunken, echogenic kidneys on ultrasound indicates chronic renal disease; renal dysfunction is virtually never reversible in these cases, and biopsy is not indicated. The majority of cases of intrinsic ARF are due to acute tubular necrosis (ATN), when the diagnosis is made on clinical grounds in >80% of cases. Renal biopsy in this setting is only indicated if there is significant doubt about the diagnosis, or the duration of renal failure is prolonged beyond 4 weeks, when a biopsy may provide useful prognostic information. Clinical scenarios where early renal biopsy in ARF may be useful are summarised in **Table 1**. Occasionally, histological examination unexpectedly identifies diseases in patients who have otherwise been asymptomatic, e.g. HIV nephropathy, systemic lupus erythematosus, multiple myeloma, thrombotic microangiopathy. This emphasises the importance of a fastidious search for systemic causes of ARF before submitting the patient to such an invasive investigation.

Contraindications to Percutaneous Renal Biopsy

- uncontrolled hypertension
- multiple bilateral renal cysts/polycystic kidney disease/renal tumour
- bleeding diathesis[1]
- hydronephrosis

_____

[1]Note that prolonged bleeding times, with normal coagulation tests, secondary to renal dysfunction can be corrected by desmopressin (see below and **Chapter 8.6**).

Table 1. Indications for early renal biopsy in patients presenting with acute renal failure

Clinical scenario	Possible diagnosis	Comments
Unexplained ARF		See text
Prolonged oliguria		See text
History of relevant drug ingestion ± eosinophilia/eosinophiluria, fever, rash	Tubulointerstitial nephritis (see **Chapter 18**)	The most common indication for early biopsy in ARF; mimics ATN; steroid therapy may shorten duration of ARF. Fever, rash and eosinophilia only present in one-third of cases
Acute/"sub-acute" decline in renal function (days to weeks) with evidence of glomerular inflammation (e.g. urinary red cell casts)	Rapidly progressive glomerulonephritis (see **Chapter 16**)	Most cases can be defined with serological techniques (e.g. ANCA, anti-GBM) but these are at present insufficient to guide therapy; the fraction & cellularity of crescents has prognostic value
Elderly patient with atherosclerotic disease ± history of angiography, surgery, etc	Atheroembolic disease/ cholesterol emboli (see **Chapter 13**)	May recover renal function after several months
Rapid decline in renal function with severe hypertension (in a patient with scleroderma)	Scleroderma renal crisis (see **Chapter 17**)	ACEI therapy may lead to recovery of renal function if renal architecture is preserved
ARF in multiple myeloma or monoclonal band in serum ± urine	Light chain nephropathy (see **Chapter 22**)	Plasma exchange is an established therapy. Note that multiple myeloma may present with ARF with no symptoms of underlying disease
ARF in the renal transplant recipient	Acute rejection, ATN, cyclosporin toxicity (see **Chapter 24**)	Provides diagnostic information relevant to treatment
Heavy proteinuria	Primary amyloidosis	Presence and type of amyloid
Severe nephritis (RPGN) associated with systemic lupus erythematosus	Diffuse proliferative GN (type IV) (see **Chapter 17**)	Biopsy identifies pattern of renal involvement in clinically active lupus nephritis & guides therapy/prognosis, e.g. presence of interstitial fibrosis, tubular atrophy & glomerular sclerosis would discourage aggressive therapy; presence of florid crescents warrants immunosuppression

- active renal or peri-renal infection
- solitary kidney (see below)
- renal artery aneurysm*
- horseshoe kidney*
- amyloidosis[2].

Note that the presence of a solitary kidney is now considered only a relative contraindication to percutaneous biopsy. Traditionally, it was felt that such kidneys were only amenable to open biopsy. However, the use of thinner biopsy needles and ultrasound guidance has rendered the percutaneous approach safe enough for use in most uni-nephric patients.

RENAL BIOPSY: TECHNICAL ASPECTS

Choice of Needle

Percutaneous renal biopsy is usually performed under local anaesthetic and ultrasound guidance. The choice of biopsy needle lies between the disposable Tru-cut™ needle and the newer spring-loaded devices. The former is hand-driven and larger (14 gauge versus 16 to 18 gauge) and is associated with a small increase in glomerular yield at the expense of a moderate increase in the risk of bleeding. The spring in the spring-loaded device may be part of the needle itself or part of a Biopty™ gun in which the passive needle sits. The advantage of the latter is a more powerful and longer needle excursion, which allows a biopsy to be taken from outside the renal capsule *per se*. However, the gun is relatively heavy and cumbersome and lends itself more to biopsy of the immobile transplant kidney rather than the mobile native kidney. When performing a native renal biopsy in a patient with ARF, we believe that the intrinsic spring-loaded device is the most suitable.

Patient Preparation for Renal Biopsy

In our unit, day case biopsies are performed unless the patient has: obesity, haemoglobin <9 g/dL, platelet count $<90 \times 10^9$/mL, abnormal clotting, or is taking warfarin. Treatment of urinary tract infections and hypertension should precede biopsy in all cases. If there is any doubt as to patient suitability, patients should remain in hospital overnight, with bed rest for 12 hours.

All patients require:

- Minimum 6 h bed-rest after biopsy.
- Full blood count, clotting screen, group and save, urea and electrolytes & MSU documented within 14 days prior to the biopsy.
- Haemoglobin >9 g/dL[3], platelets $>90 \times 10^9$/mL, normal clotting.

---

*Consider open biopsy if clinical scenario warrants the risk.
[2]Increased risk of haemorrhage.
[3]Can be lower only if staying overnight.

- Diastolic BP <95 mmHg, systolic BP <150 mmHg.
- Urine dipstick on admission — if no MSU available within last 14 days, arrange urgent microscopy.
- No aspirin for 1 week prior to biopsy. No NSAID for 24 h prior to biopsy. No warfarin.
- **Premedication:**
  - Diazepam 5–10 mg po (for anxious patients)
  - DDAVP 0.3 μg/kg iv if creatinine >300 μmol/L (DDAVP c/i in pregnancy)
  - Intravenous diazemuls or midazolam may be used if absolutely necessary
  - Fentanyl (50–100 μg) or morphine (2–10 mg) may be used for analgesia if necessary (with SaO_2 monitoring)
- IV access and SaO_2 monitoring by pulse oximetry if sedated.
- **Consent:** inform the patient that the biopsy will be performed under ultrasound guidance on the ward and that the procedure takes ~30 minutes. Discuss risks of macroscopic haematuria 1–10%; blood transfusion 0.5%; surgical/radiological intervention for bleeding <1/500; loss of kidney <1/1000 (see below).

Technique: Real Time Ultrasound Guidance

It is preferable to image the kidney and the needle as the biopsy is being performed so that there is a higher probability of obtaining tissue from the lower pole, where the risk of injuring a major blood vessel is lower. A clip with an aperture for the biopsy needle can be attached to the ultrasound probe, thereby allowing the needle to travel along a fixed path in the same plane as the ultrasound beam. The patient is usually biopsied while lying prone with one or two pillows under the abdomen and the head and shoulders resting on the bed. It is also possible to perform the biopsy with the patient sitting upright and, indeed, this approach may be easier in the obese patient.

Both kidneys are imaged, to ascertain which side is more accessible and to ensure that two kidneys are present. As the right kidney is more caudal, it is usually (but not always) easier to biopsy. An estimate is made of the depth of the kidney during deep inspiration.

Using aseptic technique, the skin overlying the chosen kidney is painted with Chlorhexidine and the skin and proposed biopsy track (down as far as the renal capsule) are infiltrated with 2% lidocaine. The most frequent mistake is a failure to use sufficient anaesthetic around the capsule. In obese patients it may be necessary to use a spinal needle to allow infiltration to the necessary depth. As a rough guide, 7–10 mL of 2% lidocaine should be instilled around the kidney.

The ultrasound probe is covered with a sterile sheath and the lower pole of the kidney is re-imaged. A small incision is made in the skin and the biopsy needle is passed through the probe clip to a point about halfway between the skin and the renal capsule.

The patient is asked to take a deep breath and to hold it while the primed needle is inserted, under direct ultrasound vision, into the lower pole. The gun is fired and the needle is withdrawn. The greatest potential for renal damage occurs if, as the needle passes through the renal capsule, the patient exhales. Therefore, it is essential to impress upon the patient the importance of keeping still as the biopsy is taken.

It is conventional to apply 2–3 min of pressure to the area after each pass, although it is doubtful that this influences the risk of bleeding from such a deep organ. The number of cores obtained depends on the question being asked (see below); however, one should not attempt more than three or four passes, or attempt a biopsy in both kidneys. The biopsy site is then covered with a small adherent dressing.

Technique: Pre-Procedure Renal Localisation

If the ultrasound machine is not set up to allow direct real-time visualisation at the time of biopsy, it is possible to perform the procedure in a "semi-blind" manner after marking the site on the skin with the aid of the ultrasound machine. In view of the weight of the apparatus this method does not lend itself well to use with the spring-loaded Biopty™ gun. The technique is identical to that described above, apart from the following points:

1. Once the site has been marked with an indelible pen, the skin cleaned and the area anaesthetised, a 22 gauge spinal needle is used to localise the kidney. With the patient holding their breath in, the needle is advanced to the approximate depth of the renal capsule. The patient is then asked to breathe normally. If the needle swings with respiration it is in the kidney. If it does not swing, the needle is advanced a small amount with the patient breath holding and the procedure is repeated.
2. Using the spinal needle as a guide, the biopsy needle is advanced with the patient holding their breath in, and movement of the needle with respiration is again demonstrated. Once the biopsy needle swings consistently, the biopsy is taken with the patient holding their breath.

Post Biopsy Observations

- Bed rest for 6 h, flat on back.
- BP every 15 min for first 2 h, every 30 min for next 2 h, then hourly for next 2 h.
- Patient can get out of bed after 6 h, and should be observed on the ward for a further 30 minutes.
- Patients at increased risk of bleeding should have 12 h bed rest.
- All urine to be collected and inspected for visible haematuria and dipstick tested for haematuria.
- Doctor should be called if BP falls >10 mmHg, or macroscopic haematuria (increase BP observations to every 10 min).

Patients should be admitted overnight if they develop macroscopic haematuria, urinary retention, severe back pain, BP falls >10 mmHg, or uncontrolled hypertension (>160/95 if over 50 years old, >150/90 if under 50 years old).

COMPLICATIONS OF RENAL BIOPSY

Haematuria and Haemorrhage

Bleeding is the primary complication of renal biopsy. It is more prevalent in biopsies done in patients with ARF in whom there is frequently a degree of uraemic platelet dysfunction. Haemorrhage may occur into the pelvi-calyceal system (leading to macroscopic haematuria), under the renal capsule (leading to acute flank pain) or into the retroperitoneum (leading to potentially life-threatening haemorrhage). Virtually all patients have microscopic haematuria (assuming renal tissue has been obtained!). Macroscopic haematuria occurs after up to 10% of biopsies and significant hypovolaemia necessitating transfusion occurs in about 1 in 200 cases[4]. The immediate appearance of blood in the urinary catheter bag always indicates a significant haemorrhage; the assistance of a urologist should be sought urgently. Similarly, acute, severe flank pain at the time of biopsy suggests brisk intra-renal or peri-renal bleeding. Obviously, further efforts at biopsy should not be attempted and urgent renal imaging should be arranged. Nephrectomy is required in less than 1 in 1000 cases.

Arteriovenous Fistulas

Intra-renal arteriovenous fistulas occur in up to 15% of cases and are diagnosed by colour-coded Doppler ultrasonography. The majority are asymptomatic and have disappeared by one year post-biopsy. Occasionally, arteriovenous fistulas present as haematuria or hypertension, and rarely as high-output cardiac failure when embolisation of the fistula may be required.

Other Complications

Flank pain persists beyond 24 h after 1 biopsy in 20 and is generally due to a blood clot in the ureter or a sub-capsular haematoma. Rarer complications include urinary infection, damage to other intra-abdominal organs and hypertension (due to persistent increase in intra-renal pressure: the "Page" kidney).

BIOPSY HANDLING[5]

For a full assessment of the changes in the renal biopsy it may be necessary to examine it by light microscopy (LM), immunohistochemistry (IH) and electron microscopy (EM). The differential diagnosis of glomerulonephritis, in particular, relies on the IH and EM findings. It is therefore necessary that the tissue obtained at renal biopsy should be allocated appropriately for these investigations, although the way in which this is done may have to be varied depending on the amount of tissue obtained at biopsy and on the methods adopted by the histopathology department. If there is any doubt as to what material is required or how it should be handled then it is essential to discuss this, before the biopsy is performed, with the pathologist who will examine it.

Light Microscopy

The tissue for LM is placed in a fixative for a number of hours before processing into paraffin (or resin) which allows thin sections to be cut and stained. The usual fixative in the UK

---

[4]Adapted from (1) Parrish AE (1992) *Clinical Nephrology*; 38: 135–141 and (2) Madaio MP (1990) *Kidney International*; 38: 529–543.
[5]For a detailed description of biopsy handling and processing refer to the following web-site: http://www.kidney-euract.org/RBpathologyconsensus.htm

is formal saline ("formalin"), a 1:10 solution of concentrated (37–40%) formaldehyde in buffered saline.

Immunohistology

This is performed routinely to assess the deposition of immunoglobulin and complement components in the kidney, particularly in glomeruli. As a minimum, most pathologists will stain for IgA, IgG, IgM and C3. Stains for C1q and C4 may also be helpful. In some cases it may be necessary to stain for kappa and lambda light chains, immunoglobulin subclasses, or to use antibodies to determine the cell types in an inflammatory or neoplastic infiltrate.

Traditionally, IH has been performed using antibodies conjugated to a fluorescent label such as fluorescein isothiocyanate (FITC), on separate cryostat sections of frozen renal tissue, and visualised using a fluorescence microscope. In many departments this is still the preferred method, since it is easy to perform and, more importantly, sensitive enough to pick up sparse deposits.

More recently, methods have been developed which allow IH to be performed on the formalin-fixed, paraffin-embedded tissue processed for LM. During this processing the antigens may become chemically altered and therefore less accessible to the antibodies used. The sections must therefore be treated before immunostaining with an antigen retrieval technique, commonly protease digestion. Following digestion, sections are incubated with a primary antibody against the immunoglobulin or other antigen of interest, followed by a secondary antibody, directed against the primary antibody, conjugated to an enzyme. This is usually horseradish peroxidase, which in the presence of an appropriate substrate will catalyse the deposition of an insoluble dye at the site of antibody localisation ("immunoperoxidase staining"). Immunoperoxidase staining is technically more demanding and less sensitive than immunofluorescence (IF), but provides a permanent record.

Electron Microscopy

The tissue for EM is pre-fixed in 3% EM-grade glutaraldehyde in 0.1 M cacodylate buffer, for 60 min, post-fixed in 1% osmium tetroxide, dehydrated in a graded series of alcohols and then critical point dried from CO_2.

In the context of ARF, the major role of EM is in the classification of glomerulonephritis, by determining the presence and distribution of immune complexes, which are seen as electron dense deposits. While a full diagnosis will be possible in many cases without EM, it is usually not possible at the time of biopsy to predict which these will be and ideally, therefore, tissue should be taken for EM in *all cases*. It is important to remember that paraffin embedding distorts tissue morphology, making it less reliable for interpretation by EM.

Handling of the Biopsy

The thin cores of renal tissue obtained by needle biopsy are very susceptible to damage by crushing or by drying, both of which may make histological interpretation difficult. Therefore it is important that great care is taken in dividing the biopsy for LM, IF and EM. In ideal circumstances this should be carried out at the bedside with the aid of a dissecting microscope. The tissue is removed gently from the biopsy needle and placed in a drop of cold normal saline. It is then viewed with the dissecting microscope to see whether glomeruli are present. The cores are then divided using a new scalpel blade so that a few glomeruli are present in the pieces for EM and IF and the rest of the tissue is placed in fixative for LM. If a dissecting microscope is not available at the bedside then it is safe to wrap the tissue in a saline soaked gauze swab and transport it immediately to the pathology department for cutting (it should *not* be placed in saline since this may introduce artefactual changes in the tissue). If a dissecting microscope is not available then the best way to ensure that glomeruli are obtained for EM and IF is to take small samples from each end of the cores. In some circumstances, it may not be possible to freeze the tissue for IF immediately. In that case it may be placed in a special transport medium containing protease inhibitors (e.g. Michel transport medium), in which it may be stored for 1–2 days if necessary. In some cases, it may also be appropriate to submit some of the tissue for microbiological culture.

Examination of the Biopsy

Each renal pathologist will have a preferred protocol for cutting and then staining the biopsy, but a number of features will be common to all. It is essential that good quality thin sections are examined, in most cases cut at several different levels.

The most common stains employed are:

1. *Haematoxylin and eosin (H&E)*
   This is useful for studying inflammatory infiltrates, tubular cytoplasm and glomerular "fibrinoid" deposits.

2. *Periodic acid-Schiff (PAS)*
   This stains the glomerular mesangium and basement membrane and is the best stain for assessment of the overall glomerular structure.

3. *Jones' silver methenamine*
   The silver stain is best for demonstrating the details of basement membrane structure and is particularly useful, for example, in showing the spikes of membranous glomerulonephritis or the double contours of mesangiocapillary glomerulonephritis.

In some cases other stains may be employed. For example the *elastic van Gieson* stain demonstrates the elastic laminae of vessels and the *Congo red* stain identifies amyloid deposits.

Examination of the biopsy is carried out in a systematic fashion with assessment of glomeruli, tubulointerstitium and vessels. One of the first tasks in the assessment of a biopsy in ARF is to decide in which of these compartments the main pathology lies. It must be appreciated that changes in the glomeruli or vessels may also produce secondary changes in the tubulointerstitium. The histological appearances of a normal kidney are shown in **Figure 1**.

GLOMERULAR CAUSES OF ACUTE RENAL FAILURE

The two major forms of glomerular injury which lead to ARF are **glomerular inflammation** (glomerulonephritis) or **glomerular thrombosis**.

Figure 1. Histology of normal kidney

(A) This low power view shows a glomerulus and surrounding tubules. At the hilum of the glomerulus the juxtaglomerular apparatus can be seen (H&E); (B) Higher power view of a normal glomerulus (H&E)

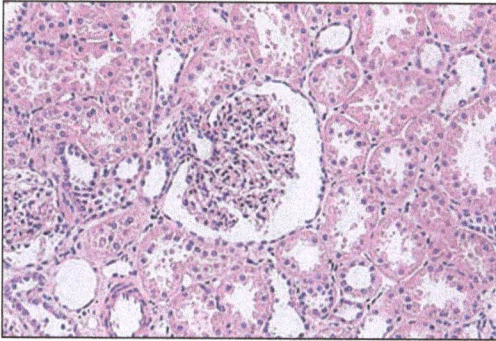

(A)

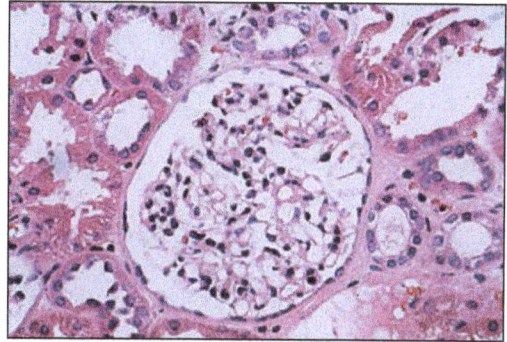

(B)

Glomerulonephritis

The forms of glomerulonephritis (GN) which are severe enough to cause ARF are characterised by a marked increase in glomerular cell number (glomerular "proliferation") and/or necrosis in the glomerulus. The clinical aspects of these important types of rapidly progressing glomerulonephritis are discussed in **Chapter 16**. An increase in glomerular cell number is conventionally known as glomerular "proliferation" although in many cases the increase is mainly due to infiltration of the glomerular tuft by inflammatory cells rather than proliferation of intrinsic glomerular cells. ARF due to glomerular damage may be characterised by increased cells in capillary lumens (**endocapillary proliferation** — see **Figure 2**) or by increased cells in Bowman's space (**extracapillary proliferation**). Increased cells in Bowman's space, which, in the setting of glomerulonephritis, consist of a mixture of inflammatory leucocytes and epithelial cells, give rise to the morphological appearance of **crescents** (**Figure 3**).

Necrosis is the term used to describe an area of disruption of the glomerular basement membrane often with nuclear fragmentation and the deposition of fibrin-rich material, which appears intensely eosinophilic in H&E sections (**Figure 4**).

Further terms which may be used to describe the changes occurring in glomeruli are:

- **Diffuse:** A lesion involving at least 50% of the glomeruli (most often >80%).
- **Focal:** A lesion involving some but not all glomeruli (<50%).
- **Global:** A lesion involving the whole glomerulus.
- **Segmental:** A lesion involving a portion of a glomerulus while leaving some capillary lumens uninvolved.

The types of glomerulonephritis which are most likely to be encountered in ARF are:

- *Diffuse endocapillary proliferative glomerulonephritis*
- *Diffuse mesangiocapillary glomerulonephritis*

Figure 2. Glomerulus from a case of diffuse endocapillary proliferative glomerulonephritis secondary to streptococcal infection

The glomerulus is markedly hypercellular and there are infiltrating mononuclear cells and neutrophil polymorphs within capillary lumens (H&E)

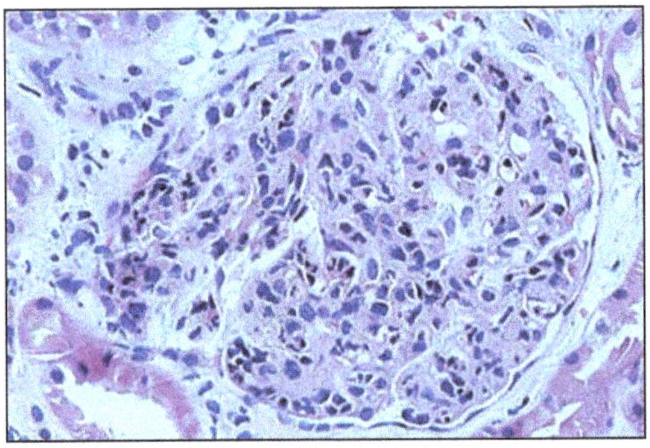

Figure 3. Glomerulus from a case of anti-GBM disease showing a large crescent (arrow, H&E)

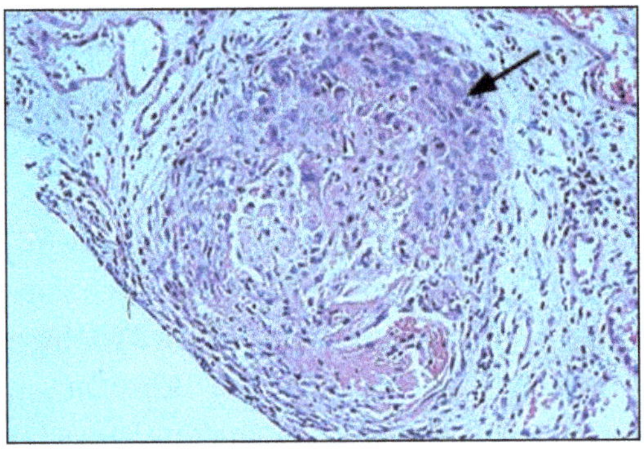

Figure 4. Glomerulus showing a prominent segmental area of fibrinoid necrosis (H&E)

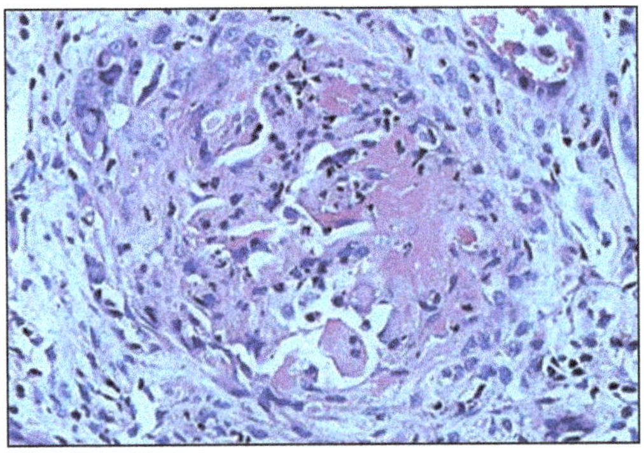

- *Focal and segmental glomerulonephritis*
- *Diffuse crescentic glomerulonephritis.*

Diffuse endocapillary proliferative glomerulonephritis

This describes a form of glomerular injury in which all, or almost all, of the glomeruli are hypercellular with an increase in cells in capillary lumens (**Figure 2**). The hypercellularity is caused both by infiltration of the glomerulus by leucocytes and by proliferation of intrinsic glomerular cells. Capillary lumens may also be occluded with swollen endothelial cells. Crescents may be present but if they are seen in more than 50% of glomeruli then the lesion is, by definition, classified as **diffuse crescentic glomerulonephritis** (see below).

Diffuse endocapillary proliferative glomerulonephritis may be seen in:

- Post-infectious glomerulonephritis.
- Cryoglobulinaemia.
- Henoch-Schonlein purpura.
- SLE — class IV.

Although these different conditions may have similar light microscopic appearances, there are differences in the immunohistochemical and ultrastructural findings (see **Table 2**).

Table 2. Differential diagnosis of diffuse proliferative endocapillary glomerulonephritis

Cause	Light microscopy	Immunohistochemistry	Electron microscopy
Post-infectious glomerulonephritis	All glomeruli affected. Glomeruli are hyper-cellular due to neutrophil/ monocyte accumulation, and increased glomerular cells	Granular capillary wall staining for C3 ± IgG. Occasional staining for IgM and IgA	Large subepithelial electron dense deposits forming conical "humps" which are *transient and disappear over a few weeks*
Cryoglobulinaemia (type II)	PAS positive deposits of cryoglobulin distend capillary lumina ("thrombi"); within the wall of arteries and arterioles result in fibrinoid necrosis	Positive immunostaining for immunoglobulins comprising the cryoglobulin deposits plus C1q, C4 and C3	Characteristic appearance of deposits as curved tubular structures clustered in bundles
Henoch-Schonlein purpura	May see FSGN or crescents	Strong mesangial IgA and C3 staining, plus staining of capillary walls	Electron dense deposits in mesangium ± capillary basement membrane
SLE	Varying picture on LM according to class. Diffuse proliferative is class IV. Commonest is class III (FSGN) — see **Table 4**	Often positive for multiple immunoglobulins and complement components (see **Table 4**)	Electron dense deposits in mesangium ± other sites (see **Table 4**)

Diffuse mesangiocapillary glomerulonephritis (MCGN)

Diffuse mesangiocapillary glomerulonephritis (also known as membranoproliferative glomerulonephritis) is divided into two main classes:

- *Type I MCGN*: deposition of subendothelial and mesangial immune complexes, which induces the extension of mesangial cells between the deposits and new basement membrane formation, producing *mesangial cell interposition* and *double contouring* on silver or PAS staining.

- *Type II MCGN*: expansion of the capillary basement membrane by material of unknown composition which has a characteristic electron dense appearance on electron microscopy (also known as "*linear dense deposit disease*").

The specific causes of Type 1 MCGN are discussed in **Chapter 16**. Both forms of MCGN most commonly present with nephrotic syndrome and/or slowly declining renal function, but ARF may occur. In both types, on LM, there is involvement of all or nearly all of the glomeruli, which show an increase in mesangial cells and matrix together with thickening of capillary walls. The enlarged glomeruli are said to have a "lobulated" appearance. Obviously, the immunohistochemical and electron microscopic features for each type will vary, as discussed above (see also **Table 3**).

Table 3. Histological features of diffuse mesangiocapillary glomerulonephritis

Type	Immunohistochemistry	Electron microscopy
TYPE 1	Coarse irregular staining for C3 on capillary walls and mesangium IgG, IgM, IgA, C1q, C4 less constant	Subendothelial and mesangial electron dense deposits. Reduplication of basement membrane around subendothelial deposits, mesangial cell interposition
TYPE 2 (Dense Deposit Disease)	Granular C3 in mesangium, sometimes along capillary walls. Usually no immunoglobulins	Linear electron dense material within the basement membrane. Also in tubular basement membranes and Bowman's capsule

Focal and segmental glomerulonephritis (FSGN)

In focal and segmental glomerulonephritis there is involvement of a proportion of the glomeruli by inflammatory lesions and, in the glomeruli involved, there is inflammation in some segments with sparing of other segments. It is possible to recognise two main patterns of involvement:

1. *Focal and segmental necrotising* — seen in the ANCA-related diseases, microscopic polyangiitis, Wegener's granulomatosis and Churg-Strauss syndrome. The glomeruli show segmental areas of capillary wall damage with the deposition of eosinophilic, fibrin-rich material ("fibrinoid necrosis"), but with little associated inflammatory cell infiltration, and with the uninvolved

glomerular segments appearing normal. Typically there is little evidence of immunoglobulin or complement deposition. It is usually not possible to distinguish between the causes on microscopy alone.

2. *Focal and segmental proliferative* — this is characterised by the presence of *segmental* glomerular endocapillary hypercellularity, often in association with immune complex deposits. There may or may not also be associated segmental fibrinoid necrosis. The segments of glomeruli away from the endocapillary hypercellularity may be normal or they may show increased mesangial cells and matrix.

Whichever of these two patterns of glomerular involvement is seen, there may also be crescent formation. It should be stressed that although the necrotising pattern is more characteristic of ANCA-associated disease, and the proliferative pattern is more usual with immune complex deposition in glomeruli, the distinction is not clear cut and the diagnosis depends on the immunohistochemical and ultrastructural findings as shown in **Table 4**.

Diffuse crescentic glomerulonephritis

If the glomerular capillary wall is severely damaged there may be activation of the coagulation system with deposition of fibrin in Bowman's space. This leads to the influx of inflammatory cells and proliferation of epithelial cells within Bowman's space forming a *cellular crescent* (**Figure 3**). In severe cases, the inflammation may lead to the rupture of Bowman's capsule with extension of the inflammatory infiltrate into the renal interstitium. As crescents age there is deposition of fibrillar material between the cells giving a fibrocellular crescent. Eventually the increased cellularity resolves leaving a lesion composed mainly of fibrous material — a *fibrous crescent*.

The presence of cellular crescents is, therefore, a reflection of the severity of glomerular inflammation rather than of a particular aetiology and any of the conditions already discussed, including diffuse endocapillary proliferative glomerulonephritis, diffuse mesangiocapillary glomerulonephritis, and focal and segmental glomerulonephritis may show crescent formation. **By convention, if crescents are present in more than 50% of glomeruli in a biopsy then the condition is referred to a diffuse crescentic glomerulonephritis.** It is important to emphasise that diagnosis of the cause involves recognition of the underlying pattern of glomerulonephritis which has led to crescent formation, using the diagnostic criteria as outlined in the preceding sections. However, crescent formation is particularly strongly associated with pauci-immune and ANCA-related glomerulonephritis and with anti-GBM disease (see **Table 3**). The percentage of glomeruli involved by crescents is often quoted, since this is an important indicator in treatment and prognosis.

Other considerations in glomerulonephritis

Glomerular inflammation may be associated with changes in the vessels and in the tubulointerstitium, and these must also be assessed. Intrarenal vessels may show necrotising vasculitis in ANCA-associated disease and in cryoglobulinaemia. Vasculitis may rarely be seen with SLE but more common is the deposition of immune complexes within arterioles without

Table 4. Differential diagnosis of focal and segmental glomerulonephritis

Disease	Immunohistochemistry	Electron microscopy	Other clinical features
ANCA associated glomerulonephritis (Wegener's granulomatosis, microscopic polyangiitis, Churg-Strauss syndrome)	No, or only scanty staining ("pauci-immune GN")	No electron dense deposits	Circulating ANCA N.B. Some patients may be ANCA negative
Idiopathic pauci-immune glomerulonephritis	No, or only scanty staining	No electron dense deposits	Regarded as renal-limited vasculitis. May be ANCA positive
Anti-GBM disease	Linear capillary wall staining for IgG ± C3. Tends to be uniform involving all glomeruli. Rarely other Igs and complement components may be present	No electron dense deposits	Circulating anti-GBM antibodies
SLE WHO classification class III <50% focal segmental necrosis WHO classification class IV >50% segmental necrosis +/− crescents	"Full house" of IgA, IgG, IgM, C1q, C4 and C3	Electron dense deposits in mesangial, subendothelial & subepithelial locations. Tubuloreticular inclusions in endothelial cells	Appropriate serology Light microscopy — varying features according to class including wire looping, haematoxyphil bodies, hyaline thrombi, double contouring
IgA nephropathy	Mesangial (± some capillary wall) IgA and C3 staining. May be smaller amounts of IgG and IgM	Mesangial electron dense deposits	Background of diffuse proliferation of mesangial cells
Henoch-Schonlein purpura	Mesangial and capillary wall IgA and C3	Electron dense deposits which may be at all 3 sites	**N.B.** Similar renal picture to IgA nephropathy but diagnosed due to additional extra-renal manifestations — vasculitic rash, GI involvement, arthralgia
Chronic bacterial infection e.g. bacterial endocarditis	Variable segmental IgG, IgM, C1q, C4 and C3	Subendothelial, mesangial and, less commonly, subepithelial deposits	May see diffuse proliferation or crescents. Longstanding cases may resemble MCGN

inflammation. It is common to see a degree of acute damage to tubules secondary to glomerular inflammation and, in some diseases, prominent tubulointerstitial inflammation may be seen.

It is important for the pathologist to give an estimate of any chronic irreversible damage the kidney has sustained since this is a good predictor of the extent to which recovery of renal function is possible. This should include the percentage of glomeruli which show segmental sclerosis, global sclerosis and fibrous crescents. The percentage of cortical tubules which are atrophic and the percentage of the interstitium showing fibrosis should also be estimated.

Glomerular Thrombosis

Glomerular thrombosis may occur in the setting of disseminated intravascular coagulation or as part of a syndrome of thrombotic microangiopathy.

- *Disseminated intravascular coagulation*

This condition may occur as a result of infection, particularly with gram-negative organisms, obstetric complications, massive tissue injury secondary to tumours, or as a result of toxins such as sustained from snake bites. There is intravascular thrombosis and consumption of coagulation factors. In the kidney, fibrin rich thrombi are found within glomerular capillary loops and sometimes within small vessels. The condition is distinguished from other causes of thrombosis such as thrombotic microangiopathy or vasculitis by the fact that there are no structural changes of the endothelium or vessel wall. In severe cases of disseminated intravascular coagulation, the kidney may show *bilateral cortical necrosis*, in which, macroscopically, there is a characteristic band of infarction within the cortex with sparing of the subcapsular area and medulla. On microscopy, in the infarcted cortex, there is widespread thrombosis of glomeruli, arterioles and small arteries resulting in almost complete necrosis within 72 hours.

- *Thrombotic microangiopathy*

The term thrombotic microangiopathy (see also **Chapter 15**) is used for a group of conditions, subdivided as follows:

— *Haemolytic uraemic syndrome*: The haemolytic uraemic syndrome has a number of underlying causes, including infection with verotoxin-producing *Escherichia coli*, pregnancy, drugs, transplant rejection and the presence of antiphospholipid antibodies. This differential diagnosis is discussed more fully in **Chapter 15**. Morphologically the condition affects the kidney only, with changes in both glomeruli and blood vessels, although in any individual case they may be more marked in one or other compartment.

— *Thrombotic thrombocytopaenic purpura*: In this condition small vessel thrombi are found throughout the body.

On light microscopy, thrombotic microangiopathy is characterised by the presence of glomerular and afferent arteriolar thrombi, arteriolar fibrinoid deposition, and loose intimal thickening of small arteries due to the accumulation of foam cells, fibrin, and red cells (**Figure 5**). The glomerular capillary walls are also thickened due to subendothelial fibrin and red cell deposition, while other glomeruli show secondary ischaemic changes, capillary loop congestion and collapse. The presence of intravascular thrombi may lead to mechanical damage to red blood cells and the

Figure 5. Thrombotic microangiopathy

The section shows an interlobular artery with marked mucoid intimal thickening. The glomeruli show tuft collapse (H&E)

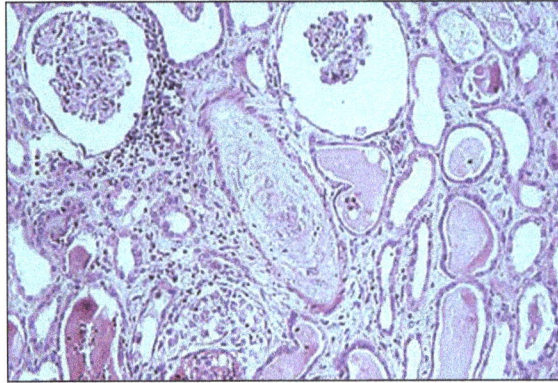

syndrome of microangiopathic haemolytic anaemia. The arteriolar fibrinoid deposition may be shown on biopsy by histochemical or immunoperoxidase staining.

VASCULAR CAUSES OF ACUTE RENAL FAILURE

Vasculitis

The most common forms of vasculitis to affect the kidney are ANCA positive vasculitides, which usually produce a picture dominated by glomerulonephritis, as described above. However, fibrinoid necrosis of larger vessels, i.e. arterioles and small arteries, may also be seen and may, in some cases, be more marked than the glomerular involvement (**Figure 6**).

Involvement of medium-sized and large vessels is also seen in:

- *Cryoglobulinaemia*

Involvement of renal arterioles and arteries is relatively common, in association with the glomerular changes (see above).

- *Classical polyarteritis nodosa*

Classical polyarteritis may affect renal vessels down to the size of large interlobular arteries and may therefore sometimes be seen in renal biopsies. The affected vessels show segmental or circumferential destruction of the wall, which is replaced by fibrin and surrounded by inflammatory cells including neutrophils and mononuclear cells. The lumen of the vessel may be occluded by thrombus.

- *Kawasaki's disease*

Kawasaki's disease may affect the main renal artery and intrarenal vessels, which show infiltration of the media and intima by neutrophils and macrophages with some fibrin deposition.

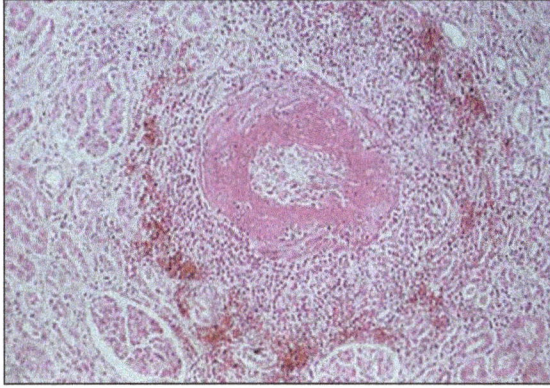

Figure 6. Necrotising arteritis

A small artery shows circumferential fibrinoid necrosis (H&E)

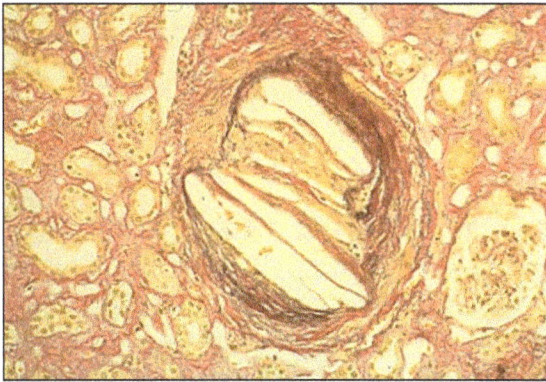

Figure 7. Cholesterol emboli in a small renal artery

In this stain the elastic of the artery wall stains black. The cholesterol itself has dissolved during processing of the section but the cleft-like spaces occupied by the cholesterol crystal are clearly seen (Elastic van Gieson)

Thrombotic Microangiopathy

This has been described above and in **Chapter 15**.

Cholesterol Emboli (see also Chapter 13)

Embolisation of material from atheromatous plaques is a relatively common cause of ARF. On renal biopsy, emboli are seen in arteries, arterioles and occasionally in glomeruli. They have the appearance of needle shaped spaces, representing cholesterol crystals, together with amorphous debris (**Figure 7**). It is important to note that cholesterol emboli dissolve after formalin fixation.

If requesting fat stains such as Sudan Black, it is important to remember that these need to be performed on fresh tissue. In some cases, a biopsy from a different site, for example a skin biopsy, may be more appropriate for diagnosis. With time there is progressive accumulation of fibrous tissue around the emboli. The kidney distal to sites of vascular obstruction shows ischaemic changes.

Acute bilateral cortical necrosis is increasingly seen in older patients with atheroembolic disease in large vessels, and those undergoing aortic aneurysm repair. Thrombosis within the atherosclerotic afferent arterioles, interlobular or arcuate arteries, may present with secondary infarction of cortical glomeruli. Chronic changes include fibrosis and calcification of the renal cortex.

TUBULOINTERSTITIAL CAUSES OF ACUTE RENAL FAILURE

Acute Tubular Necrosis

Acute tubular necrosis (ATN) is the commonest cause of ARF in clinical practice, accounting for over 60% of cases in most series. Since there is no specific treatment, it is usually diagnosed clinically, with biopsy being reserved for cases in which other (treatable) diagnoses need to be ruled out. If a biopsy is performed, ATN is observed to be a disorder of tubule destruction with no obvious anatomical lesion within the other components of the renal parenchyma. The tubule dysfunction is solely responsible for the ARF. Both ischaemic and toxic causes (**as described in Section 2**), may operate via a variety of mechanisms, including tubule obstruction, tubule lumen back-leakage, a reduction in the glomerular filtration rate, and arteriolar vasoconstriction.

Renal biopsy

- *Ischaemic cases*

Pathological changes are centred on the proximal convoluted tubule (**Figure 8**). The earliest changes observed are tubule dilatation and loss of the tubule epithelial brush border. (This may result in the proximal convoluted tubules resembling the distal convoluted tubules, and the mistaken conclusion that the distal convoluted tubules are the site of the pathology). The interstitium is oedematous and the tubule basement membrane may be damaged. Further tubule degeneration results in individual cell apoptosis and hydropic degeneration, flattening of the lining epithelium of the tubules, and loss of individual tubule epithelial cells. Shed epithelial cells may be seen in the tubule lumina, accounting for the cellular casts seen in the urine sediment on urinalysis. Regenerative changes are also seen in the tubules, namely, nuclear enlargement with prominent nucleoli, and increased mitoses. Additional features that may be present are pigment casts from haemolysis or myolysis (**Figure 9**), and very occasional mononuclear cells in the interstitium. During the recovery phase, degenerative changes subside and regenerative features supervene.

- *Toxic cases*

These tend to produce more severe necrosis of proximal convoluted tubule cells, but the tubular basement membrane remains intact. Cellular and granular casts may be more prominent, and intratubular calcification may be present.

Figure 8. Acute tubular necrosis

There is marked interstitial oedema and the tubules show flattening of the epithelium. Some tubules contain granular casts (H&E)

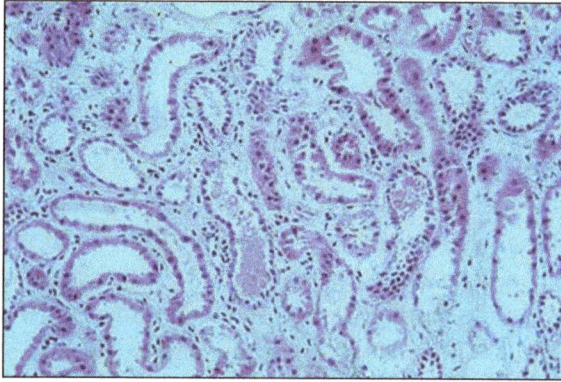

Figure 9. Acute tubular necrosis in rhabdomyolysis

Within dilated tubules there are granular pigmented casts containing myoglobin (H&E)

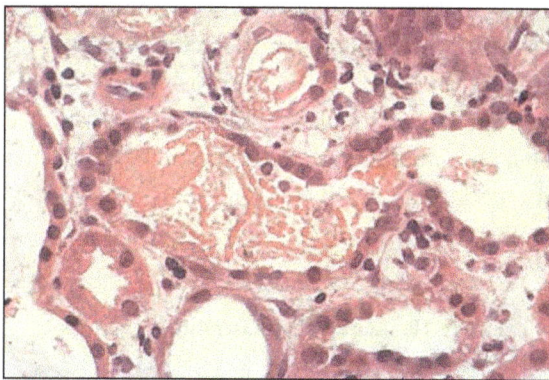

Electron microscopy

This is not routinely required to make the diagnosis. If performed it confirms the nonspecific changes of necrosis and regeneration. In ATN due to aminoglycosides, myeloid bodies may be seen intracellularly within the alyssums of proximal tubule epithelial cells.

Acute Tubulointerstitial Nephritis

Acute tubulointerstitial nephritis (TIN) is a syndrome of transient ARF, said to account for approximately 3% of ARF, though the real incidence is probably higher due to subclinical cases and patients who are not biopsied. Definitive diagnosis requires renal biopsy since the clinical presentation may mimic ATN or acute pyelonephritis.

Acute TIN results in tubule dysfunction following a primary interstitial process rather than direct tubule destruction *per se*. It is manifested by interstitial oedema and interstitial infiltration by *mononuclear* inflammatory cells, with sparing of the glomeruli and blood vessels. The specific allergic, infectious, metabolic and hereditary causes and idiopathic acute TIN are discussed further in **Chapter 18**.

- *Renal biopsy*

Renal biopsy is of use because the clinical picture in many cases is non-specific and may mimic that seen in ATN or pyelonephritis. The characteristic appearances are of interstitial oedema and a patchy infiltrate of *mononuclear cells* (**Figure 10**), which is more prominent at the corticomedullary junction, in the subcapsular zone, and around the glomeruli. These cells can also be seen invading the tubule epithelium across the basement membrane. The mononuclear cells are mainly $CD4^+$ T cells, but macrophages and some B cells are also present. Eosinophils are seen to varying degrees in drug related cases, and may also be detected on urinalysis in association with a sterile pyuria, haematuria and proteinuria. In general, it is not possible to predict the nature of the drug from the type of infiltrate (though see below). Suppurative inflammation, with a predominance of neutrophils and neutrophil casts, suggests an alternative diagnosis of acute pyelonephritis.

It is important to note that interstitial mononuclear inflammation may be seen on biopsy as a secondary component in other disorders whose main pathology is elsewhere in the nephron, particularly IgA nephropathy, SLE, microscopic polyangiitis, Wegener's granulomatosis, systemic sclerosis and cryoglobulinaemia.

Associated changes are seen in the tubular epithelium as a result of inflammation, namely patchy loss of epithelial cells, basement membrane disruption and regenerative changes. However, these changes are rarely as marked as in ATN.

Figure 10. Acute tubulointerstitial nephritis

There is a prominent infiltrate of mononuclear inflammatory cells in the interstitium and extending into tubular epithelium with tubular damage (H&E)

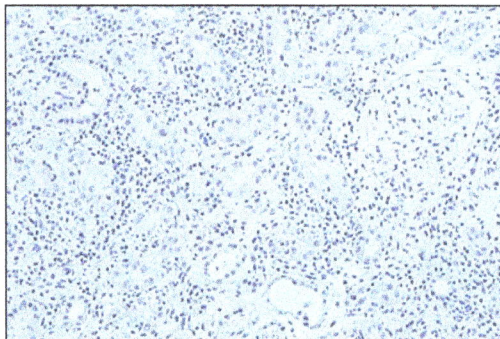

In certain cases other features may be seen on biopsy, which may give a clue to specific aetiologies:

- *Granulomas* may be seen in the interstitium and in tubular lumina in sarcoidosis, in infections (TB, fungi) as well as in some drug related cases (cephalosporins, rifampicin, lithium, cyclosporin). If infection is suspected, special stains for TB and fungi (Ziehl-Neelson and Grocott) should be requested.

- *With associated glomerulonephritis*: Acute TIN plus a minimal change glomerulonephritis may be seen with NSAIDs, ampicillin, rifampicin and lithium. Penicillamine and Sulindac have been reported to result in ATIN plus a membranous glomerulonephritis. Drugs, therefore, should be borne in mind in those cases of glomerulonephritis which present with associated tubulointerstitial changes.

Obstructive Nephropathy

Obstructive nephropathy is a relatively common cause of ARF in all age groups. Renal dysfunction occurs due to the associated hydronephrosis secondary to back pressure of accumulated fluid. For ARF to result, either lower urinary tract obstruction or bilateral upper urinary tract obstruction must be present. The specific causes at each of these sites are discussed further in **Chapter 23**.

Renal biopsy

This is not usually indicated but, if performed, will show dilatation of collecting ducts and distal convoluted tubules, with flattening of the proximal convoluted tubule brush border within 24 hours. Tubule atrophy will occur within 4 weeks if the obstruction does not resolve, followed by basement membrane thickening, interstitial scarring and glomerulosclerosis. Pyelonephritis may also be present due to superimposed infection. Prognostic features on biopsy include the degree of chronic changes; the presence of superimposed pyelonephritis; pre-existing renal disease; and the presence of renal papillary necrosis.

Acute Pyelonephritis

Acute pyelonephritis results from direct bacterial infection of the kidney, usually ascending infection from the lower urinary tract by organisms such as *E. Coli* or *S. faecalis*. Occasionally haematogenous infection is responsible due, for example, to *Klebsiella*, *Staphylococcus* or *Pseudomonas* species, especially in diabetic or immunocompromised hosts. The diagnosis is important to consider in patients who have co-existing obstructive lesions of the urinary tract, pregnancy or childhood.

Renal biopsy

Not usually indicated in straightforward cases. However if an open biopsy is performed, it will show wedge shaped areas of dense cellular infiltrate in the interstitium and tubules, with a predominance of neutrophils. There is extensive tubular destruction, with glomeruli and blood vessels being relatively spared. Neutrophils are present within tubular lumina. Microabscesses may be seen in the interstitium, and bacteria may be identified on Gram staining. Renal papillary necrosis may be a complicating feature.

Myeloma Cast Nephropathy

In multiple myeloma, light chains may form casts in renal tubules with an associated acute tubulointerstitial nephritis (see also **Chapter 22**). The casts are large, eosinophilic and may show a fractured or fragmented appearance (**Figure 11**). Multinucleated macrophage giant cells may be found adjacent to the casts. In some cases the casts may show a crystalline needle-shaped morphology. Amyloid may be present in the casts and can then be identified in a Congo red stain. The interstitium shows an infiltrate of lymphocytes and macrophages, and tubulitis may be present. Generally, the glomeruli are normal or show only non-specific ischaemic changes.

Figure 11. Myeloma cast nephropathy

There is marked tubular damage and many tubules are distended by large eosinophilic casts (H&E)

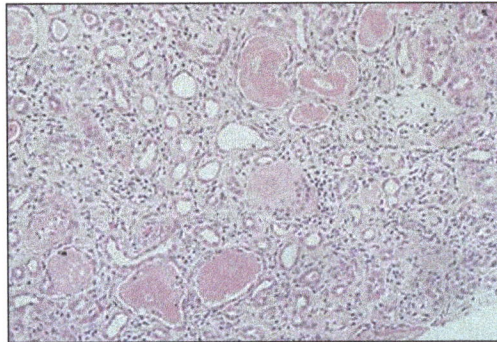

FURTHER READING

Jennette JC, Olson JL, Schwartz MM, Silva FG (eds.) (1998) *Heptinstall's Pathology of the Kidney* (5th Edition). Philadelphia: Lippincott-Raven

Madaio MP (1990) Renal biopsy. *Kidney International*; 38: 529–543

Parrish AE (1992) Complications of percutaneous renal biopsy: A review of 37 years experience. *Clinical Nephrology*; 38: 135–141

Ponticelli C, Mihatsch MJ, Imbasciati E (1998) Renal biopsy: Performance and interpretation. In: Davison AM, Cameron JS, Grünfeld J-P, Kerr DNS, Ritz E and Winnearls CG (eds.). *Oxford Textbook of Clinical Nephrology* (2nd Edition). Oxford: Oxford University Press

Regele H, Mougenot B, Brown P, Rastaldi MP, Leontsini M, Gesualdo L, Colucci T (2000) Report from Pathology Consensus Meeting on Renal Biopsy Handling and Processing, Vienna, February 25, 2000: http://www.kidney-euract.org/Rbpathology/consensus.htm

Chapter 8 _____

EMERGENCY CONSEQUENCES OF ACUTE RENAL FAILURE

8.1 Acute oliguria (pages 135–149)
8.2 Pulmonary oedema (pages 149–156)
8.3 Hyperkalaemia (pages 156–162)
8.4 Acid-base disturbances (pages 162–174)
8.5 Calcium, phosphate and magnesium disturbances (pages 174–183)
8.6 Acute uraemic (pages 183–194)

8.1 ACUTE OLIGURIA
Richard Fielding

Oliguria may be defined as a reduction in urine output to less than that required to maintain physiological homeostasis. In practice this equates to a urine output of less than 400 mL/day or approximately 0.5 mL/kg/h.

In clinical practice oliguria often results from:

1. Reduced Renal Perfusion

- Hypovolaemia (particularly post surgery).
- Reduced cardiac output (acute and chronic heart failure).

2. Intrinsic Renal Failure

- Following hypoperfusion.
- Sepsis.
- Nephrotoxins (NSAIDs, aminoglycosides, radiocontrast).
- Hepatorenal syndrome.
- Immune mediated nephritis.

3. Urinary Obstruction

For a full list of the aetiologies of ARF (and thus oliguria), see **Chapter 3**.

As a consequence of oliguria, serum urea, creatinine and potassium will rise, acidosis develops, and fluid overload ultimately ensues. Conversion of oliguria to a non-oliguric state is thus a key objective of therapy, with prevention the primary goal when possible. This section discusses the pathophysiology of oliguria and the clinical management of the oliguric patient, including the practical use of drugs such as furosemide and dopamine.

PATHOPHYSIOLOGY OF OLIGURIA

Oliguria occurs as part of the normal physiological response to hypoperfusion and has been discussed in earlier sections of this book. The mechanisms underlying ARF following ischaemic or nephrotoxic renal injury are complex and occur simultaneously. For simplicity, they can be divided into:

- Changes in GFR and intrarenal blood flow.
- Tubule cell injury, tubule obstruction and backfiltration.
- Tubule repair and recovery.

CHANGES IN GLOMERULAR FILTRATION RATE AND INTRARENAL BLOOD FLOW

Following ischaemic and nephrotoxic renal injury, the glomerular filtration rate (GFR) falls and blood flow *within* the kidney is reduced due to vasoconstriction and congestion of the intrarenal blood vessels. This leads to further reduction in GFR and exacerbates tubule damage. Furthermore, nephrons within the corticomedullary junction appear to be particularly susceptible to injury.

Under normal conditions, intrarenal blood flow and GFR are tightly autoregulated by a complex system of vasoactive mediators and autonomic nervous activity (see **Table 2**, **Chapter 1**). When mean blood pressure falls below 80 mmHg, autoregulation fails leading to vasoconstriction, with reduction in renal blood flow and GFR. Although the precise interaction of mediators remains complex and poorly understood, angiotensin II (AII), catecholamines and adenosine account for some of the intrarenal vasoconstriction. GFR is also affected by changes in the permeability of the glomerular basement membrane and obstruction within the renal tubules (**Table 1**). Glomerular permeability (K_f) depends on ionic charge of the basement membrane, number and size of slit pores and surface area. In turn, pore size is reduced by contraction of mesangial cells, stimulated by AII.

Table 1. Factors affecting GFR in acute renal injury

1. **GLOMERULAR PRESSURE (P_{GC})**
   Affected by mean arterial pressure, afferent and efferent arteriolar tone

2. **BOWMAN'S CAPSULE PRESSURE (P_{BS})**
   Affected by tubular obstruction

3. **GLOMERULAR PERMEABILITY (K_f)**
   Affected by tubuloglomerular feedback and tubular obstruction
   Affected in presence of glomerular diseases

4. **ONCOTIC PRESSURE**
   Difference between glomerular capillary (π_{GC}) and Bowman's space (π_{BS})
   Effectively unaltered in acute renal failure

$$GFR = K_f (P_{GC} - P_{BS}) - (\pi_{GC} - \pi_{BS})$$

Glomerular filtration is also affected by tubuloglomerular feedback (TGF). In an attempt to limit Na^+ and water loss, increased Na^+ delivery to the distal tubule is detected by the juxtaglomerular apparatus (JGA), which feeds back to the glomerulus to reduce GFR even further. Possible mediators for tubuloglomerular feedback include adenosine, AII and prostaglandins.

Prolonged Vasoconstriction

In experimental models of renal injury, prolonged vasoconstriction of arterioles and capillaries is seen long after the initial hypoxic or toxic stimulus has ended. This vasoconstriction prolongs renal injury and delays recovery. Possible mechanisms involve endothelins (ET) and nitric oxide (NO).

Endothelins exist in 3 isoforms (ET-1, ET-2, ET-3). ET-1 is a potent vasoconstrictor, acting predominantly on the intrarenal vasculature. Following renal ischaemia and endothelial dysfunction, endothelins are released and activate two receptors (ET_A and ET_B). Activation of ET_A on vascular smooth muscle, leads to vasoconstriction, which is partially counteracted by the vasodilator action of ET_B receptors (also present on vascular smooth muscle). During renal ischaemia, the production of ET-1 and resulting vasoconstriction may cause endothelial dysfunction, further ET-1 synthesis and prolonged vasoconstriction.

Inhibiting the synthesis and action of ET-1 has the potential to limit renal injury. Specific ET_A receptor antagonists used in experimental models of renal ischaemia have been shown to reduce vasoconstriction, tubular damage and improve renal function.

NO also plays a major role in acute renal injury. NO normally maintains vasodilatation and inhibits transcription of endothelin. In renal ischaemia, endothelial NO production is reduced, exacerbating vasoconstriction. In contrast, NO production increases within tubule cells, which may lead to peroxynitrite generation and tubule cell injury (see below).

Vascular Congestion

Vasoconstriction is also exacerbated by congestion within the intrarenal blood vessels. Although the mechanism is undetermined, activation of cell adhesion molecules such as ICAM-1, and release of leukotrienes and thromboxanes leads to aggregation of leucocytes, erythrocytes and platelets with resulting congestion and further vasoconstriction.

Hypoxia Within the Corticomedullary Junction

In the normal kidney, whilst the cortex remains well oxygenated with a PO_2 of 9 kPa, the outer medulla is relatively hypoxic at 3 kPa. This results from:

- Counter current mechanism in the vasa recta.
- Increased oxygen extraction and consumption by the thick ascending loop of Henle within the corticomedullary junction (80%) compared to cortical tubules (10%).

This renders the corticomedullary junction particularly susceptible to hypoperfusion and hypoxic injury. When the kidney is experimentally perfused with red cell depleted fluid, hypoxia occurs within 15 min with histological evidence of tubule damage to the S_3 section of the proximal tubule and medullary thick ascending loop of Henle (mTAL) which are both located at the corticomedullary junction.

The kidney attempts to conserve urinary concentrating ability whilst reducing overall oxygen demand. This is partially achieved by a preferential increase in blood flow to the nephrons at the corticomedullary junction, at the expense of blood flow to cortical nephrons. Although the overall GFR decreases, the GFR of single corticomedullary nephrons has been shown to increase. Despite these attempts at protection, the reduction in GFR, prolonged vasoconstriction and vascular congestion result in tubule injury and dysfunction.

TUBULE CELL INJURY

Following nephrotoxic or hypotensive/ischaemic renal damage, there is a spectrum of tubule cell injury ranging from "sublethal" (reversible) to "lethal" (irreversible):

"Sub-Lethal"/Reversible

- Cytoskeletal disruption.
- Loss of cell polarity with altered Na^+/K^+-ATPase sub-cellular distribution.
- Loss of cell–cell adhesion.
- Loss of cell-matrix adhesion.

"Lethal"/Irreversible

- Apoptosis.
- Necrosis.

Functional tubule cell alterations are greater than the morphological changes, resulting in severe tubule dysfunction with relatively mild disruption of tubule architecture when examined histologically. The following section describes some of the proposed mechanisms of "sublethal" injury.

Cytoskeletal Disruption and Altered Cellular Polarity

Establishment of renal tubule epithelial cell polarity is essential for maintenance of critical epithelial cell functions. Tubule epithelial cells have a highly organised cortical actin cytoskeleton which plays a major role in the regulation of many of these epithelial functions, including maintenance of polarity and cell shape, epithelial barrier function, solute transport, Cadherin-dependent cell–cell adhesion and integrin-dependent cell-matrix adhesion. Cortical actin microfilaments maintain epithelial polarity by anchoring Na^+/K^+-ATPase and other basolateral proteins to the cell membrane via actin-binding proteins such as ankyrin and spectrin. Actin-binding proteins of the ERM (ezrin-radixin-moesin) family tether apical membrane proteins of polarised epithelial cells to the cortical cytoskeleton. Disruption of the actin cytoskeleton therefore leads to loss of cell polarity, altered solute transport and dissolution of cell–cell and cell-matrix interactions.

Ischaemic renal injury causes actin microfilament disruption and loss of tubule cell polarity. Calcium influxes into the tubule cell, activating calcium dependent enzymes such as calpain and phospholipase A_2. Ischaemic injury and subsequent oxidant stress may also induce production of the inducible isoform of NO synthase (iNOS).

- **Calpain** cleaves actin-binding proteins, in particular modifying spectrin, thereby disrupting the basolateral actin network.
- **Phospholipase A_2** activation increases intracellular free fatty acids and lysophospholipids, which may contribute to changes in cell membrane integrity.
- **iNOS** increases in response to hypoxia. NO may disrupt the actin cytoskeleton, disrupt cell-matrix adhesion and increase tubule epithelial permeability.

Tubule Obstruction and Backfiltration

The tubule cell is normally anchored to the basement membrane by interaction of tubule epithelial cell basolateral β_1 integrins with matrix proteins (e.g. laminin, type IV collagen and thrombospondin). Loss of tubule cell polarity during ischaemia is associated with disassembly of cell-matrix interactions and apical redistribution of β_1 integrins. Consequently, the cell detaches from the basement membrane into the tubule lumen. Shed tubule cells aggregate into casts, which is possibly promoted by RGD (arginine-glycine-aspartic acid) domain-containing ligands, such as urinary fibronectin, that bridge integrins expressed on detached and *in situ* cells. Obstruction of the tubule by casts, with increasing tubule pressure and disruption of the tubule basement membrane is thought to cause back-leakage of glomerular filtrate into the interstitium and ultimately the venous system. This is **backfiltration**, which probably accounts for up to 40% of the observed reduction in GFR in oliguria.

TUBULE REPAIR AND RECOVERY

Following ischaemic and/or nephrotoxic injury, the kidney undergoes repair of both structure and function. The process requires recovery of cell functions, removal of tubule casts and replication of tubule cells to replace those that have lysed/detached. Within hours of tubule injury, regeneration of tubule epithelium starts under the influence of growth factors. Tubule cells appear to de-differentiate prior to re-entering the cell cycle. Mediators of regeneration are poorly understood but appear to be influenced by up-regulation and expression of series of growth factors in the tubule cells. Growth factors such as Epidermal Growth Factor (EGF), Hepatocyte Growth Factor (HGF), Transforming Growth Factor β (TGF β) and Insulin-like Growth Factor-1 (IGF-1) have been shown in experimental models to accelerate restoration of GFR and tubular histology. Possible actions of IGF-1 include:

- Increasing NO (therefore vasodilatation and renal blood flow).
- Reducing apoptosis.
- Increasing DNA synthesis and initiating transition from G0 to G1 of the cell cycle, thereby increasing proliferation and differentiation of tubule cells.

As the tubules undergo repair, glomerular filtration and renal haemodynamics are gradually restored. The medullary concentration gradient necessary for water reabsorption increases. During this restorative phase urine output increases and the patient often enters a polyuric phase, with the potential for excess urinary loss of electrolytes and water.

CLINICAL APPROACH TO THE OLIGURIC PATIENT

When faced with a patient in an oliguric state, assessment and management centres around the possible causes of oliguria. The causes of oliguria can be simplified to "pre-renal" (**Table 1**, **Chapter 3**), "post-renal" (**Table 2**, **Chapter 3**) and "intrinsic" (**Table 3**, **Chapter 3**) ARF.

This section concentrates on clinical assessment of circulating volume, optimising circulating volume and the practical use of drugs such as dopamine and furosemide to prevent and treat intrinsic renal failure. However, the importance of early identification and treatment of obstruction as a cause of oliguria should not be overlooked. A combination of clinical and ultrasound examination confirms whether the oliguria is a result of urinary obstruction. Early intervention to relieve the obstruction with nephrostomies or a bladder catheter corrects oliguria and reduces the chance of intrinsic renal failure (see **Chapter 23**).

ASSESSMENT OF EFFECTIVE CIRCULATING VOLUME

In patients with oliguria, the overall goal is to prevent and limit renal failure by ensuring "optimal" perfusion of the kidney. Renal perfusion is dependent on mean blood pressure and "effective circulating volume" of blood. Effective circulating volume (ECV) is central to renal perfusion. Unlike total body water, which can be divided into two compartments (intracellular water and extracellular water), ECV cannot be defined as a single compartment. Instead ECV is related to the pressure as well as volume within the vasculature, and is normally regulated by baroreceptors, sympathetic nerves, the renin-angiotensin system and atrial natriuretic peptide (ANP). A reduction in ECV leads to a fall in renal perfusion and oliguria, as Na^+ and water are reabsorbed.

Clinical Assessment of Effective Circulating Volume

The clinical assessment of ECV depends on signs such as blood pressure, heart rate, jugular venous pressure and peripheral temperature, as well as the clinical context.

Clinical signs consistent with reduced circulating volume include:

- Hypotension/postural hypotension.
- Tachycardia.
- Cool peripheries.
- Reduced jugular venous pressure.
- Oliguria.

Normally, ECV changes as extracellular fluid changes. This is typically seen in patients with haemorrhage following surgery or trauma, and evident by most of the clinical features above. Measurement of postural blood pressure is a sensitive method of detecting hypovolaemia, particularly in young patients who may have none of the associated signs of hypovolaemia. Heart failure also affects ECV and hence renal perfusion. In acute heart failure following myocardial infarction, the reduction in cardiac output and therefore ECV is detected by the baroreceptors, triggering Na^+ and water absorption and therefore oliguria. Improving the cardiac output (e.g. with inotropes) improves renal perfusion and urine output. In sepsis, vasodilatation leads to a reduction in ECV, although total volume of extracellular fluid remains the same. Warm peripheries, hypotension with tachycardia and hyperdynamic pulse/circulation suggests sepsis (see **Chapter 19**).

Circulating volume and renal perfusion should be easy to assess and measure. Despite clinical signs and invasive monitoring, however, assessment of ECV is often difficult. Not uncommonly, oliguria results from a combination of different aetiologies, e.g. the elderly patient with chronic heart failure, sepsis, dehydration and oliguria.

Invasive Monitoring (see also **Chapter 5**)

Where hypovolaemia is clinically apparent, the priority is to resuscitate the patient with fluid rather than delay treatment whilst establishing invasive monitoring.

When the clinical assessment of circulating volume is unclear, invasive monitoring may be helpful to:

- Assess circulating volume.
- Guide fluid replacement.
- Provide central venous access for drugs if required.

Methods of invasive monitoring include:

- Central venous pressure measurement (CVP).
- Pulmonary artery and pulmonary artery occlusion pressure (PAP and PAOP, respectively).
- Oesophageal Doppler monitoring (in mechanically ventilated patients).

CVP measurement is performed most commonly. CVP measurement may be low, normal or elevated in hypovolaemia:

- CVP <8 cm H_2O — Reduced intravascular volume.
- CVP 8–12 cm H_2O — Normal or reduced intravascular volume.
- CVP >12 cm H_2O — Increased intravascular volume (also elevated in cardiac failure, tamponade, pulmonary hypertension and tricuspid regurgitation, hypovolaemia with excess sympathetic tone).

A series of CVP measurements provides more information than one in isolation, particularly in response to intravenous fluid, provided they are consistent with other clinical measures of ECV.

Monitoring of PAP and PAOP gives more information on left-sided cardiac filling pressures. Again, PAOP may not always be reliable, and does not directly measure ECV or give information on renal perfusion. In practice, the use of PA catheters is limited to coronary and intensive care units (see **Chapters 5** and **28**).

Clinical Approach to Fluid Replacement in Acute Oliguria

Each patient should be fully assessed before, during and after fluid replacement (see also **Practice Point 1**).

(a) *Definite hypovolaemia with oliguria*

In situations where hypovolaemia and oliguria are clinically apparent (haemorrhage, burns, ketoacidosis, pancreatitis), the priority is quickly to restore circulating volume aiming to preserve renal perfusion. In practice, blood or colloid is rapidly infused to maintain a systolic blood pressure above 100 mmHg (or mean arterial pressure >70 mmHg), with the rate of infusion directed by the clinical response. A continuous infusion of up to 2–3 L/h may be initially required.

(b) *Possible hypovolaemia with oliguria*

Oliguria often occurs with few or no clinical signs of hypovolaemia. A fluid challenge is useful to help assess the circulating volume. Following a clinical assessment of ECV (pulse, postural blood pressure, JVP, peripheral temperature) 200 mL of colloid is given over 10 minutes. A rapid improvement in, for example, BP, tachycardia, or oliguria, would confirm hypovolaemia and prompt a further fluid challenge. If minimal or no change occurs, then the circulating volume may be optimal. In this situation, CVP measurements may also be useful.

- CVP <5 cm H_2O with clinical features of hypovolaemia should be corrected with colloid until the CVP measures 8–12 cm H_2O.
- CVP 5–12 cm H_2O with clinical features of hypovolaemia, again should receive a fluid challenge. Often, as fluid is replaced, sympathetic vascular tone falls. This may be seen by the trend of CVP measurements over time and in response to fluid boluses. Following a fluid challenge the CVP rises, only to fall with time as vascular tone falls. With this pattern, the aim is to continue fluid boluses until the CVP is maintained between 8–12 cm H_2O. **Note:** a **sustained** rise in CVP of ≥~4 cm H_2O following a fluid challenge suggests adequate ECV.
- CVP >12 cm H_2O or clinical signs of volume excess or cardiac failure (raised JVP, 3rd heart sound, pulmonary oedema). Intravenous fluid should be immediately stopped.

(c) *Possible cardiac failure and oliguria*

Fluid replacement should be stopped if there is clinical evidence of volume overload or cardiac failure. In the situation of cardiac failure with oliguria, treatment of the underlying cause of cardiac failure is the priority. The use of inotropes to maintain cardiac output and renal perfusion should be considered.

Following fluid resuscitation and restoration of circulating volume, oliguria may be reversed and urine output increased. Re-evaluation of the patient, CVP and fluid balance will guide further fluid replacement. The aim is to maintain the circulating volume and prevent further oliguria. This is particularly so during the recovery phase of ATN and after relief of urinary obstruction, when polyuria is common. Alternatively, oliguria persists despite restoration of the ECV and cardiac output. In this scenario, drugs such as furosemide or dopamine may be considered.

Practice Point 1. Management of oliguria

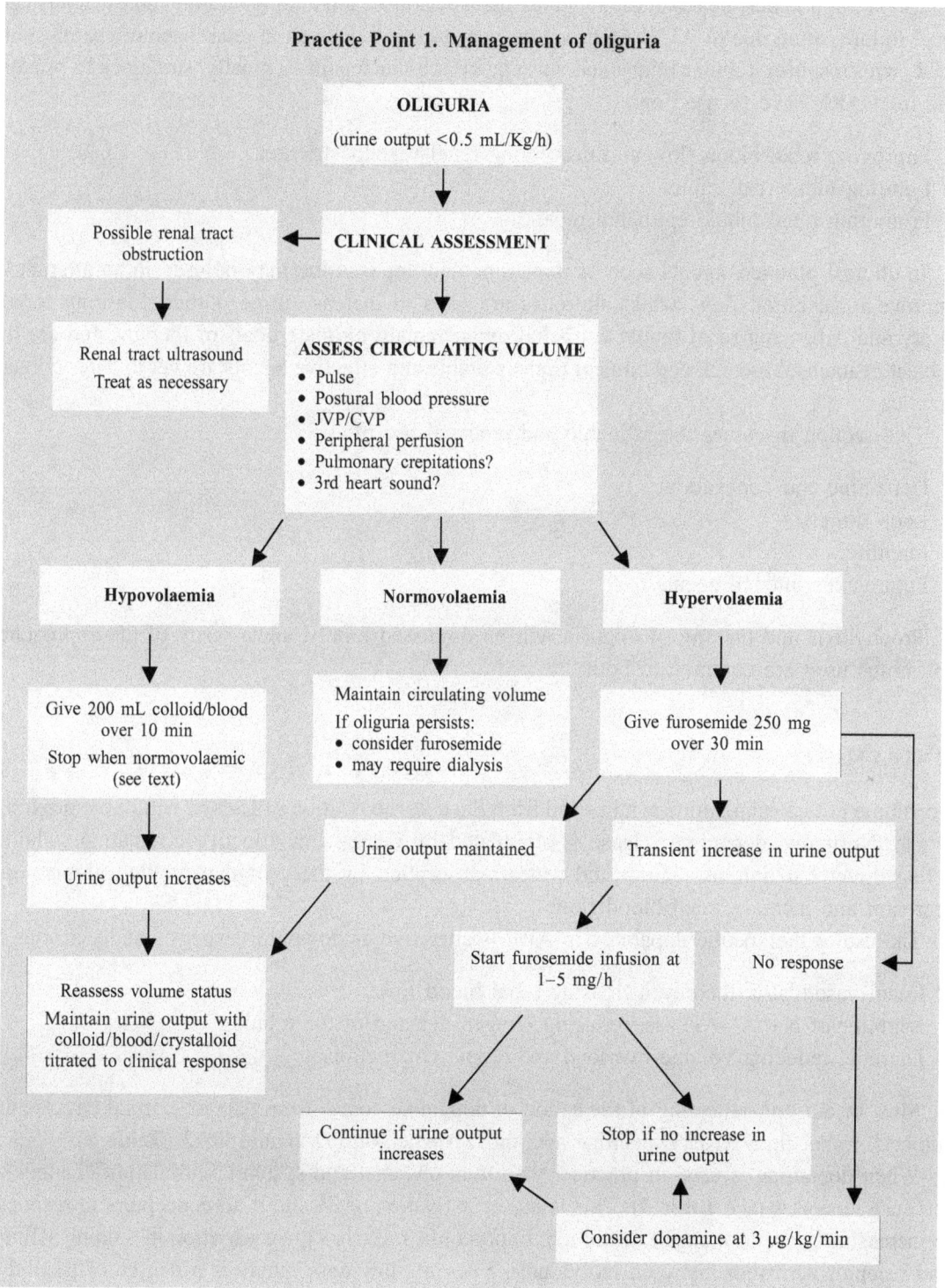

OLIGURIA

(urine output <0.5 mL/Kg/h)

CLINICAL ASSESSMENT

Possible renal tract
obstruction

Renal tract ultrasound

Treat as necessary

ASSESS CIRCULATING VOLUME

- Pulse
- Postural blood pressure
- JVP/CVP
- Peripheral perfusion
- Pulmonary crepitations?
- 3rd heart sound?

Hypovolaemia

Normovolaemia

Hypervolaemia

Give 200 mL colloid/blood
over 10 min

Stop when normovolaemic
(see text)

Maintain circulating volume

If oliguria persists:
- consider furosemide
- may require dialysis

Give furosemide 250 mg
over 30 min

Urine output increases

Urine output maintained

Transient increase in urine output

Reassess volume status

Maintain urine output with
colloid/blood/crystalloid
titrated to clinical response

Start furosemide infusion at
1–5 mg/h

No response

Continue if urine output
increases

Stop if no increase in
urine output

Consider dopamine at 3 μg/kg/min

PHARMACOTHERAPY OF ACUTE OLIGURIA

Persistent oliguria despite restoration and maintenance of the circulating volume indicates intrinsic renal failure, often due to ATN. ARF occurs as a result of changes in renal haemodynamics and GFR, with resulting tubular injury and subsequent tubular repair. Logically, strategies to prevent and treat ARF have focused on:

- Improving renal blood flow and preventing renal vasoconstriction.
- Limiting tubule cell injury.
- Promoting renal tubule epithelial repair.

In clinical practice, agents such as dopamine and dopexamine may be used in an attempt to improve renal blood flow, whilst diuretics are used to increase urine output. Limiting tubule injury and enhancing renal tubule epithelial repair remain ultimate goals of therapy, and are the subject of intense research and clinical trials; suitable and effective agents are yet to enter clinical practice.

This section discusses the rationale and practical use of:

- Dopamine and dopexamine.
- Loop diuretics.
- Mannitol.
- Future/experimental agents.

Prophylaxis and therapy of oliguria will be discussed jointly, since many of the approaches and drugs used are common to both.

DOPAMINE

Dopamine is a catecholamine synthesised from the decarboxylation of L-dopa within the proximal tubule. Normally, dopamine release is stimulated by increase in effective circulating volume, acting directly to inhibit sodium and water reabsorption by the proximal tubule, inhibit renin secretion and increase renal blood flow.

The use of therapeutic dopamine in ARF is attractive as dopamine experimentally acts as a:

- Renal vasodilator, thereby increasing renal blood flow.
- Inhibitor of Na^+/K^+-ATPase, reducing oxygen demand of the tubules.
- Diuretic, reducing volume overload and tubule obstruction.

Most of our understanding of the action of dopamine comes from data on normal euvolaemic subjects, rather than ARF. Dopamine acts on two receptors, DA1 and DA2 (**Table 2**).

When dopamine is used in practice, the effect on renal and systemic circulation changes as the dose increases (see **Table 3**). This is due to activation of $\beta1$ and α adrenoceptors in response to increasing concentrations of dopamine. Importantly, there is a great variation in binding affinity and receptor activation between individuals. Even at "low dose" there is a degree of $\beta1$ and α adrenoceptor activation, resulting in unpredictable response of the vascular smooth muscle to any given dose of dopamine. In the context of acute oliguria, the precise effects of dopamine are unclear as other mediators also affect the renal and intrarenal vasculature.

Table 2. Dopamine receptors and action		
Receptor	**Location**	**Action**
DA1	Renal vascular smooth muscle	Vasodilatation
	Proximal tubule, mTAL, collecting tubule	Reduced tubule Na$^+$ absorption
DA2	Presynaptic terminal of post ganglionic sympathetic neurons	Inhibits norepinephrine synthesis
		Vasodilatation

Table 3. Dopamine dose and effect		
Dose of dopamine	**Receptor**	**Clinical effect**
"Low dose" (0.5–3 µg/kg/min)	DA1 activation Small DA2 activation	Renal vasodilatation
"Medium dose" (3–10 µg/kg/min)	DA1 + β1 action	Increased cardiac output
"High dose" (10–20 µg/kg/min)	α1 action	Systemic and renal vasoconstriction

Evidence for the Use of Dopamine

Prevention of acute renal failure

The use of dopamine to prevent ARF has been studied in high risk groups such as patients receiving radiocontrast, or undergoing cardiac or vascular surgery. Unfortunately most studies are uncontrolled, and use small numbers of patients with variability in dopamine dose and methods to assess renal function. These factors have precluded a meta-analysis in this important area.

Only a few randomised controlled trials have been conducted. In a study of 52 patients undergoing coronary bypass surgery, low dose dopamine started at induction and continuing for 24 h post-operatively was compared to placebo. No difference in urine output or creatinine clearance was detected, although an increase in cardiac output with reduction in systemic vascular resistance was recorded in the study group. A similar study in aortic aneurysm repair showed no difference in serum creatinine or creatinine clearance at day 1 or 5 post-operatively. In 48 patients undergoing liver transplantation, there was no change in serum creatinine or GFR immediately post-operatively or at one month in those receiving perioperative dopamine. In patients with pre-existing renal impairment who received radiocontrast, low dose dopamine was not shown to improve serum creatinine when compared to placebo. Importantly renal function was shown to *deteriorate* in diabetic patients in the dopamine group.

In summary, no study at present supports the use of dopamine to *prevent* **ARF.** Possible reasons for these disappointing results may be the small numbers of patients and the low incidence of ARF in the control groups, resulting in studies under-powered to detect any benefit of dopamine. Alternatively, of course, dopamine may simply be ineffective as a prophylactic agent.

An excellent review of the dopamine studies can be found listed in the **Further Reading** section (Denton *et al.*, 1996).

Use of dopamine in established acute renal failure

Similar problems arise in studies of dopamine in established ARF. So far only small, uncontrolled studies have been conducted. Difficulties arise in comparing outcomes of these trials due to differing definitions of ARF (often made on the presence of oliguria rather than accurate measurement of GFR).

One randomised controlled trial compared the use of dopamine and furosemide in 23 patients with falciparum malaria and ARF. In patients with a creatinine between 170–350 µmol/L, the use of dopamine at 1 µg/kg/min with furosemide 200 mg every 6 h resulted in stability of serum creatinine when compared to furosemide alone or placebo.

Although there is no current evidence to support the use of dopamine in established ARF, in practice the inotropic and diuretic effects of dopamine may increase urine output, facilitating management of fluid balance and avoiding pulmonary oedema. Potential adverse effects should also be taken into account before using dopamine; these include:

- Increased cardiac output and oxygen consumption.
- Cardiac arrhythmias.
- Excessive diuresis with hypovolaemia.
- Possible increase in gut ischaemia.
- The requirement for central venous administration.

DOPEXAMINE

Dopexamine is similar to dopamine in having dopaminergic and β1 adrenergic actions. Unlike dopamine, dopexamine has no α adrenergic action. Clinical use of dopexamine results in:

- Vasodilatation, with resulting increase in cardiac output.
- Natriuresis and diuresis.
- A small increase in renal blood flow.
- Adverse effects of tachycardia, nausea and vomiting.

Limited studies in cardiac, aortic and liver transplant surgery have examined the effect of dopexamine on creatinine clearance and urine output. Dopexamine has been shown to have reno-protective properties, probably due to an increase in cardiac output rather than changes in intrarenal blood flow. Although dopexamine has not yet been shown to be superior to dopamine in improving renal function, the effective lack of α adrenergic action with dopexamine leads to a more predictable haemodynamic response and less adverse cardiovascular events than dopamine. Although dopexamine has theoretical advantages over dopamine, further studies are required to confirm any reno-protective effect of dopexamine.

LOOP DIURETICS

The use of loop diuretics in preventing and treating ARF is theoretically attractive. By inhibiting Na^+/K^+-ATPase channels, loop diuretics may:

- Reduce tubule epithelial cell oxygen demand.
- Induce a diuresis, reducing tubule lumen obstruction by casts.

In models of tubule injury, furosemide has been shown to reduce the oxygen consumption of the mTAL, increasing overall PO_2 within the kidney and reducing tubule damage. Clinical studies of furosemide are less encouraging. In patients undergoing aortic aneurysm repair, no difference in renal function has been seen. In patients with chronic renal failure receiving radiocontrast, a deterioration in renal function occurred when furosemide and hydration were used, compared to hydration alone.

In clinical practice, furosemide is often used to promote a diuresis and convert an oliguric state to a non-oliguric state. The importance of ensuring the patient has an effective circulating volume before, during and after furosemide use cannot be overemphasised. Reduction in circulating volume following furosemide is not uncommon and may have led to the reported deterioration in renal function in some clinical trials.

Uncertainty usually arises over the dose of furosemide and whether to administer as a bolus or continuous infusion. The following is a guide:

- Ensure optimal circulating volume (discussed previously).
- If still oliguric, bolus furosemide 250 mg iv over 30 minutes.
- If urine output transiently increases, either repeat bolus 250 mg or start a continuous infusion of furosemide at 1–5 mg/h to maintain a diuresis.
- If still oliguric following initial bolus, then there is no advantage in giving further furosemide.
- Assess patient for signs of volume depletion during and after furosemide, and maintain circulating volume with fluid as urine output increases.

MANNITOL

Since early laboratory studies in the 1940s, mannitol has been used in clinical practice to prevent ARF. Mannitol is an osmotic diuretic with a low molecular weight, which is freely filtered and poorly reabsorbed by the tubule. Actions of mannitol include:

- Increasing tubule fluid osmolality.
- Reducing tubule water absorption.
- Inducing net Na^+ loss.

Experimentally, mannitol has been shown to:

- Increase GFR.
- Increase renal blood flow by PGI_2 mediated afferent arteriole dilatation.

- Reduce tubule cell swelling.
- Act as a free radical scavenger.

Most studies and clinical use of mannitol have been in prevention of radiocontrast-induced ARF and in cardiothoracic surgery. Although an increase in urine output has been reported, neither prevention of ARF, nor reduction in dialysis or mortality have been demonstrated. The use of mannitol has been advocated in rhabdomyolysis, often combined in a cocktail of crystalloid and sodium bicarbonate infusions (see **Chapter 12**). Anecdotal evidence exists for its use, but again no difference in renal outcome has been demonstrated, when compared to volume replacement alone.

Several adverse features of mannitol are recognised:

- Acute expansion of the extracellular volume with precipitation of pulmonary oedema.
- Mannitol induced acute renal failure (especially when mannitol dose exceeds 200 g/day).
- Hypokalaemia, hypocalcaemia, hypomagnesaemia and hypophosphataemia.

On balance, mannitol is little used in practice due to the lack of clinical evidence and unpredictable clinical effects on circulating volume.

EXPERIMENTAL AGENTS IN THE PREVENTION AND TREATMENT OF ACUTE RENAL FAILURE

Many molecules have been studied *in vitro* and in animal models in an attempt to improve renal perfusion and enhance renal tubule repair. Clinical trials of the following agents have been conducted:

Calcium Antagonists

Interest in calcium antagonists arose when renal function was reported to improve in patients with renal transplants (possibly due to a drug effect on T-cell function). When non-transplant patients receiving radio-contrast were studied retrospectively, those patients taking calcium antagonists at the time of receiving radio-contrast had no difference in serum creatinine compared to controls.

Atrial Natriuretic Peptide (ANP)

ANP is a peptide hormone mainly produced in the cardiac atria, but also in the kidney. It binds to specific receptors on vascular smooth muscle cells and renal tubule epithelial cells and has several observable effects (see **Table 4**). A multi-centre trial of an ANP analogue (anaritide) in ATN concluded that it may be of benefit in improving dialysis-free survival in oliguric patients, but was not of benefit in those without oliguria and may be of harm through hypotensive episodes (Allgren *et al.*, 1997).

Endothelin Receptor Antagonists (ERA)

In ARF, endothelin is thought to be responsible for long lasting constriction of afferent arterioles, leading to a disproportionate decrease in GFR compared to RBF. In various experimental models of ARF, ERAs were found to be of benefit in improving renal function when used prophylactically.

Table 4. Actions of atrial natriuretic peptide			
Cardiovascular	Vasodilatation ↑ venous capacitance ↑ vascular permeability	**Adrenal**	↓ aldosterone production
Renal	↑ GFR Natriuresis Diuresis ↓ renin	**CNS**	↓ sympathetic outflow ↓ neuroendocrine function ↓ corticotrophin production ↓ salt and water intake

This has not been shown so far in humans and may be detrimental due to hypotension. There is also uncertainty over their therapeutic, as opposed to prophylactic, efficacy.

Adenosine A1 Receptor Antagonists

The phenomenon of tubuloglomerular feedback (see **Chapter 1**) also acts to reduce urine flow, and there is increasing evidence (including phase II clinical trials) for the beneficial effects of A_1 receptor antagonists to increase urine output in patients with oliguria and cardiac failure.

Other Agents

Growth factors (epidermal, hepatocyte, insulin-like), anti-ICAM antibodies and disintegrins have also been examined in animal systems, but there is as yet no place for their use in humans outside clinical trials.

8.2 PULMONARY OEDEMA

Richard Thompson and Michael Robson

DEFINITION

Pulmonary oedema is defined as an excess of extravascular lung water, which typically occupies the interstitial and alveolar lung compartments. It is a potentially life-threatening complication of ARF, which requires urgent treatment.

PATHOPHYSIOLOGY AND AETIOLOGY

In the healthy lung, there is a continuous exchange of water between the intravascular and extravascular compartments. Pulmonary oedema develops when this equilibrium is sufficiently disturbed, and the forces favouring the movement of water out of the vascular compartment

Table 5. Common causes of pulmonary oedema	
Hydrostatic oedema	**Permeability oedema — ARDS**
Increased pulmonary capillary pressure • fluid overload • left ventricular failure • mitral stenosis Decreased plasma oncotic pressure • hypoalbuminaemia	Infection Toxins Trauma Aspiration Disseminated intravascular coagulation

(capillary hydrostatic pressure, alveolar capillary permeability) exceed those favouring its return (plasma oncotic pressure, lymphatic drainage). There are numerous causes of pulmonary oedema which can be conveniently sub-divided into those resulting from predominantly hydrostatic mechanisms, in which intravascular volume reduction may be of therapeutic benefit, and causes due to increased alveolar capillary membrane permeability (**Table 5**).

In the initial stages of pulmonary oedema, fluid accumulates within the interstitial space causing the lung parenchyma to stiffen, so reducing lung compliance and increasing the work of breathing. At this stage, alveolar gas transfer is largely unaffected, and there may be few clinical signs. As the accumulation of fluid continues, the capacity of the interstitial space is exceeded and flooding of the alveoli occurs, resulting in reduced alveolar diffusing capacity. This results in hypoxia due to type I respiratory failure. Ultimately, fluid may accumulate within the pleural space, and exacerbate hypoxia through ventilation/perfusion mismatch.

As a complication of ARF, pulmonary oedema typically occurs late in the course of disease, since significant salt and water retention does not occur until the GFR decreases to below 10–20 mL/min. Furthermore, many cases of ARF result from hypovolaemia, sepsis or circulatory failure, when patients will be volume depleted rather than fluid overloaded. However, fluid overload may occur as a result of injudicious intravenous fluid therapy in the face of declining renal function. Adequate hydration is clearly essential to try and prevent incipient ARF becoming established, but fluid input must be decided upon with careful attention to urine output and clinical assessment of volume status.

CLINICAL PRESENTATION

A patient presenting with a raised serum creatinine and pulmonary oedema raises several diagnostic possibilities as shown in **Table 6**.

The clinical features of pulmonary oedema due to fluid overload in ARF are similar to those in pulmonary oedema due to other causes. Symptoms include shortness of breath, orthopnoea and blood stained sputum (rarely haemoptysis). Where clinical features may help to distinguish between causes is discussed below in **Figure 1**.

Table 6. Differential diagnosis of a raised serum creatinine and pulmonary oedema

ARF complicated by pulmonary oedema

Acute left ventricular failure complicated by ARF due to hypoperfusion (cardiogenic shock)

ARF on a background of pre-existing left ventricular failure

Chronic renal impairment and left ventricular failure (acute or chronic)

Sepsis complicated by acute tubular necrosis and ARDS

CLINICAL INVESTIGATIONS

Chest X-Ray

Although important in confirming the diagnosis, treatment must not be delayed while waiting for the chest X-ray. In contrast to the non-specific clinical features described above, the radiological features of pulmonary oedema are both more sensitive and specific, and may precede clinical signs. Typically, these radiological changes evolve through two main stages:

1. *Interstitial oedema*

Initially fluid accumulates in the perivascular interstitial tissue and the interlobular septae, resulting in loss of definition of normal vascular markings and the development of septal lines. These septal lines are more clearly seen at the lung bases, adjacent and perpendicular to the pleural surface in the lower zones (Kerley B lines). Additionally, bronchial walls become thickened resulting in peribronchial cuffing, best appreciated when perihilar bronchi are seen end-on. These changes are usually accompanied by redistribution of blood flow to the upper zones. Upper lobe blood diversion is present when the upper lobe vessels are equal to, or greater than, the size of the lower lobe vessels when measured at an equal distance from the hilum.

2. *Alveolar oedema*

As extravascular lung water increases, the alveoli fill with fluid, producing irregular areas of patchy and/or confluent consolidation. These tend to be symmetrical and may be associated with air bronchograms. In some cases, this may have a distinctive perihilar distribution ("bat's wing" pattern).

Pleural effusions may occur if excess fluid reaches the pleural space. Cardiac enlargement suggests chronic heart failure as a cause of the pulmonary oedema. It has been suggested that upper lobe diversion, septal lines and pleural effusions are more characteristic of cardiac failure than fluid overload, with the latter usually showing predominantly features of alveolar oedema. This distinction however is not absolute. In ARDS, no interstitial changes are seen and the alveolar shadowing may have a more peripheral pattern.

Arterial Blood Gases and Pulse Oximetry

Hypoxia is the cause of death in pulmonary oedema and it is vital to maintain adequate oxygenation, as discussed below. Interpretation of arterial blood gases and pulse oximetry is covered in detail in **Chapter 5**.

ECG and Cardiac Enzymes

Features of cardiac ischaemia, recent myocardial infarction or arrhythmia suggest a cardiac aetiology.

Invasive Monitoring

Central venous pressure (*CVP*, see also **Chapters 5** and **8.1**)

CVP provides a guide to circulating volume, but its usefulness should not be overstated. Although CVP measurement can provide an important guide to the rehydration of the volume-depleted patient with ARF, thus reducing the risk of iatrogenic pulmonary oedema, little additional information can be gained from CVP measurement in patients with established pulmonary oedema and a visibly elevated JVP. In common with JVP estimation, fluid overload and/or cardiac failure will elevate the CVP, whereas low CVP measurements are expected in pure LVF, hypoalbuminaemia and ARDS.

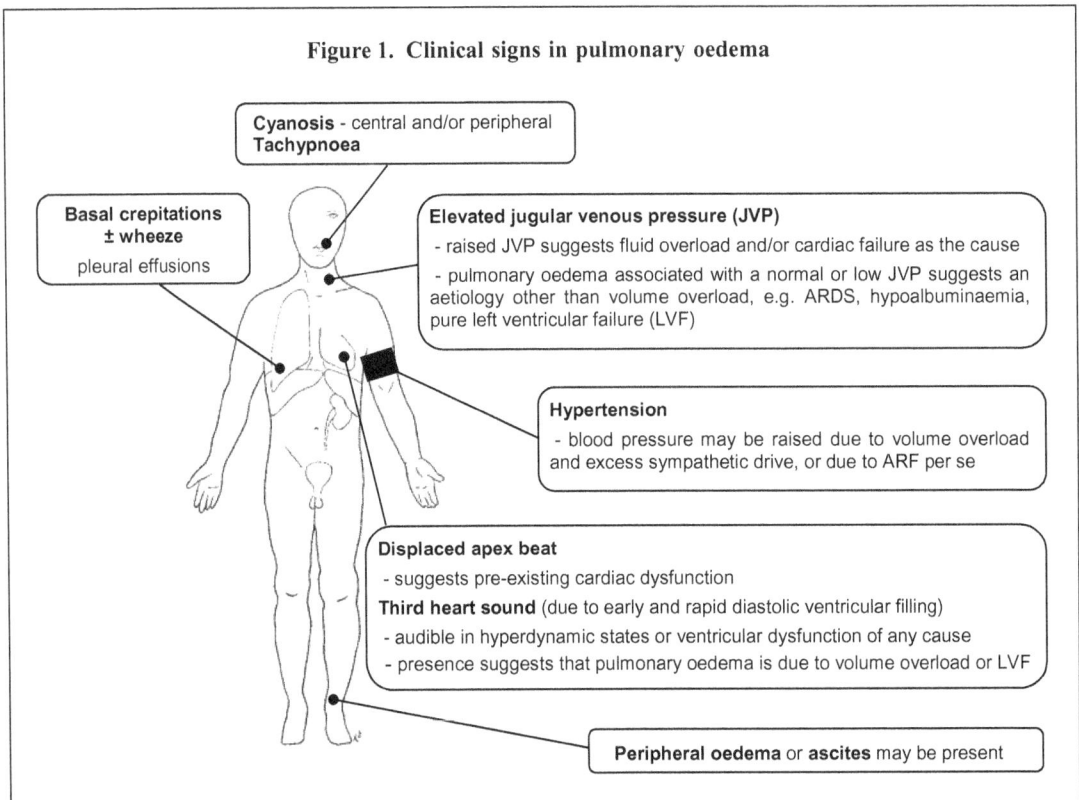

Figure 1. Clinical signs in pulmonary oedema

Cyanosis - central and/or peripheral
Tachypnoea

Basal crepitations ± wheeze
pleural effusions

Elevated jugular venous pressure (JVP)
- raised JVP suggests fluid overload and/or cardiac failure as the cause
- pulmonary oedema associated with a normal or low JVP suggests an aetiology other than volume overload, e.g. ARDS, hypoalbuminaemia, pure left ventricular failure (LVF)

Hypertension
- blood pressure may be raised due to volume overload and excess sympathetic drive, or due to ARF per se

Displaced apex beat
- suggests pre-existing cardiac dysfunction
Third heart sound (due to early and rapid diastolic ventricular filling)
- audible in hyperdynamic states or ventricular dysfunction of any cause
- presence suggests that pulmonary oedema is due to volume overload or LVF

Peripheral oedema or **ascites** may be present

Pulmonary artery catheterisation

Pulmonary artery occlusion pressure (PAOP) may be needed to differentiate between pulmonary oedema of hydrostatic origin (e.g. left ventricular failure), from that of increased pulmonary capillary permeability (ARDS) (see **Chapter 5** for details of insertion technique). ARDS is suggested by a PAOP of <15–18 mmHg. It should be noted that neither CVP nor PAOP are raised in pulmonary oedema due to hypoalbuminaemia.

TREATMENT PRINCIPLES

The immediate management of pulmonary oedema is the same irrespective of the underlying cause (see **Practice Point 2**). Since death occurs in pulmonary oedema due to hypoxia, the immediate priority is to maintain adequate oxygenation. This allows time for more specific therapies to be effective. In cases of hydrostatic pulmonary oedema, extravascular lung water can be reduced relatively rapidly by reducing venous return, either by increasing the venous capacitance (sitting the patient up or using vasodilators), or by reducing circulating volume (diuretics, venesection, haemofiltration). In cases due to increased permeability, therapy is directed at removing the insult where practical and supporting the patient until the lung recovers.

Oxygen Therapy

Since hypoxia in pulmonary oedema is predominantly the result of type I respiratory failure, raising the inspired oxygen concentration (FiO_2), and so increasing the diffusion gradient for oxygen, is usually effective. Pulse oximetry and monitoring of arterial blood gases are essential. The PaO_2 should be maintained above 8 kPa.

A number of different devices for oxygen delivery are available for use at the bedside:

- *Low-flow, variable performance oxygen mask*

Low flow oxygen masks are the simplest oxygen delivery devices (e.g. MC mask), in which an alteration of oxygen flow rate is used to vary the FiO_2. Their main disadvantage is that the actual FiO_2 is unpredictable and highly variable (24–80%). Since inspiratory flow often exceeds the rate of O_2 delivery by the mask, room air is simultaneously inspired, resulting in a reduction in FiO_2. The degree of dilution is variable, but increases with increasing ventilatory rate.

- *Nasal cannulae*

Nasal cannulae are often better tolerated, but suffer similar disadvantages to low-flow masks.

- *High-flow, fixed performance oxygen mask*

High flow oxygen masks (Venturi-type) deliver O_2 at a set concentration (24–60%). The total gas flow is sufficient to satisfy peak inspiratory flow, so no additional dilution occurs.

- *Oxygen mask with reservoir bag*

Masks with reservoir bags can be used for patients in extremis, which may allow FiO_2 >80% to be delivered. However, in such circumstances, additional respiratory support is likely to be required, e.g. CPAP or mechanical ventilation.

Practice Point 2. Treatment of pulmonary oedema in acute renal failure

Diagnosis of acute renal failure and pulmonary oedema

↓

Sit upright
Administer O_2
ABG, oximetry and CXR

↓

Origin of pulmonary oedema?

Hydrostatic   **Permeability**

Reduce circulating volume   Maintain oxygenation   Treat specific cause where practical and await improvement

↓   ↓   ↓

iv opiates
iv diuretics   Adjust FiO_2
iv vasodilators   to keep
                                   PaO_2 >8 kPa
                                   SaO_2 >92%

↓   ↓   ↓

No diuresis   Persistent hypoxia or
                                   respiratory fatigue

↓   ↓   ↓

Increase dose of   Trial
diuretic   of CPAP

↓   ↓   ↓

No diuresis   Persistent hypoxia or
                                   respiratory fatigue

↓   ↓   ↓

Urgent haemodialysis   Mechanical
or haemofiltration   ventilation

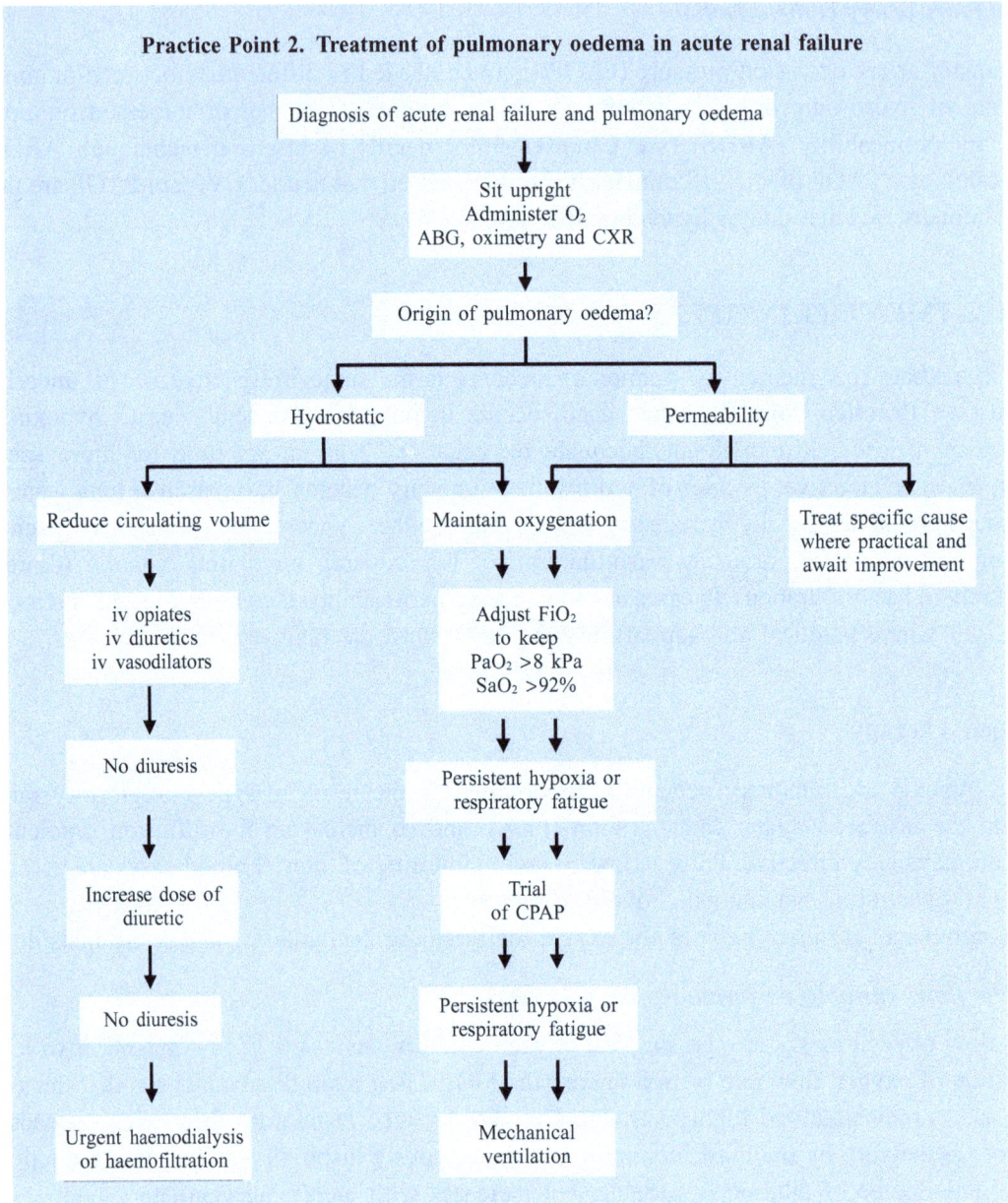

- *Continuous positive airway pressure (CPAP)*

CPAP utilises a high flow oxygen/air mixture which is delivered via wide bore tubing to a tight fitting facemask. An exhaust valve is employed to maintain a constant positive pressure at the mouth (typically 5–10 cm H_2O). This system allows the FiO_2 to be varied continuously, but accurately, while the positive pressure reduces the work of breathing. CPAP increases in intra-thoracic pressure, resulting in a decrease in venous return to the heart. Non-invasive positive pressure ventilation has been evaluated in severe pulmonary oedema and type I respiratory failure, but to date no clear additional benefit over CPAP has been demonstrated. CPAP may be started in casualty or on the ward. Preferably, however, a patient on CPAP should be monitored on a high dependency unit or ITU.

- *Mechanical ventilation*

Mechanical ventilation (i.e. referral to ITU for intubation and ventilation) will be necessary if:

— CPAP is not available.
— CPAP is not tolerated.
— Despite CPAP, the PaO_2 is not maintained above 8 kPa.
— Despite CPAP, hypercapnia or tiredness develops.

Opiates

Opiates may be useful for both anxiolytic and venodilator action. **Diamorphine hydrochloride may be given intravenously at a dose of 2.5 to 5 mg at a rate of 1–2 mg/min.** Extreme caution should be observed before administering opiates to patients in severe respiratory distress (e.g. worsening hypercapnia, falling respiratory rate).

Diuretics

Loop diuretics have dual benefit with an immediate vasodilator effect, and a slower onset diuretic effect. Conventional doses of diuretics (e.g. furosemide 10–40 mg) are unlikely to increase urine output in the context of declining renal function, oliguria and pulmonary oedema. However, large doses may be used in an attempt to produce a diuresis. **Initially furosemide, 250 mg, may be given over an hour (maximum rate 4 mg/min).** Since the peak effect occurs after 30 min, 1 h should be allowed for an effect to occur. If the urine output increases following a furosemide bolus, either repeat the 250 mg bolus or start a continuous intravenous furosemide infusion at 1–5 mg/h to maintain a diuresis. If this strategy, using high doses of diuretic, fails to produce an adequate effect, arrangements must be made for urgent fluid removal by haemodialysis or haemofiltration (see **Chapter 9**).

Vasodilators

Systemic venodilators may be of use in treating pulmonary oedema due to fluid overload or cardiac failure, since they reduce venous return by increasing venous capacitance. Additionally, their hypotensive action may be useful if hypertension is present. **Glyceryl trinitrate (GTN) may be given at a dose of 10–200 µg/min, and titrated upwards, as long as systolic blood pressure is maintained above 100 mmHg.** Sodium nitroprusside is also effective, but, since its main metabolite is toxic and is excreted by the kidneys, it should be used cautiously (maximum 72 hours). A dose of 10–200 µg/min may be used and, as with GTN, blood pressure must be monitored closely.

Venesection

This may also be a useful emergency measure if the situation is judged to be life threatening.

Haemofiltration or Haemodialysis

If diuretics are ineffective then fluid must be removed by dialysis or haemofiltration (see **Chapter 9**). Even if the patient is not in a hospital with a renal unit where dialysis is available, it may be possible to remove fluid by haemofiltration on the intensive care unit before transfer. Once stabilised, the patient can be transferred to the renal unit for further dialysis and management. If in-house dialysis or haemofiltration is not an option, there is no alternative other than to transfer. Anaesthetic expertise to ventilate the patient should be available in case this becomes necessary during the transfer.

8.3 HYPERKALAEMIA

David Throssell

DEFINITION

Severe hyperkalaemia (plasma K^+ >6.5 mmol/L) is one of the most important complications of ARF, due to the risk of life-threatening arrhythmias. This section outlines the principles of normal potassium homeostasis, and illustrates how these mechanisms are manipulated for the treatment of hyperkalaemia.

PATHOPHYSIOLOGY

98% of the total body potassium content of approximately 4000 mmol is intracellular. A high intracellular $[K^+]$ (K_{ic}) is maintained by the ubiquitous electrogenic $3Na^+/2K^+$-ATPase, which for every two K^+ ions moved into the cell pumps three Na^+ ions into the extracellular fluid (ECF). The subsequent passive movement of K^+ down its concentration gradient back to the ECF (K_{ec}) is largely responsible for the cytosol-negative resting membrane potential (RMP) found in all cells. K^+ entry into cells is promoted by catecholamines and insulin (**Figure 2**). β-adrenergic agonists probably act via direct stimulation of the $3Na^+/2K^+$-ATPase, whilst insulin stimulates the Na^+/H^+ exchanger, resulting in an increase in intracellular $[Na^+]$ which in turn drives the $3Na^+/2K^+$-ATPase.

In acidosis, most new H^+ ions are buffered intracellularly. The effect of H^+ on ECF/ICF K^+ distribution is determined by the behaviour of its accompanying anion. Organic anions (e.g. lactate) cross cell membranes freely, and in organic acidoses H^+ enters cells electroneutrally accompanied by its anion. In other forms of acidosis, in which protons enter, but anions are excluded from the cell (e.g. Cl^- in renal tubular acidosis, SO_4^{2-} and PO_4^{2-} in renal failure), electroneutrality is maintained by K^+ movement out of the cell, leading to hyperkalaemia. It follows that if hyperkalaemia accompanies organic acidoses (ketoacidosis, lactic acidosis), it must result from some feature of the illness other than acidosis (e.g. cell necrosis, renal failure), whereas in other forms of acidosis (including uraemic acidosis) hyperkalaemia is a direct consequence of H^+ excess.

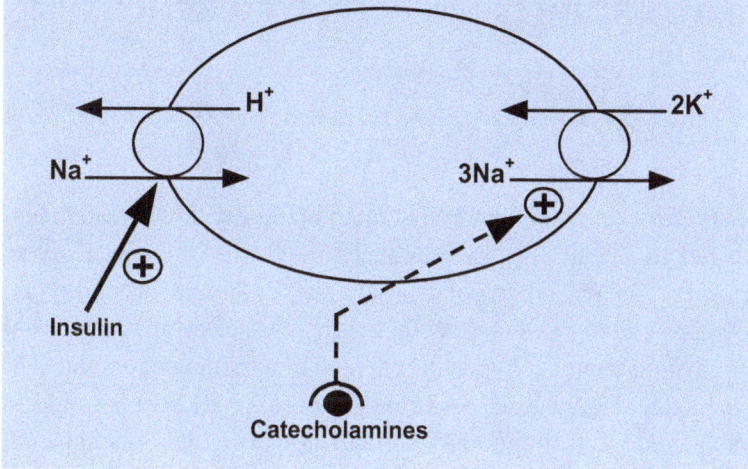

Figure 2. Hormonal influences on transcellular potassium movement

AETIOLOGY

Reduced renal K^+ excretion and the effects of H^+ on ICF/ECF K^+ distribution are the main causes of increased extracellular $[K^+]$ in ARF. Other less important but contributory factors are listed in **Table 7**. In rhabdomyolysis (see **Chapter 12**), tumour lysis (see **Chapter 21**) and haemolysis, cell breakdown releases intracellular ions including K^+ into the ECF. Blood contains approximately 60 mmol K^+/L; this K^+ is absorbed into the bloodstream after digestion of red cells during a GI bleed. Similarly, transfusion of old or inappropriately stored blood that has partially haemolysed delivers a K^+ load to the ECF. Patients treated with K^+ supplements or K^+ sparing diuretics may develop hyperkalaemia as their K^+ excretory capacity falls with the onset of ARF.

Aldosterone activates the apical Na^+ channel in the cortical collecting duct, thereby increasing Na^+ reabsorption and luminal electronegativity which promote the movement of K^+ down its electrical gradient into the tubule lumen. Angiotensin converting enzyme inhibitors (ACEIs) and non-steroidal anti-inflammatory drugs (NSAIDs) reduce angiotensin II (AII) and aldosterone activity: ACEIs act by reducing AII production from AI, and NSAIDs by inhibiting renin release

Table 7. Factors contributing to hyperkalaemia in acute renal failure

Reduced renal K^+ excretion	Drug pre-treatment with:
Uraemic acidosis	• K^+ supplements
Potassium release from:	• K^+ sparing diuretics
• muscle — rhabdomyolysis	• angiotensin-converting enzyme inhibitors
• tumours — tumour lysis	• non-steroidal anti-inflammatory drugs
• red cells — haemolysis, GI bleeding	• trimethoprim
• blood transfusion	

from the juxtaglomerular apparatus. Trimethoprim mimics amiloride by directly blocking the apical Na^+ channel. Because distal tubule Na^+ reabsorption and K^+ excretion are already inhibited in patients taking these drugs, they develop disproportionate hyperkalaemia if ARF supervenes.

CLINICAL PRESENTATION

1. Cardiac

Cardiac arrhythmias are the most important and potentially life-threatening complication of hyperkalaemia. A fall in the K_{ic}:K_{ec} ratio reduces the RMP of cardiac myocytes, decreasing conduction velocity and increasing repolarisation rates. Cardiac instability is more severe if hyperkalaemia develops quickly and is exacerbated by other electrolyte abnormalities that reduce the RMP, notably hyponatraemia, hypocalcaemia and hypomagnesaemia. The ECG changes accompanying hyperkalaemia are listed in **Table 8**, approximately in the order they appear with worsening hyperkalaemia. It is important to note, however, that sudden and life-threatening arrhythmias can occur without preceding ECG abnormalities in any patient with significant hyperkalaemia.

Table 8. ECG abnormalities in hyperkalaemia

1. Tented T waves
2. Prolonged PR and QT intervals, widened QRS complex
3. Flattened P waves
4. Sine waves
5. Ventricular fibrillation and asystole

2. Neuromuscular

By destabilising myocyte membranes, hyperkalaemia can cause muscle weakness and depressed tendon reflexes. In severe hyperkalaemia, a condition resembling Guillain-Barré syndrome has been described, which may in extreme cases cause respiratory paralysis. Sensory symptoms such as paraesthesiae are less common than motor symptoms, and the cranial nerves are usually spared because CSF is relatively protected from systemic hyperkalaemia by the blood brain barrier.

3. Metabolic

Hyperkalaemia exacerbates the metabolic acidosis (MA) accompanying acute renal impairment by two mechanisms. By competing with NH_4^+ ions on the $Na^+/K^+/2Cl^-$ cotransporter in the thick ascending limb of Henle's loop, K^+ reduces NH_4^+ reabsorption and thereby inhibits medullary concentration of NH_4^+, which is fundamental to NH_4^+ excretion in the final urine. In addition, high $[K^+]$ directly inhibits ammoniagenesis in proximal tubule cells. Because of these mechanisms, treatment of hyperkalaemia, e.g. by ion exchange resins (see below), may ameliorate MA in patients with hyperkalaemia and renal impairment.

4. Endocrine

Hyperkalaemia stimulates the secretion of insulin, glucagon and aldosterone, whilst inhibiting renin release from the macula densa. Because hyperkalaemia is also natriuretic, however, the consequent salt/water depletion may result in an increase in the final plasma [renin].

TREATMENT PRINCIPLES

Treatments for hyperkalaemia can be divided into four groups (see also **Practice Point 3**):

1. **Those which antagonise the cardiac effects of increased ECF [K⁺].**
2. **Those which promote intracellular transfer of K⁺.**
3. **Those which remove K⁺ from the body.**
4. **Those which reduce K⁺ intake.**

1. Antagonising the Cardiac Effects of Hyperkalaemia

Cardiac myocytes are stabilised by the intravenous administration of calcium salts. **10 mL of 10% calcium gluconate is infused over 2–3 min into a large vein**, and can be repeated after 5 min if ECG changes persist. Each 10 mL 10% calcium gluconate contains 2.25 mmol calcium. Calcium chloride has three times the content of elemental calcium/unit volume but is more irritant.

Important features of this treatment are as follows:

- indicated when ECG changes present or plasma [K⁺] >6.5 mEq/L
- onset of action 1–3 min
- duration of action 30–60 min
- no effect on ECF [K⁺] or K⁺ excretion
- may exacerbate digoxin toxicity.

2. Promoting Intracellular K⁺ Transfer

Three types of treatment promote the movement of K⁺ from ECF to ICF.

(a) *Insulin and dextrose infusion*

This is the mainstay of treatments promoting cellular K⁺ uptake. By upregulating Na⁺/H⁺ exchange across cell membranes, insulin increases intracellular [Na⁺] and promotes cellular K⁺ uptake by the 3Na⁺/2K⁺-ATPase (see **Figure 2**). To prevent hypoglycaemia, 2 g of glucose are administered with each unit of soluble insulin, and a standard cocktail is **50 mL 50% dextrose with 15 units soluble insulin given intravenously over 10 min**. Because of the risk of delayed

Practice Point 3. Management of hyperkalaemia in acute renal failure

Specimen haemolysed?

No — Stop K$^+$ supplements and relevant drugs

Yes — Repeat

K$^+$ >6.5 or ECG changes

Calcium gluconate 10 mL 10% i.v. → Other indications for immediate dialysis?

No → 15 units insulin +50 mL 50% dextrose i.v. ± NaHCO$_3$ if acidotic

Yes → Dialyse

Renal function progressively deteriorating → Dialyse

Renal function stable/improving and [K$^+$] satisfactory → Recheck K$^+$ regularly.
If rises again, repeat:
- Ca gluconate if indicated
- Insulin + dextrose
Add ion exchange resin po/pr

Renal function stable/improving but [K$^+$] still high → Repeat:
- Ca gluconate if indicated
- Insulin + dextrose
Add ion exchange resin po/pr

Persistent life-threatening hyperkalaemia → Dialyse

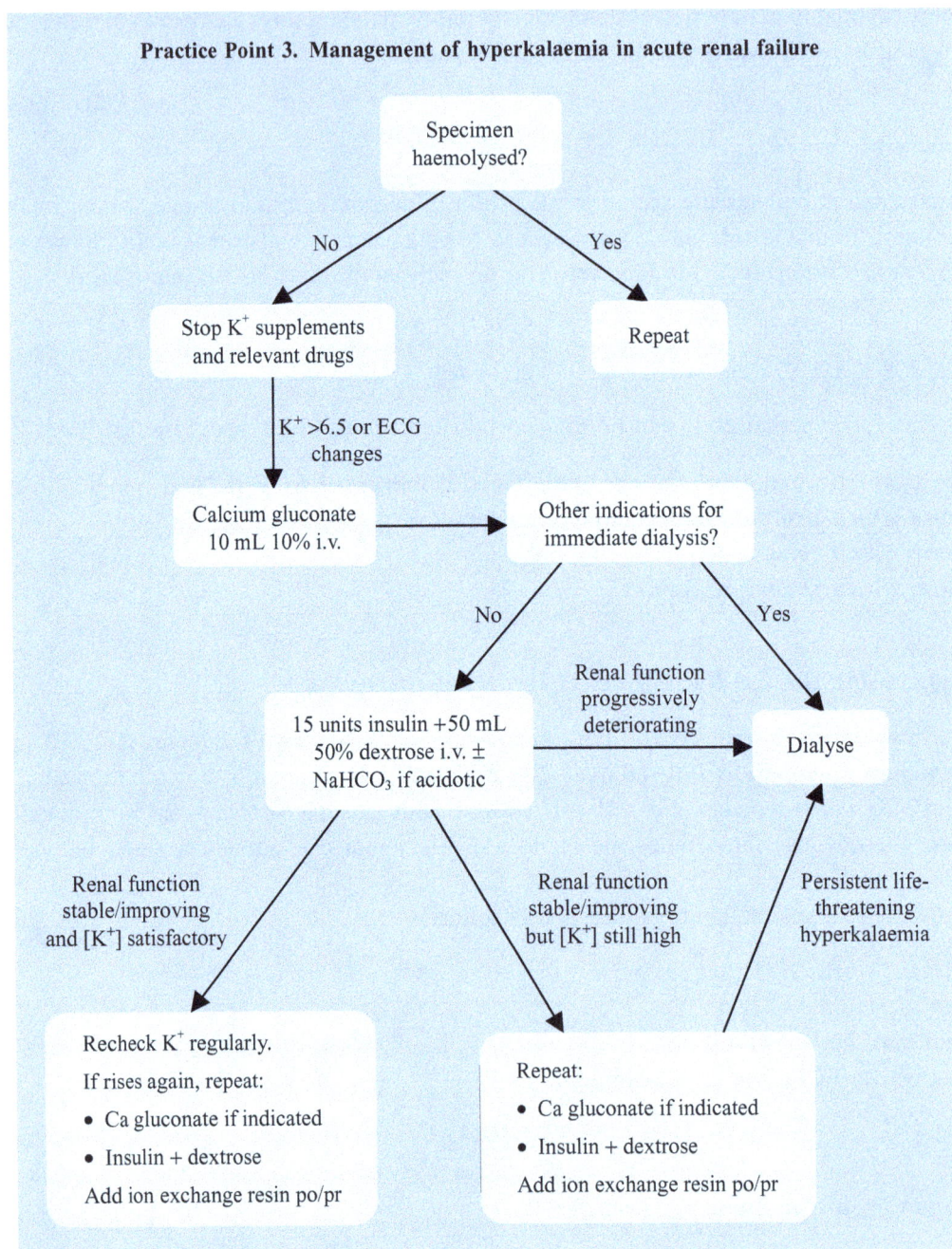

hypoglycaemia, regular monitoring of blood glucose is essential for 6 h after treatment, and is particularly important when treatment is given prior to transfer to a referral centre. Treatment is best avoided in patients about to dialyse, since intracellular movement of K$^+$ may reduce its clearance via the extracorporeal circuit.

Important features of this treatment are as follows:

- onset of action 15–45 min
- duration of action 4–6 h

- expected decrease in plasma [K$^+$] 0.6–1.5 mEq/L
- delayed hypoglycaemia reported in up to 75% of patients.

(b) *Sodium bicarbonate infusion*

By neutralising extracellular H$^+$ in acidotic and hyperkalaemic patients, intravenous NaHCO$_3$ may promote Na$^+$/H$^+$ exchange across cell membranes, thereby increasing intracellular [Na$^+$] and upregulating the 3Na$^+$/2K$^+$ exchanger. Studies in chronic haemodialysis patients have shown no significant effect of administered NaHCO$_3$ on plasma [K$^+$], but degrees of hyperkalaemia were mild-moderate and the findings may not apply to patients with ARF.

If NaHCO$_3$ solution is administered to hyperkalaemic patients, its use is best restricted to those with mixed venous [HCO$_3^-$] <20 mEq/L, who are neither hypocalcaemic nor hypernatraemic. **It should not be relied upon as monotherapy. 300–600 mL of isotonic NaHCO$_3$ solution (1.26%, 150 mmol each of Na$^+$ and HCO$_3^-$/L) are given intravenously over 15–30 minutes.**

In the setting of hyperkalaemic cardiac arrest, give 50 mL 8.4% NaHCO$_3$ and repeat as necessary (monitor arterial pH, see **Chapters 5** and **8.4**).

Important features of NaHCO$_3$ treatment for hyperkalaemia are as follows:

- onset of action 5–15 min
- duration of action 60–120 min
- dangers of treatment include:
  — salt/water overload
  — overshoot alkalosis
  — reduction in plasma free [Ca^{2+}] causing tetany
  — precipitation of Ca salts if co-administered with calcium gluconate/chloride

(c) *β-adrenergic agonists*

Since these agents directly stimulate the 3Na$^+$/2K$^+$-ATPase, they have been used intravenously and by nebuliser in the treatment of hyperkalaemia. Their onset, efficacy and duration of action are similar and additive to those of insulin and dextrose treatment but, because of their potential to induce tachyarrhythmias in patients already predisposed to cardiac instability, their use is not recommended.

3. Removing K$^+$ from the Body

(a) *Cation exchange resins*

Calcium and sodium polystyrene sulphonate (Calcium resonium and Resonium A) are ion exchange resins which exchange cations (predominantly K$^+$) for calcium and sodium respectively. The exchanged K$^+$ ions are subsequently excreted with the stool.

Administration is either oral, in a dose of 15 g three to four times daily, or rectally as a suspension of 30 g resin in 100 mL 2% medium viscosity methylcellulose and 100 mL water (retained for 9 hours).

Always co-prescribe osmotic laxatives, e.g. lactulose 10–20 mL 8 hourly. Approximately 1 mEq of K^+ is excreted for each gram of resin administered. Important features of this treatment are as follows:

- onset of action 30–60 min rectally, 2–4 h orally
- duration of action 4–6 h
- dangers of treatment include:
  — constipation
  — hypercalcaemia (Ca Resonium)
  — salt/water overload (Resonium A)
  — hypomagnesaemia

(b) Dialysis

In the absence of functioning kidneys, haemodialysis is the most efficient means of removing body K^+, and can clear 35 mmol K^+/h using a dialysate $[K^+]$ of 1–2 mmol/L. Peritoneal dialysis removes K^+ at approximately 20% of this rate. If possible, glucose-free dialysate should be used to discourage movement of K^+ into cells from which it is released post-dialysis, causing a rebound in plasma $[K^+]$. If glucose-free dialysate is used, particularly in patients previously treated with insulin and dextrose, regular blood glucose monitoring is mandatory.

Of note, certain forms of ARF are associated with severe, early, and often refractory hyperkalaemia. These include rhabdomyolysis (see **Chapter 12**), tumour lysis syndrome (see **Chapter 21**) and massive haemolysis (see **Chapter 12**).

4. Diet

All patients with ARF should be prescribed a low-potassium diet (see **Appendix B**).

8.4 ACID-BASE DISTURBANCES
David Throssell

NORMAL ACID-BASE HOMEOSTASIS

Metabolism of a typical mixed Western diet generates 1 mEq H^+/kg body weight/day. H^+ generated by amino acid (AA) breakdown constitutes the main source of acid produced by normal metabolism. Since animal protein is rich in cationic and sulphur-containing AAs, and vegetables and fruit have a high content of organic acids, net acid generation is less in vegetarian than carnivorous diets.

H^+ released into the circulation from the liver is buffered by the bicarbonate buffer system (BBS):

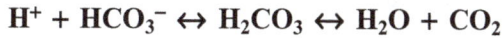

$$H^+ + HCO_3^- \leftrightarrow H_2CO_3 \leftrightarrow H_2O + CO_2$$

As a result, $[HCO_3^-]$ falls and pCO_2 rises. Assuming ventilation is normal, the CO_2 is rapidly exhaled by the lungs. The HCO_3^- deficit is repaired more slowly by new HCO_3^- production in the kidneys, and equilibrium is thus maintained.

Renal tubule cells produce new HCO_3^- by two mechanisms: deamination of glutamine with excretion of the resulting NH_4^+ ions in the urine, and conversion of CO_2 to H^+ and HCO_3^- with excretion of the resulting H^+ as titratable acid ($H_2PO_4^-$). Since one new HCO_3^- is generated for each NH_4^+ or $H_2PO_4^-$ appearing in the urine, renal net HCO_3^- production and therefore net acid excretion (NAE) can be defined as:

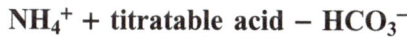

$$NH_4^+ + \text{titratable acid} - HCO_3^-$$

Under steady state conditions in a healthy subject, urine NAE is equal to the net H^+ generated by hepatic metabolism of dietary constituents. In metabolic acidosis (MA), NAE is increased by upregulation of ammoniagenesis to rates of up to five times normal.

INVESTIGATION OF ACID BASE DISORDERS

Acid base disorders associated with ARF can be characterised using the following measured and derived indices:

1. Arterial Blood Gas Measurement

Normal ranges for the three indices important in the analysis of acid-base disorders are as follows:

$$
\begin{array}{ll}
\text{Arterial blood pH:} & 7.40 \pm 0.04 \\
[HCO_3^-]: & 24 \pm 2 \text{ mmol/L} \\
\text{PaCO}_2: & 4.7\text{--}6.0 \text{ kPa (35--45 mmHg)}
\end{array}
$$

The four classical acute acid — base disorders are characterised by the following combinations of these parameters:

$$
\begin{array}{ll}
\text{Acute metabolic acidosis:} & \text{low pH; low } [HCO_3^-], \text{ low PaCO}_2 \\
\text{Acute metabolic alkalosis:} & \text{high pH; high } [HCO_3^-], \text{ high PaCO}_2 \\
\text{Acute respiratory acidosis:} & \text{low pH; high normal } [HCO_3^-], \text{ high PaCO}_2 \\
\text{Acute respiratory alkalosis:} & \text{high pH; low normal } [HCO_3^-], \text{ low PaCO}_2
\end{array}
$$

If the primary disturbance is metabolic (reflected by an abnormal $[HCO_3^-]$), a compensatory respiratory change (reflected by an altered $PaCO_2$) moves the pH towards 7.40. Conversely, a primary respiratory abnormality (reflected by an abnormal $PaCO_2$) is accompanied by a compensatory metabolic change (evidenced by an altered $[HCO_3^-]$) which also moves the pH nearer normal. As already discussed, metabolic acidosis is the commonest acid-base disorder in patients with ARF. Since respiratory acid-base abnormalities may co-exist with MA (*vide supra*), it is important to establish in any patient with MA whether the accompanying fall in $PaCO_2$ is appropriate to the degree of acidosis. If it is not, a superadded respiratory acid-base disorder must be present. In uncomplicated MA, each 1 mmol fall in $[HCO_3^-]$, should be accompanied by a fall in $PaCO_2$ of approximately 0.15 kPa. A smaller fall indicates co-existing respiratory acidosis, whilst a greater fall indicates respiratory alkalosis. A consequence of this observation is that patients with underlying MA may have respiratory acid-base disorders despite a $PaCO_2$ which falls within the normal range.

2. The Plasma Anion Gap

Because plasma is an electroneutral solution, there is no difference (gap) between its content of cations and anions, and the term anion gap (AG) is therefore a misnomer. AG refers to the **apparent** excess of cations over anions when only those electrolytes included in a standard biochemical profile are considered, and other ("unmeasured") ions are ignored. It is defined as $([Na^+] + [K^+]) - ([Cl^-] + [HCO_3^-])$.

Since

$$\textbf{sum of anions = sum of cations}$$

then

$$[Cl^-] + [HCO_3^-] + [\textbf{unmeasured anions}] = [Na^+] + [K^+] + [\textbf{unmeasured cations}]$$

and

$$[UA] - [UC] = ([Na^+] + [K^+]) - ([Cl^-] + [HCO_3^-])$$

Since

$$\textbf{Anion gap (from above)} = ([Na^+] + [K^+]) - ([Cl^-] + [HCO_3^-])$$

then

$$\textbf{Anion gap} = [\textbf{unmeasured anions}] - [\textbf{unmeasured cations}]$$

By quantifying the physiologically important unmeasured anions and cations (i.e. those excluded from a standard biochemical profile), an expected value for the anion gap can be therefore be calculated (**Table 9**). (Note that in North American texts, $[K^+]$ is usually excluded from the calculation, giving an expected anion gap of 12 ± 2 mEq/L.) Since this expected value assumes normal concentrations of the unmeasured anions and cations listed in **Table 9**, it must be corrected for abnormalities in any of their levels. For practical purposes, hypoalbuminaemia is the only common biochemical abnormality which significantly affects the anion gap: for each 10 g/L fall in serum [albumin], the expected value for the anion gap should be reduced by 4 mEq/L. A second, but less common cause of a reduced AG is IgG myeloma, in which the myeloma protein acts as an unmeasured cation.

Table 9. Quantification of anion gap

Unmeasured anions (mEq/L)		Unmeasured cations (mEq/L)	
Protein	14.5	Ca^{2+}	5
Phosphates	2	Mg^{2+}	1.5
Sulphates	1		
Organic acids	5		
Total	22.5	Total	6.5

Anion gap = unmeasured anions − unmeasured cations
= 22.5 − 6.5 (in normal subjects)
= **16 (±2) mEq/L**

Patients with MA can be divided into two groups based on their AG. In those with a normal AG, the fall in $[HCO_3^-]$ is by definition accompanied by an equal rise in $[Cl^-]$ (i.e. the anion accompanying new H^+ is Cl^-). Such normal anion gap acidoses usually result from excessive HCO_3^- losses or impaired acid excretion. In all other patients, the anion accompanying new H^+ is not Cl^-, and the AG is therefore raised. Overproduction of organic acids is the usual cause: the H^+ is buffered by HCO_3^-, causing a reduction in plasma $[HCO_3^-]$, and the accompanying organic anion accounts for the increased anion gap. Causes of normal (hyperchloraemic) and high AG acidoses are listed in **Tables 10** and **11**.

In patients with a high AG acidosis, comparison of the fall in plasma $[HCO_3^-]$ with the rise in anion gap can identify mixed acid-base disorders as follows:

$\uparrow$AG = $\downarrow[HCO_3^-]$ (within 5 mEq/L): simple high AG acidosis
$\uparrow$AG < $\downarrow[HCO_3^-]$ (by ≥ 5 mEq/L): mixed high AG MA + normal AG MA
$\uparrow$AG > $\downarrow[HCO_3^-]$ (by ≥ 5 mEq/L): mixed high AG MA + metabolic alkalosis

Table 10. Causes of metabolic acidosis with normal anion gap

1. **Renal causes**
   - early/mild renal failure
   - renal tubular acidosis
   - ureterosigmoidostomy/ileal conduit

2. **Gastrointestinal causes**
   - diarrhoea
   - vomiting with achlorhydria

3. **Administered substances**
   - fluid (dilutional acidosis)
   - Cl^- — containing acid
   - nonchloride — containing acid with rapid renal clearance of anion

Table 11. Causes of metabolic acidosis with high anion gap
Ketoacidosis
Uraemic acidosis
Lactic acidosis
Ingestion of toxins:
• salicylates
• methanol
• ethylene glycol
• chronic paraldehyde ingestion

Uraemic acidosis is typically accompanied by a high anion gap. The acidosis reflects impaired HCO_3^- reabsorption and reduced NH_4^+ production and excretion, whilst the high anion gap results from impaired excretion of inorganic and organic anions, predominantly sulphates and phosphates. In mild ARF or early CRF the retention of H^+ ions, which results from tubule dysfunction, may exceed the retention of anions, which is a function of decreased GFR. Such patients will have a hyperchloraemic acidosis rather than the high anion gap MA more typical of uraemia.

3. The Plasma Osmolar Gap

Plasma osmolality (P_{osm}) can be calculated as follows:

$$P_{osm} \text{ (mOsm/L)} = (2 \times \text{[Na]}) + \text{[urea]} + \text{[glucose] (all in mmol/L)}$$

Under normal circumstances, measured P_{osm} (evaluated by a physicochemical technique such as freezing point depression) should exceed calculated P_{osm} by no more than 10 mOsm/L (the "osmolar gap"). An increased osmolar gap suggests either that the measured $[Na^+]$ is spuriously low (e.g. when measured by flame photometry in a hyperlipidaemic sample) or that an additional (unmeasured) low molecular weight solute is present. Since a spuriously low $[Na^+]$ is rarely a problem with modern analytical techniques, a high osmolar gap implies the presence of an unmeasured solute, usually an alcohol. The combination of a high anion gap acidosis (due to carboxylic acid products ± lactic acidosis) and a high osmolar gap (due to the alcohols themselves) is typical of poisoning with ethanol, methanol and ethylene glycol, which should then be sought by specific assays.

4. Specific Organic Acid and Toxicological Assays

When the investigations outlined in **1–3** (above) suggest ketoacidosis, lactic acidosis, or poisoning with ethanol, methanol or ethylene glycol, the respective diagnoses should be confirmed with specific organic acid and toxicological assays. In the presence of a high AG MA and a high osmolar gap, the demonstration of calcium oxalate crystals on urine microscopy is pathognomonic of ethylene glycol poisoning.

PATHOGENESIS OF ACID-BASE DISORDERS IN ACUTE RENAL FAILURE

Since the kidney is the organ responsible for new HCO_3^- generation, it is not surprising that the predominant acid-base disorder in patients with ARF is MA due to reduced or absent net acid excretion (NAE). Because ammoniagenesis in surviving nephrons can be upregulated fivefold, MA becomes significant when the GFR falls to approximately 20% of normal. In addition to this almost invariable abnormality, specific causes and consequences of ARF can produce further acid-base disturbances which, when superimposed on the underlying MA, result in a mixed metabolic picture (**Table 12**). These will now be discussed in turn.

Table 12. Acid-base disorders in acute renal failure

1. **Metabolic acidosis**
   Normal anion gap (mild ARF)
   High anion gap due to:
   - decreased GFR
   - ± endogenous organic acid accumulation
   - ± breakdown products of toxins

2. **Mixed metabolic acidosis and metabolic alkalosis**
   Uraemic acidosis +
   - vomiting
   - aggressive diuresis
   - excessive HCO_3^- replacement

3. **Mixed metabolic acidosis and respiratory alkalosis**
   Uraemic acidosis +
   - septic shock
   - hepatorenal syndrome
   - salicylate intoxication

4. **Mixed metabolic acidosis and respiratory acidosis**
   Uraemic acidosis +
   - alveolar underventilation

METABOLIC ACIDOSIS

1. Endogenous Organic Acid Accumulation

(a) *Lactic acidosis*

Normal subjects generate (and therefore in steady state break down) approximately 15–30 mEq/kg of lactic acid (LA) daily. In the extreme situation of total anoxia, when ATP requirements must be met entirely by anaerobic glycolysis, rates of lactic acid production approximate to 70 mEq/min. This contrasts with estimated maximum rates of LA breakdown (which occurs by oxidation or glycogenesis in liver, kidneys and muscle) of approximately 12 mEq/min. Lactic

Table 13. Causes of lactic acidosis

Type A: accompanied by tissue hypoxia
Shock:
- cardiogenic
- septic
- hypovolaemic
- anaphylactic

Severe hypoxaemia:
- respiratory failure
- CO poisoning

Ischaemic injury to specific tissues:
- prolonged convulsions/exhaustive exercise
- ischaemic necrosis (e.g. bowel infarction)

Type B: impaired lactate metabolism without hypoxia
Drugs and toxins:
- biguanides (metformin, phenformin)
- alcohols (ethanol, methanol, ethylene glycol)
- sugars (fructose, sorbitol, xylitol)
- cyanide, nitroprusside
- salicylates

Hereditary enzyme defects:
- glucose 6-phosphate deficiency
- fructose 1,6-diphosphatase deficiency
- pyruvate carboxylase deficiency
- pyruvate dehydrogenase deficiency

Common but unrelated causes:
- diabetes mellitus
- liver failure
- renal failure
- leukaemias, lymphomas, tumour lysis

acidosis (usually defined as high anion gap MA accompanied by plasma [lactate] ≥ 4 mmol/L) may result either from relative tissue hypoxia (type A) or from a number of unrelated conditions which interfere with lactate metabolism (type B) (**Table 13**). Because of the disparity between potential rates of LA generation and metabolism, type A lactic acidosis, which develops during tissue hypoxia due to hypoxaemia, hypotension or tissue underperfusion, represents the most severe and dangerous form of MA, and carries a poor prognosis if tissue hypoxia cannot be rapidly corrected. Because of the clinical contexts in which it arises, this type of LA is frequently accompanied by ARF. In contrast, type B LA, which usually results from congenital, acquired or drug-induced hepatic dysfunction, causes less profound acidosis and is less strongly associated with ARF. Causes of type B LA are listed in **Table 13**.

(b) *Ketoacidosis*

Ketoacidosis results from relative or absolute insulin deficiency, accompanied by increased levels of hormones with anti-insulin actions (adrenaline, glucagon, glucocorticoids). Insulin deficiency and "anti-insulin" excess promote mobilisation of fatty acids from adipocytes, and after transfer to the liver these are metabolised to Acetyl CoA. Deficiency of ADP resulting from this fatty acid catabolism inhibits the breakdown of Acetyl CoA via the citric acid cycle, which is usually the predominant mechanism, and it is metabolised instead to ketoacids (acetoacetate, β hydroxybutyrate and acetone).

Factors contributing to the development of the two most clinically important varieties of ketoacidosis, diabetic and alcoholic, are as follows:

1. *Diabetic ketoacidosis*

- insulin deficiency in newly diagnosed DM
- omission of insulin during intercurrent illness in established DM
- upregulation of "anti-insulin" hormones during intercurrent illness

2. *Alcoholic ketoacidosis*

- following starvation with consequent glycogen depletion, inadequate gluconeogenesis and low insulin levels
- hypovolaemia due to vomiting, reduced fluid intake and alcohol-induced diuresis. Resulting α-adrenergic response inhibits insulin release from pancreatic β cells
- increased hepatic production of Acetyl CoA, and subsequently ketoacids, during ethanol breakdown
- if conscious level falls, decreased clearance of ketoacids by brain (which is normally responsible for approximately 50% of ketoacid breakdown)

Both diabetic and alcoholic ketoacidosis are strongly associated with ARF for several reasons:

- Both are characterised by profound salt/water depletion which predisposes to ARF.
- A reduction in conscious level, particularly in alcoholic ketoacidosis, predisposes to compartment syndromes and rhabdomyolysis.
- 25% of ketoacids generated in the liver are metabolised by the kidneys. Renal failure may therefore exacerbate ketoacidosis by reducing rates of ketoacid breakdown.
- Patients with established diabetic nephropathy have a lower threshold for developing ARF during concurrent illness.

In alcohol abusers, lactic acidosis may be superimposed on ketoacidosis because:

- Ethanol metabolism generates NADH which promotes conversion of pyruvate $\rightarrow$ lactate.
- Thiamine is an essential cofactor for pyruvate dehydrogenase, which converts pyruvate (and indirectly lactate) to Acetyl CoA. Glucose administered to thiamine-deficient alcoholics is metabolised to lactic acid which cannot be metabolised and therefore accumulates.
- Severe salt-water depletion may cause hypotension, tissue hypoxia and increased lactic acid production.

Patients with combined alcoholic ketoacidosis and lactic acidosis may cause diagnostic difficulties. Vomiting is often profuse and the consequent metabolic alkalosis may mask the expected fall in HCO_3^-. In addition, the high NADH:NAD ratio resulting from ethanol metabolism promotes conversion of acetoacetate (the substrate for the nitroprusside reaction used in stick tests for ketones) to β hydroxybutyric acid (which does not react with nitroprusside). Tests for ketonuria and ketonaemia may therefore be only weakly positive or even negative. Diagnostic pointers to this combination include:

- A very high anion gap which markedly exceeds any fall in plasma $[HCO_3^-]$.
- A plasma lactate level which is elevated (normal range 0.6–1.7 mmol/L) but insufficient to fully account for the rise in anion gap.
- Negative or weakly positive urine or plasma nitroprusside reaction.
- If alcohol has been consumed recently, elevated plasma ethanol and high plasma osmolar gap.

2. Breakdown Products of Toxins

Methanol and ethylene glycol, whilst themselves harmless, are metabolised to the toxic products formic acid and glycolic acid/oxalic acid respectively. Poisoning with these agents should be suspected when a high anion gap acidosis is accompanied by a high osmolar gap in a patient with low or undetectable plasma ethanol levels. As with alcoholic ketoacidosis, poisoning with either agent may be accompanied by lactic acidosis. Tubule precipitation of calcium oxalate frequently causes ARF after ethylene glycol ingestion, and the presence of oxalate crystals on urine microscopy can confirm the diagnosis before the results of specific assays are available. ARF is less common in methanol poisoning, in which damage to the CNS and optic nerve is more significant.

The affinity of alcohol dehydrogenase for ethanol is 100 times greater than that for either methanol or ethylene glycol. If poisoning with these agents is recognised early, treatment with ethanol, which competitively inhibits their metabolism, can be instituted and may prevent blindness or renal failure. Alternatively, treatment with the new alcohol dehydrogenase inhibitor, fomepizole, early in the course of ethylene glycol poisoning prevents renal injury by inhibiting the formation of toxic metabolites (see also **Chapter 11**).

MIXED METABOLIC ACIDOSIS AND METABOLIC ALKALOSIS

The relative severity of the two components of this combined metabolic disorder determines the final plasma $[HCO^-_3]$. In predominant acidosis, the $[HCO^-_3]$ is low; in predominant alkalosis, it is high; and if the abnormalities are of equal size, it is normal. The latter situation may cause diagnostic difficulty because there is no *prima facie* acid base disorder. It should be suspected when a patient with renal failure has a normal plasma $[HCO^-_3]$ but a high anion gap. The anion gap remains high because it is not influenced by the causes of metabolic alkalosis (MAL) which accompany ARF.

1. Uraemic Acidosis + Vomiting

Vomiting and uraemia may co-exist in patients in whom:

- severe vomiting or large nasogastric aspirates cause salt/water depletion sufficient to induce renal failure
- uraemia ± associated pathologies cause severe vomiting

Although hypokalaemia is usual in patients with severe or prolonged vomiting, it is largely due to kaliuresis and is therefore absent in patients with co-existing renal failure.

2. Uraemic Acidosis + Aggressive Diuresis

Because diuretics increase urinary Na^+, K^+, Cl^- and water losses, but do not cause bicarbonaturia, patients who are overdiuresed have a contracted ECF volume with a high plasma $[HCO^-_3]$ ("contraction alkalosis"). This alkalosis is maintained by upregulation of ammonia excretion by hypokalaemia and by increased proximal tubular HCO_3^- reabsorption due to stimulation of the apical sodium hydrogen antiporter (NHE3) by angiotensin II (AII). High AII levels result in turn from renin released in response to a low ECF volume.

Patients developing ARF due to overdiuresis, or the continued consumption of diuretics when fluid intake is reduced due to intercurrent illness, may develop combined MA and MAL. Whilst the MAL will respond to salt and water replacement, acidosis will persist unless the ARF is pre-renal and can be prevented from progressing to established acute tubular necrosis by intravenous fluid replacement.

3. Uraemic Acidosis + Excessive NaHCO₃ Replacement

In contrast to **1** and **3** above, this combination is characterised by a normal or high ECF volume. It arises when MA, usually lactic acidosis or ketoacidosis, is treated inappropriately or excessively with intravenous $NaHCO_3$ in patients who already have, or subsequently develop, ARF.

MIXED METABOLIC ACIDOSIS AND RESPIRATORY ALKALOSIS

This condition is characterised by low plasma $[HCO^-_3]$, a $PaCO_2$ which is less than expected for the degree of acidosis, and a pH which reflects the relative severity of the two metabolic abnormalities.

1. Uraemic Acidosis and Septic Shock (see **Chapter 19**)

Endotoxaemia causes hyperventilation and consequent respiratory alkalosis. Since septic shock is a common cause of ARF, the two pathologies frequently co-exist and may cause a mixed acid-base disorder.

2. Hepatorenal Syndrome (see Chapter 25)

Liver failure stimulates respiration via sympathetic nerve activity and possibly endotoxaemia. Patients with the hepatorenal syndrome may therefore have mixed MA and respiratory alkalosis.

3. Salicylate Intoxication

The metabolic consequences of inadvertent or intentional salicylate poisoning [usually from aspirin ingestion but occasionally from ingestion of methylsalicylate (oil of wintergreen)] are complex and include:

- Respiratory alkalosis:
  — the dominant acid base abnormality in adults
  — caused by direct stimulation of respiratory centre
- High anion gap metabolic acidosis due to:
  — salicylic acid (minor contributor)
  — lactic acid, due to inhibition of Kreb cycle enzymes
  — ketoacids formed by stimulation of lipolysis, vomiting and poor food intake
  — ARF if this supervenes

In children, high anion gap MA is the predominant acid-base disorder. A respiratory acidosis may occur when very severe poisoning damages the respiratory centre. A MAL occurs due to profuse vomiting.

In adults, the usual acid base abnormality is a dominant respiratory alkalosis accompanied by mild metabolic acidosis. If ARF supervenes, the metabolic acidosis becomes more significant.

Features of salicylic acid toxicity which predispose to the development of ARF include:

- Salt/water depletion due to:
  — vomiting caused by salicylate-induced stimulation of chemosensitive trigger zone
  — sweating and tachypnoea due to uncoupling of oxidative phosphorylation (conversion of ADP $\rightarrow$ ATP) with consequent increase in heat generation, O_2 consumption and CO_2 production
  — bicarbonaturia, with consequent natriuresis
  — aminoaciduria due to $\uparrow$ plasma [AA] secondary to aminotransferase deficiency
  — glycosuria if hyperglycaemia results from upregulation of hepatic glycogenolysis
- Glomerular afferent arteriolar vasoconstriction due to inhibition of vasodilatory prostaglandins

MIXED METABOLIC ACIDOSIS AND RESPIRATORY ACIDOSIS

Because hyperventilation and consequent hypocapnia are the normal physiological response to MA, co-existing respiratory acidosis is present whenever the $PaCO_2$ is suppressed less than would be anticipated for the ongoing pH (see "diagnosis"). In some circumstances, therefore, respiratory acidosis can be present when the $PaCO_2$ falls within the normal range.

Mixed MA and respiratory acidosis may accompany ARF when the underlying cause of ARF also causes respiratory dysfunction (e.g. Wegener's granulomatosis) or when a complication of

ARF affects ventilation (e.g. uraemic coma causing respiratory depression). "Double acidosis" is potentially life-threatening and must be treated aggressively, usually by assisted ventilation in the first instance, followed by treatment of the MA as appropriate.

TREATMENT OF ACID-BASE DISORDERS IN ACUTE RENAL FAILURE

1. Metabolic Acidosis

Since high anion gap uraemic acidosis occurs only in association with significant renal impairment (see above) many patients with ARF and MA require renal replacement therapy. Most authors therefore list significant acidosis (pH <7.2) as an indication for dialysis in ARF, particularly if it is associated with hyperkalaemia. MA due to any concomitant organic acid accumulation will be corrected by dialysis, but the underlying cause (shock, severe hypoxaemia or local ischaemic injury in type A lactic acidosis, and relative insulin deficiency in ketoacidosis) must also be addressed as necessary.

Treatment of methanol and ethylene glycol poisoning

When treating these patients, **always obtain advice from the local poisons information centre**.

As discussed previously, poisoning with methanol and ethylene glycol should be treated with **ethanol** which, by acting as a preferential substrate for alcohol dehydrogenase, reduces the production of toxic metabolites. Administration is as a 5–10% solution in 5% dextrose or 0.9% saline, aiming for therapeutic levels of 100–150 mg/dL. As an approximate guide, a bolus of 0.6 g/kg is followed by an infusion of 0.07 g/kg/h (in non-drinkers) — 0.15 g/kg/h (in habitual drinkers). In severe poisoning (plasma concentration >100 mg/dL) methanol can also be effectively removed by haemodialysis. In such patients, methanol metabolism can be inhibited by the addition of ethanol to the dialysate (to achieve a concentration of 100 mg/dL) or administration as an infusion via the venous bubble trap.

Alternatively, **fomepizole** may be used for the treatment of ethylene glycol poisoning. Fomepizole is given by intravenous infusion over 30 min, initially 15 mg/kg followed by 10 mg/kg every 12 h for 4 doses, then 15 mg/kg every 12 h until plasma ethylene glycol concentration is below 200 mg/L (3.2 mmol/L).

2. Mixed Metabolic Acidosis and Metabolic Alkalosis

Restoration of ECF volume in hypovolaemic alkalosis reduces plasma $[HCO_3^-]$ which, if urine output is restored, falls further because of bicarbonaturia. In established oligoanuric renal failure treated by dialysis, persistent alkalosis is very uncommon since ECF volume is usually normal or high, and losses of HCl via vomiting are rarely sufficient to negate uraemic acidosis. An exception is patients treated for prolonged periods by continuous haemofiltration, who may develop alkalosis due to continuous generation of HCO_3^- from buffers (usually lactate) in the replacement solution. Such iatrogenic alkalosis can be treated by using a replacement solution with a lower concentration of buffer, slowing the rate of filtration (assuming other biochemical indices are satisfactory), or alternating buffered with buffer-free replacement solutions.

Patients with established ARF and hypervolaemic alkalosis due to inappropriate $NaHCO_3$ therapy should be ultrafiltered and dialysed against fluid with a reduced concentration of HCO_3^- or acetate.

3. Mixed Metabolic Acidosis and Respiratory Alkalosis

Hepatic failure and septic shock associated with ARF are managed by standard techniques: in true hepatorenal syndrome the only effective treatment is liver transplantation. Patients with salicylate intoxication and a good urine output should be alkalinised (aiming for a urine pH of ≥ 7.5), although this may be constrained by an already high plasma $[HCO_3^-]$ due to respiratory alkalosis. A high pH promotes dissociation of salicylic acid into H^+ and salicylate. Urinary excretion of salicylate anions, which unlike salicylic acid are not reabsorbed by non-ionic diffusion, is therefore increased, and non-ionic diffusion of aspirin into the CSF is reduced. Although 50% protein-bound, aspirin is usefully cleared by haemodialysis which is indicated when blood aspirin levels exceed 80 mg/dL, when symptoms are life-threatening (e.g. development of coma or convulsions) or when ARF supervenes.

4. Mixed Metabolic Acidosis and Respiratory Acidosis

In the presence of uraemic acidosis, significant respiratory acidosis (which as already discussed may occur without a large increase in $PaCO_2$) should be treated aggressively, if necessary by assisted ventilation.

8.5 CALCIUM, PHOSPHATE AND MAGNESIUM DISTURBANCES
Anthony Dorling

INTRODUCTION

Calcium and phosphorus are important elemental constituents of the body, comprising 2% and 1% respectively of total body weight (i.e. an average 70 kg human contains 1.4 kg of calcium and 0.7 kg of phosphorus). The majority of this is stored within bone as hydroxyapatite $[Ca_{10}(PO_4)_6(OH)_2]$ and other calcium phosphate complexes. In contrast, magnesium is a trace constituent, comprising 0.04% total body weight (or 26 g/70 kg); like calcium and phosphate, the majority of magnesium is stored within the mineral lattice of bone.

Although each of these elements has distinct physiological roles, they share similar mechanisms of absorption from the gut, storage in the skeleton and excretion through the kidneys. The plasma concentrations of calcium, phosphate and magnesium, which are normally maintained within a narrow range by sophisticated homeostatic mechanisms, are invariably deranged in ARF, with potentially serious consequences.

MECHANISMS OF HOMEOSTASIS

A detailed discussion of the regulation of calcium, phosphate and magnesium balance is beyond the scope of this chapter. However, a broad understanding of the mechanisms by which plasma concentrations are maintained is essential in order to appreciate the derangements which occur with ARF. **Note** that renal handling of calcium, phosphate and magnesium is covered in **Chapter 2**.

There are five important points to highlight:

1. Excretion of calcium, phosphate and magnesium is primarily by the kidneys. Under normal conditions, the bulk of filtered substrate is reabsorbed and only 1–2% of filtered calcium ($\approx$5 mmol), 3% of magnesium ($\approx$5 mmol) and 5–20% of phosphate (average 30 mmol) passes into the urine daily.
2. Under equilibrium conditions in adults, the daily amount of calcium, phosphate and magnesium absorbed by the gut is equal to that excreted by the kidneys. It therefore follows that when excretion is deranged in ARF, it is important to regulate the amount of calcium and phosphate, that is, ingested and absorbed.
3. Bone is the major storage organ for calcium and phosphate (and to a lesser extent magnesium). Under equilibrium conditions in adults, the daily turnover from amorphous calcium and phosphate is modest and release of calcium and phosphate equals uptake into bone. Magnesium is similarly influenced. This equilibrium is disordered in renal failure.
4. Homeostasis is controlled by two principal hormones, vitamin D and parathyroid hormone (PTH), both of which have multiple actions on calcium, phosphate and magnesium regulation, as discussed below. In humans, the precise physiological role of calcitonin in maintaining plasma concentrations of calcium and phosphate is unresolved. The metabolism of both PTH and vitamin D is disordered in ARF.
5. Plasma phosphate concentration has an important bearing on calcium homeostasis as follows:

   (a) Plasma concentrations of both are limited by precipitation of insoluble calcium phosphate when the $[Ca^{2+}] \times [PO_4^{2-}]$ product exceeds 5.5 ($\mu M \times \mu M$).
   (b) Phosphate has an indirect influence on $[Ca^{2+}]$ through vitamin D and PTH metabolism (inhibits 1α-hydroxylation of vitamin D — see below).

This interrelationship means that hyperphosphataemia is usually accompanied by hypocalcaemia.

HORMONAL CONTROL OF HOMEOSTASIS

1. Parathyroid Hormone (PTH)

PTH is a polypeptide hormone manufactured, stored and secreted by parathyroid cells, which is released primarily in response to reductions in plasma calcium concentration. The other factors which influence parathyroid cells are:

(a) **Raised vitamin D levels** suppress PTH via a direct effect on the parathyroid glands and indirectly through the influence on plasma calcium concentration.

(b) **Plasma magnesium concentration:** PTH is suppressed by raised plasma magnesium concentration, although this is probably of little physiological importance. Paradoxically, magnesium deficiency results in hypoparathyroidism and hypocalcaemia, reflecting the crucial role of magnesium in the action of many intracellular enzymes — in this case probably adenylate cyclase, which is an important "second messenger" involved in PTH release.

Plasma phosphate has no direct influence on the parathyroid glands but will influence PTH secretion indirectly through changes in plasma calcium.

The primary physiological purpose of PTH is to maintain plasma calcium concentration within a fairly narrow range. Its actions are to:

- increase the release of calcium and phosphate from the skeleton
- increase the tubular reabsorption of calcium
- reduce the tubular reabsorption of phosphate, thereby increasing renal phosphate excretion
- increase the 25-hydroxylation of vitamin D in the kidneys, thereby increasing intestinal absorption of calcium, magnesium and phosphate[1]

2. Vitamin D

Vitamin D is actually two related compounds, ergocalciferol (vitamin D_2) which is absorbed from the gut, and cholecalciferol (vitamin D_3) which is manufactured in the skin from 7-dehydrocholesterol. In their basic state, neither has significant biological activity. These forms undergo hydroxylation in the liver by the enzyme D-25-hydroxylase to become 25-hydroxyvitamin D (D_2 and D_3), which represent the major storage forms of these vitamins[2]. These 25-hydroxyvitamin D moieties are further hydroxylated to 1,25 $(OH)_2$ vitamin D (D_2 and D_3) in the kidney by 25-hydroxyvitamin D-1α-hydroxylase and it is this form which has optimal biologic activity[3]. Most humans have more vitamin D_3 than D_2, but each moiety has the same potency.

The 1α-hydroxylation of vitamin D is regulated by:

- PTH (increases conversion).
- plasma calcium concentration (reduces conversion).
- plasma phosphate concentration (reduces conversion)

The major physiological effects of 1,25 $(OH)_2$ vitamin D are to:

- enhance the absorption of calcium, phosphate and magnesium from the intestine
- stimulate the release of calcium and phosphate from the skeleton
- inhibit PTH secretion

---

[1]Under most conditions, phosphate absorption from gut is passive and dependent only the intraluminal concentration of phosphate. Vitamin D dependent absorption is only important in conditions of dietary phosphate deprivation.
[2]25-hydroxyvitamin D is much less biologically active than 1,25 $(OH)_2$ vitamin D.
[3]25-hydroxyvitamin D can also be hydroxylated to 24,25 $(OH)_2$ vitamin D by 25-hydroxyvitamin D-24-hydroxylase which is found in kidney and many other tissues, although the precise biologic function of this metabolite has not been fully defined.

Practice Point 4. Hypermagnesaemia

Plasma magnesium: normal range 0.7–1 mmol/L

Clinical manifestations of acute severe hypermagnesaemia (>2 mmol/L)

- general — nausea, vomiting, lethargy, vasodilatation
- neuromuscular — confusion, respiratory depression, weakness, absent tendon reflexes, complete paralysis (>9 mM)
- cardiovascular — hypotension, bradycardia, heart block, cardiac arrest

All manifestations are exacerbated by hypocalcaemia (<1.8 mmol/L)

Management of hypermagnesaemia in acute renal failure

- No specific treatment required unless symptoms or signs of hypermagnesaemia
- Aggressive rehydration and correction of pre-renal renal failure (see treatment of hypercalcaemia). Diuretics enhance renal excretion of magnesium; give 120 mg furosemide IV when rehydrated*
- Stop administration of magnesium-containing compounds
- 10 mL of 10% calcium gluconate by slow IV infusion (5 min) if there are cardiovascular or neuromuscular manifestations
- Haemodialysis with magnesium-free dialysate if in established renal failure

*Not usually needed.

CALCIUM/PHOSPHATE/MAGNESIUM DISTURBANCES IN ARF

Plasma magnesium concentrations tend to rise in ARF, but usually result in no specific symptoms unless accompanied by an abnormally high ingestion of magnesium-containing compounds, such as antacids or laxatives. However, the effects and symptoms of hypermagnesaemia are exacerbated by hypocalcaemia. Magnesium excess should be considered in any patient with ARF with nausea, vomiting, confusion, or lethargy, especially when there is associated respiratory depression and absent tendon reflexes. Hypermagnesaemia rarely requires treatment (see **Practice Point 4**). If required, haemodialysis with a magnesium-free dialysate is the only effective way of reducing plasma magnesium but, in the short term, intravenous calcium gluconate should be given to antagonise the physiological consequences of hypermagnesaemia.

There are several patterns of calcium and phosphate disturbance associated with ARF:

(1) Hyperphosphataemia with Hypocalcaemia.
(2) Acute Renal Failure Associated with Hypercalcaemia.
(3) Acute Renal Failure Associated with Hypophosphataemia.

(1) Hyperphosphataemia with Hypocalcaemia

Except in the special circumstances described in **(2)** and **(3)**, an abrupt decline in GFR is always accompanied by some degree of hyperphosphataemia and hypocalcaemia. These changes occur in experimental animals with both oliguric and non-oliguric ARF, and it is clear from these models that the degree of biochemical derangement of calcium and phosphate concentrations reflects the severity of the renal failure.

Pathophysiology

The factors contributing to hyperphosphataemia are:

(a) **Reduced renal excretion** in the face of normal or enhanced intestinal absorption or increased endogenous loading of phosphate.
(b) **Secondary hyperparathyroidism** (which develops within several days) leading to release of phosphate from bone.

In addition, there are a number of conditions associated with ARF where gross hyperphosphataemia, due to massive release of phosphate from intracellular stores (e.g. in rhabdomyolysis, occurs as part of the primary problem.

The factors leading to hypocalcaemia are:

(a) **Hyperphosphataemia** itself, through the precipitation of insoluble calcium phosphate (when the solubility product of calcium and phosphate is exceeded), and reduced hydroxylation of vitamin D.
(b) **Intracellular uptake** in severely damaged tissues.

Clinical presentation

Experimental studies and clinical observations indicate that the hyperphosphataemia of renal failure can exacerbate the degree and severity of the renal damage, particularly when accompanied by hypovolaemia, hyperuricaemia or myoglobinuria. The acceleration in decline of renal function is thought to be due to precipitation of amorphous calcium phosphate crystals in the renal tubules, causing a tubulointerstitial nephritis.

The other predominant consequence of severe hyperphosphataemia is acute precipitation of calcium phosphate complexes in other soft tissues, including blood vessels and major organs, especially the heart and lungs. This is a serious complication in patients with chronic renal failure and uncontrolled hyperphosphataemia. Acutely, hyperphosphataemia may manifest in the skin as intense pruritus and papular eruptions, and arrhythmias can occur as a result of deposition within the conducting tissue.

The hypocalcaemia associated with ARF is often asymptomatic because, as total plasma calcium falls, the concentration of free Ca^{2+} ions is maintained by dissociation from plasma proteins (due to the accompanying acidosis and severe uraemia). However, tetany, arrhythmias and seizures can occur and represent the severe manifestations of hypocalcaemia.

Treatment principles (see **Practice Points 5** and **6**)

In situations where the occurrence of severe hyperphosphataemia is predictable, for instance after major tissue injury or prior to oncologic treatment of large tumour bulks, ARF can often be

Practice Point 5. Hyperphosphataemia

Plasma phosphate: normal range 0.8–1.5 mmol/L

Systemic conditions associated with severe hyperphosphataemia (plasma phosphate >3 mmol/L)
- tumour lysis syndrome: especially haematologic and lymphoid malignancy, particularly if large tumour bulk, but has been reported with adeno, small cell and squamous cell carcinomas (see **Chapter 21**)
- rhabdomyolysis and ischaemia-reperfusion states (see **Chapter 12**)
- severe haemolysis
- severe tissue injury, including bowel infarction and pancreatitis
- iatrogenic (rapid IV infusion/phosphate enemas)

Clinical manifestations of hyperphosphataemia
- usually asymptomatic
- acute precipitation of calcium phosphate crystals when [Ca]∗[PO$_4$] product >5.5
  — acute pruritus
  — arrhythmias
  — interstitial nephritis/acute nephrocalcinosis and worsening ARF

Management
- prevent or treat the primary condition causing hyperphosphataemia
- rehydrate if pre-renal ARF: monitor CVP, IV colloid if BP <100 mmHg systolic, N Saline (0.9%) to maintain diuresis, infuse at 1 L every 4–6 h
- dietary restriction of phosphate intake and oral phosphate binders with food (calcium carbonate 0.5–1 g with meals)
- haemodialysis

prevented by ensuring adequate hydration and maintaining a good diuresis and phosphaturia. Similarly, appropriate volume expansion in patients with reduced circulating volume and pre-renal failure is critical, particularly in those patients with massive hyperphosphataemia, to enhance renal perfusion, maintain GFR and increase phosphate excretion.

The aim of therapy once ARF is established is to normalise plasma concentrations of calcium and phosphate by achieving a balance between the amount of calcium and phosphate entering the plasma pool and that leaving it. Dietary restriction of phosphate intake is important, as are oral phosphate binders such as calcium carbonate to limit the amount of phosphate absorbed through the gut. These measures are still important in those conditions associated with endogenous release of intracellular phosphate, such as rhabdomyolysis (see **Chapter 12**).

Dialysis is the only effective means of removing phosphate once renal failure is established. Approximately 30 mmol of phosphate is removed during each four hour haemodialysis session, most of this during the first two hours, by which time plasma phosphate levels have usually fallen to normal. Plasma concentrations rebound after dialysis due to slow intercompartmental redistribution, which for phosphate is approximately 10 times slower than for urea. Regular, rather than prolonged, dialysis sessions are therefore the most effective way to remove phosphate.

Practice Point 6. Hypocalcaemia

Plasma calcium: normal range 2–2.5 mmol/L
Calcium corrected for albumin = measured calcium + [(40-serum albumin in g/L) × 0.02]

Clinical manifestations of acute hypocalcaemia
There is no close correlation between corrected [calcium] and manifestations of hypocalcaemia, because it is ionised [calcium] which is important

- neuromuscular — paraesthesiae, hyperreflexia, carpopedal spasm, tetany*, seizures
- cardiovascular — hypotension, bradycardia, prolonged QT on ECG, arrhythmias, cardiac failure

Management
- Be wary of precipitating tetany during correction of acidosis
- 10 mL of 10% calcium gluconate (2.2 mmol) by slow IV injection if there are neuromuscular or cardiac manifestations. Repeat once if required
- Persistent manifestations may require continuous infusion. Give 2 mL of 10% calcium gluconate per kg, diluted in 500 mL 5% dextrose, over 6 h to raise plasma calcium by 0.5–0.75 mmol/L
- If established renal failure give oral vitamin D supplementation, e.g. 1α calcidol 0.25 µg daily

*Chovstek (tapping facial nerve) and Trousseau (carpal spasm 3 min after cuff occlusion) signs reveal latent tetany, but may be absent in clinically significant hypocalcaemia. Chovstek's may be positive in 10–25% with normocalcaemia.

The hypocalcaemia of ARF rarely requires specific treatment, unless there are signs of severe symptomatic hypocalcaemia, when intravenous calcium gluconate should be given and oral supplements of 1α-hydroxylated vitamin D started, to increase calcium absorption from the gut (see **Practice Point 6**).

Recovery phase

Transient hypercalcaemia and hypomagnesaemia are common in the diuretic phase during recovery from ARF, especially when severe hyperphosphataemia has been a feature, but these rarely require treatment. Delayed hypercalcaemia, presenting several weeks after recovery, has been reported.

(2) Acute Renal Failure Associated with Hypercalcaemia

There are a number of pathological conditions, predominantly malignant, in which ARF associated with acute hypercalcaemia can arise (see **Table 14** for examples). In these conditions, the ARF may be aetiologically related to the raised plasma calcium (although other mechanisms may contribute to the ARF).

The effects on the kidneys of an acutely raised plasma calcium include:

(a) Renal vascular vasoconstriction.
(b) Reduction in the ultrafiltration of plasma calcium (if associated with a raised PTH).

Table 14. Examples of conditions associated with hypercalcaemia and renal failure

Malignancies	**Granulomatous disease**
solid tumours (with or without bony metastatic disease)	tuberculosis
lung (squamous cell)	sarcoidosis
breast	
ovarian	**Drugs**
pancreatic	thiazide diuretics
	lithium
haematologic malignancy	
multiple myeloma	**Endocrine**
Hodgkin's disease	hyperparathyroidism
	phaeochromocytoma

(c) Reduction in tubule sodium reabsorption, resulting in renal sodium and potassium wasting, polyuria and often nocturia; combined with the nausea and vomiting that often accompanies acute hypercalcaemia, dehydration and pre-renal ARF can occur.

(d) Precipitation of calcium in the renal tubules leading to obstruction and interstitial nephritis.

The other clinical features of acute hypercalcaemia include anorexia, constipation, abdominal pain, confusion and somnolence. Plasma phosphate concentration is usually reduced in these conditions. The focus of investigation should be to identify the cause of the hypercalcaemia.

Treatment principles (see **Practice Point 7**)

Ultimately, the underlying cause of the hypercalcaemia will need to be treated. However, the initial phase of treatment should be aimed at limiting the effect of hypercalcaemia on the kidneys and reducing plasma calcium concentrations. The mainstay of treatment is to rehydrate with suitable intravenous fluids, usually saline, and reverse any pre-renal ARF. Treatment of hypophosphataemia with phosphate replacement should normally not be considered until renal function has been stabilised and measures to lower plasma calcium have been initiated. Broadly speaking, reducing plasma calcium can be achieved in one of three ways:

- **Enhance the excretion of calcium.**
- **Enhance calcium uptake into bone/reduce release from bone.**
- **Reduce absorption of calcium from the gut.**

• *Enhancing calcium excretion*

In patients without established ARF, rehydration with saline will enhance calcium excretion because of the inter-relationship with sodium excretion. Only once rehydration is satisfactory is it appropriate to consider loop diuretics to enhance further renal calcium excretion. Thiazides, by enhancing distal tubule calcium reabsorption, are contraindicated in hypercalcaemia. Dialysis, which may be indicated for ARF, is an effective means of removing plasma calcium if low calcium dialysates are used.

Practice Point 7. Hypercalcaemia

Concentration (mmol/L) and associated symptoms

- **Mild** <3.0 — few symptoms, if any
- **Moderate** >3.0–3.5 — polyuria, polydypsia, nocturia, nausea, anorexia, constipation
- **Severe** >3.5 — as with moderate hypercalcaemia, plus vomiting, abdominal pain, somnolence, confusion, depression, renal failure, coma

Factors indicating that urgent treatment is required

- severe dehydration with hypotension (systolic <100 mmHg)
- pre-renal ARF
- confusion/somnolence
- corrected calcium >3.5 mmol/L

Treatment protocol for severe hypercalcaemia

- IV rehydration if BP <80 mmHg systolic
  - Insert CVP line and give 500 mL colloid stat — repeat until BP >100 mmHg
  - Use N saline (0.9%) when hypotension corrected — give 1L 4–6 hourly depending on CVP and urine output
- IV furosemide only once dehydration corrected
  - Give 120 mg stat and continue at 40 mg 4–6 hourly if patient making urine
  - Rehydration/furosemide will cause calcium to fall by up to 1 mmol/L in 24 h
- Specific therapy — tailor according to suspected cause (see text)
  - prednisolone 30 mg/day orally
  - salmon calcitonin 8 U/kg 6 hourly s/c or IM OR 10 U/kg daily IV in N/Saline
  - disodium pamidronate IV, dose according to level of hypercalcaemia: 30 mg if <3 mmol/L, 60 mg if 3–4 mmol/L, 90 mg if >4 mmol/L, maximum infusion rate of 60 mg/h, maximum dose per treatment of 90 mg

MONITOR

- postural BP/urine output
- CVP if severe dehydration, systolic BP <80 or pre-renal renal failure
- serum electrolytes
  - correct K^+ and Mg^{2+} as indicated
  - both tend to fall as hypercalcaemia is corrected

- *Enhancing calcium uptake into bone/reducing release from bone*

Calcitonin rapidly (i.e. within hours) enhances the net uptake of calcium into bone, but has a limited duration of action (3–4 days) due to the development of resistance. Bisphosphonates are especially useful for longer lasting reduction of hypercalcaemia, particularly that associated with bony metastatic malignancy. However, their action is often delayed for 24 h or more, so they should be used in conjunction with other measures during the initial period.

- *Reducing absorption of calcium from the gut*

Steroids are effective at reducing the absorption of calcium from the gut and are particularly good at treating hypercalcaemia associated with granulomatous disease, where abnormal metabolism of vitamin D contributes to increased calcium absorption (i.e. in sarcoidosis or vitamin D intoxication), or hypercalcaemia due to haematologic or lymphoid malignancy (e.g. multiple myeloma). However, the maximum effect of steroid therapy usually takes a week or so. Other treatments that are effective at reducing serum calcium, but not routinely used in patients with renal failure, include mithramycin, gallium nitrate and oral phosphate.

(3) Acute Renal Failure Associated with Hypophosphataemia

There are two particular circumstances (both rare) where ARF may be associated with hypophosphataemia.

These are:

(a) Rhabdomyolysis. Although rhabdomyolysis is typically associated with hyperphosphataemia due to PO_4^{2-} release from damaged muscle, profound hypophosphataemia (<0.48 mmol/L) may in itself predispose to muscle necrosis, rhabdomyolysis and myoglobinuric ARF. A typical patient is usually an alcoholic with phosphate deficiency and a pre-existing myopathy. The hypophosphataemia can develop after IV glucose administration. Rhabdomyolysis is discussed in detail in **Chapter 12**.

(b) Following intravenous infusion of large doses of fructose or xylitol, which cause uncontrolled utilisation of intracellular phosphate (ATP), lactic acidosis, and acute hepatic and renal injury.

In both these situations, plasma hypophosphataemia may be masked by the accompanying ARF.

8.6 Acute Uraemia
Rachel Hilton

DEFINITION

Uraemia literally means urine in blood. The term was defined by Bergstrom as "a toxic syndrome caused by severe glomerular insufficiency associated with disturbances in tubular and endocrine functions of the kidneys. It is characterised by retention of toxic metabolites, derived mainly from protein metabolism, and associated with changes in volume and electrolyte composition of the body fluids and excess or deficiency of various hormones".

PATHOPHYSIOLOGY

Uraemic Toxicity

The clinical manifestations of uraemia are associated with the retention and accumulation of metabolites normally excreted by the kidneys, and are largely relieved by dialysis. At least some "uraemic toxins" are likely to be derived from protein metabolism, since increased protein intake or catabolism accentuates uraemic symptoms, which may be alleviated by protein restriction. However, attempts to identify specific uraemic toxins among the myriad of compounds that accumulate in uraemic blood and tissues have been largely unsuccessful.

Bergstrom and Furst (1983) proposed a number of stringent criteria that a putative uraemic toxin should satisfy:

1. It should be chemically identified and accurately quantifiable in biological fluids.
2. Its concentration in tissue or plasma from uraemic subjects should exceed that present in non-uraemic subjects.
3. Its concentration should correlate with specific uraemic symptoms that disappear when the concentration is reduced to normal.
4. Toxic effects of the compound in a test system should be demonstrable at the concentration found in tissue or fluids from uraemic patients.

Very few substances meet all of these criteria, often for technical reasons.

Compounds that accumulate in uraemic blood and tissues are called uraemic retention solutes, and may be arbitrarily subdivided according to their molecular weight. Substances with a low molecular weight of up to 300 Da are readily dialysable, and these include urea (MW 60 Da) and creatinine (MW 113 Da). Middle molecules with a molecular weight of 300–15,000 Da are poorly dialysable, and these include parathyroid hormone (MW 9,424 Da) and β_2-microglobulin (MW 11,818 Da). Large molecular weight substances (MW >15,000 Da), such as myoglobin, are non-dialysable. Factors other than molecular weight may also affect the ease of removal of a substance by dialysis, including electrostatic charge, steric configuration, degree of protein binding and compartmentalisation.

Small Molecules

The strongest case for the role of low molecular weight solutes in uraemia comes from the repeated observation that symptoms promptly abate upon initiation of dialysis. Although the following sections emphasise the role of organic retention compounds, it should not be forgotten that water and various inorganic ions, such as H^+, Na^+, K^+, Mg^{2+}, Al^{3+} and PO_4^{2-}, may also cause toxic and even life-threatening effects if not adequately controlled.

Urea

Urea is the principal end product of protein metabolism, its rate of excretion correlating with the protein catabolic rate and therefore, in the metabolically stable patient, with protein intake. The role of urea as a uraemia toxin has been extensively explored. In one classic study it was demonstrated that dialysis against dialysate containing high urea concentrations worsens uraemic symptoms. Urea can also be shown to have a number of toxic effects *in vitro*, such as inhibition of the red cell NaK2Cl co-transport system, decreased cellular cAMP production, and inhibition of inducible nitric oxide synthase and apoptosis in macrophages. In most of these models, however, the development of toxic effects requires urea concentrations well above those that would be observed in clinical practice. It is not yet clear, therefore, to what extent urea may itself contribute to uraemic toxicity as opposed to serving as a mirror for the retention of other, as yet unidentified, low molecular weight toxic substances.

Nevertheless, urea is unequivocally recognised as a useful marker of uraemic solute retention. A direct correlation can be observed between urea kinetics and morbidity in patients undergoing dialysis, as both urea clearance and the time average concentration of urea in the plasma of patients on dialysis have been correlated with patient outcome in well-designed clinical studies. Urea clearance is now widely used for quantifying the dose of dialysis.

Guanidines

The guanidines are structural metabolites of arginine, synthesised in the liver, and include such uraemic retention solutes as creatinine and methylguanidine. Creatinine is a water-soluble metabolite of creatine and a precursor of methylguanidine. Although creatinine progressively accumulates in renal failure, and *in vitro* has been shown to block chloride channels and to reduce myocardial cell contractility, there is no convincing evidence of its toxicity at concentrations encountered in clinical practice.

Other guanidines have been postulated to have a role in the uraemic syndrome, including methylguanidine and guanidinosuccinic acid, which are present in uraemic sera at levels that are toxic *in vitro*. They have a variety of effects, including suppression of the natural killer cell response to interleukin 2 and inhibition of neutrophil superoxide production.

Arginine is a precursor in the synthesis of nitric oxide, which is an endogenous vasodilator and mediator of cell signalling in macrophages and other cells. Some guanidine compounds, as arginine analogues, are strong competitive inhibitors of nitric oxide production, the most specific of these being asymmetric dimethylarginine (ADMA). This compound is present at significantly increased levels in uraemia, and has been implicated in the development of hypertension.

Other small molecules

Several other groups of small molecular weight compounds have been proposed as uraemic toxins, and these are shown in **Table 15**. Some of these are derived from naturally occurring amino acids by the action of intestinal bacteria. Although many of these compounds can be shown to interfere with biochemical and metabolic processes, toxic effects are, with few exceptions, generally observed at higher concentrations than those found in uraemic sera.

Middle Molecules

It has long been observed that the severity of uraemic symptoms correlates poorly with urea and creatinine concentrations, particularly in patients who are treated with peritoneal dialysis. These patients have fewer uraemic symptoms, and it has also been claimed that they are at less risk than haemodialysis patients for the development of peripheral neuropathy, despite lower clearance of small molecules. Such observations led to the hypothesis that this manifestation of uraemic toxicity relates to the accumulation of higher molecular weight substances, which are more readily cleared by peritoneal dialysis than by haemodialysis, probably because of the greater permeability of the peritoneal membrane.

Table 15. Major uraemic retention products and their main toxic effects (from Vanholder, 1997)

Urea	Inhibition of red cell NaK2Cl co-transport
	Decreased cAMP production
	Increased 2,3-DPG binding to haemoglobin
	Inhibition of macrophage inducible nitric oxide synthase
Creatinine	Chloride channel blockade
	Reduced contractility of myocardial cells
Guanidines	Inhibition of natural killer cells
	Inhibition of neutrophil superoxide production
	Induction of seizures
	Inhibition of nitric oxide synthesis
Nitric oxide	Hypotension
	Uraemic bleeding
Aliphatic and aromatic amines	Uraemic encephalopathy
Indoxyl sulphate	Decreased drug-protein binding
	Inhibition of deiodination of thyroxine
Oxalate	Deposition of calcium oxalate in tissues
Parathyroid hormone	Increased cellular calcium uptake
	Interference with various biochemical functions
β_2-microglobulin	Amyloidosis
Polyamines	Inhibition of erythroid colony formation
	Accelerated atherosclerosis
Purines	Disturbance of neurotransmission
	Inhibition of calcitriol production and metabolism
Phenols and indoles	Inhibition of cellular respiration
	Inhibition of phagocytic respiratory burst
Phosphates	Itching
	Hyperparathyroidism
Urofuranic acids	Inhibition of drug-protein binding
	Neurological abnormalities
Homocysteine	Proliferation of vascular smooth muscle
	Enhanced thrombogenicity

The search for these so called middle molecules has led to the identification of several compounds of the appropriate molecular weight (300–15,000 Da) in uraemic sera, but only a few of these compounds have been chemically characterised. β_2-microglobulin, parathyroid hormone and advanced glycosylation end products all conform to the structural definition of middle molecules.

β_2-microglobulin

β_2-microglobulin (MW 11,815 Da) is a component of the HLA class I complex, and is normally excreted by the kidneys when this complex is degraded. β_2-microglobulin therefore accumulates in patients with renal failure and is the major constituent of the amyloid-like deposits present in dialysis-related secondary amyloidosis. This may develop as early as 1–2 years after the initiation of dialysis.

Parathyroid hormone

Parathyroid hormone (PTH, MW ±9,000 Da) is recognised as a major uraemic toxin, although its increase in concentration in renal failure is due to increased secretion rather than decreased renal clearance. Excess PTH causes an increase in intracellular calcium and, in animal models of uraemia, has been implicated in the aetiology of anaemia, platelet dysfunction, encephalopathy, neuropathy, cardiomyopathy, and glucose intolerance. In humans with renal disease, PTH has been causally linked to uraemic neuropathy and to a number of uraemic symptoms, such as pruritus.

Advanced glycosylation end-products

Recently, cross-linked advanced glycosylation end products (AGEs) have been proposed to be uraemic toxins. These are formed by the non-enzymatic reaction of glucose and other reducing sugars with free amino groups, and accumulate in uraemic patients due to a combination of enhanced generation due to oxidative or carbonyl stress and diminished clearance by the kidneys. AGEs retain their reactivity and may subsequently combine with circulating and tissue macromolecules. They have been implicated in the formation of dialysis-associated amyloidosis, can inactivate nitric oxide and can affect the function of the calcitriol receptor. They may also have a role in the vasculopathy and macrophage dysfunction of uraemia.

Large Molecules

The normal kidney can remove molecules up to 40,000 Da in size. Such substances may accumulate in renal failure and are not efficiently removed by dialysis. High-molecular-weight fractions of uraemic plasma ultrafiltrate can inhibit metabolic processes *in vitro*, but few substances have been well characterised.

Cystatin C (MW 13.3 kDa) is a cysteine-protease inhibitor, and Clara cell protein (CC16, MW 15.8 kDa) is a phospholipase A_2-inhibitor protein, with an immunosuppressive role in the respiratory tract. Serum concentrations of both these molecules are elevated in renal failure. Leptin is a 16 kDa plasma protein that suppresses appetite and induces weight loss in mice, and accumulates in renal failure. This has been implicated in the anorexia of uraemia, as there is a reverse correlation in uraemia between leptin and nutritional indices such as serum albumin and lean body mass.

In spite of extensive research into the nature and behaviour of a wide range of compounds having a potential pathophysiological role in the uraemic syndrome, there has so far been little influence on the therapy of uraemia. The identification of toxic substances with clinically significant effects would be of great importance and could have therapeutic implications, with the potential to develop metabolic manipulations, pharmacological therapy or dialysis membranes designed to eliminate specific substances.

Other middle and large molecules

Three proteins with clear inhibitory effects on specific polymorphonuclear cell functions have been characterised by amino acid sequence analysis:

1. Granulocyte inhibiting protein I (GIP I; MW 28,000 Da), inhibits chemotaxis, oxidative metabolism and intracellular bacterial killing.
2. Granulocyte inhibiting protein II (GIP II; MW 9,500 Da), inhibits granulocyte glucose uptake and respiratory burst activity.
3. Degranulatory inhibiting protein (DIP; MW 14,000 Da), inhibits spontaneous and stimulated polymorph degranulation.

CLINICAL PRESENTATION

The uraemic syndrome has a wide spectrum of clinical manifestations, involving many different systems of the body as shown in **Table 16**. The kidney has a substantial reserve capacity and clinical symptoms of renal failure do not generally develop until the GFR is reduced to 15 mL/min or less. **The clinical features of the syndrome are most dramatically manifest in anuric ARF.** Conversely, in patients with chronic renal failure, the onset of uraemic symptoms may be rather insidious, often occurring relatively late in the course of their disease. In such patients the manifestations of severe uraemia should rarely be seen, other than in untreated patients with terminal renal failure.

Gastrointestinal Manifestations

Gastrointestinal manifestations are amongst the earliest and most typical of uraemic symptoms. Anorexia is the earliest symptom, followed by nausea and vomiting, typically in the morning. In more advanced uraemia, stomatitis, oesophagitis, gastritis, colitis and, more seldom, pancreatitis may occur, and gastrointestinal bleeding is not uncommon. Uraemic fetor, with a characteristic urine-like odour to the breath, may occur in association with a bitter or metallic taste in the mouth.

Neurological Manifestations

The development of renal failure may be accompanied by uraemic encephalopathy and, less commonly, peripheral neuropathy, either alone or in combination. Uraemic encephalopathy is a term used to describe the non-specific neurological symptoms of uraemia, which respond to dialysis treatment. Symptoms range from minor cognitive changes to the development of disorientation and coma. In severe uraemia, muscle cramps, fasciculations, twitching or myoclonus may occur.

Table 16. Clinical manifestations of the uraemic syndrome

System	Symptom or complication
Cardiovascular system	Hypertension and left ventricular hypertrophy Accelerated atherosclerosis Congestive cardiac failure, cardiomyopathy Acquired valvular heart disease Pericarditis Dysrhythmias
Respiratory system	Pleural effusion, pulmonary oedema
Gastrointestinal system	Anorexia, nausea and vomiting Stomatitis, oesophagitis, gastritis GI bleeding Ascites
Nervous system	Fatigue Encephalopathy Hiccups Peripheral and autonomic neuropathy Restless legs, myoclonic jerks
Musculoskeletal system	Muscle cramps, proximal myopathy Renal bone disease
Haematology	Anaemia Platelet dysfunction, prolonged bleeding time
Immunology	Increased susceptibility to infection
Endocrinology	Glucose intolerance Impaired insulin metabolism Hyperparathyroidism, defective vitamin D metabolism Growth retardation Sexual dysfunction
Skin	Pruritus Soft tissue calcification and necrosis
Fluid and electrolyte	Peripheral oedema Hyperkalaemia Hyponatraemia Hyperphosphataemia Hypocalcaemia Metabolic acidosis
Miscellaneous	Weight loss Uraemic fetor Hypothermia Altered lipid metabolism

Uraemia is also associated with abnormalities of the peripheral nervous system, most commonly a distal symmetrical mixed motor and sensory neuropathy, usually affecting the lower limbs. This typically occurs in the context of chronic, rather than acute, uraemia. Sensory symptoms, such as paraesthesiae, burning dysaesthesiae and pain, usually precede motor symptoms, which occur at a more advanced stage. Motor dysfunction can lead to muscle atrophy and, ultimately, paralysis. Autonomic dysfunction may occur in up to 50% of patients, manifest as postural hypotension, particularly troublesome during dialysis.

Cardiovascular Manifestations

The majority of uraemic patients retain sodium and water, which may lead to peripheral or pulmonary oedema, hypertension, cardiac failure, pleural effusions and ascites. Other complications include accelerated atherosclerosis, left ventricular hypertrophy and cardiomyopathy. Uraemic pericarditis may occur, causing chest pain with or without a friction rub. In some patients fibrinous pleuritis with pleuritic pain and a pleural rub may coexist with pericarditis.

In experimental uraemia, diminished responsiveness of cardiac α and β receptors has been observed, perhaps related to uraemic autonomic neuropathy. There is decreased diastolic compliance due to myocardial interstitial fibrosis, which is associated with activation of myocardial interstitial cells.

Haematological Complications

Normochromic, normocytic anaemia is extremely common and is due to deficient renal production of erythropoietin. Other contributory factors include gastrointestinal haemorrhage, multiple blood samplings, haematinic deficiency and haemolysis. It has also been postulated that retained uraemic toxins may cause erythropoetin resistance.

Bleeding complications can occur in both acute and chronic renal failure, leading to gastrointestinal or skin haemorrhage and bleeding at sites of surgery and trauma. Spontaneous organ bleeding is unusual. The haemorrhagic tendency defect is multifactorial, and primarily related to a qualitative impairment in platelet function, manifested by a prolonged bleeding time.

Three key pathogenetic factors have been postulated: a circulating toxin that accumulates in uraemia, abnormal prostaglandin metabolism, and anaemia. Platelet function can be restored by incubation in normal, rather than uraemic, serum which supports the concept of a circulating toxin. A possible candidate is nitric oxide, recently implicated as an important mediator of defective coagulation in uraemia. Abnormal prostaglandin metabolism is another potential contributory factor. Some workers have observed reduced platelet synthesis of thromboxane A_2, a potent promoter of platelet aggregation, in uraemia. Alternatively, the pronged bleeding time could reflect an endothelial abnormality; uraemic vascular endothelium releases increased amounts of prostacyclin, which could diminish platelet adhesion to the vascular wall. Finally, anaemia per se may play a role; raising the haematocrit, either by blood transfusion or by the administration of recombinant human erythropoetin, can frequently normalise the bleeding time. This is probably a flow-dependent phenomenon, reflecting the fact that a low haematocrit increases the laminar nature of blood flow, thus diminishing platelet-endothelial interaction. Anaemic patients who have normal renal function may also have prolonged bleeding times.

Musculoskeletal Manifestations

Skeletal abnormalities develop slowly, becoming clinically apparent after some time on dialysis. In the setting of the acute uraemic syndrome this is usually of minor importance. However, if renal recovery is not anticipated, prophylactic measures should be instituted to avoid the otherwise inevitable onset of renal osteodystrophy. Occasionally, severe secondary hyperparathyroidism may present as proximal muscle weakness.

Cutaneous Manifestations

Pruritus and excoriations are common problems in uraemia, and may be intractable. Secondary hyperparathyroidism has been implicated in the aetiology of uraemic itching. The skin becomes dry and atrophic, often with a characteristic "muddy" discoloration, particularly in sun-exposed areas. This is due to an accumulation of β-melanocyte-stimulating hormone, which is normally excreted by the kidneys and is poorly dialysable. Precipitation of urea crystals on the skin, "uraemic frost", is exceptionally rare, except in very severe uraemia.

INVESTIGATIONS

The assessment of a patient with ARF requires a careful history, physical examination and urinalysis, review of previous records and a recent drug history. If the patient is known to have impaired renal function then the diagnosis of uraemia is usually straightforward. Few of the typical symptoms are specific for uraemia, however, and clinical signs and symptoms may not develop until the GFR is reduced to around 15 mL/min or less. Serum urea levels may be used as a crude guide, uraemic symptoms usually becoming apparent when the serum urea rises above 25–30 mmol/L. Patients with diabetes, with smaller body mass and with a rapid rise in blood urea are likely to be more susceptible. Reducing the level of serum urea, either by conservative treatment or by dialysis, usually alleviates uraemic symptoms.

It is of paramount importance to distinguish between acute and chronic renal failure, as the approach to these patients differs greatly. This is not always straightforward. The history is often of great help, whereas physical examination and laboratory tests may be inconclusive. Factors suggestive of chronicity include long duration of symptoms, nocturia, absence of acute illness, presence of anaemia, hyperphosphataemia, hypocalcaemia, neuropathy, band keratopathy, and radiological evidence of renal osteodystrophy. However, it should be noted that anaemia, hyperphosphataemia, and hypocalcaemia may also complicate acute renal failure.

Most chronic renal diseases ultimately lead to reduction of renal size and loss of cortical thickness; renal ultrasonography should therefore be performed in all patients with renal failure to assess kidney size and exclude obstruction. Renal size can, however, be normal or increased in a variety of chronic renal diseases, such as diabetic nephropathy, amyloid and polycystic kidney disease. Renal biopsy may be necessary for diagnosis if renal size is preserved, but it is rarely helpful in patients with small scarred kidneys and is associated with an increased risk of bleeding (see **Chapters 6** and **7**).

COMPLICATIONS

Certain complications are life-threatening and require immediate therapy. Severe fluid retention may lead to congestive heart failure and pulmonary oedema, and requires immediate treatment with loop diuretics (see **Chapter 8.2**). Hyperkalaemia and metabolic acidosis should be diagnosed promptly and corrected. In the presence of acidosis, hyperkalaemia may be treated by correcting acidosis with sodium bicarbonate. Potassium may also be lowered acutely by intravenous insulin and glucose. An ion-exchange resin may then be given orally or rectally to eliminate potassium (see **Chapter 8.3**). Acute dialysis treatment is indicated if fluid, acid-base and electrolyte balances cannot be adequately controlled by the above measures, or for severe uraemia complicated by pericarditis or encephalopathy (see **Chapter 9**).

TREATMENT PRINCIPLES

Correction of Reversible Factors

A number of factors may exacerbate pre-existing renal failure, such as volume depletion, accelerated hypertension, urinary tract infection or obstruction, drugs and toxins such as non-steroidal anti-inflammatory agents, systemic infections and hypercalcaemia (**Table 17**). These factors should be sought and corrected to preserve residual renal function. The volume status should be carefully evaluated in all patients and optimised by administration of appropriate fluid in order to optimise blood pressure, tissue perfusion and GFR (see **Chapters 8.1** and **10**).

Under certain circumstances, protein catabolism may be increased, thus exacerbating uraemic symptoms without affecting the GFR. For example, metabolic acidosis accelerates the rate of muscle protein breakdown. Volume status permitting, sodium bicarbonate should therefore be

Table 17. Potentially reversible causes leading to exacerbation of renal failure or uraemic symptoms

Exacerbation of renal failure	Hypovolaemia
	Hypotension
	Hypertension
	Nephrotoxic agents
	Urinary or systemic infection
	Urinary tract obstruction
Exacerbation of underlying systemic disease	Systemic vasculitis
	Lupus nephritis
Inappropriate diet	Excessive protein
	Inadequate calories
Increased catabolism	Intercurrent infection
	Corticosteroids
Metabolic derangement	Hypercalcaemia
	Acidosis

given to maintain the serum bicarbonate above 22 mmol/L. Other such reversible or avoidable factors include concurrent corticosteroid treatment, intercurrent infection and inadequate energy intake.

Diet

Patients are often highly catabolic and require a high calorie intake (50 kCal/kg body weight). Excessive dietary protein, however, enhances production of nitrogenous waste products and increases uraemia. Restriction of dietary protein can have an important role in management, provided that good nutrition is maintained. The objective of dietary modification in renal failure is to provide sufficient calories to avoid catabolism and starvation ketoacidosis, while minimising production of nitrogenous waste. This is best achieved by restricting dietary protein intake to protein of high biologic value (i.e. rich in essential amino acids) at approximately 0.5 g/kg/day and by providing most calories in the form of carbohydrate (approximately 100 g/day). Potassium-containing foods should be reduced or totally eliminated (see also **Appendix B**).

Dialysis

If the above measures fail to control uraemic features, or if the blood urea rises above 40 mmol/L, dialysis in the form of haemodialysis or peritoneal dialysis should be instituted (see **Chapter 9**). Absolute indications to initiate dialysis are signs of pericarditis, pulmonary oedema not responsive to diuretics, therapy-resistant hyperkalaemia and uraemic encephalopathy.

Correction of Bleeding Tendency

No specific therapy is required in asymptomatic patients. However, attempted correction of the haemostatic defect is indicated in patients who are bleeding or who are being prepared for a surgical procedure, including diagnostic renal biopsy. The therapeutic modalities that are available are shown in **Table 18**.

Table 18. Correction of prolonged bleeding time in uraemia		
Therapy	**Dose**	**Duration of action**
Dialysis	1–2 treatments	Variable
Cryoprecipitate	10 units IV every 12–24 h	8–24 h
DDAVP	0.3 µg/kg IV over 15–30 min in 50 mL N/Saline	4–8 h; tachyphylaxis after 1–2 doses
Blood transfusion/ erythropoietin	To raise haematocrit to >30%	Prolonged if haematocrit remains elevated
Conjugated oestrogens	0.6 mg/kg/day IV for 5 days	Peak action at 5–7 days; duration >2 weeks

Partial or complete correction can be achieved by dialysis in up to two-thirds of patients, probably due to removal of some circulating toxin or toxins. Alternatively, administration of cryoprecipitate probably acts by replenishing a pro-coagulant factor to increase platelet aggregation. Factor VIII:von Willebrand factor complexes (FVIII:vWF) have been implicated, although no quantitative or qualitative defect in FVIII:vWF has been identified in uraemia. These multimers act by increasing platelet adhesion to the vessel wall. Although an efficient mode of correction, the delayed onset of action (8–24 h), the obligate volume of fluid and concerns about transmission of infectious diseases have limited the usefulness of cryoprecipitate. The conventional mode of treatment of uraemic bleeding is the intravenous administration of 1-deamino-8-D-arginine vasopressin (DDAVP), which is a long-acting analogue of antidiuretic hormone. This is thought to act by transiently releasing endogenous stores of large FVIII:vWF multimers from endothelial cells. The effect is maximal within 1 h and lasts 4–8 h, but is of limited use if bleeding is prolonged, since tachyphylaxis occurs after one or two doses, probably due to depletion of endothelial stores of FVIII:vWF multimers. Two other modalities that may be useful are raising the haematocrit to 30%, by blood transfusion or erythropoetin, and the administration of conjugated oestrogens. The effect of conjugated oestrogens is longer acting, with a peak effect at 5–7 days and duration of more than 2 weeks. The mechanism of action is unclear. It is obviously important to discontinue any medications with antiplatelet activity, such as aspirin.

OUTCOME

The mortality rate for ARF approximates 50% and has changed little in the past three decades, in spite of significant advances in supportive care, perhaps reflecting a tendency for more aggressive intervention in an ageing population. Mortality rates are higher in older patients and in those with multiple organ failure. With appropriate management, death is usually a consequence of the primary disease and rarely directly due to uraemia.

FURTHER READING

Oliguria

Allgren RL, Marbury TC, Noor Rahman S, *et al.* (1997) Anaritide in acute tubular necrosis. *The New England Journal of Medicine*; 336: 828–834

Bellomo R, Chapman M, Finfer S, *et al.* (2000) Low-dose dopamine in patients with early renal dysfunction: A placebo-controlled randomised trial. ANZICS Clinical Trials Group. *Lancet*; 356: 2139–2143

Better OS, Rubenstein I, Winaver JM, *et al.* (1997) Mannitol therapy revisited (1940–1997). *Kidney International*; 51: 886–894

Denton MD, Chertow GM, Brady HR (1996) "Renal-dose" dopamine for the treatment of acute renal failure: Scientific rationale, experimental studies and clinical trials. *Kidney International*; 40: 4–14

Edelstein CL, Ling H, Schrier RW (1997) The nature of renal cell injury. *Kidney International*; 51: 1341–1351

Firth JD (1998) The clinical approach to the patient with acute renal failure. In: Davidson AM, Cameron JS, Grunfield J-P, *et al.* (eds.). *Oxford Textbook of Clinical Nephrology* (2nd Edition). Oxford: Oxford University Press; pp. 1557–1582

Glynne PA, Lightstone L (2001) Acute renal failure. *Clinical Medicine*; 1: 266–273

Galley HF (ed.) (1999) Critical care focus. 1: Renal failure. London. BMJ Books
Lieberthal W (1997) Biology of acute renal failure: Therapeutic implications. *Kidney International*; 52: 1102–1115
Star RA (1998) Treatment of acute renal failure. *Kidney International*; 54: 1817–1831

Pulmonary Oedema

Ingram RH, Braunwald E (1992) Pulmonary edema: Cardiogenic and noncardiogenic. In: Braunwald E (ed.). *Heart Disease* (4th Edition). Philadelphia: WB Saunders; pp. 551–568
Leach RM, Bateman NT (1993) Acute oxygen therapy. *British Journal of Hospital Medicine*; 49: 637–644

Acid-Base Disturbances

Brent J, McMartin K, Phillips S, et al. (1999) Fomepizole for the treatment of ethylene glycol poisoning. *The New England Journal of Medicine*; 340: 832–838

Calcium, Phosphate and Magnesium Disturbances

Chan JCM, Gill Jr JR (eds.) (1990) *Kidney Electrolyte Disorders*. New York: Churchill-Livingstone

Acute Uraemia

Alvestrand A, Stenvinkel P (1997) The uraemic syndrome. In: Jamison RL and Wilkinson R (eds.). *Nephrology*. London: Chapman & Hall; pp. 467–477
Bergstrom J (1985) Uraemia is an intoxication. *Kidney International*; 17: S2–S4
Bergstrom J, Furst P (1983) Uraemic toxins. In: Drukker W, Parsons FM, Maher JF (eds.). *Replacement of Renal Function by Dialysis*. Boston MA: Martinus Nijhoff; 354
Ritz E, Stefanski A, Rambausek M (1997) The role of the parathyroid glands in the uraemic syndrome. *American Journal of Kidney Diseases*; 26: 808–813
Teschan PE (1994) Uraemia: An overview. *Seminars in Nephrology*; 14: 199–204
Vanholder R, De Smet R, Hsu C, et al. (1994) Uraemic toxicity: The middle molecule hypothesis revisited. *Seminars in Nephrology*; 14: 205–218
Vanholder R (1997) Uraemic toxins. *Advances in Nephrology*; 26: 143–163
Vanholder R, De Smet R (1999) Pathophysiologic effects of uraemic retention solutes. *Journal of the American Society of Nephrology*; 10: 1815–1823

Chapter 9 _____

RENAL REPLACEMENT THERAPY IN ACUTE RENAL FAILURE

9.1 INDICATIONS FOR RENAL REPLACEMENT THERAPY
Paul Stevens

Acute renal failure (ARF) is characterised by a rapid, potentially reversible decline in renal excretory function occurring over a period of hours or days. The **classical indications** for renal replacement therapy (RRT) therefore revolve around replacing this excretory function until such time as the kidney recovers. Historically, the only 2 techniques widely available have been intermittent haemodialysis (HD) and peritoneal dialysis (PD). The last 20 years however have seen the reinvention of old techniques and a proliferation of new techniques, in particular the development of continuous renal replacement therapy (CRRT). These developments in RRT have opened up a field of **alternative indications (Table 1)**.

Classical Indications for Renal Replacement Therapy

There is good consensus among nephrologists with regard to the classical indications for RRT (**Table 1**). There is less consensus over when to begin RRT. Life-threatening hyperkalaemia and pulmonary oedema in the setting of ARF are clear indications to start RRT, but the level of azotaemia at which to start is controversial. Although uraemic symptoms and complications merit treatment, there is a reluctance to introduce RRT in patients with non-oliguric ARF, partly based on the supposition that the introduction of RRT will result in oliguria and a poorer survival. There has been no study addressing the question of when to start treatment and the question of whether or not early dialysis is deleterious has never been answered. Intuitively, the longer deranged metabolism and volume overload persist the more likely a patient is to develop complications. The author advocates intervention with RRT once ARF has become established, basing this decision on an overall picture of loss of renal excretory function rather than the level of uraemia alone. Experience suggests that early intervention allows better control of fluids and solutes and enables improved nutrition.

Table 1. Classical and alternative indications for renal replacement therapy	
Classical	Hyperkalaemia
	Metabolic acidosis
	Uraemia (encephalopathy, pericarditis, uraemic bleeding)
	Pulmonary oedema
	Hyponatraemia
	Drug overdose/poisoning with dialysable agents
Alternative	Nutritional support
	Cardiac failure
	Acute respiratory distress syndrome
	Hyperthermia
	Sepsis/septic shock
	Pancreatitis
	Hepatic failure

Alternative Indications for Renal Replacement Therapy

These have grown up around the Continuous RRT (CRRT) techniques and are predominantly intensive care based indications (see **Chapter 28**). In the intensive care unit (ICU), RRT should be regarded as part of the organ support system for patients with multi-organ failure, and lends itself to making volume provision for adequate nutrition, treating refractory left ventricular failure and enabling easier correction of electrolyte and acid-base disturbance. Two areas are more controversial, acute respiratory distress syndrome and sepsis.

Acute respiratory distress syndrome (ARDS)

There are 3 potential mechanisms through which RRT may prove beneficial in ARDS:

- Removal of inflammatory mediators.
- Reduction of extravascular lung water.
- Reduction of carbon dioxide formation by deliberate induction of hypothermia.

   Preferential lowering of extravascular lung water with ultrafiltration as compared with diuresis has been demonstrated in ARDS and a trend towards improved outcome (which did not reach statistical significance) has also been reported.

Sepsis

Mediators of the systemic inflammatory response syndrome (SIRS), sepsis and septic shock include a number of middle molecular weight compounds such as TNF, IL-1, IL-6, IL-8, complement and platelet activating factor (PAF). The highly porous synthetic membranes used for CRRT lend themselves to elimination of such compounds through filtration and adsorption (see **Chapter 9.5**). Although substantial removal of cytokines by membrane adsorption and convection has been demonstrated, no prospective studies have indicated that this has any impact on serum cytokine concentrations. Neither have any studies to date shown that removal of these substances has a positive effect on patient survival.

Other indications

Patients with left ventricular failure can respond very well to RRT. In these patients, cardiac failure leads to activation of renal compensatory mechanisms resulting in retention of salt and water and refractory extracellular fluid expansion. Ultrafiltration offloads the ventricle, downregulates the renal compensatory mechanisms and allows diuresis to return in those patients who respond.

In hepatic failure, CRRT is the preferred modality, but patients with hepatorenal syndrome from chronic liver failure should not be treated unless there is a plan for liver transplantation. In those who are treated, dialytic support should be initiated early and aggressively (see **Chapter 25**).

Core temperature reduction can be a side effect of RRT. Cooling has been shown to lead to increased peripheral vascular resistance and less cardiovascular instability with preservation of cardiac output. Previous studies have also shown a reduction in oxygen consumption with deliberate cooling by the use of RRT.

CRITERIA FOR COMMENCING RENAL REPLACEMENT THERAPY

The broader application of RRT to **alternative**, non-renal areas has a small but developing literature. Most applications have still to undergo prospective validation and much of the evidence is still anecdotal. This is not surprising; what is surprising, is that the use of RRT for the **classical** renal indications is almost as anecdotal and there are no scientifically established criteria for the initiation of RRT. Bellomo and Ronco have proposed a set of criteria for initiation of RRT (**Table 2**). They recommend that the presence of one criterion is sufficient to initiate therapy in a critically ill patient, the presence of 2 makes it mandatory.

Table 2. Criteria for initiation of renal replacement therapy	
Oliguria (urine output <200 mL/12h)	Anuria (urine output <50 mL/12h)
Hyperkalaemia (K$^+$ >6.5 mmol/L)	Severe acidosis (pH <7.1)
Uraemia (blood urea >30 mmol/L)	Clinically significant organ oedema
Uraemic encephalopathy	Uraemic pericarditis
Uraemic neuropathy/myopathy	Severe dysnatraemia (Na$^+$ >160 or <115 mmol/L)
Hyperthermia	Drug overdose with a dialysable toxin

From: Bellomo R, Ronco C (1998) Indications and criteria for initiating renal replacement therapy in the intensive care unit. *Kidney International*; 53(S66): 106–109.

9.2 CHOICE OF MODALITY

Paul Stevens

INTRODUCTION

Intermittent HD (IHD) has been available for the treatment of ARF for the last 50 years and peritoneal dialysis (PD) for even longer. PD was the first continuous treatment modality and although the concept of continuous HD dates back to the beginning of the clinical practice of HD, it is only in the last 20 years that the blood-based CRRT techniques have developed and become widely available. With the widespread availability of CRRT, use of PD in ARF has become restricted to situations where low efficiency dialysis is required or where anticoagulation is contraindicated.

There are a plethora of dialysis techniques for the nephrologist to choose from (**Table 3**), and in making the choice, a number of factors have to be considered. These include: *patient factors*, *technique factors* and *survival factors*.

Table 3. Renal replacement therapy modalities	
Intermittent therapies	**Continuous renal replacement therapies**
Intermittent haemodialysis (IHD)	Peritoneal dialysis (PD) — continuous ambulatory peritoneal dialysis (CAPD) — continuous cycling peritoneal dialysis (CCPD) — continuous equilibrium peritoneal dialysis (CEPD)
Intermittent haemofiltration (IHF)	Continuous arteriovenous/venovenous haemofiltration (CAVH/CVVH)
	Continuous arteriovenous/venovenous haemodialysis (CAVHD/CVVHD)
	Continuous arteriovenous/venovenous haemodiafiltration (CAVHDF/CVVHDF)
	Continuous high flux haemodialysis (CHFD)
*Sustained low efficiency dialysis (SLED)	
*Intermittent isovolaemic haemodialysis combined with slow continuous haemofiltration (SCUF)	
*These techniques combine intermittent and continuous features and are associated with good haemodynamic stability.	

PATIENT FACTORS AFFECTING CHOICE OF MODALITY

There may be clear patient contraindications to choice of modality. For example, patients who are hypercatabolic following abdominal surgery are unlikely to be suitable for PD.

The **underlying disease process** and the **indications for dialysis** are therefore important considerations:

1. The Underlying Disease Process and Choice of RRT Modality

Patients with isolated ARF are likely to be cardiovascularly stable and not particularly catabolic. Any form of RRT may be used, but in practice it is logical to use a simple, efficient, cheap intermittent therapy such as IHD. Supervention of other organ failure changes the picture. For example, in cardiovascularly unstable patients, IHD is relatively contraindicated. However, intermittent haemofiltration (IHF) would be well tolerated and has the advantage of retaining simplicity. On the other hand, the coexistence of ARF and cerebral oedema, or ARF in the setting of hepatic failure, makes **any** form of intermittent therapy contraindicated and the choice lies between the different continuous therapies available. Patients with combined renal and respiratory failure are likely to require large volumes of fluid, and tight control of extracellular volume status will aid weaning from ventilation. These patients are also more likely to be cardiovascularly unstable and are best managed with CRRT.

2. The Indications for Dialysis and Choice of RRT Modality

The indications for dialysis are a major factor in choice of modality. If the requirement is for highly efficient rapid solute removal then IHD is the logical choice. In patients with very high urea levels rapid solute removal may be contraindicated and a low efficiency intermittent or continuous technique may be utilised. On the other hand, if the main indication is fluid removal in a cardiovascularly unstable patient then some form of CRRT is the treatment of choice.

3. Location of the Patient and Duration of Treatment

The requirement for patient mobility is also a major consideration in choice of modality. Continuous techniques do not lend themselves to treks around hospital departments for various investigations and interventions. Patients on the ICU are more likely to be treated with CRRT by rote, those on the ordinary ward are more likely to receive IHD, IHF or PD. Choice of modality under these circumstances is strongly influenced by local expertise and availability.

TECHNIQUE FACTORS AFFECTING CHOICE OF MODALITY

The characteristics of the differing techniques make it possible to select that technique most suited to a patient's needs. Considerations include solute and water clearance, complications, and ease of application and cost.

Solute and Water Clearance

Most patients with ARF require a RRT technique that efficiently clears solutes, precluding the use of low efficiency techniques such as PD and unpumped arteriovenous haemofiltration. Although

Table 4. Solute clearance with different dialysis modalities

Technique	Regimen	Urea clearance (mL/min)	Urea clearance (L/day)
Haemodialysis	4 h	160	38
Peritoneal dialysis	4 × 2 L exchanges 1 litre ultrafiltration	6.3	9
CAVH/CVVH	Ultrafiltration rate 500 mL/h	8	11.5
	Ultrafiltration rate 1.3 L/h	22	31.7
CAVHD/CVVHD	Dialysate flow rate 1 L/h Ultrafiltration rate 300 mL/h	22	31.7
CAVHDF/CVVHDF	Dialysate flow rate 1 L/h Ultrafiltration rate 600 mL/h	27	38.9
CHFD	Dialysate flow rate 6 L/h Ultrafiltration rate 200 mL/h	42	60.5

IHD is the most efficient technique, its intermittent nature means that, even when performed on a daily basis, the daily urea clearance of some continuous techniques is at least as good, and in some cases better (**Table 4**). CRRT may therefore control peak urea concentrations better than IHD, despite being less efficient.

A similar issue arises when comparing IHD with CRRT for the treatment of drug overdoses. Plasma levels of drugs which are easily dialysed, but have a large volume of distribution, are rapidly reduced during HD but often rebound after HD. CRRT results in gradual drug elimination — the same daily clearance will allow a greater mass of the drug to be removed and a lower peak level. The optimal RRT modality for substances with a large volume of distribution, which are renally excreted, may therefore be a combination of IHD followed by CRRT.

With all dialysis techniques, the magnitude of the reduction in intravascular volume is related to the rate of ultrafiltration and the rate of plasma refilling. Cardiovascularly unstable patients and those with hypoalbuminaemia, sepsis, multiple organ failure or autonomic dysfunction are more likely to become hypotensive at lower ultrafiltration rates. Removal of a given volume of fluid by IHD performed for 4 h daily (or less frequently) cannot be achieved as readily as by CRRT, where the same volume of fluid can be removed with a net fluid removal rate one-sixth or less than that required with IHD. The greater the patient's intravascular volume excess, the greater the indication for choosing some form of CRRT.

Complications of RRT and Ease of Application

When deciding on the optimal RRT modality, haemodynamic stability is of paramount importance in patients with ARF. There is evidence to suggest that haemodynamic instability delays recovery from ARF. We have found a reduction in the period of dialysis dependence in patients with severe ARF, when changed from pure IHD to a combination of isovolaemic IHD (for solute removal) combined with interdialytic slow continuous ultrafiltration (SCUF) (for fluid removal). This effect was most likely to have been through improved cardiovascular stability. In the treatment of acute liver failure and ARF this becomes even more important because haemodynamic instability adversely influences intracranial pressure (see **Chapter 25**). For the same reasons patients with ARF and brain injury are best managed with CRRT.

A risk of bleeding is a relative contraindication for CRRT employing extracorporeal blood circuits. This may be one indication for PD; IHD with no heparin is also a suitable alternative.

Membranes used in CRRT are of at least intermediate biocompatibility. The influence of biocompatibility on outcome in ARF is still controversial. There are compelling reasons why more biocompatible membranes should confer an advantage but the case for their exclusive use in ARF is far from proven (see **Chapter 9.5**).

Modern blood-based CRRT techniques have the same requirement for machines and trained nursing staff as IHD. Intermittent therapies allow more intensive use of resources in terms of numbers of patients treated, and are less likely to be subject to blood circuit complications than CRRT. IHD is also significantly cheaper, as the dialysers/filters employed in CRRT are more expensive, and CRRT employs the use of pharmacologically prepared dialysis and substitution fluids.

SURVIVAL FACTORS AFFECTING CHOICE OF MODALITY

Many studies have compared patient survival with RRT technique. Early studies were retrospective, comparing CRRT with historical controls treated with IHD. When corrected for severity of illness (utilising a "severity of illness" score) some of these studies suggest a survival advantage with CRRT in critically ill patients. These results should be interpreted with caution, as the magnitude of the effect of each scored illness on survival is never accurately reflected. Comparison of mortality with the different RRT techniques can only be through a properly randomised prospective study in which the only difference between treatment groups is the modality of dialysis. Correction must also be made for the dose of *delivered* dialysis. The sample size required to demonstrate a difference in mortality, from choice of modality alone, would be very high. There are difficulties too with using overall mortality as the end-point as it is entirely possible that a survival benefit may be confined to subgroups of patients such as those with haemodynamic instability and those with acute liver failure. Audit of the gradual introduction of CRRT to one ICU in the United Kingdom saw survival from combined renal and respiratory failure rise from 25% with IHD during 1983–1984, to 48% with isovolaemic haemodialysis combined with SCUF between 1984–1986, and to 54% with CAVHD from 1986–1988 — uncontrolled but thought-provoking data.

RECOMMENDED CHOICE OF MODALITY

The first considerations are the availability of the technique and the local expertise. The particular indication for treatment together with the complexity of the patient then combine to dictate the choice of treatment (**Table 5**). An important point is that this may change with the patient's situation, emphasising the need for therapy to be tailored to the individual patient's needs.

Table 5. Choice of renal replacement modality

Indication	Clinical condition	Suggested modality
Uncomplicated ARF	Stable, non-catabolic Stable, catabolic	Haemodialysis, peritoneal dialysis Haemodialysis
ARF & fluid overload	Stable Unstable	Haemodialysis, CRRT CRRT
ARF & raised intracranial pressure	Stable and unstable	CRRT
ARF & respiratory failure	Stable Unstable	Haemodialysis, CRRT CRRT
Septic shock		CRRT
ARDS	Stable and unstable	CRRT
Electrolyte abnormalities		Haemodialysis, CRRT
Drug overdose/poisoning		Haemodialysis and/or CRRT

9.3 ACUTE HAEMODIALYSIS

Paul Stevens

INTRODUCTION

In 1913, Abel and his colleagues predicted the use of dialysis for the treatment of ARF after successfully removing salicylate from dogs by using a device to circulate blood through collodion tubes surrounded by a jacket filled with normal saline. However, it was not until Kolff and Berk introduced and used the first practical artificial kidney in 1944 that this prediction became reality. The impact of the availability of dialysis was graphically demonstrated during the Korean War in 1952. Mortality from traumatic ARF was reduced from 91% to 65% with the introduction of dialysis, allowing Teschan to observe that "ARF was a wasting disease, often complicated by infections, poor wound healing, bleeding and anaemia". Although comparative results from civilian practice were less impressive, nevertheless the introduction of dialysis dramatically reduced the proportion of ARF patients dying of renal causes.

Although many aspects of acute HD have since become widely accepted, anecdotal practice has enjoyed a free reign in this area of nephrology, and controversy still exists. This section reviews the basic principles of HD, considers some of the controversial areas, including dialysis prescription and choice of membrane, and discusses anticoagulation for HD and the complications of HD.

BASIC PRINCIPLES OF HAEMODIALYSIS

The aims of HD are solute and water removal, and correction of electrolyte abnormalities and acid-base disturbance. These aims are accomplished by a combination of diffusive and convective processes taking place simultaneously within the artificial kidney.

The Haemodialysis Circuit (Figure 1)

The major components of the HD circuit include the patient, circulatory access, connecting lines to the artificial kidney (dialyser), and a dialysate delivery system. The dialyser is a membrane separation device allowing transfer of solute and water between blood and dialysate (and vice versa). Dialysate, an osmotically balanced solution of electrolytes, dialysis buffer and glucose, is separated from blood by a semi-permeable membrane (SPM). Conventionally, blood and dialysate flow through the dialyser in opposite directions in order to maintain solute concentration gradients between the 2 sides of the membrane throughout its length. Dialysate is generated from a mixture of water and dialysis fluid concentrate (plus or minus bicarbonate depending on the dialysis

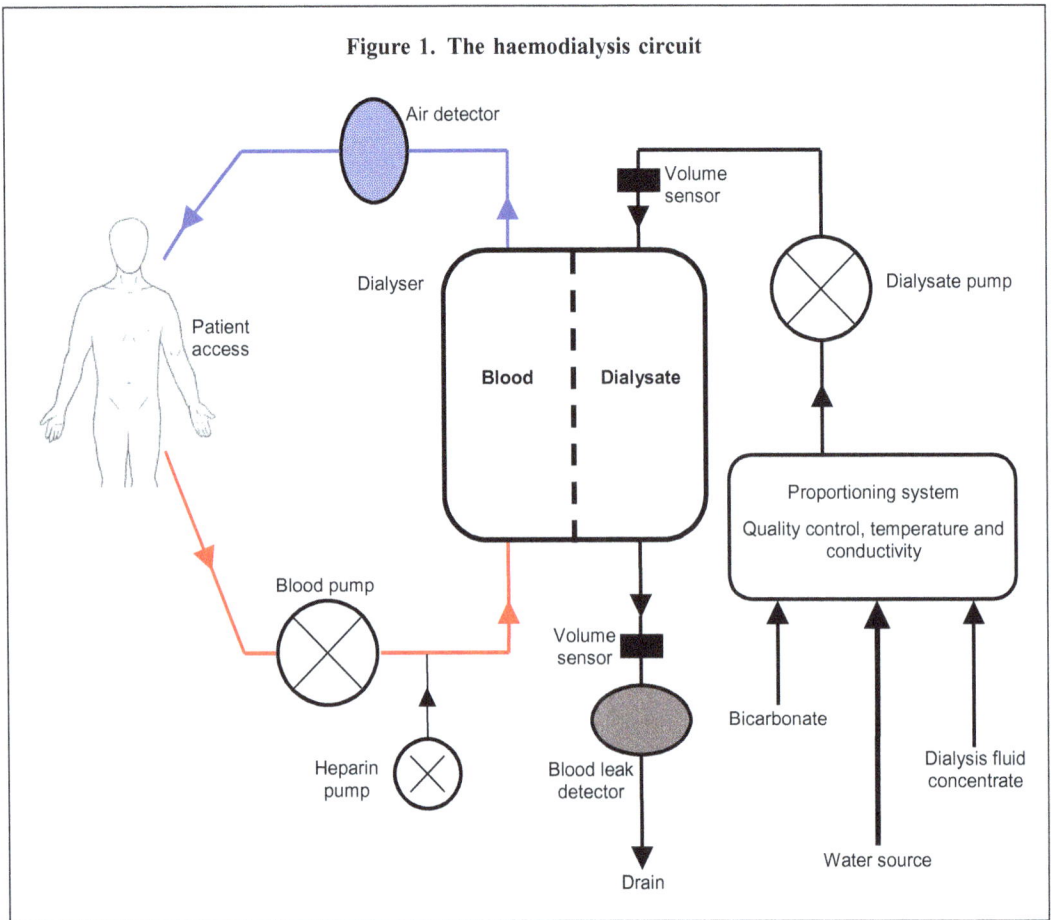

Figure 1. The haemodialysis circuit

buffer selected). Generation of dialysate, the composition of which is designed to resemble plasma water, is controlled by a proportioning system, which also acts to control concentration (conductivity) and temperature within pre-set limits. As blood flows in a laminar fashion over the membrane, waste products of metabolism and ions permeate the membrane. Mass transfer of solute is predominantly dependent on diffusion, but some transfer of solute will also occur in association with water movement (convection). Water transport is usually accomplished through creation of a pressure difference across the membrane (transmembrane pressure or TMP). Water transport will also take place if there is an osmotic pressure difference between blood and dialysate (this underlies the principle of fluid removal in peritoneal dialysis, described in **Chapter 9.4**).

Diffusion

Diffusion describes the movement of solute from an area of high concentration to one of lower concentration. The mass transfer of solute is dependent on its rate of diffusion. In dialysis, this is determined by a number of factors including the characteristics of the solute, the dialysis membrane itself, and the rate of delivery and removal of solute (**Table 6**).

Table 6. Factors governing diffusive solute transport in haemodialysis	
Solute factors	Membrane factors
• Size	• Type
• Charge	• Porosity and thickness
• Protein binding	• Surface area
Rate of solute delivery (blood flow) and rate of removal (dialysate flow)	Duration of dialysis
• Concentration gradient between blood and dialysate	

Convection

Convection describes the bulk movement of water and solute to produce an ultrafiltrate of plasma, solute being dragged across the membrane by the movement of water. The ease with which solute is dragged across a given membrane is described by its sieving coefficient — the ratio of its concentration in ultrafiltrate to its concentration in plasma (see also **Chapter 9.5**). Positive pressure in the blood compartment of the dialyser, together with negative pressure suction to the dialysate compartment, establishes the transmembrane pressure (TMP), which is the driving force for ultrafiltration (UF). Formation of ultrafiltrate is also dependent on solute and membrane characteristics (**Table 7**). The relative contribution of convection to solute removal during HD varies with the molecular weight of the solute and the rate of UF. The larger a molecule is, the greater the contribution of convection to its overall clearance.

Table 7. Factors governing convective solute transport in haemodialysis

Sieving coefficient of solute
- Size of solute
- Solute charge
- Protein binding

Transmembrane pressure
- Blood flow rate
- Oncotic pressure
- Negative hydrostatic pressure (dialysate compartment)

Membrane factors
- Type of membrane
- Water permeability
- Surface area

Duration of treatment
Concentration of solute in blood

Figure 2. Schematic representation of dialysis

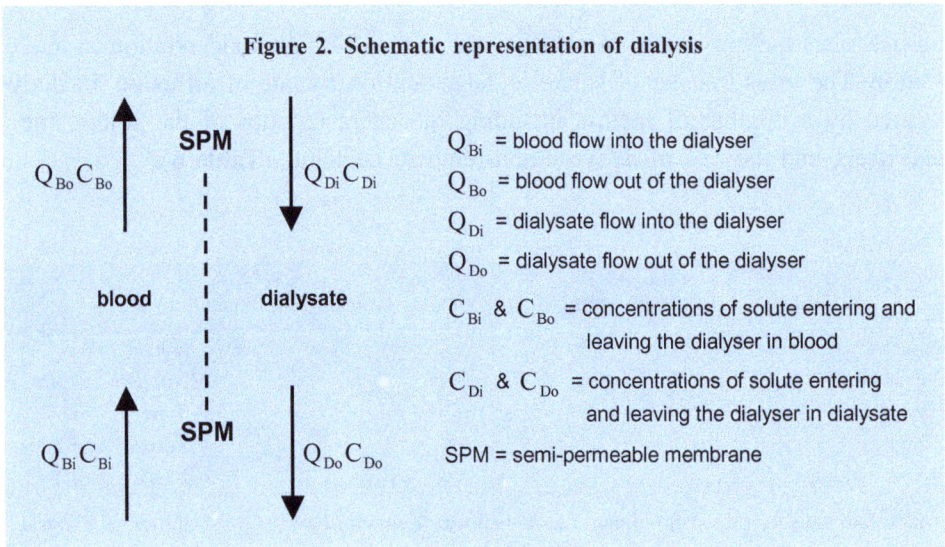

Q_{Bi} = blood flow into the dialyser
Q_{Bo} = blood flow out of the dialyser
Q_{Di} = dialysate flow into the dialyser
Q_{Do} = dialysate flow out of the dialyser
C_{Bi} & C_{Bo} = concentrations of solute entering and leaving the dialyser in blood
C_{Di} & C_{Do} = concentrations of solute entering and leaving the dialyser in dialysate
SPM = semi-permeable membrane

Clearance

The overall clearance of a solute by dialysis is equal to the sum of its diffusive and convective clearance. For any given dialyser this will depend on blood and dialysate flow rates, the ultra-filtration rate, and the concentrations of solute in blood and dialysate (**Figure 2**).

For simplification, it can be assumed that the total amount of solute entering the dialyser equals the amount leaving. Solute entering and leaving the dialyser in blood or dialysate is a product of its respective concentration and flow rate. It follows that

$$Q_{Bi}C_{Bi} + Q_{Di}C_{Di} = Q_{Bo}C_{Bo} + Q_{Do}C_{Do} \qquad (1)$$

also

$$Q_{Bo} = Q_{Bi} - Q_{UF} \text{ and } Q_{Do} = Q_{Di} + Q_{UF}$$

therefore

$$Q_{Bi}C_{Bi} + Q_{Di}C_{Di} = (Q_{Bi} - Q_{UF})C_{Bo} + (Q_{Di} + Q_{UF})C_{Do} \tag{2}$$

Equation (2) can be rewritten in terms of the solute flux attributable to diffusion plus the solute flux attributable to convection. Again the amount of solute leaving the blood compartment is assumed to equal that entering the dialysate compartment, thus

$$Q_{Bi}(C_{Bi} - C_{Bo}) + Q_{UF}C_{Bo} = Q_{Di}(C_{Do} - C_{Di}) + Q_{UF}C_{Do} \tag{3}$$

The left-hand side of **Equation (3)** is the net solute flux from blood, which if divided by the concentration gradient will give the net solute clearance from the blood compartment, thus

$$\text{Clearance (from blood)} = \frac{Q_{Bi}(C_{Bi} - C_{Bo})}{(C_{Bi} - C_{Di})} + \frac{Q_{UF}C_{Bo}}{(C_{Bi} - C_{Di})} \tag{4}$$

It can be seen that in the absence of UF, solute clearance becomes proportional to blood flow, and for small solutes (molecular weight up to 300 Daltons — see **Table 8**) this is a linear relationship up to blood flows of 200 mL/min (**Figure 3**).

The right hand side of **Equation (3)** is the net flux of solute into the dialysate; when divided by the concentration gradient, the net solute clearance into the dialysate compartment is expressed by

$$\text{Clearance (into dialysate)} = \frac{Q_{Di}(C_{Do} - C_{Di})}{(C_{Bi} - C_{Di})} + \frac{Q_{UF}C_{Do}}{(C_{Bi} - C_{Di})} \tag{5}$$

In the absence of UF, solute clearance is proportional to dialysate flow, a relationship which is linear up to dialysate flows of 500 mL/min.

Table 8. Sizes of molecules and mode of clearance in haemodialysis		
	Molecular weight (Daltons)	**Mode of solute clearance**
Small solutes Urea, creatinine, electrolytes Bicarbonate, phosphate, oxalate, homocysteine	<300	Diffusion
Middle molecules Vitamin B_{12}, inulin, lipid A, Advanced glycosylation end-products, β_2-microglobulin, PTH, leukotrienes, Thromboxane, prostaglandins, PAF, Ubiquitin, vancomycin	300–12,000	Diffusion Convection
Large molecules Tumour necrosis factor, interleukins	12,000–50,000	Convection (Adsorption)

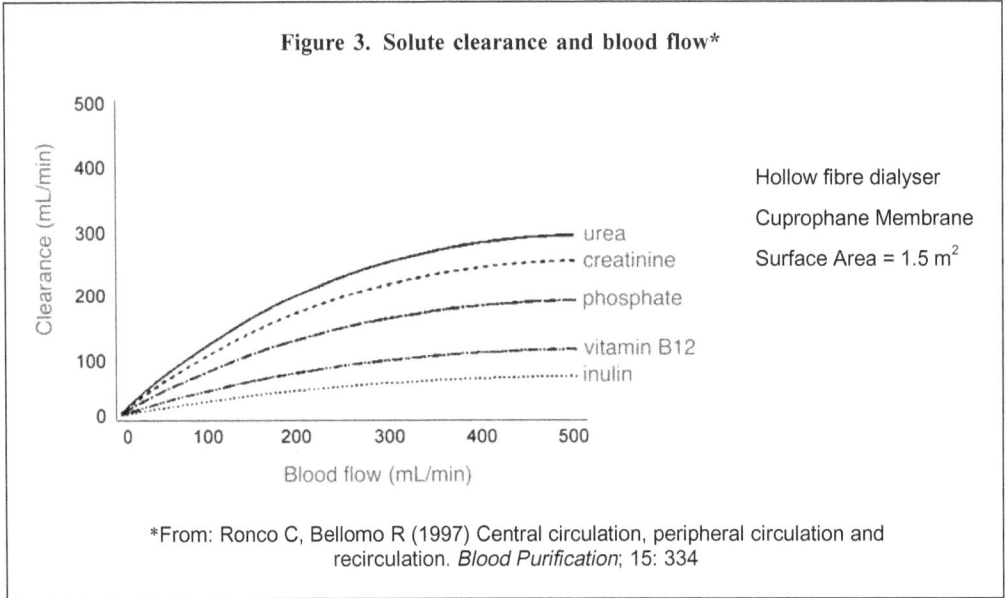

Figure 3. Solute clearance and blood flow*

Hollow fibre dialyser

Cuprophane Membrane

Surface Area = 1.5 m^2

urea
creatinine
phosphate
vitamin B12
inulin

*From: Ronco C, Bellomo R (1997) Central circulation, peripheral circulation and recirculation. *Blood Purification*; 15: 334

Ultrafiltration (see also **Chapter 9.5**)

Ultrafiltration (UF) is the process by which fluid is removed during HD. Every dialyser has a membrane UF coefficient (K_m) which is a reflection of membrane surface area and membrane porosity. The total UF volume during a period of dialysis is therefore determined by:

$$\text{Ultrafiltration volume (mL)} = K_m \times TMP \times t$$

which gives

$$Q_f \text{ (mL/h)} = K_m \times TMP$$

where Q_f is the UF rate (mL/h), K_m is the membrane UF coefficient (derived from the ratio Q_f/TMP and expressed as [(mL/h) $\times$ (m^2/mmHg)]), t is the duration of dialysis in hours and TMP is the transmembrane pressure measured in mm Hg (derived from $P_b - P_{uf} - \pi$).

P_b is the positive (hydrostatic) pressure in the blood compartment and favours UF

P_{uf} is the hydrostatic pressure in the dialysate compartment; it is a negative pressure and thus favours UF

π is the oncotic pressure in the blood compartment and opposes UF

   The main purpose of UF in dialysis is the therapeutic removal of fluid, both to treat fluid overload and to make room for hyperalimentation and drug administration. Modern HD machines are volumetrically controlled (see **Figure 1**), allowing tight control of UF rates; this is an important consideration, as modern membranes have high hydraulic (water) permeability. The TMP during dialysis is automatically adjusted to achieve the desired UF rate. The total volume of ultrafiltrate generated during HD is usually small (1–3 L/session) in comparison to haemofiltration techniques (see **Chapter 9.5**), and the contribution of convective removal to small solute clearance in HD is therefore minimal. One exception to this is in the use of acetate free biofiltration, in which there is a significant convective component. This HD technique associates diffusive removal of solute with a higher UF rate of 5 to 8 L/session (to allow for post-dialyser reinfusion of a bicarbonate solution).

DIALYSERS, MEMBRANES, BIOCOMPATIBILITY & DIALYSATE

Dialysers in clinical use are either hollow fibre in structure (the most common) or flat plate. The structure has altered very little over the years although changes and improvements have been made in the manufacturing process, the geometry and structure of the membrane, and the sterilisation process. These changes have been driven by the continuing search for more efficient methods of dialysis, by the requirements of biocompatibility and by the perceived need to remove middle molecules.

Dialyser Structure

Both hollow fibre and flat plate dialysers consist of a polyurethane shell surrounding an arrangement of hollow fibres or parallel plates suspended in dialysate. Hollow fibre dialysers contain bundles of thousands of fibres similar in structure to capillaries, each fibre having an internal diameter varying between 175–250 µm, depending on the requirements of the RRT technique. In parallel plate dialysers each membrane sheet is laid on top of the other; blood and dialysate flow in parallel but separate compartments between the sheets.

Two important considerations are the priming volume and the membrane surface area. Higher membrane surface areas are desirable but lead to higher priming volumes and thus a greater risk of haemodynamic instability. Priming volumes vary between 60–120 mL, to which dialysis lines add a further 100–150 mL, resulting in a total priming volume of 160–370 mL, an important practical consideration in patients with ARF. Hollow fibre dialysers allow a better compromise between priming volume and membrane surface area than flat plate dialysers. Dialysers with higher surface areas generally have higher urea clearances but urea clearance is also dependent on the porosity and thickness of the dialyser membrane. In ARF, dialysers with urea clearances of less than 300 mL/min are generally used to ensure that rates of solute flux are not too high (see **Complications of acute HD**).

Dialysis Membranes and Biocompatibility

Dialysis membranes may be broadly divided into 4 categories: *cellulose, substituted cellulose, cellulosynthetic* and *synthetic* (see **Table 9**).

The various different membranes have differing biocompatibility (**Table 10**). The word biocompatibility derives from the Greek *bios*, meaning life, and the Latin *compatibilis*, meaning mutually tolerant of. In relation to HD, biocompatibility describes the interactions between blood and the various components of the dialysis process, and thus encompasses blood-dialyser and line interactions, anticoagulation, dialysate composition, and sterilisation procedures. Membranes represent the largest area of contact with blood and are therefore the most important aspect of biocompatibility.

Table 9. Membranes used in dialysers for haemodialysis

Membrane category	Membrane
Cellulose	Cuprophane
Substituted cellulose (surface hydroxyl groups substituted with acetate)	Cellulose acetate Cellulose diacetate Cellulose triacetate
Cellulosynthetic (surface hydroxyl groups substituted with diethylaminoethyl)	Hemophan
Synthetic	Polysulfone Polyamide Polyacrylonitrile (PAN) Polymethylmethacrylate (PMMA) Ethylvinylalcohol copolymer (EVAL)

Table 10. Biocompatibility of membranes used in clinical practice

Membrane	Reduction in WBC (%)	Peak level of C3a (ng/mL)
Cuprophane ETO sterilised	66	7,039
Cuprophane steam sterilised	60	4,667
Polycarbonate	41	1,577
Ethylvinylalcohol copolymer	52	3,785
Cellulose acetate	39	2,690
Hemophan	20	2,252
Polysulfone	10	1,205
PMMA	8	814
PAN flat plate	10	415
PAN hollow fibre	10	230

Redrawn from Schiffl H, Küchle C, Lang SM (1997) Clinical consequences of blood flow-dialyser membrane interactions in ARF. *Blood Purification*; 15: 366–381.

The contact of blood with artificial surfaces leads to a number of important consequences (**Table 11**), the clinical significance of which is a continuing source of controversy. Observations in experimental models suggest that the use of more biocompatible membranes would improve survival from ARF and reduce the period of dialysis dependence. Similar results have been reported from studies in human ARF, which suggest that dialysis with more biocompatible (synthetic) membranes in comparison with cuprophane reduces the period of dialysis dependence, reduces catabolism, is associated with fewer infective complications during the period of ARF, and results in improved survival. Other studies, however, found no difference in outcome between

Table 11. Consequences of blood contact with artificial surfaces

1. Humoral consequences	Comments
Activation of the kallikrein-kininogen system	
Activation of the coagulation cascade and activation of platelets	$\Rightarrow$ thrombin generation, thrombin formation and dialyser clotting
Complement activation via the alternative pathway	Extent determined by: • binding of regulatory proteins — factor B promotes activation — factor H inhibits activation — factor D modulates factor B • design of the dialyser • heparin dosage • host factors

2. Cellular consequences	Comments
Mast cells	Histamine release
Monocytes	$\uparrow$ transcription of IL-1 & TNF Up-regulation of adhesion receptors Elaboration of reactive oxygen species
Neutrophils	Transient pulmonary sequestration De-granulation & release of enzymes Elaboration of reactive oxygen species Up-regulation of adhesion receptors

the 2 types of membrane, supporting the view that the severity of the underlying disorder (and perhaps also the skill of the centre) outweighs the importance of dialyser membrane bioincompatibility in the prognosis of ARF.

A fascinating experimental development in membrane technology, which may have future applications in human ARF, is the tissue-engineered kidney. This utilises porcine renal proximal tubule cells grown as confluent monolayers along the inner surface of polysulfone hollow fibres — the bioartificial renal tubule assist device. The combination of this device connected in series with a synthetic haemofilter has been shown successfully to replace the filtration, transport, metabolic, and endocrinological functions of the kidney in acutely uraemic dogs (Humes *et al.*, 1999).

Choice of Dialysate

Dialysate supplied by the proportioning system is produced from a combination of water, dialysis concentrate and bicarbonate. Dialysate flows during HD are generally ≥ 500 mL/min, exposing patients to a significant quantity of water during HD. This water therefore needs to be of high

Table 12. Dialysate composition	
	Concentration (mmol/L)
Sodium	135–155
Potassium	0–4
Calcium	1.25–1.75
Magnesium	0–0.75
Chloride	90–120
Glucose	0–10
Bicarbonate	25–40
or	
Acetate*	30–35

*Not recommended.

biochemical and microbiological quality, particularly as bacterial cell wall fragments such as lipid A are more easily able to backfiltrate across modern HD membranes.

The composition of dialysate (**Table 12**) is monitored by the proportioning system and may be varied within certain limits through adjustment of the machine or by using different strength concentrate, depending on the clinical circumstances and the patient's pre-dialysis biochemistry. The usual choice of buffer is bicarbonate. Acetate buffered haemodialysis is gradually disappearing from clinical practice, particularly in ARF. This stems from observations that accumulation of acetate during HD leads to a number of adverse reactions including peripheral vasodilatation, systemic hypotension, and a decrease in left ventricular function. Loss of carbon dioxide into the dialysate during acetate buffered dialysis is also said to lead to a fall in $PaCO_2$ and a resultant loss of respiratory drive leading to hypoxia.

Acetate-free biofiltration employs a dialysate of similar composition to standard haemodialysis but is totally devoid of acetate (bicarbonate buffered dialysate still contains 3 mmol/L of acetate). Reinfusion of sodium bicarbonate solution (166 mmol/L) post-dialyser is employed to replace bicarbonate and correct acidosis.

ANTICOAGULATION IN ACUTE HAEMODIALYSIS

Although subject to the same considerations as anticoagulation in chronic HD, patients with ARF are more likely to suffer from coagulopathies and thrombocytopenia, and are more likely to be subject to surgical and interventional procedures. As with any other extracorporeal circulatory technique, the aim is to anticoagulate the extracorporeal circuit, not the patient. The type of anti-coagulation available ranges from standard heparinisation to no anticoagulant at all (**Table 13**). Choice will be dictated by clinical circumstances, local skills and experience.

Regardless of technique, anticoagulation begins with good dialyser preparation. Meticulous flushing of the dialyser with 2 L of heparinised saline (use 10,000 IU/L), ensuring that all the bubbles are removed and allowing the dialyser to soak in heparinised saline for a few hours, pays dividends in terms of prevention of dialyser clotting. Adequate vascular access is important to ensure good blood flow (see **Chapter 9.6**); lipid infusions during dialysis should be avoided.

Method	Regimen	Advantages	Disadvantages
Standard heparinisation	500–2,000 IU bolus to the dialyser Followed by 5–10 IU/kg/h maintenance	Simplicity of use Easily reversed	Risk of thrombocytopenia
Regional heparinisation	1,000–2,000 IU bolus 5–20 IU/kg/h to arterial side of dialyser with 10–20 mg/h protamine to the venous side	Reduced risk of bleeding	Protamine requirements variable Requires frequent readjustment of heparin/protamine ratio Possibility of rebound bleeding
Low molecular weight heparin	Dalteparin 35 IU/kg bolus Followed by 5–10 IU/kg/h maintenance	Reduced risk of bleeding	Difficult to monitor
Prostacyclin	Start infusion at 2–8 ng/kg/min, systemically 30 min before dialysis and continue during dialysis ± low dose heparin at 2–4 IU/kg/h	Good dialyser patency	Difficult to monitor Short half-life Risk of hypotension and hypoxia Abdominal cramps
Nafamostat mesylate	0.1 mg/kg/h	Good potential	Limited experience
Regional citrate	100–180 mL/h 4% trisodium citrate to arterial side of the dialyser Needs calcium-free dialysate and infusion of 0.5 mL/h 5% calcium chloride to the venous limb	Reduced risk of bleeding Good dialyser patency	Labour intensive Risk of hypocalcaemia Risk of metabolic alkalosis
Saline flush	25–30 mL isotonic saline flush to arterial side of dialyser every 15–30 min	Lowest risk of bleeding	Labour intensive Risk of dialyser clotting

Table 13. Anticoagulation for acute haemodialysis

Heparin

Standard heparinisation

For patients at low risk of bleeding standard heparinisation protocols may be followed. Alternatively, a minimal heparin protocol involving 500 IU boluses to the dialyser every 30 min may be used. Anticoagulation may be monitored at the bedside using activated clotting times, aiming for 200–250 sec (normal 90–140) or 160–180 sec for tight heparinisation. Alternatively, the activated partial thromboplastin time (APTT) may be used, adjusting heparin infusions to maintain the APTT between 35–45 seconds. The risk of haemorrhage increases with the age of the patient, coexistent liver or cardiac failure, poor general condition and a history of recent bleeding. Although bleeding is the major complication, heparin may also cause vascular thrombosis and thrombocytopenia. Heparin binds to platelet factor IV forming an epitope to which antibodies develop. These antibodies are reported to develop in 20–30% of patients, but only 1–3% develop significant thrombocytopenia. However, up to two-thirds of these patients develop thromboembolic sequelae, and patients identified as having heparin-induced thrombocytopaenia should receive no further heparin.

Regional heparinisation

Regional heparinisation has the theoretical advantage of anticoagulation of the HD circuit alone. However, because protamine has a shorter half-life than heparin, rebound anticoagulation may occur. Other side-effects of protamine include anaphylaxis, hypotension, leucopoenia and thrombocytopaenia. Monitoring is labour intensive, requiring frequent adjustment of infusion rates, and unless a centre has good experience it is probably best avoided.

Low molecular weight heparin

Low molecular weight heparins have a more predictable anticoagulant effect and have less impact on platelet function. They are also less likely to cause thrombocytopaenia, but because of cross-reactivity, should not be used in patients who have had heparin-induced thrombocytopaenia. One drawback is that their elimination varies with kidney function, although their use in intermittent HD should not lead to significant accumulation. Dosage should be adjusted to keep anti-factor Xa activity between 0.3–0.6 IU/kg.

Prostacyclin (see also **Chapter 9.5**)

Prostacyclin, with or without low dose heparin, can provide adequate anticoagulation and is particularly useful in patients with coagulopathy and/or thrombocytopaenia. The 2 potential major problems, particularly with higher doses of prostacyclin (>5 ng/kg/min), are hypotension and hypoxia (**Figure 4**). However, prostacyclin has a short half-life and these changes are readily reversible. Patients may also complain of abdominal cramps at higher infusion rates.

Regional citrate anticoagulation

Citrate administered to the arterial limb of the HD circuit binds calcium and prevents clotting. Citrate entering the body is metabolised to bicarbonate releasing the bound calcium thus preventing systemic anticoagulation. In theory therefore, citrate is the ideal agent for anticoagulation of the extracorporeal circuit. Unfortunately, there are a number of problems that offset this. To achieve desired levels of anticoagulation, a substantial quantity of trisodium citrate has to be infused. This in turn may lead to hypernatraemia and metabolic alkalosis (from metabolism of citrate) unless suitable correction is made. To reduce the amount of calcium in the circuit, a calcium-free dialysate must be used together with a post-dialyser infusion of calcium (see also **Chapter 9.5**). Even then, there is a risk of hypocalcaemia in patients unable rapidly to metabolise the citrate load.

Figure 4. Prostacyclin related hypoxia during haemodialysis

Illustrates the short half-life of prostacyclin, arterial oxygen levels recovering within 30 min of cessation of infusion

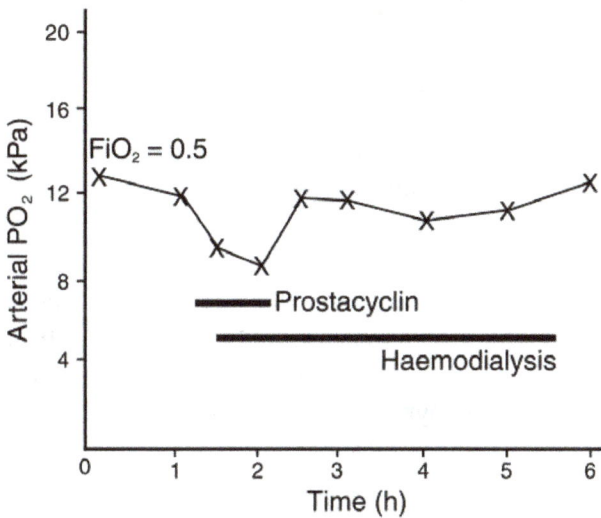

No anticoagulation

An alternative is to use no anticoagulation other than diligent dialyser preparation. Patients at significant risk of bleeding, or those with coagulopathies and/or thrombocytopaenia, may be effectively managed without anticoagulation providing blood flow rates of ≥ 250 mL/min and saline flush protocols are observed. The technique relies on delivering 25–30 mL boluses of isotonic saline to the arterial limb of the circuit every 15–30 min throughout dialysis. Although labour intensive, when properly performed the dialyser clotting rate is only 1–2% making it the method of choice in experienced hands.

Others

Nafamostat mesylate is a serine protease inhibitor and acts on the same factors as antithrombin III. It has a very short half-life which diminishes the risk of systemic anticoagulation. Experience to date is limited. Another inhibitor of thrombin is **Hirudin**, which has no cross reactivity with heparin or low molecular weight heparins, making it an attractive proposition in heparin-induced thrombocytopenia. It is administered as a single bolus at the start of dialysis. Again experience is limited and it has a prolonged half-life in renal failure.

COMPLICATIONS OF ACUTE HAEMODIALYSIS

Complications related to acute HD may be related to the dialysis technique, to the dialysis circuit, or to the dialysis access (see **Chapter 9.6**). Those related to the dialysis circuit include disconnection of dialysis lines, blood leaks secondary to membrane rupture, use of inappropriate dialysate and air embolism. In practice, all of these are uncommon, and are also detected by the monitoring devices included within modern HD machines. Important technique-related complications include hypotension, dialysis dysequilibrium, arrhythmias, effects on nutrition, and bleeding secondary to anticoagulation (see above).

Dialysis-Related Hypotension and Arrhythmias

During dialysis, urea and other small solutes rapidly diffuse into dialysate leading to a fall in plasma osmolality. This results in movement of water from the extracellular compartment into the intracellular compartment. At the same time, UF causes water to move into the dialysate compartment; the resultant fall in plasma volume and failure of plasma refilling leads to hypotension (**Figure 5**). The contribution of solute flux and water flux to dialysis hypotension was beautifully shown by Bergstrom *et al.* (1976). In cardiovascularly unstable chronic HD patients he demonstrated that isolated UF without dialysis conferred haemodynamic stability. Dialysis without UF in the same patients also conferred haemodynamic stability. In practice most patients can tolerate UF rates of up to 0.4 mL/min/kg body weight, particularly if dialysate sodium levels are kept at 140 mmol/L. **With UF rates above 0.4 mL/min/kg the incidence of dialysis hypotension rises exponentially** (Ronco & Bellomo, 1997). Rapid solute and water flux may also contribute to cardiac arrhythmias in patients with myocardial disease. These may be severe enough to result in cessation of dialysis, otherwise the treatment is that of the underlying arrhythmia.

Figure 5. Movement of solute and water during (A) haemodialysis and during (B) isolated ultrafiltration

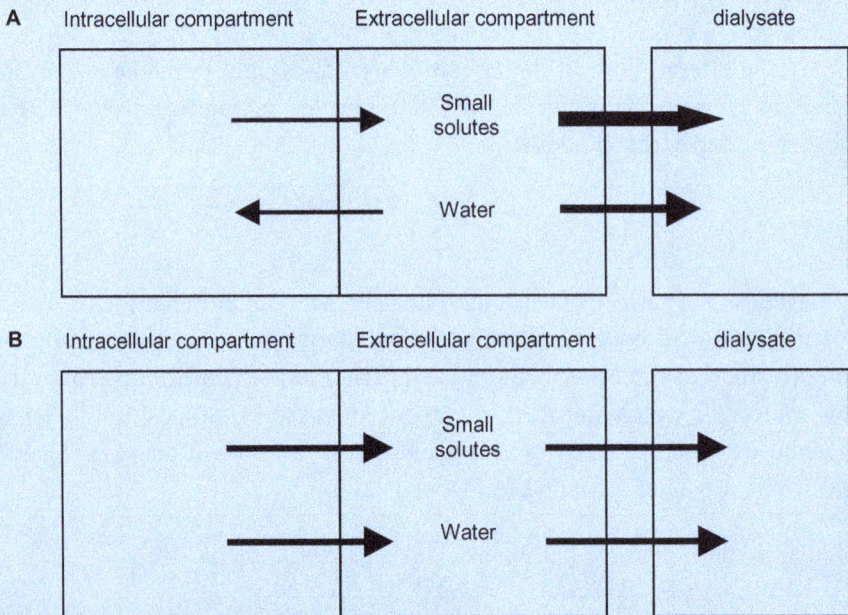

Table 14. Symptoms and signs of dialysis dysequilibrium	
Mild to moderate	Muscle cramps, anorexia, dizziness
	Headache, nausea, disorientation, restlessness, blurred vision, asterixis
Severe	Confusion, seizures, coma, death

Dialysis Dysequilibrium Syndrome

The same solute and water fluxes leading to hypotension during the dialysis process conspire to produce dialysis dysequilibrium. Movement of water into brain cells induces cerebral oedema and the neurological manifestations of dialysis dysequilibrium (**Table 14**). Patients with urea levels of >60 mmol/L are particularly susceptible. Other risk factors include extremes of age, severe metabolic acidosis, and pre-existing cerebral disease. The mainstay of treatment is prevention by gentle frequent dialysis early in the course of the illness. A dialyser with a low urea clearance should be used with blood flow rates of 150 mL/min for only 2 h of dialysis to begin with. Patients with significant fluid overload should be treated by isolated UF *followed* by the short period of dialysis.

Effects on Nutrition (see **Appendix B**)

Effects on nutrition may occur through nutrient losses in dialysis and through the catabolic effect of the dialysis process. Less biocompatible membranes are associated with greater induction of protein catabolism. During HD the average loss of free amino acids has been reported to be 5–8 g/dialysis. An additional 4–5 g of peptide-bound amino acids are also lost, amounting to a total loss of 10–13 g/dialysis. If glucose-free dialysate is used roughly 28 g of glucose is removed during 4 h of dialysis. The addition of glucose to dialysate (11 mmol/L) results in a gain of approximately 23 g of glucose by the patient.

Air Embolism

Although air detection devices in the HD circuit have made this a rare complication, it can also occur through disconnection of central venous catheters and can be fatal unless rapidly diagnosed and treated. The rate and volume of air entering the circulation determine the significance of air embolism. It is estimated that 300–500 mL entering at a rate of 100 mL/sec is a fatal human dose. Symptoms range from none at all to immediate cardiovascular collapse and are dependent on the patient's position. Patients sitting up may lose consciousness and convulse, whilst those lying down may complain of shortness of breath, cough and chest tightness. It should be considered in any patient on HD sustaining sudden cardiorespiratory or neurological dysfunction. Treatment involves clamping the venous line and stopping dialysis. The patient should be placed supine on their left side in the head down position. Oxygen should be given (100% at 10 L/min); it may be necessary to aspirate air from the right ventricle.

DIALYSIS PRESCRIPTION IN ACUTE RENAL FAILURE

Dialysis prescription in ARF encompasses duration and frequency of HD for solute clearance and correction of acid-base and electrolyte disturbances (dialysis adequacy), and control of volume status for prevention of fluid overload and facilitation of nutritional support.

Dialysis Adequacy in ARF

Normal glomerular filtration is of the order of 170–180 L/day, a value we cannot hope to achieve in normal clinical practice with any existing dialysis technique. The question therefore becomes how much dialysis is adequate? In chronic renal failure this has received considerable attention over the years and a clear inverse relationship between dialysis adequacy and morbidity and mortality has been established. Measurement of dialysis adequacy in patients with chronic renal failure has been based on urea kinetic modelling, urea being chosen because it reflects dietary protein intake and protein catabolic rate, and is also a reflection of the efficiency of small solute clearance. Although there are recognised indications for renal replacement therapy in ARF (see **Chapter 9.1**), guidelines for intensity and frequency are anecdotal and practice varies considerably. In the 1970s, it was proposed that keeping blood urea levels below 30 mmol/L would reduce the incidence of uraemic complications (Kleinknecht *et al.*, 1972). This view was challenged in the 1980s by a study showing that keeping urea and creatinine levels at 21 mmol/L and 470 µmol/L respectively between dialyses, compared with patients with corresponding levels of 35 mmol/L and 800 µmol/L, had no effect on mortality and morbidity (Gillum *et al.*, 1986).

In recent years it has been suggested that the development of ARF is itself associated with increased mortality over and above the severity of the underlying illness. Reports have also suggested that survival amongst patients with ARF and comparable severity of illness scores is better in those with higher Kt/V urea levels, rekindling interest in measurement of dialysis adequacy in ARF. These studies suggest that in the absence of a defined target for optimal dialysis in ARF there should be some quantification of the dose of dialysis in these patients, particularly as there is no current consensus on either dose or the method used to assess it.

Kt/V is defined as the dialyser clearance of urea, K (mL/min), multiplied by the duration of dialysis, t (minutes), divided by the volume of distribution of urea in the body, V (mL). The volume of distribution V approximates to total body water and is assumed to be 0.6 × body weight in males and 0.55 × body weight in females. There are inherent problems with measurement of Kt/V in ARF patients and a number of factors need to be taken into consideration when considering measurement of dialysis adequacy in these patients (**Table 15**).

Problems with Measurement of Urea Kinetic Modelling in Acute Renal Failure

Catabolism

In chronic HD it is reasonable to assume that a steady state exists, where urea production equals urea removal. In ARF this is not the case and the extent of protein catabolism differs widely among patients. The amount of protein breakdown is comparatively low in patients without underlying catabolic disorders, such as drug-induced nephrotoxicity, but when ARF is associated

Table 15. Factors influencing interpretation of dialysis adequacy in ARF

Measurement of UKM	Catabolic rate
	Single-pool versus double-pool urea kinetics
	Blood-based versus dialysate-based kinetics
	Total body water in ARF
Prescribed versus delivered dialysis in ARF	Dialyser clotting
	Catheter recirculation
	Early termination of dialysis
	Patient weight

with sepsis, trauma, surgery and shock, catabolism is markedly increased. Biochemically, hypercatabolism is expressed by a disproportionately increased level of blood urea nitrogen and by increased urea nitrogen appearance exceeding 5 g/day, frequently as high as 20–30 g/day. Urea nitrogen appearance equals the sum of daily losses of urea nitrogen plus the change in body urea nitrogen. The practical consequence is an increase in time averaged urea concentration (TAC_{urea}). Knowledge of the TAC_{urea} allows estimation of protein catabolic rate and may be calculated by the following equation:

$$TAC_{urea} = \frac{Td(C_1 + C_2)}{2(Td + Id)} + \frac{Id(C_2 + C_3)}{2(Td + Id)}$$

where C_1 and C_2 are the pre- and post-dialysis urea levels, C_3 is the urea level just prior to the next dialysis, Td is the dialysis time and Id is the interval between dialyses. A TAC_{urea} of 18 mmol/L is roughly equivalent to a Kt/V of 1.2.

Single pool versus double pool urea kinetics

Blood-based calculation of UKM is more accurate when it is based on post-dialysis measurements, which take into account the post-dialysis rebound in blood urea levels — so called double pool urea kinetics. The 30-minute post-dialysis increase in urea level reflects equilibration of urea between tissue and blood; measured Kt/V using single pool urea kinetics in HD is therefore always higher than with double pool urea kinetics. In hypotensive, peripherally vasoconstricted ARF patients receiving inotropic blood pressure support it is likely that changes in regional blood flow ensure that the distribution of urea becomes multicompartmental, making calculation of double pool urea kinetics an oversimplification.

Dialysate-based urea kinetics

More recently interest has focussed on assessing dialysis adequacy in ARF by measuring dialysate-based urea kinetics. This approach measures the amount of urea removed in dialysate during dialysis expressed as a percentage of total body urea, the solute removal or reduction index (SRI):

$$SRI = \frac{100\% \times total\ urea\ in\ dialysate}{pre\text{-}dialysis\ urea \times total\ body\ water}$$

Measurement of SRI relies on accurate measurement of urea in spent dialysate and accurate measurement of dialysate volume but avoids the problems of urea compartmentalisation and of blood recirculation (see below). Evanson *et al.* (1998) found that Kt/V assessed by SRI was significantly lower than single pool and double pool Kt/V.

Total body water

Measurement of Kt/V by SRI still relies on estimates of total body water based on a patient's weight. These estimates are likely to be inaccurate in patients with ARF who often have markedly increased extracellular volume, leading to over estimates of delivered dialysis dose, accentuating the discrepancies between prescribed and delivered dialysis dose.

Prescribed versus Delivered Dialysis in Acute Renal Failure

A number of studies have looked at prescribed dialysis dose versus delivered dialysis dose in ARF. Regardless of whether delivered dialysis dose is assessed by blood-based or dialysate-based urea kinetics, delivered dose has been shown to be 75% or less of that prescribed. Factors implicated include patient weight, catheter recirculation, low flux dialysers, dialyser clotting, and premature termination of dialysis because of hypotension (see **Complications of acute haemodialysis**).

Catheter recirculation (see also **Chapter 9.6**)

Catheter recirculation averages 8–10% but has been shown to vary depending on the access site and the length of catheter. It may be simply evaluated by the low-flow method. At constant flow conditions (usually a blood flow of 200 mL/min or greater) simultaneous samples are taken for urea estimation from the arterial and venous ports of the HD blood lines (A and V); the pump speed is then turned down to 50 mL/min for 30 sec and a further sample is taken from the arterial port (A_1). Blood recirculation may be calculated by

$$Recirculation\ (\%) = \frac{100 \times (A_1 - A)}{(A_1 - V)}$$

In well functioning internal jugular and subclavian lines blood recirculation is only 2–4% but in femoral venous lines this may increase to as much as 22% in the shorter catheters (13.5–15 cm). Longer femoral catheters (19.5–24 cm) have recirculation rates of 10–12%. Catheter recirculation will be increased by reversal of lines (using the "venous" limb of the catheter to take blood and the "arterial" limb to return). Reversed lines increase recirculation in internal jugular and subclavian catheters by up to 12% with a resultant decrease in dialysis delivery.

Patient weight

In studies considering delivered versus prescribed dialysis dose in ARF, multivariate analysis has shown patient weight to be the single most important factor. Statistical modelling suggests that for every 10 kg increase in predialysis weight the chance of delivering a Kt/V of less than 1.2 increases by 1.95 times (Evanson *et al.*, 1998). This is further illustrated by computer-based modelling of dialysis prescription to achieve a desired level of metabolic control, the marker of which is the TAC_{urea} for HD (or steady state urea level for continuous renal replacement therapy). Data from 20 critically ill patients with ARF who received uninterrupted continuous renal replacement therapy for at least 5 days were used to generate blood urea nitrogen versus time curves for simulated patients of varying dry weights. By using urea kinetic modelling, the number of HD sessions per week required to achieve a TAC_{urea} of 21, 28 and 35 mmol/L at varying patient weights was predicted (**Figure 6**). Each HD was assumed to last for 4 h and to provide a urea clearance of 180 mL/min. The model predicted that even with daily HD it would not be possible to achieve a TAC_{urea} of 21 mmol/L in patients over 80 kg body weight.

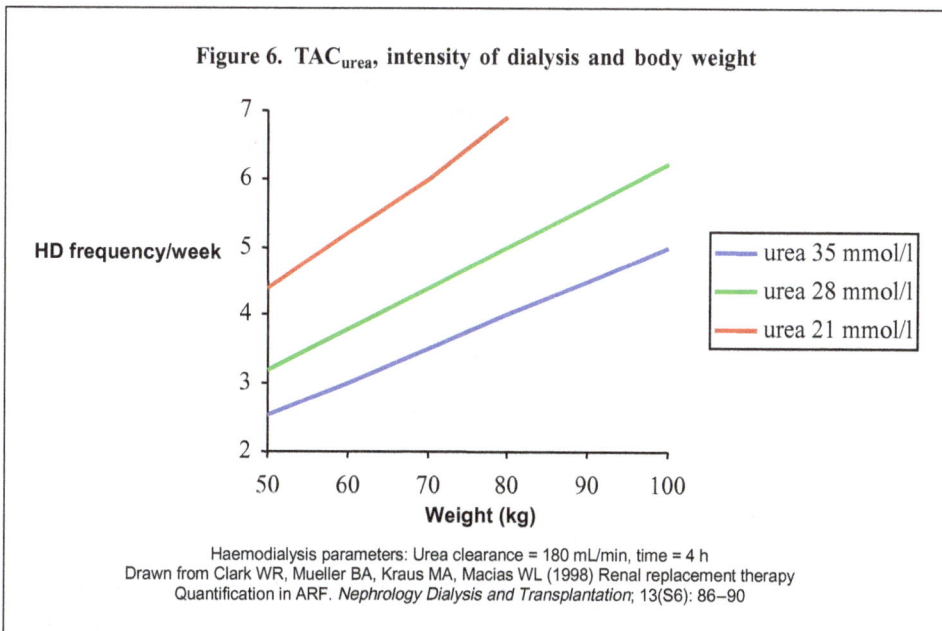

Figure 6. TAC_{urea}, intensity of dialysis and body weight

Haemodialysis parameters: Urea clearance = 180 mL/min, time = 4 h
Drawn from Clark WR, Mueller BA, Kraus MA, Macias WL (1998) Renal replacement therapy Quantification in ARF. *Nephrology Dialysis and Transplantation*; 13(S6): 86–90

Daily versus Intermittent Haemodialysis

In a recent study, Schiffl *et al.* (2002) report that daily intermittent HD is superior to conventional (alternate-day) HD in critically ill patients with ARF and a clinical diagnosis of acute tubule necrosis. Daily HD was associated with better control of plasma urea and creatinine, fewer hypotensive episodes during HD, a lower UF volume during each session, more rapid recovery of renal function, and significantly higher survival rates (28% mortality, 14 days after last HD, versus 46% in conventional HD arm). There was a greater incidence of sepsis, respiratory failure, gastrointestinal bleeding and progression from non-oliguric to oliguric ARF, in the conventional HD group. It should be noted that the delivered dialysis dose in this study was less than that prescribed, predominantly because most of the patients included were hypercatabolic, with high rates of urea generation. Importantly, the mean blood urea nitrogen levels were significantly higher in the alternate-day HD group, which, unsurprisingly, had more uraemic complications than the daily-HD group. This suggests that undertreatment in the conventional HD group may have been a more important factor in outcome than the frequency of dialysis. In addition, it appears that the patients enrolled in this study were less severely ill than those in previous studies that yielded far less impressive outcome data. Nevertheless, there is an increasing body of evidence that suggests alternate day HD is inadequate therapy for patients presenting with ARF.

Practice Point 1. Acute haemodialysis

1. Ensure circulatory access is adequate. Avoid short femoral venous catheters and reversal of lines because of increased recirculation

2. Choose a HD technique suited to a patient's needs. Where available use techniques conferring haemodynamic stability such as acetate free biofiltration or sustained low efficiency dialysis

3. Use a membrane of at least intermediate biocompatibility. Larger patients will require (and tolerate) larger surface area membranes yielding higher urea clearances

4. Remember that the larger the dialyser the greater the priming volume. In patients at risk from haemodynamic instability consider using a 4.5% human albumin solution prime to avoid a sudden drop in blood volume when the patient is connected to the HD circuit

5. Standard heparinisation provides well established, easy to manage, cheap anticoagulation for patients not at risk from bleeding. Choose and become familiar with different types of anticoagulation regimen and their potential problems so that you can easily switch from standard heparinisation to an alternative when the clinical situation dictates

6. Dialysate fluid should be bicarbonate buffered or acetate free. Different dialysis concentrates are available and the choice of dialysate composition should be dictated by a patient's predialysis biochemistry. Dialysate sodium levels of ≥140 mmol/L are associated with less haemodynamic instability. The biochemical composition and microbiological purity of dialysate delivered to the dialyser should be periodically checked

7. Use blood flow rates of 150 mL/min and dialysis times of 2 h with low flux dialysers for the first dialysis, particularly in patients with urea levels of over 50 mmol/L. Blood flow rates may be increased over subsequent dialyses to 200–250 mL/min. Dialysate flow rates of 500 mL/min are adequate for most purposes

8. The duration and frequency of dialyses should be guided by measurement of dialysis adequacy. Evidence suggests that delivered dialysis in ARF is significantly less than prescribed. Recent evidence also suggests that survival may be improved by more intensive dialysis. Aim to achieve a TAC_{urea} of <25 mmol/L. Most catabolic patients will need daily dialysis, usually of at least 4 h duration

9. Ultrafiltration rates of 0.3–0.4 mL/min/kg are generally acceptable, above this the incidence of hypotension increases exponentially. Use isolated ultrafiltration and sequential ultrafiltration and dialysis in haemodynamically unstable patients

10. In patients beginning to recover from ARF, the measured TAC_{urea} will fall and the frequency of dialysis may be reduced

Removal of Fluid with Haemodialysis

Treatment of fluid overload and removal of fluid to make room for nutrition and drug infusions is equally as important as solute removal in ARF but is frequently hampered by haemodynamic instability (see **Complications of HD**). In patients dialysing for the first time, assessment of the amount of fluid to be removed involves rigorous clinical assessment of the patient, guided where feasible by invasive pressure monitoring, and close attention to fluid intake and output charts together with changes in weight (where recorded). Once dialysis has been instituted, patients must be weighed daily to assess interdialytic weight gain. Patients unable to get out of bed should either be managed on weigh-beds or have a weight monitoring system in place under the bed. Although volume management is easier in patients with non-oliguric renal failure the patient must be considered as a whole when making decisions about fluid removal. In those patients with, or at risk from, respiratory failure, removal of fluid should not be influenced by any consideration of preservation of urine output. There are adjuncts available to inform clinical judgement, e.g. on line monitoring of haematocrit, and where present these should be used.

The volume of fluid to be removed and the duration of treatment time will determine the rate of fluid removal desired. The rate of fluid removal achieved will be highly dependent on the haemodynamic stability of the patient but is also influenced by solute removal, as previously discussed. Ultrafiltration rates above 0.3–0.4 mL/min/kg body weight are associated with frequent hypotension during HD. One way to minimise this is to use sequential isolated ultrafiltration and dialysis without ultrafiltration. Alternatively a different dialysis technique such as acetate free biofiltration or sustained low efficiency dialysis (SLED) may be employed. In SLED, dialysis times are extended to ≥8 h because low dialysate flows of only 100 mL/min are employed. Slow removal of solute allows greater haemodynamic stability and increased treatment time allows a lower ultrafiltration rate.

9.4 ACUTE PERITONEAL DIALYSIS
Edwina Brown

Peritoneal dialysis (PD) was often the treatment of choice and/or the only treatment available for the management of ARF in the early days of dialysis. In recent years, with the increased availability of HD and the use of CRRT techniques in intensive care units, PD has fallen out of favour as a means of dialysing patients with ARF. Although acute PD techniques have many disadvantages compared to HD/CRRT, some advantages still remain (**Table 16**).

PD can often be quite temperamental and therefore difficult to establish. Experienced nursing is required in terms of avoiding infection, ensuring good catheter function and knowledge of how to use cycling machines. However, the same is also true of HD, so where the expertise is present, peritoneal dialysis is a useful modality in the treatment of ARF, particularly for patients with poor cardiac function in whom HD could potentially be dangerous. It is also a useful backup if there are restricted HD facilities.

Table 16. PD in acute renal failure	
Advantages	**Disadvantages**
Gentle, slow dialysis thereby minimising risk of disequilibrium syndrome	PD catheters cannot be inserted in patients who are at risk of having multiple intra-abdominal adhesions
Can be done manually (although risk of infection increased cf. to when cycling machine used)	Contraindicated after aortic aneurysm surgery because of risk of infecting graft
Fluid removal very gradual so minimal cardiovascular stress	Cannot be done for first few days after laparotomy because of likelihood of fluid leak
PD can therefore be more safely carried out than HD in patients with poor cardiac function	Impairs movement of diaphragm so relative contraindication in patients on ventilators or with respiratory problems
Can be done in patients with poor vascular access	

PRINCIPLES OF PERITONEAL DIALYSIS

In PD, solute and fluid exchange occurs between peritoneal capillary blood and dialysis solution in the peritoneal cavity. The "membrane" lines this cavity and consists of a vascular wall, interstitium, mesothelium and adjacent fluid films.

Small molecular weight solute transfer occurs according to the physical laws of diffusion, as described in **Chapter 9.3**. Thus if the concentration of substance X is higher in blood than dialysate, movement of X will be from blood to dialysate. However, the longer the dialysate is allowed to dwell in the peritoneum, more X will pass into the dialysate, thereby reducing the concentration gradient and hence the rate of passage of X. The concentration gradient could also be in the other direction. Thus, if Y is more concentrated in dialysate than blood, then movement of Y will be from dialysate to blood.

Fluid movement in PD is determined by osmosis. Thus fluid will move across the peritoneal membrane from the compartment with the lower to that with the higher osmotic pressure. By using this principle, fluid removal in PD is achieved by increasing the osmotic pressure. As discussed later, this is achieved by increasing the dialysate dextrose concentration. This movement of fluid induces a movement of solutes by convection or "solvent drag" in the absence of a concentration gradient. This is important for middle-sized molecular weight solute transfer.

Efficiency of PD, as with HD, depends on:

* total time on dialysis — dependent on the type of PD (see below)
* dwell time of each exchange
* blood flow
* surface area
* permeability of the peritoneal membrane
* dialysate flow
* ultrafiltration rates.

Peritoneal surface area is similar to the surface area of the skin and ranges between 1.7 and 2.0 m^2 in an adult; thickness varies according to the area examined. Effective peritoneal surface for dialysis depends on the blood supply. Blood flow through the peritoneum is not as easily controllable as in HD. The adequacy of PD is reduced when blood flow is reduced in low cardiac output states associated with hypotension and heart failure. In low cardiac output states, less membrane will be perfused, thereby reducing dialysis efficiency. Blood flow through the peritoneal capillaries can be increased by vasodilators. Indeed, use of intravenous or intraperitoneal vasodilators in experimental animals has been shown to increase PD clearances. Their use in patients is limited by hypotension.

Membrane permeability, or effective pore size, depends on ultrastructural differences (and changes over time) in the various components, particularly the capillaries and mesothelium.

Ultrafiltration (UF) is the difference between the volume of dialysate drained out of the peritoneum and the volume infused. By using labelled albumin, it has been shown that the intraperitoneal volume increases rapidly over the first 2 h, before declining. The actual UF rate is governed mainly by the osmotic pressure gradient, which is controlled by osmolar concentration of the dialysate fluid and the membrane permeability. The peritoneal membrane is not a true semipermeable membrane so passage of fluid is not determined entirely by the total number of solute particles on either side of it. Rather, the membrane is partially permeable, so flow is also a function of the number of molecules of large, relatively impermeable solutes. This factor is important for the development of new fluids to achieve UF.

Transfer of fluid from the peritoneum into the vascular tree occurs, as well as the UF into the peritoneal cavity discussed above. Both the peritoneal lymphatics and absorption of fluid across the capillaries according to Starling's forces play a role in the reabsorption of dialysate from the peritoneum. This phenomenon is clinically important. UF rate varies from individual to individual and in some instances can be negative, i.e. the net balance is for dialysate to be retained, particularly during a long dwell.

Different amounts of solute and fluid are transferred with different dwell times of dialysate. This is summarized in **Table 17** — for ease of understanding, two examples of membrane permeability (low and high permeability) are given.

From **Table 17**, it can be seen that PD is more efficient using rapid exchanges with short dwell times for patients with high membrane permeability, and long dwell times for patients with low membrane permeability. Different types of PD have evolved to maximise the efficiency of PD in terms of both solute (clearance) and fluid (ultrafiltration) transfer, and for the social convenience of the patient.

Table 17. Solute (low molecular weight) and water removal during PD using different dwell times

Dwell time	Low permeability membrane	High permeability membrane
Short, 1–2 h	Solute + Water +	Solute ++ Water +++
Medium, 4–6 h	Solute ++ Water +++	Solute +++ Water +
Long, 10–12 h	Solute +++ Water ++	Solute ++++ Water +/−

Intermittent Peritoneal Dialysis (IPD)

IPD was the original form of PD and was developed mainly for the treatment of ARF at a time when HD was not so readily available and continuous haemofiltration had not been developed. IPD is still a useful modality of dialysis in ARF, particularly for patients who are cardiovascularly unstable. It is a "gentle" form of dialysis allowing slow correction of electrolyte imbalances, thereby avoiding problems with disequilibrium.

Dialysis usually takes place for 24 h twice a week (minimum), utilising rapid exchanges each of 1–2 h duration, though a single dialysis episode can be longer to correct fluid overload or major electrolyte abnormalities. The exchanges are usually done via an automatic cycling machine, but they can be (and were historically) done manually. The regimen commonly used is 24 L of dialysate over 24 h with 2 L exchanges of 2 h duration (10 min for running in, 70 min dwell time and 20 min for draining). Smaller volume exchanges (usually 1 L) are used for the first week of a new catheter to avoid leakage of peritoneal fluid through the exit site. Although this regimen maximises ultrafiltration by using short exchanges, solute transfer is rarely sufficient for long term management. Fluid swings between the vascular and peritoneal compartments can be a problem, and dialysis adequacy is usually poor, particularly in catabolic patients. IPD is therefore restricted to being a temporary form of dialysis.

Continuous Ambulatory Peritoneal Dialysis (CAPD) and
Continuous Cycling Peritoneal Dialysis (CCPD)

Other types of PD such as CAPD or CCPD are mainly used for patients maintained on chronic PD. They may be used as part of the management of ARF if the episode is prolonged but are not part of the management of the acute phase. Both require long dwells of full volume exchanges (2–2.5 L) and therefore cannot be performed with a brand new catheter. Furthermore, IPD is the most efficient form of PD in the short term, allowing quicker correction of biochemical abnormalities and fluid overload.

INSERTION OF PERITONEAL DIALYSIS CATHETERS

PD catheters can be inserted either percutaneously, using a Seldinger technique as described in **Practice Point 2**, or surgically. In ARF, the patient is often too sick for a general anaesthetic and the catheter needs to be used immediately or soon after insertion. The catheter is therefore most commonly inserted percutaneously. The complications of PD catheter insertion are detailed in **Table 18**.

PRESCRIBING PERITONEAL DIALYSIS IN ARF

As with HD, the aim of PD is to correct electrolyte abnormalities, normalise the acid-base status, remove nitrogenous waste products, and remove excess fluid. Unlike HD, though, the PD regimens used in ARF are quite different to those used as maintenance dialysis for the

Practice Point 2. Insertion of peritoneal dialysis catheters

Preoperative management prior to insertion of PD catheter

i. Powerful laxative, e.g. sodium picosulfate with magnesium citrate (Picolax®, 1 sachet), should be given the night before catheter insertion — this decreases risk of bowel perforation and eases placing of catheter intraperitoneally. In an emergency, though, this is not always possible

ii. Prophylactic antibiotics should be given approximately 1 h prior to catheter insertion. Traditionally, this has been iv vancomycin, but this should now be avoided to lessen the risk of emergence of vancomycin-resistant bacteria. A recommended alternative is 1.5 g cefuroxime iv

iii. The patient should empty their bladder immediately before catheter insertion or a bladder catheter should be passed (to avoid accidental bladder perforation)

Percutaneous Seldinger insertion technique

This technique is simple to learn, can be done by physicians at the bedside on the ward, and obviates the need for theatre time and general anaesthesia. As the incision site is very small, the catheter can be used immediately with a smaller risk of fluid leak. It is preferable to move the patient to a "clean" room, such as the treatment room, or a room designated for this purpose in the PD unit. The nurse assisting should have experience with PD. Talk through with the patient exactly what will happen at each stage of the procedure — sedation is only mild so patient is often aware of what is going on.

1. The patient should be lying flat with one pillow if possible

2. Give SLOWLY iv sedation — e.g. metoclopramide 10 mg + pethidine 50 mg + diazepam 5–20 mg

3. Anaesthetise area 2–3 cm below umbilicus injecting down towards peritoneum and make a 2–3 cm horizontal incision in the midline

4. Insert introducing needle — it is safest to use a needle with a plastic outer sheath which can be advanced over the sharp inner needle; if in the peritoneum, the plastic sheath should be advanced easily. The inner needle is then removed. This technique minimises risk of bowel perforation (see **Table 18**)

5. Attach sterile giving set to introducing needle and run in approximately 500 mL warm saline — minimises risk of bowel perforation (see **Table 18**)

6. Advance guide-wire through the introducing needle. The wire should feed in very easily. *If there is any resistance to inserting the guide-wire, the technique should be abandoned.* The most common cause for this is a loop of bowel loaded with faeces, or the existence of adhesions

7. Remove outer sheath of introducing needle

8. Use rigid dilator over guide-wire to make a track for the catheter

9. Insert a larger dilator with a "peel-away" sheath over the guide-wire trying to angle it down into the pelvis. Remove the guide-wire and dilator together leaving the sheath

10. Insert the catheter through the sheath which is then peeled off

11. Make sure that the first Dacron cuff is buried in the skin incision site

12. Make the exit site (the spot should be marked). It should be at least 3 cm from the site where the distal cuff will be in the subcutaneous tunnel, to avoid subsequent extrusion of the cuff through the exit site

13. Use as small an incision as possible to make the exit site, to avoid fluid leakage and the need for sutures

14. Attach a tunnelling device to the catheter to create the subcutaneous tunnel and bring out the catheter

15. Attach a connector (usually made of titanium) to the catheter, and then a short line to the connection device to enable dialysate bags to be attached. The actual devices will vary depending on the manufacture of the dialysate bags

16. Suture the original insertion site. Sutures are not needed, and should be avoided at the exit site as they increase the risk of early exit site infection

Table 18. Complications of peritoneal catheter insertion

Complication	Diagnosis	How to avoid	Management
Bladder perforation	Urine drains from catheter	Ensure that bladder is empty prior to catheter insertion	Resite PD catheter Catheterise bladder for several days
Bowel perforation	Solid particles in PD effluent Abdominal pain with multiple Gram negative organisms in PD fluid	Bowel evacuation prior to catheter insertion Run in 500–1,000 mL fluid prior to catheter insertion if using "blind" technique Avoid "blind" percutaneous technique if high risk of adhesions Do not persist with percutaneous technique if there is resistance to advancing guide-wire	Laparotomy to identify and repair perforation. It is often possible to leave the PD catheter *in situ* Appropriate antibiotics
Intraperitoneal bleed	Blood in PD effluent Change in patient's haemodynamic status depending on amount of blood loss	Same as above "Blind" percutaneous technique should not be used in patients known to have bleeding disorder	Conservative management if haemodynamically stable. Heparinise catheter to avoid its clotting If patient unstable, laparotomy required
Fluid leak	Fluid draining from exit site	Make all incisions as small as possible Limit volume of PD exchanges if using catheter early	Drain out PD fluid Avoid any further PD until exit site healed
Exit site infection	Red exit site with or without pus	Prophylactic antibiotics	Appropriate antibiotics

chronic patient (see **Table 19**). The acute patient is more likely to be symptomatically uraemic, fluid overloaded and to have electrolyte problems. To increase the efficiency of PD, dialysate flow rates need to be optimised. This can be done by increasing exchange volume and exchange frequency. When the catheter is new, exchange volume and dwell time, however, need to be limited to avoid fluid leakage. For these reasons, intermittent peritoneal dialysis (IPD) is usually used for patients with ARF. IPD is usually used for two 24 h periods a week (see before).

Table 19. The variables to be considered when prescribing intermittent peritoneal dialysis

Duration of dialysis	Usually for 24 h for each session
	Session can be extended if needed to optimise biochemical or fluid control
	Session can be interrupted, e.g. for an X-ray, and missed time "made up" when patient reconnected
Volume of dialysate	Usually 24 L used over 24 h
Exchange volume	1 L for first week of new catheter
	1.5 L for second week
	Can be increased to 2 or 2.5 L thereafter depending on size of patient
Exchange frequency (or dwell-time)	Dwell-time determines time available for diffusion and ultrafiltration
	Depends on exchange volume, so shorter dwell-time with smaller volume exchanges
	• to enable total volume of dialysate to be cycled over 24 h period
	• small volumes are used when catheter is new, and shorter cycles are needed to minimise period of raised intra-abdominal pressure to minimise risk of fluid leakage
Ultrafiltration requirements	Ultrafiltration is determined by osmotic gradient between plasma and dialysate
	Osmotic gradient is determined by dextrose concentration of dialysate
	If no fluid removal required use only 1.36% dextrose
	Ratio of hypertonic (2.27 or 3.86%) dextrose to isotonic (1.36%) dextrose prescribed depends on amount of fluid needed to be removed
	Amount of ultrafiltration achieved varies from patient to patient so start gradually (e.g. 5 L 1.36% and 5 L 2.27%) and increase dextrose concentration as needed
	Weigh patient (when peritoneum empty) to assess net fluid loss

COMPLICATIONS OF PERITONEAL DIALYSIS

The complications of PD (see **Table 20**) are often mechanical, and can usually be avoided or easily managed by nursing/medical staff with expertise in PD. To the inexperienced, PD can often be a frustrating experience. The other major complication is infection, either of the exit site or peritonitis. As already discussed, dialysis-related complications, such as disequilibrium or hypotension due to excessive or too rapid fluid removal, are much less common with PD compared to HD.

MONITORING OF EFFICACY OF PERITONEAL DIALYSIS

There are no established guidelines as to how to measure or monitor adequacy of acute PD. Standard clinical observations are used to monitor the patient. As many standard PD cycling machines do not measure ultrafiltration, the fluid status of the patient should be determined clinically and by regularly weighing the patient (preferably when the peritoneum is empty). Dialysis adequacy can be assessed by improvements in biochemical parameters such as plasma

Table 20. Complications of peritoneal dialysis

Complication	Management
Poor catheter function	Flush catheter with 20 mL saline to clear any fibrin, blood clot (from recent insertion)
	DO NOT TRY TO TRY TO DRAW BACK ON CATHETER WITH SYRINGE AS THIS MAY "SUCK" OMENTUM INTO CATHETER AND BLOCK IT
	Obtain abdominal X-ray to detect constipation ± catheter migration
	Give aperient or enema in first instance, if clinically possible
	Drainage may depend on patient position, e.g. may improve if patient lying on particular side
Poor ultrafiltration	May be related to poor drainage (see above)
	Increase number of hypertonic bags
	If ultrafiltration inadequate despite using predominantly hypertonic fluid, consider HD
Fluid leakage	Avoid using full volume exchanges with new catheter
	Discontinue dialysis for 2–3 days if possible to allow healing of exit site
	If not possible and/or when dialysis recommenced use small volume (1 L) exchanges
Exit site infection	Most likely due to *Staphylococcus aureus* so commence treatment with flucloxacillin orally
	Change antibiotic treatment if necessary when cultures and sensitivities are available
Peritonitis	Diagnosed by dialysis effluent becoming cloudy with >50 WBC/cu mm on microscopy
	Start antibiotic treatment at once, i.e. before cultures and sensitivities are available
	Not possible to use daily intraperitoneal antibiotics, as is usual with peritonitis treatment for chronic PD
	Need to cover Gram +ve and −ve organisms
	Most commonly used regimens are based on vancomycin and gentamicin (or other aminoglycoside)
	Antibiotics are best administered as a loading dose in 1 L dialysate intraperitoneally and allowed to dwell for 4–6 h
	• Vancomycin 30 mg/Kg
	• Gentamicin 0.6 mg/Kg
	IPD session should then be completed to "wash out" infection
	Monitor blood levels of both antibiotics and repeat dose as needed
	Continue with one or both antibiotics, or change antibiotics, to complete 2 week treatment period depending on sensitivities of cultures
	If not possible to have breaks in PD, or if PD discontinued for some reason, antibiotics can be given intravenously

urea, creatinine, bicarbonate, sodium and potassium. Increasing urine output and a drop in pre-dialysis plasma creatinine from one session to the next suggest that renal function may be improving. Dialysis can then be discontinued and, when clinically indicated, the PD catheter is removed.

9.5 CONTINUOUS RENAL REPLACEMENT THERAPIES
Lui Forni

Continuous renal replacement therapies (CRRT) provide the mainstay of renal replacement in the critically ill. Whereas arterial blood pressure and systemic vascular resistance tend to fall during HD, several studies have shown that both of these parameters are maintained, or even increased, when a similar volume of fluid is removed by continuous haemofiltration, as the rate of fluid and solute removal is slow.

CRRT may be diffusion-based (dialysis) or convection based (filtration). CRRT is usually the treatment of choice in the ICU (see **Chapter 28**), although, with the advent of high dependency units, CRRT may be adapted to provide treatment over shorter periods, to accommodate for changes in nursing staffing levels. Although slow continuous dialysis is occasionally practised, this section focuses on filtration based CRRT.

With regard to solute clearance, CRRT techniques are as efficient as conventional HD in removing solutes over the course of 24 to 48 hours. Although the clearance rate of small solutes (such as urea) is slower per unit time, the rates of removal are similar over a longer time-scale. Over a 24 h period, the clearance is similar to a single run of conventional HD and indeed improved clearance is seen over 48 h with CRRT techniques. CRRT also has the advantage of effectively removing excess fluid in hypotensive patients, whereas HD is frequently limited by further hypotension in this setting. It should be emphasised that hypotension can still occur if too much fluid is removed, or if fluid is removed too quickly.

Another proposed advantage of CRRT is the removal of immunomodulatory substances produced by septic or highly catabolic patients (see **Chapters 9.3** and **19**). Conventional HD utilises less porous membranes than CRRT techniques, which are less efficient in removing substances of larger molecular weight, such as inflammatory mediators. In theory, removal of such substances might lead to improved patient outcome, but to date there are few data to support this.

HAEMOFILTRATION: BASIC PRINCIPLES

Movement of fluid across a semipermeable membrane occurs through osmosis, which can be enhanced by the generation of a pressure gradient across the membrane, the process of ultrafiltration (**Figure 7A**).

As discussed briefly in **Chapter 9.3**, ultrafiltration (UF) is governed by:

$$Q_f = K_m \times TMP \qquad (1)$$

where Q_f is the UF rate in mL/h and K_m is the membrane UF coefficient expressed in $(mL/h) \times (m^2/mmHg)$.

Haemofiltration involves the removal of water through UF and the consequent removal of solutes by frictional forces between water and solutes (so-called solvent drag). This results in the transport of small and middle molecular weight solutes (<5,000 Da) through the haemofilter membrane. The transport of solutes with water flow is termed convection (**Figure 7B**), and the clearance of solutes will depend principally on the qualities of the membrane used and its UF coefficient [**Equation (1)**]. Haemofilter membrane filters are highly permeable and contain pores of a known dimension. These pores will allow convection of solutes **smaller** than that of the pore size through the membrane. Therefore all solutes below the pore size are handled by the haemofilter in an almost identical manner. A principal difference between filtration and dialysis is that an idealised replacement fluid is required in filtration to prevent excessive fluid removal. The use of the replacement fluid will lower by dilution the plasma concentration of those solutes not present in the replacement fluid. This process is summarised in **Figure 7C**. A diagrammatic representation of haemofiltration is shown in **Figure 8**.

The process of UF is enhanced by the addition of pumps to generate a positive pressure within the blood compartment (P_b) and a negative pressure within the filtrate channel (P_{uf}), generating a pressure gradient across the membrane: the transmembrane pressure (TMP) which is expressed as:

$$TMP = P_b - P_{uf} - \pi \qquad (2)$$

where P_b is the hydrostatic pressure of the blood, P_{uf} is the hydrostatic pressure in the ultrafiltrate, and π is the oncotic pressure of the blood.

The solute filtration flux (Q_f), which describes the movement of solute across a semipermeable membrane in which the solute is "carried" with solvent (convection), occurs as a result of a TMP gradient, and is given by:

$$TMP = Q_f (P_b - P_{uf} - \pi) \qquad (3)$$

From **(1)**, it follows that an increase in generated TMP will increase UF from the blood to the filtrate. Consequently an increase in pump speed will increase blood flow (and hydrostatic pressure), or an increase in the filtrate pump speed will increase filtrate flow, both leading to an increase in the TMP and hence UF. Several factors will influence the efficiency of this process (see below).

During continuous haemofiltration the efficiency of solute removal is determined by the UF rate and the sieving coefficient. The sieving coefficient (SC) defines the ability of a solute to cross a membrane and is derived from the ratio of the solute concentration in the ultrafiltrate to the solute concentration in the plasma. Therefore a solute that freely permeates the membrane would have a SC of 1.0. A solute that is not filtered would have a SC of 0. A sieving coefficient of 0 may be due to the molecular weight of the solute (i.e. too large to be filtered) or the solute may be extensively protein bound. During continuous arteriovenous haemofiltration, the arterial

Figure 7. Diagrammatic representation of the main processes involved in haemofiltration. A. Ultrafiltration; B. Convection; C. Haemofiltration

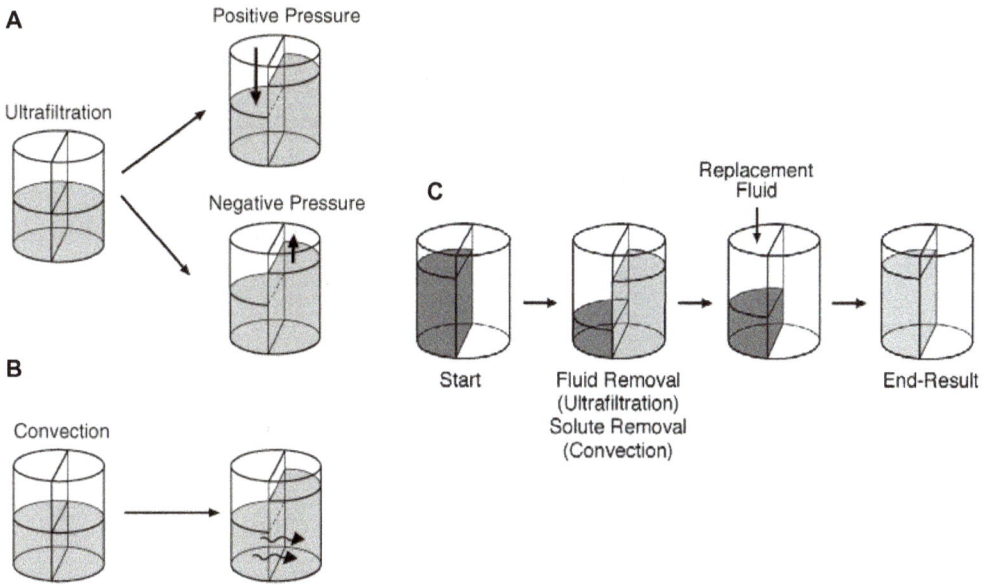

A

Ultrafiltration

Positive Pressure

Negative Pressure

B

Convection

C

Start

Fluid Removal
(Ultrafiltration)
Solute Removal
(Convection)

Replacement
Fluid

End-Result

Figure 8. Diagrammatic representation of haemofiltration

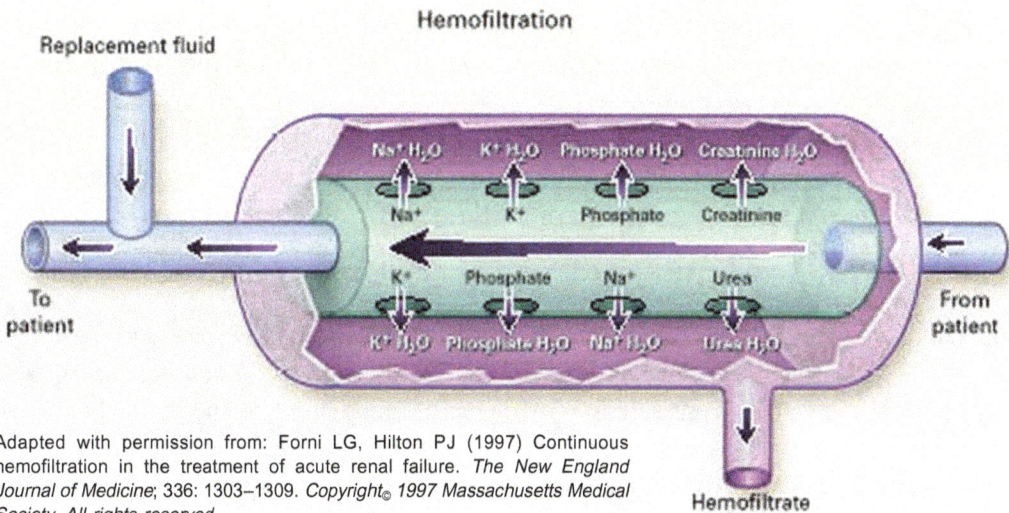

Hemofiltration

Replacement fluid

To patient

From patient

Hemofiltrate

and venous concentrations may be different throughout solute removal, and therefore it is more accurate to calculate the sieving coefficient during continuous arteriovenous haemofiltration from the average of the arterial [A] and venous [V] concentrations. This is given by:

$$SC = [UF] \div ([A] + [V] \div 2) \tag{4}$$

where [UF] represents the solute concentration in the ultrafiltrate. As outlined, in continuous haemofiltration, there is **no** solute loss by diffusion. Consequently the venous concentration will be equal to arterial if the sieving coefficient is 1. If the sieving coefficient is less than 1, more water than solute will be removed and therefore the venous concentration will be slightly greater than the arterial concentration. In practice this difference is not clinically significant for most solutes, and it can be assumed that the arterial and venous concentrations are the same, as in continuous venovenous haemofiltration (CVVH). Hence the above equation can be simplified to:

$$SC = [UF] \div [A] \tag{5}$$

Water accounts for approximately 93% of the plasma. If we assume this as being 100% (the difference can be ignored clinically) then the rate of clearance of a solute will be the product of the SC, which is constant during continuous arteriovenous or venovenous haemofiltration, and the UF rate:

$$\text{Rate of solute clearance} = SC \times \text{ultrafiltration rate} \tag{6}$$

As a consequence, an increase in the rate of UF will also increase the solute clearance.

Haemodiafiltration (HDF) refers to a combination of dialysis and filtration. Solute loss primarily occurs by diffusion but >25% may occur through convection. The addition of HD to the haemofiltration system undoubtedly achieves higher clearances of smaller solutes than haemofiltration alone. The initial introduction of haemodiafiltration was driven by the need to increase clearances obtained using continuous arteriovenous haemofiltration (CAVH). Such systems do not employ a blood pump, the UF rate being governed solely by the blood pressure. The addition of a dialysis circuit increases diffusional clearance of solutes, although in contrast to conventional HD the dialysate flow is less than the blood flow. Hence in CAVHDF clearance of low molecular weight solutes is limited by the dialysate flow, whereas in conventional HD the dialysate flow is greater than blood flow and hence clearance is blood flow dependent.

CONTINUOUS RENAL REPLACEMENT THERAPY NOMENCLATURE

Arteriovenous systems involve the use of an arterial catheter to allow blood to flow into the extracorporeal circuit and a venous catheter for the blood return. As a consequence, this relies entirely on the systemic blood pressure to provide the filtration pressure and herein lies the major disadvantage of these systems when applied, in particular, to the ICU. Although arteriovenous access is relatively simple to set up and does not require an extracorporeal blood pump it does require arterial puncture, with its attendant risk of arterial embolisation and exsanguination if the system becomes disconnected. The patients who require continuous therapies tend to be relatively hypotensive and tolerate any fall in blood pressure poorly. Also, in severe peripheral vascular disease, blood flow may be erratic.

Venovenous systems involve both catheters or, more conventionally, one dual lumen catheter being inserted in a great vein. This dictates that a blood pump is required in order to circulate blood through the extracorporeal circuit. These systems do not require arterial access, involve less systemic anticoagulation, often use only one dual lumen catheter, and have faster and more reliable blood flows than arterial based systems.

Continuous Arteriovenous Haemofiltration (CAVH)

CAVH employs the arterial pressure to generate the transmembrane potential and removes fluid and solutes by UF and convection. It is the original and simplest form of the technique. However, the efficiency of solute removal is generally quite low in that it relies on the mean arterial blood pressure and this is often suboptimal in the critically ill. Low blood flow is also associated with frequent clotting of the extracorporeal circuit, and prolonged arterial cannulation often results in problems at the arterial puncture site. CAVH often results in clearances as low as 10–15 mL/min and therefore 24 h/day operation or the addition of enhancing techniques is often required to ensure adequate metabolic control.

Continuous Arteriovenous Haemodiafiltration (CAVHDF)

CAVHDF employs the addition of a dialyser circuit and therefore combines diffusion and convection to remove small solutes. This compensates in part for the inadequacies of CAVH, although the equipment needed is considerably more complex and the other disadvantages of CAVH are not eliminated.

Continuous Venovenous Haemofiltration (CVVH)

CVVH incorporates an occlusive pump into the filtration circuit. Consequently UF is not governed by the arterial pressure but is generated by the blood pump speed; thus the limitations imposed by the arterial pressure are removed. Consequently, solute clearance is directly controlled by the physician. Such circuits incorporate safety devices to detect low inflow pressure as well as the presence of air in the circuit. Filtration rates up to and exceeding 100 mL/min can be achieved although such rates are rarely required. Given the clear advantages of CVVH over other continuous techniques it has widespread use in ICUs.

Continuous Venovenous Haemodiafiltration (CVVHDF)

CVVHDF utilises venovenous access and a blood pump as in CVVH but with the addition of a dialyser circuit as was introduced to enhance the technique of CAVH. This has the advantage of enhanced small solute clearances, as discussed above. CVVHDF is considered by many to be the technique of choice for managing ARF in catabolic critically ill patients (see **Chapter 28**). Addition of dialysis to haemofiltration (i.e. haemodiafiltration) achieves higher clearances and improved biochemical control. Equivalent clearance rates may be achieved by high volume haemofiltration, although this has the disadvantage that returning large volumes of replacement fluids to the patient is prone to error and is more labour intensive (less of a problem with the newer automated machines — see below). There are no data to support the use of one over the other; in practice, choosing between CVVHDF and high volume haemofiltration comes down to factors such as machine availability, and ICU staffing levels and expertise.

Slow Continuous Ultrafiltration (SCUF)

SCUF is strictly a dehydrating procedure and as such solute removal is minimal. Access can be arteriovenous or venovenous. SCUF is primarily used when the fluid removal goals are modest. Slow continuous UF with dialysis is also occasionally practised, which adds diffusive clearance to the dehydrating process.

Continuous High Flux Dialysis (CHFD)

Patients with ARF complicated by sepsis and multi-organ failure produce large amounts of middle molecular weight molecules (500–5,000 Da, e.g. cytokines). Although CVVHDF provides adequate urea clearance, the clearance of middle molecules is low because of low membrane permeability or poor diffusion of these molecules. Convection is therefore necessary and can be achieved by using synthetic membranes with greater sieving capacity. CHFD combines a modified continuous HD (CVVHD) circuit with a highly permeable dialyser, i.e. diffusion + convection. It has the advantage that it provides urea clearances of up to 60 L/24 h, and adequate middle and large molecule clearances, while avoiding the need for large quantities of replacement fluids (the dialysate acts as both dialysis and replacement fluid). CHFD is not widely available at present.

Continuous Equilibrium Peritoneal Dialysis (CEPD)

CEPD is a long-dwell procedure similar to CAPD. A semipermanent PD catheter is placed. Initially rapid exchanges are used to achieve fluid and solute balance in similar fashion to acute peritoneal dialysis. This is followed by longer dwell times to maintain metabolic balance (see **Chapter 9.4**).

TECHNICAL ASPECTS OF CVVH

Overview

Figure 9 outlines the general components of a fully automated CVVH system which may be viewed as consisting of a blood circuit, filtrate circuit and a replacement fluid circuit. Blood is removed from the patient via the "take" port of the venous catheter. This is anticoagulated, and the blood pump then generates blood flow through the haemofilter and blood is returned through the "return" lumen. A blood flow detector in line with the blood pump will detect a fall in blood pressure which indicates access delivery failure; this may be referred to as the "arterial" pressure sensor. Problems with the filter, such as clotting, are not detected by the blood flow sensor but will be detected by the venous pressure sensor which is located in the post-filter venous drip chamber. A fall in venous pressure indicates decreased flow to the venous side and if the blood

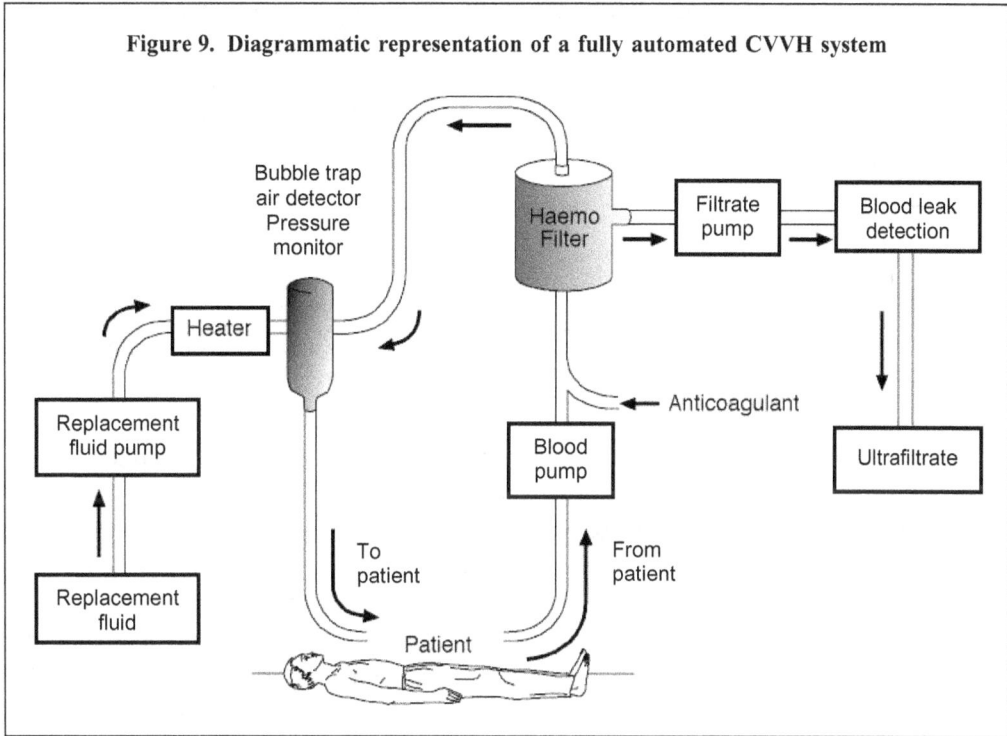

Figure 9. Diagrammatic representation of a fully automated CVVH system

flow to the filter is normal the decreased venous flow is often due to clotting in the filter. However, clotting usually occurs in the drip chamber before it occurs in the filter and this will lead to a rise in venous pressure. This will necessitate changing the tubing and the haemofilter.

The UF circuit consists of a second pump, which by increasing the negative hydrostatic pressure in the filtration circuit, increases UF through a rise in the TMP. The filtration rate may be varied between 0 and 30% of the blood flow rate. Any further increase in filtration rate results in excessive haemoconcentration which shortens filter life significantly. This enables a desired amount of plasma water to be removed per hour, as the amount of ultrafiltrate produced can be monitored. A third pump regulates the amount of replacement fluid mixed with the blood via a heater into the venous drip chamber. The replacement fluid may be added prior to blood entering the filter (pre-dilution) in certain circumstances.

Venous Access (see also **Chapter 9.6**)

The preferred site of access is the right internal jugular vein, followed by the left internal jugular vein. The subclavian approach, although often used in the ICU, is probably a last resort given that the patient may need long term dialysis and this route is associated with long term problems such as stenosis. As discussed earlier, in CVVH the low venous pressure dictates the addition of an extracorporeal blood pump to circulate blood through the extracorporeal circuit. Venovenous access is best achieved with a double lumen catheter to reduce the complications seen with individual catheters for the "give" and "take" lines. Examples include the Quinton Mahurkar catheter (11.5 French) and the Vascath Flexicon (10.8 French). More recently, high flow triple lumen catheters have been introduced. This includes the Vygon Trilyse-Cath™ which is a 12 French catheter with two main lumens (11G and 12G) as well as a smaller distal lumen (16G) ideal for drug delivery and pressure monitoring. Catheters of this type allow blood flow rates (Q_b) of up to 320 mL/min and although some dual lumen catheters may have up to 20% recirculation the continuous nature of CVVH leads to high enough clearances that this may be ignored.

Extracorporeal Blood Pump

Many different blood pumps can be used for continuous haemofiltration, including the Gambro AK-10, Hospal BSM-22 and the Baxter BM-11. The use of an extracorporeal pump necessitates the integration of pressure alarms on both the "arterial" ("take") and "venous" ("give") lines as well as an air detection system. Fully automated systems, as outlined above, have additional roller pumps to control the UF rate. These systems are capable of generating blood flows (Q_b) as high as 700 mL/min. From **Equation (2)** the transmembrane pressure (TMP) produced at such flow rates can lead to an UF rate in excess of 2 L/h. New generation machines, such as the Gambro AK 200 include on line facilities which prepare replacement fluids as needed and are fully automated. This system is able to perform all modes of CRRT and can produce ultrafiltrate rates of up to 4.0 L/h; it also has the facility for profiling of sodium, bicarbonate and UF rate. The Prisma (Hospal) machine, which produces ultrafiltrate rates of up to 2.0 L/h, has a dialysate delivery system with an integrated UF control apparatus, allowing both CVVH and CVVHDF. These machines are relatively simple to use, allow flexibility of treatment over 24 h and reduce nursing staff workload.

Haemofilters

An impressive array of filters is available commercially. These differ principally in the composition of the membrane which may be cellulose-based or synthetic. Cellulose based membranes (cellulose acetate, cuprophan and hemophan) have a low permeability coefficient to water, i.e. low-flux. The synthetic membranes such as polysulphone, polyamide and polyacrylonitrile are higher flux (higher K_m). Therefore the synthetic membranes are more suited to convective therapies in that they have a higher sieving coefficient for solutes over a larger molecular weight range than their cellulose based counterparts.

Filters that are best suited to convective treatments alone include polyamide filters such as the Gambro FH66 and FH77. These consist of bundles of 8–12,000 polyamide hollow fibres and provide an effective surface area of 0.6 and 1.4 m^2 respectively. The FH66 is used for uncomplicated slow CVVH whereas the larger FH77 is used in grossly hypercatabolic states where more rapid filtration rates may be required. Where the filter is being used for both convective and diffusive treatments then polysulphone membranes such as the Fresenius are preferred.

Issues relating to membrane biocompatibility have been discussed in **Chapter 9.3**.

Anticoagulation

Anticoagulation is required to maintain patency of the extracorporeal circuit during continuous therapies and heparin provides adequate anticoagulation in most cases. The aim is to prolong filter life without producing significant systemic anticoagulation; various manoeuvres prior to commencing CVVH may reduce heparin requirements. These include:

- Adequate flushing of the filter with at least 2 L of saline containing 5,000 i.u. of heparin per litre.
- Maintaining a filtration fraction of no greater than 20% thereby avoiding significant haemoconcentration.
- Use of pre-dilution techniques if necessary (see below).

Before commencing CVVH, a bolus of heparin (1,000–2,000 i.u.) is given down the "take" port of the venous catheter, the dose depending on the platelet count and the APTT. A continuous infusion of 300–500 i.u./h is then commenced. The APTT is measured after 2 h, from a sample taken from the "give" line in the circuit. The aim is for an APTT value of 1.5–2 times control. The heparin dose should be increased in patients with evidence of clotting within the circuit. Conversely, the dose should be reduced where there is overt bleeding or severe thrombocytopaenia. In some cases, heparin free filtration can be performed, although this invariably leads to a reduction in filter life. Patients with very low levels of antithrombin III and heparin cofactor II may be prone to premature clotting of the filter despite regular heparin therapy and this may be corrected by infusing fresh frozen plasma or, if available, antithrombin III concentrate.

An alternative anticoagulant is low molecular weight heparin (LMWH) which may cause less bleeding and less thrombocytopaenia than unfractionated heparin. To date, no significant studies have been performed using LMWH as anticoagulant in CRRT. Evidence from intermittent HD does not suggest that the use of LMWH confers any major advantages, and at present the main clinical indication for their use is in the patient with heparin induced thrombocytopaenia. Moreover, the use of LMWH has distinct disadvantages. Firstly, they are costly. Secondly, monitoring the degree of anticoagulant activity is unreliable using the APTT, and therefore monitoring heparinoid or anti-factor Xa levels may be necessary, which may not be locally available and is expensive.

An alternative approach to anticoagulation is the use of sodium citrate which chelates ionised calcium, thereby inhibiting the calcium dependent clotting factors IXa, Xa and VIIIa, even in the presence of intrinsic stimuli. This approach uses an infusion of sodium citrate into the "take" limb of the extracorporeal circuit and, given its mode of action, dictates that intravenous calcium must also be infused systemically to maintain the ionised serum calcium concentration. This is achieved through infusion of 5% calcium chloride into the venous return line at a rate adjusted according to the plasma calcium concentration. The major potential problems with citrate anticoagulation include hypercalcaemia and hypocalcaemia, hypernatraemia (due to the hypertonic sodium citrate solution) and acid base disturbance. Metabolic alkalosis may ensue through citrate metabolism to bicarbonate. However, of more concern is the critically ill patient with deranged liver function. In these patients citrate metabolism may be impaired, leading to lactate intolerance and eventual lactic acidosis. Therefore it is imperative that the patient is able to metabolise citrate before therapy is commenced.

The inhibitor of platelet aggregation, prostacyclin (Flolan™) may also be used for regional anticoagulation under certain circumstances including:

- Patients who are actively bleeding.
- Patients with a platelet count $<80 \times 10^9/L$.

- Where there is suspicion of an intracerebral bleed.
- Presence of coagulopathy.

Table 21 outlines a schedule for the use of prostacyclin anticoagulation. Side effects include headache, facial flushing, tachy or bradycardia and hypotension. In the hypoxic ventilated patient one may also see increased pulmonary shunting with worsening hypoxia. Initially an infusion of 2.5 ng/kg/min for 30 min is used, over which time the patient is observed for hypotension and deteriorating gas exchange (see also **Chapter 9.3**). If this period is uneventful the dose is increased to 5.0 ng/kg/min for a further 30 min before haemofiltration is commenced. As well as the side effects listed above the use of prostacyclin is also limited by expense.

Table 21. Preparation/dosing of prostacyclin infusion

50 mL of normal saline containing 100 μg of prostacyclin is used (2 μg/mL)

Dosing is then dependent on body weight:

Bodyweight (kg)	Flow rate (mL/h) for initial 30 min	Flow rate (mL/h) thereafter
30	2.5	4.5
40	3.0	6.0
50	4.0	7.5
60	4.5	9.0
70	5.0	10.0
80	6.0	12.0
90	6.5	13.0
100	7.5	15.0

Initial dose corresponds to approximately 2.5 ng/kg/min.

Observe for hypotension and deteriorating oxygenation.

CHOICE OF BUFFERING SYSTEM IN CRRT

Why Buffer?

During haemofiltration, water and all solutes of plasma up to a molecular weight of approximately 15–20 kDa are removed, although the absolute cut off depends on the filter type used. Among the solutes removed is the bicarbonate ion. The effect that this may have on the plasma bicarbonate concentration is easily calculated. If we consider a patient with a plasma bicarbonate of 25 mmol/L being haemofiltered at a filtration rate of 30 mL/min, the haemofilter will remove 45 mmol of bicarbonate per hour and, if progressive acidosis is to be prevented, these bicarbonate ions must be replaced or regenerated. The replacement solutions used in most haemofiltration systems contain physiological amounts of sodium, chloride, calcium and magnesium but not bicarbonate. The bicarbonate ion is replaced with an alternative such as sodium lactate for two principal reasons. Firstly, mixtures containing equivalent bicarbonate concentrations have a short shelf life. When stored in plastic containers the bicarbonate ions are partially converted to carbonate with loss of CO_2 by diffusion through the walls of the containers. Secondly, a mixture of physiological concentrations of calcium and bicarbonate leads to a precipitate of calcium carbonate, as this exceeds its solubility product.

Lactate is an acceptable substitute for bicarbonate provided that it is efficiently metabolised to CO_2 and water, as this effectively generates "new" bicarbonate ions through the tricarboxylic acid cycle. Over a 24 h period, lactate buffered CVVH will result in a net loss of up to 1,000 mmol of bicarbonate and therefore the substitution fluid must provide adequate substrate to replace these losses as well as to buffer ongoing acid production. With normal hepatic function an individual is able to metabolise approximately 100 mmol of lactate per hour, hence generating an equimolar amount of bicarbonate. In the acutely ill patient, this may not be the case and therefore an alternative buffering agent should be used. This may be either bicarbonate based replacement fluid (see below) or so-called lactate free replacement fluid, where sodium bicarbonate is infused independently of the haemofiltration circuit.

Choice of Replacement Fluid

Table 22 outlines the constituents of some commercially available replacement fluids which differ principally in their potassium concentrations as well as the buffer employed. The choice of replacement fluid is governed by local practice. In the case of low potassium or potassium free fluids this must be added to the replacement fluids (**Table 23**). The advantage of potassium free solutions is that they may be used in all individuals and the amount of potassium added will depend on the individual's requirements. This can be corrected for potassium intake by other means such as TPN.

Table 22. Constituents of commercially available replacement fluids (5000 mL volume)						
Constituent	Gambro HF21	Gambro HF22	Gambro HF25	Fresenius HF02	Hospal Haemovex No2	Hospal[1,2] Haemosol B0
Na$^+$ (mmol/L)	140	140	140	140	142	140
K$^+$ (mmol/L)	1.0	0	4.0	0	0	0
Ca^{++} (mmol/L)	3.25	3.25	3.25	2.00	2.00	1.75
Mg^{++} (mmol/L)	1.5	1.5	1.5	1.0	0.75	0.5
Cl$^-$ (mmol/L)	100.75	100.75	100.75	111	103	109.5
Lactate (mmol/L)	45	45	45	0	45	3
Acetate (mmol/L)	0	0	0	35	0	0
Glucose (g/L)	1.96	1.96	1.96	0	0	0
Osmolarity (mOsm/L)	300	300	300	290	292.2	287

[1]Replacement fluid used for bicarbonate buffered haemofiltration (see text). 250 mL 5.88% bicarbonate is added to each 4750 mL bag prior to use, to yield a final bicarbonate concentration of 32 mmol/L.
[2]Note: low lactate fluids are available (e.g. Monosol, lactate ~30 mmol/L) for use in patients who develop a metabolic alkalosis using standard lactate-buffered bags ("over-buffering").

Table 23. Regimen for addition of KCl to potassium free containing replacement fluids

The following table outlines the amount of KCl in mmol to be added to 4.5 dm^{-3} of potassium free replacement fluid and is meant as a guide. The concentration per litre is also given for simplicity

Serum K$^+$ (mmol/L)	KCl to be added to each bag	Final [K$^+$] (mmol/L)
3.0–3.5	20 mmol	4.44
3.6–4.0	18 mmol	4.00
4.1–4.5	16 mmol	3.56
4.6–5.0	14 mmol	3.11
5.1–5.5	12 mmol	2.67
5.6–6.0	10 mmol	2.22
>6.1	None	0

Electrolyte balance can be calculated and adjusted accordingly while the patient is receiving CVVH. For example, at an UF rate of 1 L/h with a serum potassium of 4.0 mmol/L, this equates to a total loss of 96 mmol K$^+$ in 24 h (24 L × 4 mmol). If a steady state K$^+$ concentration is required with no other supplementation then 4.0 mmol/L can be added to the replacement fluid. If TPN were then started on this patient, containing 75 mmol K$^+$ in 3 L, then the overall K$^+$ deficit would be 21 mmol. In this case, in order to maintain fluid balance, 21 L of replacement fluid would be given, hence the K+ needed would be 1 mmol/L.

One problem that may be encountered with purely convective therapies is hypophosphataemia and most patients will require phosphate supplementation at some stage.

Pre- and Post-Dilution

This refers to the infusion site with respect to the haemofilter. Post-dilution is the more traditional approach to haemofiltration. During post-dilution the blood is concentrated in the filter reaching its maximum concentration at the end of the filter. The blood is then diluted to the required volume with replacement fluid. In pre-dilution techniques the blood is diluted in the "take" lumen before the filter. Clearly, if the same volume is used for pre-dilution as post-dilution the overall clearance must be reduced. The clearance during pre-dilution is given by **Equation (7)**:

$$\frac{Q_B \times Q_{UF}}{Q_B + Q_{INF}} \tag{7}$$

where Q_B is blood flow through the filter (mL/min), Q_{UF} is the UF volume (mL/min) and Q_{INF} the volume of infused replacement fluid (mL/min). This formula is a simplification of the formula derived from plasma water flow. For clinical purposes it is more convenient, although overestimates clearance by ~6%. The advantage of pre-dilution is that it may decrease the incidence of clotting in the filter and therefore may reduce the amount of anticoagulant used. However, this must be balanced against the higher clearances obtained using post-dilution techniques for the same volume of replacement fluid, and hence increased expense. Fluid balance is also more complex with pre-dilution techniques.

BICARBONATE BUFFERED HAEMOFILTRATION

The use of bicarbonate based buffering systems was first described in 1990. The catalyst for its development was the recognition of a group of patients who appeared to deteriorate rather than improve when commenced on CVVH. This was apparent through hypotension, worsening acid-base parameters, increasing inotrope requirements and eventual circulatory collapse. These patients were found to have lactic acidosis.

Lactic Acidosis

Lactic acidosis is the most commonly encountered cause of metabolic acidosis (see **Chapter 8.4**), and the mortality associated with its development remains high. Renal support is almost always necessary in patients who develop lactic acidosis and multi-organ failure. Given that haemofiltration is the treatment of choice for such individuals, attention must be paid to the choice of substitution fluid. As discussed above, lactate is an acceptable substitute for bicarbonate provided it is efficiently metabolised. Under conditions where lactate cannot be efficiently metabolised (e.g. liver failure) then continuous haemofiltration with continued donation of lactate through the substitution fluid will result in a worsening of acid-base parameters and a deterioration in the patient's condition.

Technical Aspects of Bicarbonate Buffered Haemofiltration

Bicarbonate buffered solutions are usually prepared locally and consist of 4.5 dm^{-3} bags of either isotonic NaCl (154 mmol/L) or isotonic $NaHCO_3$ (139 mmol/L). The infusion ratio is determined by the severity of the acidosis. The rate of bicarbonate donation can be adjusted either by varying the $NaCl/NaHCO_3$ ratio or by varying the rate of haemofiltration. Using this system, donation rates of between 1 and 2 mmol/min for prolonged periods can be achieved in order to maintain a normal plasma pH. The incompatibility of both calcium and magnesium salts with such replacement fluids necessitates that they are infused separately from the haemofiltration circuit.

Selection criteria

Three groups of patients may benefit from bicarbonate buffered haemofiltration:

1. Patients with established lactic acidosis, defined as a blood lactate of >5 mmol/L accompanied either by an arterial pH <7.2 or a requirement for >60 mmol $NaHCO_3$/h to maintain a stable arterial pH.
2. Patients who are intolerant of lactate buffered haemofiltration. When treated with a lactate-based haemofiltration fluid (lactate concentration 45 mmol/L) they show a rise in blood

lactate of >5 mmol/L. Note that patients with a high initial blood lactate concentration who do not show an excessive increment in blood lactate can safely be treated by lactate-based haemofiltration. In these cases, the hyperlactataemia is a result of overproduction rather than a failure of lactate metabolism, and this is not associated with the development of progressive acidaemia.

3. Patients with profound acidaemia (e.g. pH <7) and severe shock and/or cardiac failure, in whom rapid reversal of the acidosis is required.

A theoretical limit is reached when sodium bicarbonate is being administered at 150 mmol/L and at the maximum rate of practical filtration of the machine (~100 mL/min). The net donation rate of bicarbonate ions under these conditions would be approximately 13 mmol/min.

Techniques now being developed allow the use of bicarbonate-containing substitution fluids to be used in place of lactate-based solutions (see **Table 22**). However, these "physiological" bicarbonate replacement fluids do not allow adequate treatment of severe lactic acidosis, given the restraints on the bicarbonate concentration in the replacement fluid. In such cases, additional bicarbonate will need to be infused independently of the extracorporeal circuit. Bicarbonate buffered haemofiltration does not cure lactic acidosis but represents an efficient means of ensuring that the acidosis itself is not fatal, and buys time for attempts to be made to correct the underlying cause.

CVVH PRESCRIPTION IN ACUTE RENAL FAILURE

In general, the metabolic control of ARF requires urea clearance rates of ~20 L/day. Filter flow is usually between 100–200 mL/min. Filtrate is usually removed at 1–2 L/h and fluid balance is adjusted by varying the fluid replacement rate (1 L/h UF rate = clearance of 17 mL/min). These filtration rates can usually be achieved with mean arterial blood pressures >50–70 mmHg. Higher clearances are achieved by increasing haemofiltration volumes (making fluid replacement more complicated) or by adding dialysis (CVVHDF), as discussed earlier. Adding 1 L/h dialysate flow rate to 1 L/h UF rate will increase the clearance to 34 mL/min. At present there are few data concerning dose of CVVH/CVVHDF for ARF and no consensus on how the dose of RRT should be measured. A recent study demonstrated that increasing the UF rate (35 versus 20 mL/h/kg) in CRRT improved the survival of critically ill patients with ARF (Ronco *et al.*, 2000). These data suggest that CVVH "dose" may be important in determining outcome, but further studies are required.

TROUBLESHOOTING

Some of the major problems which may be encountered when performing CVVH are outlined below, together with potential solutions!

Raised Venous Pressure

- Often due to increase in resistance of blood return to patient.
- Check blood lines are not kinked/occluded/clamped.

- Check clotting time.
- Check for clots in the bubble trap.
- If venous pressure persistently >200 mmHg change filter.

Low Venous Pressure

- Increase blood flow rate via pump speed.

Arterial Pressure Alarm

- Check patient's blood pressure.
- Check arterial ("take") line.
- Check patency of access; consider swapping "take" and "return" ports.
- Consider vessel spasm.

Access Vessel Spasm

- Causes "juddering" of the bloodlines.
- Slow blood flow rate (to ~100 mL/min).
- Is the patient hypovolaemic?

Air Alarm

- Adjust level in bubble trap (if possible).
- Occasionally caused by spasmodic blood flow; consider reducing blood flow.
- Additions to the circuit:
  — TPN/drugs given to the circuit must go into the venous line/return line
  — Blood sampling is performed from the take/arterial line before the site of anticoagulant infusion

Coloured Ultrafiltrate

- Pink or red ultrafiltrate may suggest a blood leak, therefore change filter.
- Yellow ultrafiltrate may reflect hyperbilirubinaemia or drug infusion.
- Brown ultrafiltrate is seen with myoglobinaemia.

Hypophosphataemia

- May be supplemented via TPN, enteral route or intravenously.
- IV infusion of 10 mL Addiphos (20 mmol) plus 10 mL 5% dextrose at 3 mL/h.

Progressive Acidosis

- Measure serum lactate if on lactate buffered replacement fluid.
- Reduce filtration rate and consider bicarbonate buffered or lactate free replacement fluids.
- Search for underlying cause!

DRUG PRESCRIBING DURING CONTINUOUS REPLACEMENT THERAPY

CRRT are often employed in the critically ill and as such a knowledge of the clearance of drugs by this technique is essential. Many factors influence the clearance of drugs by haemofiltration and these are outlined in **Table 24** (see also **Appendix A**).

Table 24. Factors controlling drug removal during continuous renal replacement therapy	
Volume of distribution	Ultrafiltration volume
Degree of protein binding	Drug membrane interaction
Protein polarisation	Plasma half-life of drug
Sieving coefficient	Presence of dialysis

The efficiency of the removal of drugs or any other solute is related to the UF rate and the sieving coefficient. Several factors may affect the sieving coefficient, including:

Membrane Type

The sieving coefficient for several drugs differs depending on the type of membrane used. Polyacrylonitrile or polyamide membranes have different drug interactions than polysulfone membranes.

Drug Charge

Drug charge can affect both convective and diffusive transport depending on the nature of the drug-membrane charge interaction. The charge effect can alter the removal of drugs including aminoglycosides, cephalosporins and penicillins. Some drugs may also bind to membranes; this is seen with the aminoglycoside antibiotics.

Molecular Size

The molecular size of most drugs is smaller than the maximum size freely removed by convection during haemofiltration and therefore tends not to be an important determinant of drug removal. However, drug size is important with diffusive loss during dialysis-based techniques.

Protein Binding

The major determinant of drug removal by haemofiltration is binding to plasma proteins which are not filtered, so only unbound drug can be removed. The degree of protein binding of a drug is influenced by several factors including:

- pH
- molar concentration of drug and protein
- bilirubin
- heparin
- free fatty acids
- presence of displacing drugs.

The relative importance of these factors depends on the drug in question.

Equations (4) and **(5)** outlined the calculation of the sieving coefficient. This may be expanded when considering drug removal by haemofiltration according to:

$$SC = AUC - UF \div AUC - P \qquad (8)$$

where AUC-UF and AUC-P represent the areas under the time-drug concentration curves for the ultrafiltrate and the plasma, respectively.

Total Drug Removal

Calculation of the total amount of drug removed during haemofiltration allows dose modification where needed. The drug removal may be calculated by measuring the drug concentration either in the ultrafiltrate or, more commonly, in the plasma. If the drug in question is measured in the ultrafiltrate the amount of drug removed (in mg) is given by:

$$\text{[Ultrafiltrate] (mg/L)} \times \text{UF rate (L/min)} \times \text{Time of procedure (min)} \qquad (9)$$

Alternatively the plasma level may be used to calculate the ultrafiltrate concentration:

$$\text{[Ultrafiltrate]} = \text{[Plasma] (mg/L)} \times \text{unbound fraction} \qquad (10)$$

The unbound fraction is given by:

$$\text{Unbound fraction} = (100 - \% \text{ bound}) \div 100 \qquad (11)$$

The available protein binding data have been obtained from studies in healthy people. Unfortunately these data are not readily available although some pharmacokinetic data may be available from the manufacturers. Therefore the amount of drug removed (mg) can be calculated from:

$$\text{[Plasma] (mg/L)} \times \text{unbound fraction} \times \text{UF rate (L/min)} \times \text{time of procedure (min)} \qquad (12)$$

The plasma sample should be taken at steady state, ideally halfway between maintenance doses after at least three half-lives.

The above formulas are, unfortunately, applicable only for the small number of drugs for which plasma levels are easily obtainable. In most cases, it is necessary to estimate the average steady state plasma concentration from the dosing regimen and rate of clearance through:

$$\text{Average [drug]} = \text{dosing rate (mg/min)} \div \text{Clearance (mL/min)} \qquad \textbf{(13)}$$

The dosing rate is either the dose divided by the dosing interval if given intermittently or the infusion rate for a drug given by continuous intravenous infusion.

9.6 VASCULAR ACCESS
Richard Baker and Paul Glynne

INTRODUCTION

Catheters used for gaining central vascular access should:

- be safe and easy to insert
- be ready for immediate use following insertion
- require low maintenance and be economical to use as a disposable catheter
- enable high blood flow rates during dialysis.

Two devices currently fulfil these criteria — the *double lumen dialysis catheter* and *the silastic, cuffed, tunnelled catheter*. Double lumen catheters are usually used for short-term access. However, tunnelled catheters should be considered at an early stage if recovery of renal function is likely to be delayed (approximately one third of cases of ARF). Formerly, Scribner shunts were used for acute vascular access but their usage is now largely restricted to patients with chronic renal failure with difficult vascular access.

DOUBLE LUMEN CATHETERS

There is a range of dialysis catheters made from different plastics. All these catheters share common features which include:

- rigidity at room temperature to facilitate insertion but softer at body temperature to prevent vessel trauma
- proximal and distal lumens separated by a minimum of 2 cm to prevent access recirculation[1]
- a continuous path for blood to permit high blood flow rates and heparin-free dialysis

---

[1]More detailed information about double lumen catheters and access recirculation can be found in **Sections 9.3** and **9.5** of this chapter.

- ease of insertion into subclavian, internal jugular and femoral sites
- insertion using a modified Seldinger technique to minimise vessel trauma
- maximal blood flow of 300 mL/min.

SILASTIC CUFFED TUNNELLED CATHETERS

These catheters may be dual lumen catheters (e.g. Permcath®), or alternatively they may consist of two single lumen catheters (e.g. Tesio® catheters). These devices are more difficult to insert and usually require either fluoroscopic screening or surgical insertion. The advantages of these catheters, once inserted, include:

- higher blood flow rates (>400 mL/min)
- lower infection rates
- less thrombogenic than other plastic dual lumen catheters
- good long term survival — up to 70% one year catheter survival.

CHOICE OF ACCESS SITE

Temporary dual lumen catheters are commonly inserted in three sites (**Figures 10** and **11**). Internal jugular lines may be inserted from a high (#1) or low (#2) approach as shown in **Figure 10**. As an alternative, the subclavian (#3) or femoral (#4) routes may be used.

The choice of route is largely dependent on the experience of the operator but the following points should be borne in mind:

Internal Jugular Route

- Favoured neck approach — low risk of pneumothorax and late stenosis.
- Suitable for ambulant patient.
- Uncomfortable for a conscious patient.

Subclavian Route

- Suitable for ambulant patient.
- Least favoured route due to high risk of late stenosis (up to 40%).
- Highest risk of complications.

Femoral Route

- Technically the easiest route with lowest complication rate.
- Can be used immediately without requiring check X-ray.
- Easiest to insert if patient unable to lie flat (e.g. pulmonary oedema).
- May be particularly useful in intensive care setting when "neck congestion" occurs.
- Ideal in bacteraemic patients, i.e. new catheter for each dialysis session.

Figure 10. Anatomy of internal jugular and subclavian vein line insertion sites

#1 — high internal jugular vein approach
#2 — low internal jugular vein approach
#3 — subclavian vein approach

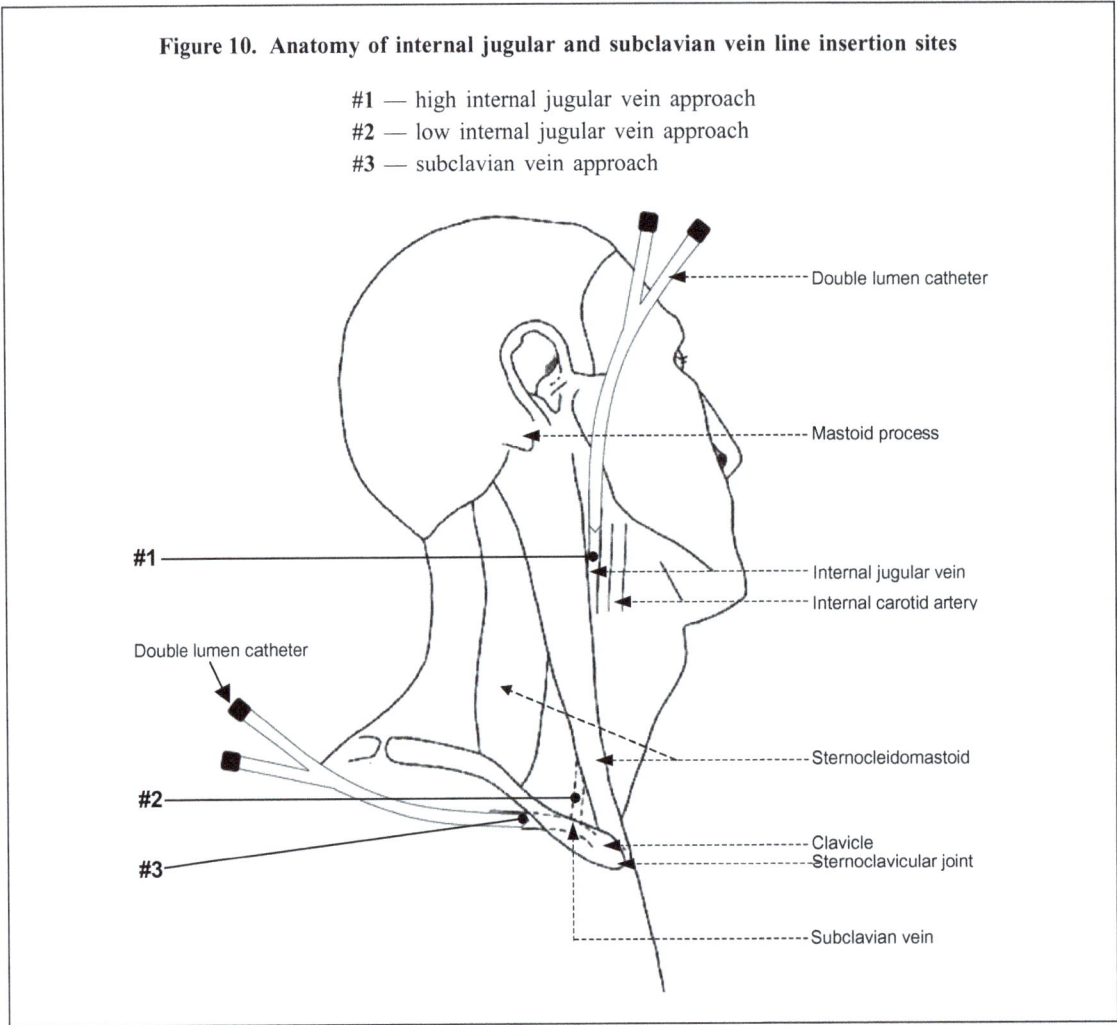

- Not suitable for an ambulant patient except for one-off usage.
- Requires longer catheter (>20 cm) to minimise recirculation (see **Chapter 9.3** and **9.5**).

COMPLICATIONS OF INSERTION

Early Complications

Internal jugular route

- Puncture of the carotid artery — subsequent dialysis should be postponed or performed in a "heparin-free" fashion. Haematoma in this area may cause tracheal compression.
- Recurrent laryngeal palsy — usually self-limiting associated with the local anaesthetic.
- Horner's syndrome — rare but caused by damage to sympathetic trunk.
- Pneumothorax/haemothorax — much rarer than with subclavian route.
- Great vessel/cardiac puncture — rarer due to relatively straight path of catheter.

Figure 11. Vascular access

Top half — Diagrammatic representation of internal and subclavian line positions
Lower half — anatomy of femoral line insertion

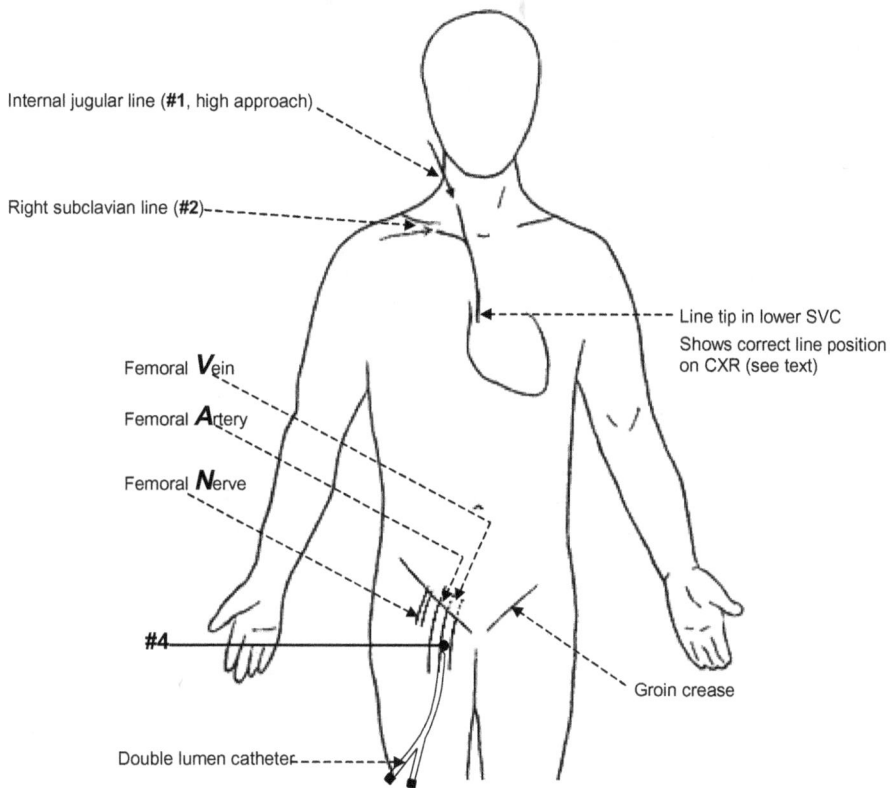

Internal jugular line (**#1**, high approach)

Right subclavian line (**#2**)

Line tip in lower SVC
Shows correct line position on CXR (see text)

Femoral **V**ein

Femoral **A**rtery

Femoral **N**erve

#4

Groin crease

Double lumen catheter

- Air embolism — catheter should be occluded during insertion.
- Thoracic duct perforation — on left side only.

Subclavian route

- Puncture of the subclavian artery — subsequent dialysis should be postponed or performed in a "heparin-free" fashion.
- Cardiac arrhythmias — associated with insertion of guide-wire or inappropriately long catheter.
- Pneumothorax — may require chest drain.
- Haemothorax — may require chest drain.
- Brachial plexus injury.
- Puncture of SVC with mediastinal haemorrhage — life threatening — may require surgical intervention.
- Cardiac rupture with tamponade — life threatening — may require surgical intervention.
- Air embolism — catheter should be occluded during insertion.

Practice Point 3. Line insertion techniques

Internal jugular route	Subclavian route	Femoral route
Prepare trolley with all necessary items for line insertion		
15 cm catheter to position in SVC on the right; use longer line on the left side		25 cm line, to prevent recirculation
Patient must be fully supine, possibly with head down tilt on the bed if the patient is dry. This is because the internal jugular vein must be dilated	Patient must be fully supine, possibly with head down tilt if the patient is dry (subclavian v. must be dilated) A rolled towel or alternatively a bag of saline is placed between the patients shoulder blades to keep the shoulders back on the mattress. Turn patient's head 45° away from the insertion side	Lay the patient flat on the bed; not necessary to be fully supine
Wash hands and put on sterile gown and gloves Create sterile field around insertion site, shaving off any hair and using drapes as required		
Two routes may be used for approaching the IJV (**Figure 10–#1 & #2**). The high approach is safer. The low approach is only recommended to those either experienced or using some form of ultrasound or fluoroscopic guidance, due to the proximity of right dome of the pleura Locate insertion site just lateral to the pulsations of the carotid artery, and medial to the sternocleidomastoid muscle, at the midpoint of a line drawn between the mastoid process and the suprasternal notch (see **Figure 10–#1**)	Locate insertion site approximately at a point where the inner third of the clavicle joins the middle third (see **Figure 10–#3**). There is usually a pronounced bend in the clavicle at this point	Locate insertion site approximately 1cm medial to the pulsations of the femoral a. and 2–3 cm below the groin crease (see **Figure 11–#4**). This allows the needle to track subcutaneously towards the groin crease and keeps the actual line entry site away from the groin area, reducing risk of line contamination
Infiltrate around insertion site with 2% lidocaine and wait 5 min to allow anaesthetic to take effect Skin puncture is performed using a 22-gauge needle attached to a 10 mL syringe half-filled with normal saline		
Advance the needle at an angle of 45° to the skin, aiming for the ipsilateral nipple	Advance needle under the clavicle towards the bag lying under the shoulder blades. After a short distance and once the needle is under the clavicle the direction of approach is changed. Once under the clavicle advance needle behind it aiming directly at the suprasternal notch	A short subcutaneous track is made with the needle travelling in a cephalic direction before aiming deeper toward the vein which is approximately 1 cm medial to the pulsations of the femoral a.

- Apply gentle suction to the needle while approaching the vein; syringe should fill with dark red, non-pulsatile blood (bright red pulsatile blood indicates arterial puncture — withdraw syringe and apply firm pressure for 10 mins)
- Once cannulated, withdraw needle and approach vein with the 18-gauge needle supplied with the catheter set
- Once located remove syringe and pass guide-wire down needle for approximately 15 cm (use mark on the guide-wire)
- Only advance the wire if it passes freely, otherwise withdraw and resite needle
- Remove needle over the guide-wire while making sure not to let the wire move relative to the skin
- Make a small cut with a scalpel at the point of entry through the skin to allow the dilator to be inserted
- Pass the dilator over wire to enlarge vein track — fix the wire relative to the skin while advancing the dilator
- Remove the dilator over the wire again securing the wire relative to the skin
- Pass the catheter over the wire — it should advance with minimal trauma
- Check that both ports aspirate freely and fill with heparinised saline (1,000 u/mL) — check dead space volume on packet
- Secure the catheter to the skin with a suture either side of the lumen, clean area around site and cover with dressing

Confirm position of the catheter tip in the lower SVC on chest X-ray prior to use

Femoral route

- Puncture of the femoral artery — requires direct pressure to achieve haemostasis; subsequent dialysis should be postponed or performed in a "heparin-free" fashion.
- Groin or retroperitoneal haematomas — caused by puncture through both layers of vessel.

There is little doubt that the placement of temporary dialysis catheters is greatly assisted by the use of ultrasound guidance, where available. Ultrasound guides have been shown to increase the success rates for catheter insertion and reduce complications.

Later Complications

Infection

Line-related sepsis may manifest itself as a localised exit site infection or a systemic bacteraemia with or without shock. Bacteraemia generally originates from contamination of the catheter lumen or the migration of bacteria from the skin. Consequently, skin flora (commonly *S. aureus* and *S. epidermidis*) are responsible for most infections. However, diptheroids, gram-negative organisms and fungi may also be involved, particularly in immunocompromised hosts or in patients already receiving antibiotic treatment. Regular review of inserted catheters is the most important preventive measure, and central lines should be changed at least once a week to reduce the risk of infection. Although the risk of line-related sepsis is less with tunnelled catheters, clinicians should be aware that this does occur and be prepared to intervene. Line infection necessitates prompt catheter removal and preferably a short catheter free interval. Before any antibiotic therapy is started, blood cultures (one set from the line and one set peripherally) should be taken. In addition, swabs from the catheter exit site and the catheter tip, should also be sent for culture. The choice of antibiotic should be discussed with the microbiology team but depends upon the patient's immune status/clinical condition, the causative pathogen and the likelihood of drug-resistant organisms being involved, such as Methicillin-resistant *Staphylococcus aureus*. In the immunocompetent host, an IV glycopeptide antibiotic (e.g. vancomycin) is a reasonable first line choice but this should be changed if the drug-sensitivity patterns subsequently indicate that an alternative, such as flucloxacillin, would be as effective. When the causative organism is of low-virulence, such as *S. epidermidis*, simply removing the catheter may be sufficient, but IV antibiotic treatment for 48 h should be given if the infection is more severe (e.g. with systemic features). If the infection is caused by *S. aureus*, IV antibiotic treatment for 2 weeks is indicated and careful clinical review for disseminated septic foci and endocarditis should be performed at the end of this time. Treatment of the systemically unwell patient with severe line-related sepsis is discussed further in **Chapter 19**.

Thrombosis

Central venous catheters predispose to the development of thromboses in the central veins. This association is particularly common using the subclavian route, with thrombosis rates of up to 50% in some studies. As a result, the subclavian route is best avoided for acute dialysis access since thrombosis may jeopardise future formation of fistulae or A–V grafts. One possible mechanism underlying catheter-induced thrombogenicity is that rapid blood flow through the dialysis catheter causes turbulence which leads to vascular endothelial proliferation and eventually stenosis. Treatment options include thrombolysis, angioplasty and stenting, but long term prognosis is not favourable as most vessels eventually become partially or fully occluded. Some renal units use prophylactic subcutaneous heparin or low molecular weight heparin to offset this risk.

FURTHER READING

Choice of Modality

Abramson S, Singh AK (1999) Continuous renal replacement therapy compared with intermittent hemodialysis in intensive care: Which is better? *Current Opinions in Nephrology and Hypertension*; 8: 537–541

Conger J (1998) Dialysis and related therapies. *Seminars in Nephrology*; 18: 533–540

Dillon JJ (1999) Continuous renal replacement therapy or haemodialysis for ARF? *The International Journal of Artificial Organs*; 22: 125–127

Acute Haemodialysis

Abel JJ, Rowntree LG, Turner BB (1913) On the removal of diffusible substances from the circulating blood of living animals by dialysis. *Journal of Pharmacology and Experimental Therapeutics*; 5: 611–623

Bergstrom J, Asaba H, Furst P, Oules R (1976) Dialysis, ultrafiltration, and blood pressure. *Proceedings of the European Dialysis and Transplant Association*; 13: 293

Clark WR, Mueller BA, Kraus MA, Macias WL (1998) Renal replacement therapy quantification in ARF. *Nephrology Dialysis and Transplantation*; 13(S6): 86–90

Evanson JA, Himmelfarb J, Wingard R, et al. (1998) Prescribed versus delivered dialysis in ARF. *American Journal of Kidney Diseases*; 731–738

Evanson JA, Ikizler TA, Wingard R, et al. (1999) Measurement of the delivery of dialysis in ARF. *Kidney International*; 55: 1501–1508

Gillum DM, Dixon BS, Yanover MJ, et al. (1986) The role of intensive dialysis in ARF. *Clinical Nephrology*; 25: 249–255

Himmelfarb J, Tolkoff-Rubin N, Chandran P, et al. (1998) A multicenter comparison of dialysis membranes in the treatment of ARF requiring dialysis. *Journal of the American Society of Nephrology*; 9: 257–266

Humes HD, Buffington DA, MacKay SM, et al. (1999) Replacement of renal function in uremic animals with a tissue-engineered kidney. *Nature Biotechnology*; 17: 451–455

Jorres A, Gahl GM, Dobis C, et al. (1999) Haemodialysis-membrane biocompatibility and mortality of patients with dialysis-dependent ARF: A prospective randomised multicentre trial. *Lancet*; 354: 1337–1341

Ronco C, Bellomo R (1997) Central circulation, peripheral circulation and recirculation. *Blood Purification*; 15: 334–345

Schiffl H, Küchle C, Lang SM (1997) Clinical consequences of blood flow-dialyzer membrane interactions in ARF. *Blood Purification*; 15: 366–381

Schiffl H, Lang SM, Fischer R (2002) Daily haemodialysis and the outcome of acute renal failure. *N Engl J Med*; 346: 305–310

Smith LH, Post RS, Teschan PE, *et al.* (1955) Post-traumatic renal insufficiency in military casualties II. Management, use of an artificial kidney, prognosis. *American Journal of Medicine*; 18: 187–206

Continuous Renal Replacement Therapies

Chatoth DK, Shaver MJ, Marshall MR, *et al.* (1999) Daily 12-hour sustained low-efficiency hemodialysis (SLED) for the treatment of critically ill patients with ARF (ARF): Initial experience. *Blood Purification*; 17: 29

Davenport A, Will EJ, Davidson AM (1993) Improved cardiovascular stability during continuous modes of renal replacement therapy in critically ill patients with acute hepatic and renal failure. *Critical Care Medicine*; 21: 328

Forni LG, Hilton PJ (1997) Continuous hemofiltration in the management of ARF. *The New England Journal of Medicine*; 336: 1303–1309

Golper TA (1992) Indications, technical considerations, and strategies for renal replacement therapy in the intensive care unit. *Journal of Intensive Care Medicine*; 7: 310

Golper TA, Wedel SK, Kaplan AA, *et al.* (1985) Drug removal during CAVH: Theory and clinical observations. *International Journal of Artificial Organs*; 8: 307

Hilton PJ, Taylor J, Forni LG, Treacher DF (1998) Bicarbonate-based haemofiltration in the management of ARF with lactic acidosis. *Quarterly Journal of Medicine*; 91: 279–283

Kronfol NO, Lau AH, Colon-Rivera J, *et al.* (1986) Effect of CAVH membrane types on drug sieving coefficients and clearances. *ASAIO Transactions*; 32: 85

Manns M, Sigler MH, Teehan BP (1998) Continuous renal replacement therapies: An update. *American Journal of Kidney Diseases*; 32: 185

Ronco C (1993) Continuous renal replacement therapies for the treatment of ARF in intensive care patients. *Clinical Nephrology*; 40: 187

Ronco C, Bellomo R (1998) Renal replacement methods in ARF. In: Cameron S, Davison AM, Grunfeld J-P, *et al.* (eds.). *Oxford Textbook of Clinical Nephrology* (2nd Edition) 1583–1606. Oxford: Oxford University Press

Ronco C, Bellomo R, Homel P, *et al.* (2000) Effects of different doses in continuous veno-venous haemofiltration on outcomes of acute renal failure: A prospective study. *Lancet*; 356: 26–30

SECTION 3

THE DISEASES

Chapter 10

SHOCK AND ACUTE RENAL FAILURE
Susan Crail and Stephen Morgan

The "shocked" state results from an inability of the circulation to supply sufficient oxygen and nutrients for the needs of vital organs and tissues or to remove toxic metabolites. The term was first used medically in the eighteenth century in descriptions of gunshot wounds and in the following century was used for the effects of fluid loss in cholera. The need for manoeuvres such as volume replacement in haemorrhagic shock was not really recognised until the nineteenth century, and the use of blood and plasma for the treatment of blood loss only became widely used during World War II.

There are many possible causes of shock all of which lead to the same fundamental problem — inadequate tissue perfusion. Tissue hypoxia, if not corrected rapidly, can lead to organ failure including acute renal failure (ARF). Different organs have differing abilities to deal with hypoxia. The brain will begin to die within minutes but the kidney may eventually recover from several hours of oxygen deprivation. Indeed, the capacity of renal tubule epithelial cells to regenerate following ischaemic injury is what permits organ donation.

Sustained renal hypoxia, however, leads to cell damage with the development of acute tubular necrosis (ATN). The causes of ATN may be sub-divided as shown in **Table 1**. In all of these cases, the fundamental problem is ischaemic tubule injury (see **Chapter 8.1**).

This chapter discusses the underlying pathophysiology and management of shock, and its prevention. Many protocols exist to aid the management of shock and ATN and it is unlikely that it would be possible to formulate a single didactic protocol with which everyone would agree. Before describing the changes in the kidney in shock, it is first necessary to understand what happens in the normal physiological state.

Table 1. Types of shock	
Hypovolaemic shock	Due to loss of circulating volume. Losses may be exogenous (e.g. haemorrhage) or endogenous (e.g. capillary leak)
Cardiogenic shock	Pump failure. Most commonly seen post-myocardial infarction
Obstructive shock	May be regarded as a subtype of cardiogenic shock. Caused by impediment to flow of blood from the heart
Distributive shock	Sepsis syndrome (see **Chapter 19**); anaphylaxis

RENAL HAEMODYNAMICS (see also **Chapter 1**)

Blood flow through the kidney is approximately 20–25% of the total cardiac output, i.e. 1.1 L/min, with the majority being through the renal cortex (normally >90%). The glomerular filtration rate (GFR) is 125 mL/min. With a normal haematocrit of 0.45, renal plasma flow (RPF) is $0.55 \times 1.1 = 605$ mL/min. The filtration fraction is calculated from GFR/RPF = 125/605 which is approximately 20%. Blood flow through an organ is defined as change in pressure/total organ vascular resistance.

In the kidneys, there are two sets of arterioles and two sets of capillaries — glomerular and peritubular. This makes the renal vasculature unusual. Normally, resistance in the afferent and efferent arterioles is approximately equal and accounts for most of the total vascular resistance in the kidneys. The two sets of capillaries are separated by the efferent arterioles and the hydrostatic pressure in the second (peritubular) set of capillaries is much lower than in the first. This low peritubular capillary pressure is crucial for tubular reabsorption of fluid, while the high glomerular pressure is needed for effective glomerular filtration. The afferent arteriole is largely under the control of the vasodilator nitric oxide (NO). If NO synthesis is blocked, significant changes in the resistance of the afferent arteriole may be seen with little effect on the efferent arteriole.

As described in detail in **Chapter 1**, the renal circulation is capable of **autoregulation**, i.e. it is able to maintain relatively constant blood flow over changes in a mean renal arterial pressure range of ~80–180 mmHg. Autoregulation is an adaptive process that prevents major changes in renal blood flow due to arterial pressure fluctuations. It also prevents excessive changes in salt and water excretion by avoiding dramatic alterations in GFR. Autoregulation is only possible in the face of a limited range of arterial pressures. Below a mean arterial pressure (MAP) of 70 mmHg, virtually no blunting of the effects of hypotension is possible and below 20–30 mmHg renal artery perfusion stops. This means that in a patient who is not chronically hypertensive, a MAP of >70 mmHg needs to be maintained to maintain renal function. Renal blood flow (RBF) and GFR can be altered even within the autoregulatory range by other factors such as angiotensin II and the sympathetic nervous system (see **Table 2**, **Chapter 1**).

The renal response to volume depletion is initially afferent arteriolar vasodilatation followed by efferent arteriolar vasoconstriction in an attempt to maintain sufficient pressure to allow glomerular filtration. Cortical filtration is affected earliest with maintenance of juxtamedullary glomerular filtration. Blood flow in the outer medulla is maintained by adenosine, prostaglandin and nitric oxide production.

Whatever the cause of shock, there is a final common pathway resulting in cell death. The major factors in this process are:

Circulatory Changes in Shock

Cardiac output falls as a result of reduced ventricular preload with a compensatory increase in systemic vascular resistance, rise in pulse rate and vasoconstriction. The increase in sympathetic activity as circulatory failure occurs leads to diversion of blood flow to essential organs. Clinical measurements of systemic blood pressure will not detect changes in regional blood flow so that the early organ damage of hypoperfusion may begin unnoticed. A rise in heart rate almost always precedes a drop in systemic blood pressure but, in the later stages of severe hypovolaemic shock, a paradoxical bradycardia may be seen. As a result of the decrease in peripheral blood flow, blood stasis develops. As this becomes established, tissue acidosis develops with endothelial damage, and plasma can leak from the vascular compartment into the interstitial space. This further compounds the reduction in ventricular preload.

Neurohumoral Changes

Many neurohumoral changes take place throughout the body; the precise role of each component is not yet clear. The changes include:

- Increased ADH, ACTH, beta endorphin and growth hormone.
- Activation of the renin-angiotensin system.
- Release of polypeptide kinins from kininogens causing vasodilatation and capillary permeability.
- Production of arachidonic acid products, prostaglandins and leukotriene antagonists.
- Complement activation.

Cellular Changes

An early fall in cellular ATP, consequent upon tissue ischaemia, disrupts ion-pump activity causing cell swelling and death.

Different organs vary in their capability to survive hypoxia. Tubule cells may survive for 1–2 h at 37°C but neurones will die much more rapidly. Even within organs, susceptibility to hypoxia varies, an example being the tubule cells of the kidney which undergo ischaemic necrosis long before glomerular necrosis occurs. This is attributed to the relatively hypoxic renal medulla, even in the normal state, together with the high O_2 demands of metabolically active tubule epithelial cells, particularly those of the proximal tubule.

AETIOLOGY OF HYPOVOLAEMIC SHOCK

The causes of hypovolaemic shock may be divided up in the manner listed in **Table 2**. It is rare for only one pathology to contribute to the aetiology of ATN in a critically ill patient; often there are other contributory factors such as the development of sepsis, pigment nephropathy and use of nephrotoxic drugs (see **Chapter 28**).

PATHOPHYSIOLOGY OF ACUTE TUBULAR NECROSIS

Necrosis of tubule cells is not the only aspect of renal damage seen in shock. Most damage is seen in the straight S_3 segment of the proximal convoluted tubule (PCT) and the medullary thick ascending limb, as they have the lowest blood flow and are most sensitive to ischaemia. The changes, described in detail in **Chapter 8.1**, include:

Table 2. Causes of hypovolaemic shock

Obvious	Blood loss	Intra-operative losses, acute trauma, post-partum, gastrointestinal bleed
	Vomiting	Intestinal obstruction, infection, diabetic autonomic neuropathy
	Diarrhoea	High output stomas, infection (*Clostridium difficile* toxin), inflammatory bowel disease
	Fistulas	Enterocutaneous
	Polyuric states	Recovery period of ATN, hypercalcaemia, hyperglycaemia, diuretics
Occult	High insensible losses	Pyrexia, sweating, hyperventilation
	Plasma loss	Burns, exfoliative dermatitis, erythrodermic skin disease
	Intestinal obstruction	Intraluminal fluid accumulation
	Pancreatitis	Ileus, vomiting, similar picture to septic shock
	Ascites	Maldistribution of fluid due to hypoalbuminaemia, portal venous hypertension
	Hypoalbuminaemia	Malnutrition, nephrotic syndrome, liver disease

1. Tubule Cell Injury

Cell necrosis or apoptosis occurs depending on the severity of the injury. The straight (S_3) segment of the proximal tubule is the most sensitive to injury, due to the relative hypoxia of the region in which these segments lie.

2. Disruption of the Actin Cytoskeleton

Ischaemia disrupts the actin cytoskeleton leading to:

- Abnormal solute transport due to loss of cell polarity with apical translocation of the basal Na^+/K^+-ATPase; this may result in sodium being pumped into the cell, and thus cell swelling.
- Loss of cell–cell adhesion with loss of epithelial barrier functions.
- Loss of cell-matrix adhesion with cell shedding into the tubules and cell–cell clumping (cellular cast formation).

3. Tubule Lumen Obstruction

Shed tubule cells express adhesion molecules which mediate homotypic cell aggregation leading to tubule obstruction. Tubule cells may also complex with Tamm-Horsfall protein to form obstructing cellular casts.

4. Vascular Congestion Related to Inflammatory Changes within the Microcirculation

- Endothelial cell (EC) injury, swelling and plugging.
- EC adhesion molecule expression and leucocyte adherence/plugging.
- Leucocyte recruitment into renal parenchyma with consequent inflammation.

The evolution of ATN can be divided into three time periods:

1. Initiation phase lasting from hours to days.
2. Established phase, usually lasting for about two weeks but may be prolonged.
3. Recovery phase which may be early or delayed.

During the initial and established phases RBF is decreased by approximately 50%, but GFR is decreased to 5–10% of normal levels. ATN is potentially preventable during the initiation phase. However, during the established phase, even if RBF is restored using such methods as volume replacement and dopamine, little effect is seen on the GFR. This suggests there is regional maldistribution of blood flow with medullary hypoxia, which appears to be related to an imbalance between endothelin and NO. Persistent hypoxia then leads to the pathological changes described above.

In the recovery phase of ATN, damaged tubule cells (**not** having undergone apoptosis/necrosis) can regain function. Survivor cells replicate to cover denuded basement membrane. Consequently, approximately 95% of patients with ATN will regain clinically useful renal function.

CLINICAL RECOGNITION OF THE SHOCKED PATIENT

It is important to recognise and rapidly institute management of shock before end organ damage becomes established and irreversible. It is essential to identify those patients at risk of shock; this usually follows a typical clinical prelude as discussed above and in **Chapter 3**. Basic clinical observations often give the first clues and subsequent interventional techniques may confirm it.

1. Heart Rate

This is the first easily measured parameter to alter in hypovolaemic shock. Pulse rate increases to maintain cardiac output and allow blood pressure/organ perfusion to be maintained.

2. Systemic Blood Pressure (see also **Chapter 5**)

This can be maintained, in an otherwise fit individual, until approximately 25% of the circulating volume has been lost. In most clinical situations, it is only possible to measure blood pressure using non-invasive methods but, in the ICU, invasive blood pressure monitoring via a directly transduced arterial line allows continuous readout of levels allowing more rapid assessment of response to treatment (see **Chapter 28**). **Note**, absolute blood pressure readings may be misleading — a value of 120/60 mmHg may be appropriate for a young fit person but in someone who is normally hypertensive it may reflect hypotension, with hypoperfusion of organs such as the kidneys which adapt to chronically elevated blood pressure.

3. Urine Output (see also **Chapter 4.2**)

Insertion of a urinary catheter from which hourly output readings can be taken is essential in the management of a patient at risk of becoming shocked. Minimum acceptable urine output is generally accepted as 0.5 mL/kg/h.

4. Hypoxia

Inadequate tissue perfusion leads to tissue hypoxia. The patient will become tachypnoeic as the body attempts to compensate. Tachypnoea will also occur as a response to the evolving metabolic acidosis, as lactate is generated in oxygen-starved tissues.

5. Central Venous Pressure (CVP) Monitoring

The CVP is a guide to circulating volume and filling pressure of the right ventricle. It is most useful in the shocked patient in measuring the response to a fluid challenge rather than to measure absolute values. CVP readings will be affected by factors such as myocardial failure and increased pulmonary vascular resistance as well as by operator variability and patient position.

6. Pulmonary Artery Occlusion Pressure (PAOP) Catheters

These measure pulmonary arterial pressure (PAP) and left atrial filling pressure. They are usually only available for use on the ICU and require medical and nursing staff who have been trained in their use. Recently there have been movements away from the use of these catheters as some studies have identified increased morbidity and mortality associated with their use. Whether this is due to inadequate training of staff in the interpretation of results and their manipulation is still unclear.

Information which can be obtained from use of these catheters can be divided into:

- **Pressures** — CVP and PAP can be transduced directly and continually. PAOP can be obtained intermittently. From these values, filling pressures for both sides of the heart can be measured allowing calculation of volume status and ventricular function.
- **Cardiac output** — this can be calculated using the thermodilution method and can be used in determining need for inotropes.
- **Oxygen delivery** and **consumption**.

Various clinical conditions affect the relationship between the PAOP and left ventricular end diastolic pressure (LVEDP), thereby limiting the usefulness of readings obtained. These include:

- Heart rate — particularly severe tachycardia which will lead to recording of relatively high readings.
- Mitral and/or aortic valve disease.
- Increased pulmonary vascular resistance, e.g. pulmonary embolus.
- Impaired ventricular compliance — left ventricular hypertrophy, acute MI, restrictive pericarditis.
- Positive pressure ventilation.

Further discussion of the use of pulmonary artery catheters and other invasive monitoring procedures can be found in **Chapters 5** and **28**.

DIAGNOSIS OF ACUTE TUBULAR NECROSIS

Laboratory investigations and clinical observations can be used in confirming the cause of ARF in a shocked patient. Clinical findings have been discussed in the previous section. In this section, we consider laboratory investigations which may be used to back up the suspicion of shock-associated ARF and also interventional procedures which may be of help.

Urinalysis

(i) Biochemistry — In pre-renal failure with intact tubule function, the body attempts to conserve sodium and water. Sodium is avidly reabsorbed by tubules which are still intact in an attempt to compensate for the low-flow state. In established ATN by contrast, tubule compensatory mechanisms are lost and the usually little urine that is made will be of lower osmolality and higher sodium concentration. Thus, the concentration of sodium and the ratio of urine to plasma osmolality can help to distinguish pre-renal from renal and post-renal failure (see **Table 3**, **Chapter 4.2**). In the clinical setting, the usefulness of urinalysis is limited as the patient may be oliguric and unable to provide a suitable urine sample, may have received IV fluids, or may have been given a diuretic before samples are obtained. The most urgent need in a hypovolaemic patient is to begin fluid resuscitation as soon as possible.

(ii) Microscopy — Urine microscopy is used to look for red cell morphology, and for the presence of casts and crystals. In shock-associated ARF, the presence of non-dysmorphic red cells can indicate bleeding from the renal pelvis, ureters or bladder. However, the presence of red cells should also prompt thoughts of glomerulonephritis or tubulointerstitial nephritis. The presence of white cells or bacteria is obviously of use in diagnosing sepsis. There are various types of tubule casts which indicate the cause of ARF. These are described in **Chapter 4.2**.

Haematology and Biochemistry (see also **Chapters 4.3** and **4.4**)

A patient with pre-renal failure will usually have a full blood count and serum chemistry that reflect a hypovolaemic state:

- **Urea** (mmol/L):**creatinine** (μmol/L) **ratio** — in a normal person this is roughly 1:20. With intravascular volume depletion, the ratio drops and may become 1:5–10.
- **Haematocrit** — raised in dehydration. Anaemia can develop rapidly in ARF, so changes in haematocrit are not always helpful in distinguishing between acute and chronic disease.

Role of Renal Biopsy

In general, renal biopsy is not necessary in the management of shock-associated ARF. In patients who have atypical features of ARF suggesting pathology other than ATN, biopsy may be undertaken to exclude causes such as acute glomerulonephritis and tubulointerstitial disease. Renal biopsy may also have a role in the patient who fails to recover renal function weeks after the initial precipitating insult to see if there are histological features of recovery or cortical necrosis.

To **summarise**, a combination of clinical suspicion following typical precursor events (e.g. G.I. bleed), physical examination, urine biochemistry and microscopy, and typical serum biochemistry are usually sufficient to make the diagnosis of ATN.

MANAGEMENT OF SHOCK

Expansion of plasma volume with restoration of blood pressure is necessary and is often the first step before definitive management of the underlying cause can be instituted (see **Practice Point 1**).

1. Replacement Fluids

The debate about the optimum type of replacement fluid in hypovolaemia continues. In comparing the benefits of crystalloids and colloids, it is difficult to provide any robust statistical evidence of the benefit of one over the other.

The exact choice of fluid depends to an extent on the cause of hypovolaemia. In acute haemorrhage, blood is needed but there is no need to replace all blood loss with blood. Viscosity of blood and hence microcirculatory flow is optimum at a haematocrit level of approximately 30%. Other colloids can therefore be used in addition during fluid resuscitation in haemorrhagic shock. Colloid solutions determine the oncotic pressure regulating fluid shifts across the vascular cell membrane and, therefore, much lower colloid volumes are needed to restore intravascular volume in comparison to crystalloids. In fluid loss due to diarrhoea or severe dehydration, however, crystalloids are indicated in order to restore both intravascular and interstitial fluid deficiencies. Crystalloid solutions such as saline and Ringer's lactate are distributed into the intravascular and interstitial spaces. Electrolytes do not cross the cellular membrane readily, so crystalloid solutions determine the osmotic pressure regulating electrolyte shift across the cell membrane. Crystalloids reduce colloid oncotic pressure and therefore predispose to pulmonary and peripheral oedema particularly in uraemic or septicaemic patients.

(a) *Human albumin solutions*

Until recently, albumin solutions were often used in fluid resuscitation. Whilst the half-life of transfused albumin is much shorter than that of endogenous albumin, it does have a relatively sustained effect on intravascular volume. A major review article published in the British Medical Journal in July 1998, looked at the effect of administration of human albumin solution (HAS) in a variety of critically ill patients. It found no evidence that administration of HAS reduced mortality and some evidence that it in fact increased mortality. Various explanations have been forwarded to try and explain this, including a detrimental effect on coagulation due to interference with platelet aggregation and increased inhibition of factor Xa by antithrombin III. There may also be increased leakage of albumin into extravascular spaces causing oedema formation due to increased permeability of capillary membranes in critically ill patients. This is likely to be due to direct cellular damage and the action of pro-inflammatory cytokines. Consequently, most hospitals have reduced or discontinued their use of albumin in acute hypovolaemic states. Other

Practice Point 1. Management of hypotension

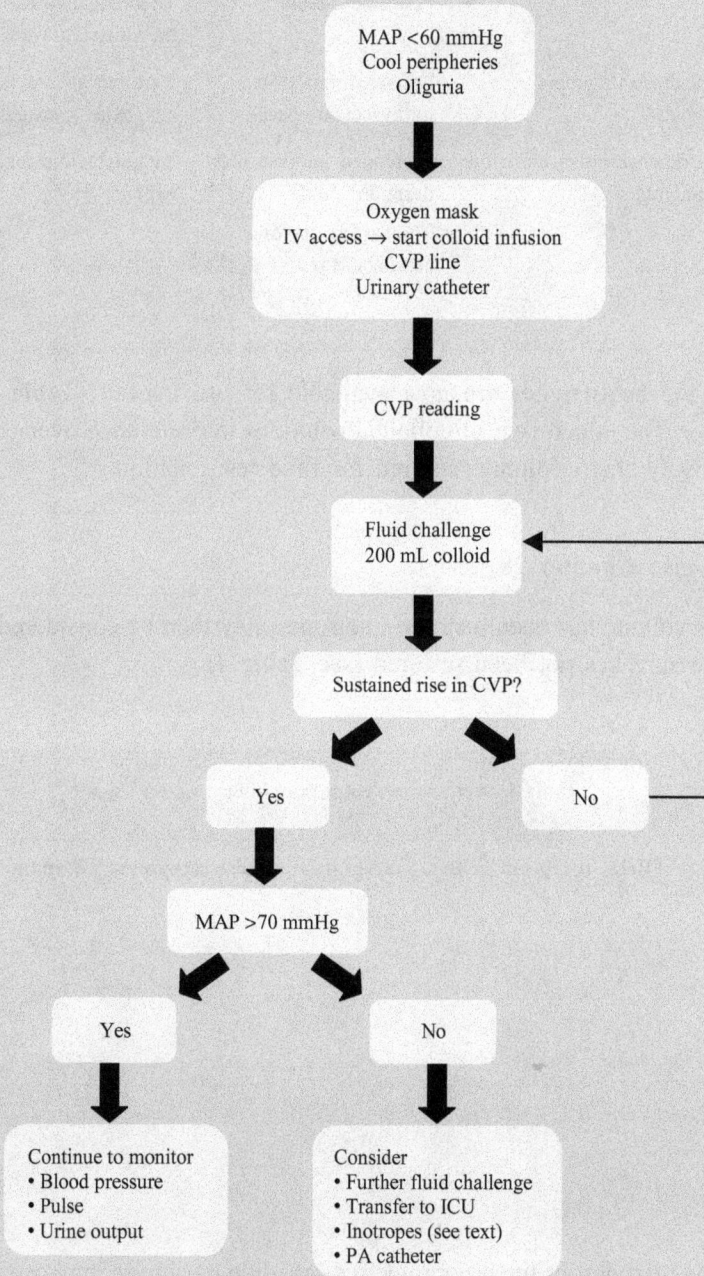

MAP <60 mmHg
Cool peripheries
Oliguria

↓

Oxygen mask
IV access → start colloid infusion
CVP line
Urinary catheter

↓

CVP reading

↓

Fluid challenge
200 mL colloid

↓

Sustained rise in CVP?

Yes   No

MAP >70 mmHg

Yes   No

Continue to monitor
• Blood pressure
• Pulse
• Urine output

Consider
• Further fluid challenge
• Transfer to ICU
• Inotropes (see text)
• PA catheter

Table 3. Available colloid solutions			
Solution	Description	For	Against
Gelatins	Small molecular weight	Relatively cheap Few side-effects	Rapid elimination Theoretical risk of prion disease transmission
Dextrans	Sucrose polymers	Longer duration in intravascular space	Rare but severe side effects — anaphylaxis, coagulation disturbances
Hydroxyethyl starch solutions	Branched polysaccharide polymers	Prolonged intravascular duration Thought to decrease capillary leaks	Anaphylactoid reaction, expensive

solutions such as the hetastarches are now available for use instead (**Table 3**) but these are relatively expensive. The added cost of colloidal solutions in preference over crystalloid may be offset by the relatively small volume required for fluid resuscitation.

2. Inotropes (see also **Chapter 28**)

Once intravascular volume has been restored, inotropes may then be considered if an acceptable systemic blood pressure has not been restored (see **Table 4**).

Table 4. Actions of sympathomimetic agents				
Drug	Beta$_1$ receptors	Beta$_2$ receptors	Alpha receptors	Dopamine receptors
Dopamine	++	0	+ to ++	++
Epinephrine	++	++	+	0
Norepinephrine	++	0	++	0
Isoprenaline	++	++	0	0
Dobutamine	++	+	+	0
Dopexamine	++	++	0	++

(a) *Dopamine*

Dopamine has long been part of the renoprotective schedule used in many hospitals and has been discussed at length in **Chapter 8.1**. The theoretical benefits of low-dose dopamine on renal blood flow have led to its widespread use in the management of ARF. Controlled clinical trials have failed to show any overall beneficial effects on outcome in ARF; however, its diuretic effects may be useful in fluid balance control so it may still be used in the overloaded patient. If it does not work within 24 h, it should be stopped.

(b) *Dobutamine and dopexamine*

Generally the agents of choice in cardiogenic shock. They are discussed further in **Chapter 28**. They are not used in hypovolaemic shock as they cause vasodilatation and further lowering of blood pressure. Dopexamine has, however, been used in regimens attempting to prevent ARF, for example in major elective surgery. Some preliminary studies have suggested that it may have a renoprotective effect, but further large scale studies are needed and its routine use cannot be recommended.

(c) *Norepinephrine*

Norepinephrine has on occasion been blamed as a cause of ARF due to its vasoconstrictive properties. However, especially in septic shock (**Chapter 19**), it is probably the most beneficial agent in improving renal perfusion due to its ability to raise systemic vascular resistance, and thus MAP, and thereby restore renal perfusion.

(d) *Epinephrine*

Epinephrine is a powerful positive inotrope. The dose delivered can be titrated to achieve a suitable cardiac output. Epinephrine and norepinephrine are best used in patients with a pulmonary artery catheter *in situ* to monitor response, and to ensure that occult hypovolaemia does not develop during treatment, masked by the inotropes.

3. Diuretics

Diuretics such as furosemide and mannitol are often advocated in the management of ARF. Epidemiologic studies suggest that non-oliguric ATN is associated with a lower risk of dialysis dependence and greater chance of recovery than oliguric ATN. Although this may simply reflect a lesser degree of injury in the non-oliguric variant, efforts are generally made to improve urine output in those with shock and ARF, not least to minimise attendant risks of pulmonary oedema. Even if urinary output is not restored, experimental evidence suggests that use of a loop diuretic will reduce tubule epithelial cell ATP and oxygen requirements, as it blocks the chloride exchange pump in the loop of Henle. There is, however, little clinical evidence to support this assertion. Furosemide has been used in the dose range 250–1,000 mg/day, either as boluses or as infusions at a rate of 10 mg/h.

To date, no consistent evidence has shown benefit from diuretics and, in the authors' opinion, they may be detrimental by predisposing to further renal damage through hypovolaemia. Mannitol also involves fairly large fluid volumes and may lead to fluid overload in ATN.

4. Other Methods

If all of these interventions are failing, the outlook for the patient is poor. Regular reassessment of the patient is essential. Other interventions which may be considered include intra-aortic balloon pump and LV assist (for cardiogenic shock). These are only available in specialist ICUs and will not be discussed here.

ACUTE RENAL REPLACEMENT THERAPY IN SHOCK (see also Chapter 9)

In established ARF, renal replacement therapy (RRT) becomes necessary to allow removal of toxic metabolites and sufficient plasma water to allow for nutritional support. Other indications for renal replacement therapy in the intensive care setting include:

- Uraemia.
- Hyperkalaemia.
- Refractory fluid overload.
- Severe metabolic acidosis.

We prefer to initiate RRT in critically ill patients as soon as a diagnosis of established ATN has been made and before they become profoundly uraemic. The aim of RRT in the acutely unwell patient is to mimic the physiology of their native kidney as closely as possible until recovery occurs. There are possible pitfalls in the prescription of renal replacement therapy such as:

- Inadequate correction of biochemical abnormalities.
- Inaccurate fluid balance.
- Further ischaemic insults to the kidney due to hypotensive episodes.
- Prolongation of duration of oligoanuria — not proven but widely believed.
- Haemorrhage due to anticoagulation.
- Complement activation due to membrane bioincompatibility (i.e. the foreign dialyser membrane surface activates the complement cascade).

Current techniques available for RRT on the ICU are discussed further in Chapters 9 and 28.

OUTCOME OF PATIENTS WITH SHOCK-ASSOCIATED ATN

The overall survival of patients with ARF has changed very little over the last two decades. Part of this is attributed to changes in the demographics of people accepted for treatment — many more elderly patients and those suffering with multi-organ failure are now treated aggressively. Recent government figures have been published comparing mortality rates on intensive care units but, in looking at these, differences in patient composition must also be considered. Tertiary referral units where procedures such as heart valve surgery are carried out may have higher mortality figures as they treat the sicker patients. Difficulties in statistical interpretation also stem from the fact that ARF is a syndrome, not a disease with a single cause, and its outcome is therefore subject to many variables. In addition, people with ATN often either start with or develop other organ pathologies which will affect outcome.

The APACHE II (acute physiology and chronic health evaluation) scoring system has been used widely in an attempt to predict chances of survival in patients admitted to intensive care units. However, its predictive capacity in those with ARF has been questioned. ARF in the ICU setting is often part of multi-organ failure and is frequently associated with sepsis. The APACHE II scoring system does not take into account the cause of ARF, only its existence. Survival in patients with ATN due to nephrotoxins and those with ATN due to ischaemia can be shown to have very different survival and mortality rates. For example, a group in New Jersey (Weisberg *et al.*, 1997) found a mortality rate of 10% at 21 days in a group of patients with nephrotoxin-induced ATN versus 30% in a similar group with ischaemia-induced ATN. Similarly, dialysis-free survival was 66% in the nephrotoxic group versus 41% in the ischaemic group.

Recommendations proposed by the UK Renal Association and the Intensive Care Society suggest that approximately 90% of patients with isolated ARF requiring renal replacement therapy should survive to hospital discharge. However, if there is combined severe acute renal and respiratory failure the survival rate drops to about 45%, and in multi-organ failure, only 5–15% of patients survive to discharge.

FURTHER READING

Cochrane Injuries Group Albumin Reviewers (1998) Human albumin administration in critically ill patients: Systematic review of randomised controlled trials. *British Medical Journal*; 317: 235–240

Hinds CJ, Watson D (1996) *Intensive Care, A Concise Textbook* (2nd Edition). London: WB Saunders Company Ltd

Weisberg LS, Allgren RL, Genter FC, Kurnik BR (1997) Causes of acute tubular necrosis affects its prognosis. The Auriculin Anaritide Acute Renal Failure Study Group. *Archives of Internal Medicine*; 157: 1833–1838

Chapter 11

TOXINS AND DRUGS AND ACUTE RENAL FAILURE
Afzal Chaudhry

TOXIC NEPHROPATHIES: DEFINITION

The term "Toxic Nephropathy" describes those renal disorders that are caused by exposure to radiocontrast media, therapeutic and recreational drugs, and other environmental chemicals. The possibility that a nephrotoxic agent may be responsible for renal injury should be considered in all patients presenting with acute renal failure (ARF). This is true for every type of ARF, whether it be glomerular, tubulointerstitial or vascular in aetiology. Drug toxicity may also contribute to the development of ARF in patients with other diagnoses, e.g. glomerulonephritis (GN). The condition is often underdiagnosed; as many as a quarter of all cases of ARF are now due in some way to drug toxicity. Furthermore, toxic nephropathies are not without long-term sequelae; up to 25% of patients are left with chronic renal impairment, with 12.5% mortality. The incidence of toxic nephropathies has risen over the last 20 years, reflecting both the increasing use of diagnostic and therapeutic agents as well as greater awareness of their nephrotoxic potential.

PATHOPHYSIOLOGY

Toxic nephropathy can occur as a result of:

(1) altered renal blood flow ("functional")
(2) direct renal cell damage ("direct")
(3) immune-mediated renal cell injury ("allergic").

(1) "Functional" Nephrotoxicity

"Functional" ARF is secondary to altered regulation of glomerular filtration, and is predominantly determined by variations in pre- and post-glomerular arteriolar resistance. Mechanisms underlying "functional" nephrotoxicity include the following:

- Inhibition of the renin-angiotensin system, in situations where the system has become vital to the maintenance of glomerular filtration, leads to the development of ARF.
- Alterations in the balance of vasoconstrictor agents (e.g. thromboxanes and endothelins) and vasodilatory agents (e.g. prostaglandins) can lead to ARF in susceptible individuals.
- Direct vascular damage and endothelial swelling with thrombosis may cause ARF.

- Excessive volume depletion associated with diuretic use can lead to a reduction in glomerular filtration rate (GFR) and ARF.

"Functional" ARF is usually rapidly reversible upon cessation of the nephrotoxic insult.

(2) "Direct" Nephrotoxicity

ARF results from direct renal cell injury caused by the nephrotoxic agent. Renal tubule epithelial cells are the major targets of nephrotoxic damage. **Table 1** lists a number of mechanisms by which nephrotoxins may cause cellular injury. A given nephrotoxic agent may induce cell injury via multiple mechanisms. In addition, impairment of tubule solute and water reabsorption following tubule injury may lead to afferent arteriolar constriction following up-regulation of transforming growth factor β (TGFβ).

(3) "Allergic" Nephrotoxicity

This is discussed in **Chapter 18** — acute tubulointerstitial nephritis (TIN). Rarely, severe glomerulonephritis may also result from drug allergy.

Table 1. Biochemical mechanisms of nephrotoxin induced cellular injury

Mechanism	Consequences
Direct changes in plasma membrane permeability	
Altered phospholipase activity	Abnormal plasma membrane structure
	Inhibition of normal membrane reconstitution
Cytoskeletal alterations	Loss/redistribution of membrane enzymatic components
	Altered area available for trans-membrane transport
Altered plasma membrane transporter function	Changes in cell volume, shape and homeostasis
Perturbation of intracellular calcium homeostasis	Activation of calcium-dependent degradative enzymes
	Loss of mitochondrial oxidative phosphorylation
Disturbance of normal lysosome function	Intracellular release of degradative lysosomal enzymes
Oxygen free radical production	Lipid bilayer peroxidation and loss of function
	Loss of cytoprotective glutathione
	Chromosome and DNA breakage

SITE OF TOXIC EFFECT

Nephrotoxic agents in the systemic circulation reach the kidneys in high concentrations, since they receive between 20–25% of the resting cardiac output. The processes of glomerular filtration, proximal tubule secretion and reabsorption serve to concentrate toxins within the tubule lumen.

Consequently, renal tubule cells are exposed to toxic concentrations of many circulating drugs and chemicals. Nephrotoxic agents exert their effects at one or a number of discrete regions along the length of the nephron, producing characteristic clinical syndromes. The site-selective nature of the damage is determined by a multitude of factors, which include:

- regional differences in intra-renal blood flow
- the localisation and specificity of various transport mechanisms
- the balance of bioactivation and detoxification reactions
- the degree of activity of regenerative/repair mechanisms.

Glomerular Injury

Direct glomerular damage is rare. Injury may be a result of direct toxicity to glomerular capillary endothelial cells, e.g. mitomycin C induced haemolytic uraemic syndrome. Toxins may act as antigens or as haptens, leading to the deposition of immune complexes within the glomerulus, e.g. gold or penicillamine induced membranous GN. Certain drugs are also associated with ANCA-positive vasculitis and crescentic nephritis (e.g. propylthiouracil, hydralazine).

Proximal Tubule Injury

Proximal tubule damage is the most common manifestation of nephrotoxic injury. The reasons for this are as follows:

- Tubular transport of heavy metals, organic anions and cations, peptides, low molecular weight proteins and glutathione conjugates occurs within the proximal tubule.
- The enzymes cytochrome P-450 and cysteine conjugate β-lyase are almost exclusively localised to the proximal tubule. Bioactivation-dependent nephrotoxicity will therefore localise to this region of the nephron.
- The outer medullary S_3 segment of the proximal tubule is particularly susceptible to ischaemic injury that may result from toxin-induced hypoperfusion (see above — "functional" nephrotoxicity). This reflects the high O_2 requirements of this tubule segment, in a region of the kidney that already exists in a state of low O_2 tension (see **Chapter 1**).

Medullary Injury

Low O_2 tension within the renal medulla renders this region particularly susceptible to changes in renal blood flow, e.g. NSAIDs.

Intratubular Obstruction

In addition to intratubular obstruction caused by the aggregation of sloughed epithelial cells, precipitation of the nephrotoxic agent within the tubule may obstruct urine flow, e.g. aciclovir. This is usually pH dependent, and may often be avoided by the administration of intravenous fluids.

Distal Tubule and Collecting Duct Injury

Tubule dysfunction in this region of the nephron leads to disorders of concentration, electrolyte imbalance and acidification defects. Exactly which of a number of different mechanisms is involved depends on the particular nephrotoxic agent. In some cases, the precise mechanism of toxicity is unknown. Amphotericin B causes relatively specific distal tubule toxicity.

CLINICAL ASSESSMENT OF THE PATIENT

Clinical History and Examination (see also **Chapter 4.1**)

Important, but rarely truly diagnostic because of the wide spectrum of clinical presentations in toxic nephropathy. Rash and fever raise the suspicion of a drug-induced TIN (see **Chapter 18**).

Drug History

Questioning should be extended to cover use of recreational drugs, topical solutions/creams/ointments and herbal remedies. Questions should also be asked as to the possibility of environmental and/or occupational exposure to any form of chemical agent.

Laboratory Investigations

Investigations of particular relevance to specific nephrotoxins are described in the appropriate sections, later in this chapter. Detailed descriptions of laboratory investigations in ARF are given in **Chapter 4**.

Renal Biopsy

Although histopathological confirmation may provide the greatest evidence for the role of the suspected toxin in the development of ARF, such evidence is not always conclusive. Further, renal biopsy is often not undertaken, particularly if the deterioration in renal function has followed a pattern and time course consistent with the known renal effects of the suspected toxin. Rather, the diagnosis is made retrospectively following improvement in renal function after withdrawal of the toxin.

TREATMENT PRINCIPLES

A number of general principles, discussed below, apply when considering how best to **prevent** toxic nephropathy. With regards to the treatment of **established** toxin/drug induced ARF, renal dysfunction is often reversible following withdrawal of the offending drug. Other specific treatments are detailed in the appropriate section of this chapter — "Nephrotoxicity of Specific Agents".

Prevention of Toxic Nephropathies

Identification of "at-risk" patients

Patients who are particularly susceptible to the nephrotoxic effects of a particular agent benefit from early identification, closer monitoring and early intervention to protect them from toxic side effects. General risk factors for the development of a toxic nephropathy include:

- Volume depletion and/or the use of diuretics.
- Concurrent administration of another potential nephrotoxic agent.
- The presence of concurrent diseases, e.g. diabetes mellitus, systemic sepsis and multiple myeloma.
- Pre-existing renal disease.
- Advanced age.
- Peak serum concentration of the particular agent, cumulative dose and duration of exposure.

Adequate patient hydration

Careful and regular assessments of intravascular volume status are essential (see **Chapter 8**) since hypovolaemia is a major risk factor for the development of nephrotoxicity.

Restricting the use of nephrotoxic agents

Wherever possible, the number of potential nephrotoxins administered at any one time should be minimised. This is especially true if several agents are known to act synergistically to cause renal damage.

Assessment of renal function

Serial measurements of renal function are essential. For many agents, nephrotoxic effects are completely reversible provided that the agent is withdrawn at an early enough stage. Note that rising drug levels, rather than suggesting an impending nephrotoxic effect, may in fact be indicative of an already declining GFR.

Specific therapeutic manoeuvres

Specific therapies known to minimise nephrotoxicity should be used if possible, e.g. once daily gentamicin; sodium loading and cisplatin; urinary alkalinisation and sulphonamides, methotrexate, or uric acid (tumour lysis syndromes — see **Chapter 21**).

Immune-mediated nephrotoxicity (see also **Chapter 18**)

This is difficult to prevent as its occurrence is sporadic and unpredictable. Once detected, the offending agent should be withdrawn immediately. Drug rechallenge, even at a lower dose, is

Table 2. Nephrotoxic agents and their mechanisms of nephrotoxic injury

Mechanism of injury	Site of injury	Nephrotoxic agent
Altered intra-renal haemodynamics	Intra-renal vasculature (in particular the efferent arteriole)	ACEI, amphotericin B, cyclosporin A, NSAIDs, radiocontrast agents
Direct tubule toxicity	Proximal tubule	Aminoglycosides, foscarnet, cisplatin, heavy metals, chloroform, radiocontrast agents
	Thick ascending limb of the Loop of Henle	Aminoglycosides, amphotericin B, cyclosporin A, radiocontrast agents
	Distal tubule and collecting duct	Amphotericin B, pentamidine, NSAIDs, lithium
Tubulointerstitial nephritis (see **Chapter 18**)	Renal interstitium	Penicillins, cephalosporins, fluoroquinolones, sulphonamides, nitrosoureas, NSAIDs, lithium
Medullary and papillary necrosis	Medullary papillae	NSAIDs
Intratubular precipitation and obstruction	Non-specific	Aciclovir, sulphonamides, methotrexate, chemotherapy (tumour lysis syndromes)
Tubule toxicity secondary to rhabdomyolysis (see **Chapter 12**)	Non-specific	Cocaine, ecstasy, other recreational drugs of abuse
Thrombotic microangiopathy (see **Chapter 15**)	Renal arterioles & glomerular capillaries	Cyclosporin A, mitomycin C
Unknown (? Immune complex or autoimmune mediated)	Glomerular	Gold, penicillamine, propylthiouracil, hydralazine

unwise since a second exposure to the nephrotoxin is likely to result in more severe renal injury than that which occurred during the initial exposure.

Table 2 classifies the nephrotoxic agents discussed in this chapter according to the mechanism by which they induce renal dysfunction.

NEPHROTOXICITY OF SPECIFIC AGENTS

Note, for drug prescribing in ARF refer to **Appendix A**.

ANGIOTENSIN CONVERTING ENZYME INHIBITORS (ACEI)

By far the most common manifestation of ACEI induced renal dysfunction is that of ARF secondary to abrupt and marked changes in intra-renal haemodynamics. In certain situations

Table 3. Clinical states associated with increased activity in the renin-angiotensin system

Bilateral renal artery stenosis, or unilateral stenosis in a single functioning kidney

Conditions leading to reduced renal blood flow

- congestive cardiac failure
- hypovolaemia
- sepsis
- nephrotic syndrome

Sodium depletion

Hepatic cirrhosis

(listed in **Table 3**), angiotensin II mediated vasoconstriction of the glomerular efferent arteriole plays a crucial role in the maintenance of an adequate GFR. The use of an ACEI in these circumstances causes efferent arteriolar vasodilatation leading to a fall in both glomerular capillary pressure and filtration fraction — this results in reversible ARF.

Whenever renal function declines following the introduction of an ACEI, the possibility of underlying renal artery stenosis should be considered. Although toxicity may be limited by appropriate changes to the patient's fluid and sodium balance, a persistent and/or progressive decline in renal function may necessitate permanent drug withdrawal. ACEI have also been reported to cause both acute TIN and a form of membranous GN.

ANTI-BACTERIAL THERAPY

Aminoglycosides

The use of aminoglycoside antibiotics is often limited by nephrotoxicity. Despite attempts to reduce toxicity by methods such as dose determination by nomogram, shortened dosage regimens and regular monitoring of serum drug levels, between 5 and 26% of patients will still suffer some degree of aminoglycoside induced renal dysfunction.

Clinically, patients usually present with transient polyuria (probably secondary to the inhibition of chloride ion transport in the thick ascending limb of the loop of Henle), followed by the onset of non-oliguric ARF. The presence of brush border enzymes (e.g. alkaline phosphatase, γ-glutamyl transferase) may be detected early in the development of renal injury, and is subsequently accompanied by glycosuria, proteinuria, and even leucocyturia. Electrolyte abnormalities including hypocalcaemia, hypokalaemia, and hypomagnesaemia may also be seen. Although renal dysfunction is usually reversible, recovery may be delayed up to 6 weeks, and may also be incomplete, particularly in those patients with pre-existing renal disease. Risk factors for the development of toxicity are listed in **Table 4**.

Histological examination demonstrates initial damage to the brush border followed by the appearance of myeloid bodies within the lysosomes and, later, tubule cell necrosis. Myeloid bodies result from the accumulation of undegraded phospholipid within the lysosomes secondary

Table 4. Risk factors for the development of aminoglycoside induced nephrotoxicity

High drug dose

Long duration of therapy

Volume depletion or the use of diuretics

Concurrent administration of another potential nephrotoxic agent, e.g. amphotericin B, ACEI, cyclosporin A, or radiocontrast media

Sodium or potassium depletion

Systemic sepsis

Pre-existing renal disease

Advanced age

to inhibition of intracellular phospholipases by the aminoglycoside. The mechanisms of aminoglycoside cytotoxicity are poorly understood, but may include:

- altered lysosomal membrane permeability leading to intracellular leak of lysosomal contents
- interference with the activity of intracellular enzymes and signalling pathways
- reduced mitochondrial respiration.

With regards to prevention of toxicity, there is considerable evidence that once daily administration protocols have reduced the incidence of nephrotoxicity, without significant loss of treatment efficacy, compared with more traditional multiple daily dosing regimens. In addition, monitoring of drug levels is essential (see **Appendix A**). Note that once ARF ensues, once daily administration regimes are not indicated. Further, it is clear that careful optimisation of fluid balance prior to the commencement of therapy, along with regular assessments of renal function prior to, during and after drug therapy, all help to reduce the incidence of toxic effects. However, for the time being, it is likely that aminoglycoside induced nephrotoxicity will remain a significant clinical problem.

Fluoroquinolones

Several of these drugs, ciprofloxacin in particular, have been reported to cause an acute TIN which is usually non-oliguric in nature. Skin rashes are, however, uncommon. Withdrawal of the drug usually leads to a rapid return to baseline renal function.

Penicillins/Cephalosporins

Only rarely, given their widespread usage, do penicillins or cephalosporins cause any significant degree of nephrotoxicity. When it does occur, by far the most common clinical presentation is that of a typical interstitial nephritis.

Sulphonamides

Although acute TIN is now the most common manifestation of sulphonamide induced nephrotoxicity, intratubular precipitation with concomitant tubule obstruction may still be seen, especially when urinary pH is <pH 5.5. Such precipitation may be prevented by adequate hydration and urinary alkalinisation.

Vancomycin

The incidence of vancomycin induced nephrotoxicity (most often due to acute tubular necrosis) has fallen considerably since various impurities have been removed from the available formulations, and is now reported to be in the region of 5% when the drug is used alone. There is some evidence however that vancomycin may potentiate aminoglycoside induced nephrotoxicity.

Macrolides

Azithromycin is associated with the development of acute TIN (see **Chapter 18**).

Trimethoprim

Trimethoprim may cause an increased creatinine:urea ratio because it competes for proximal tubule secretion of creatinine. It also has an amiloride-like effect (see **Chapter 2**) which may lead to hyperkalaemia.

ANTI-FUNGAL THERAPY

Amphotericin B

The therapeutic effect of amphotericin B is dependent upon its ability to interact with the sterol components of plasma membranes (affecting particularly the cells of the distal tubule and collecting duct), altering cell permeability by the formation of aqueous pores. The nephrotoxic effects of amphotericin B are mediated not only by this direct cytotoxicity, but also by renovascular vasoconstriction with subsequent renal ischaemia. Toxicity has been reported in up to 80% of patients treated with amphotericin B, and sodium depletion seems to be a particularly strong predisposing factor. Initial tubule injury results in nephrogenic diabetes insipidus, renal tubular acidosis and hypokalaemia. In most cases, renal function rapidly returns to baseline following discontinuation of therapy. Treatment can often be restarted following a modest dose reduction. Alternatively, liposomal amphotericin, which has a substantially lower incidence of nephrotoxicity because it is not extensively filtered at the glomerulus, may be considered.

Pentamidine

Pentamidine is now most frequently used for the treatment of Pneumocystis pneumonia in patients with HIV infection. Whilst it is rare for nebulised pentamidine to cause any significant renal injury, intravenous administration is associated with nephrotoxicity in between 25 and 65% of cases due to the direct tubular toxicity of the drug. Renal failure usually begins within the first week of treatment, is non-oliguric in nature and is reversible, with recovery beginning a few days after the discontinuation of therapy. Initial mild proteinuria and glycosuria may be accompanied by hypomagnesaemia, hypocalcaemia and hyperkalaemia if the treatment is continued. The severity of the renal injury is increased in the presence of other nephrotoxic agents such as aminoglycosides, amphotericin B, and cyclosporin A.

ANTI-VIRAL THERAPY

Aciclovir

The use of aciclovir has become increasingly widespread for the treatment of herpes infections, and topical formulations are now available without prescription. Non-oliguric renal failure is the most common clinical presentation and urinalysis often reveals mild proteinuria and microscopic haematuria. Higher doses, and in particular the rapid administration of intravenous boluses, can lead to the sudden intratubular precipitation of the drug, accompanied by needle-shaped crystals in the urine and occasional episodes of flank pain. Withdrawal of the drug normally leads to a full recovery within several days. Again, adequate hydration, particularly in patients with pre-existing renal disease, reduces toxicity.

Note that ganciclovir, used for the treatment of cytomegalovirus (CMV) infections, is not nephrotoxic.

Foscarnet

Foscarnet, a known tubule toxin, is used in the treatment of both CMV and herpes infections, and is available in both intravenous and topical formulations. Although the incidence of foscarnet induced ARF is extremely high (66% in one review), such renal failure is usually reversible. Nevertheless, on occasions, affected patients may require temporary dialysis. Electrolyte abnormalities may also occur — most frequently hypocalcaemia, although hypercalcaemia, hypo- and hyper-phosphataemia, and hypomagnesaemia have all been recorded. Adequate hydration with intravenous saline appears to be extremely effective in reducing nephrotoxicity.

ANTI-REJECTION THERAPY

Cyclosporin A

The introduction of cyclosporin A has proven to be one of the most important advances with regard to prolonging the longevity of many solid organ transplants. Unfortunately, some form of nephrotoxicity is seen in nearly all patients treated with the drug. Almost all cases of cyclosporin A induced toxicity fall into one of the three following categories.

Acute renal failure

Within the kidney, cyclosporin A causes vasoconstriction of both the afferent and efferent arterioles leading to a dose dependent fall in both renal blood flow and GFR. Both endothelins and thromboxanes have been implicated in the pathogenesis of vascular resistance alterations. At higher doses, such vasoconstrictor changes may result in the development of ARF, but renal function usually rapidly returns to baseline following either dose reduction or discontinuation of therapy.

Thrombotic microangiopathy (see also **Chapter 15**)

On occasions, a thrombotic microangiopathy with fibrinoid necrosis and hyaline change is seen affecting the renal arterioles and glomerular capillaries. The pathogenesis of this lesion is poorly understood.

Chronic renal failure

Chronic use of the drug may produce an obliterative arteriopathy associated with tubule atrophy and a characteristic "striped" interstitial fibrosis. This is clinically manifest as hypertension, mild proteinuria, tubule dysfunction, and renal failure which may be irreversible and progressive.

Careful attention to serum cyclosporin levels, with regular and accurate assessments of renal function, seem to be the most effective methods for reducing the incidence of nephrotoxicity. Even so, in the long term, renal damage may be unavoidable. There is some evidence that the use of calcium channel blocking agents not only helps to protect against early renal damage induced by renal vasoconstriction, but also may help to prevent the more progressive and chronic interstitial damage seen with continued drug use.

ANTI-RHEUMATIC THERAPY

Gold Salts/Penicillamine

Proteinuria, sometimes within the nephrotic range, is the most common clinical manifestation of gold induced nephrotoxicity. In the vast majority of cases (up to 90%), histological examination demonstrates a membranous nephropathy with sub-epithelial electron deposits. Minimal change disease accounts for the remaining 10%.

As with gold, penicillamine induced nephrotoxicity usually presents as proteinuria, with membranous nephropathy being the most common pathological lesion. Proteinuria usually occurs within the first 6 to 18 months of treatment although it may only develop after several years, or even after the drug has been discontinued. On occasions, penicillamine has been reported to cause a lupus-like syndrome and even a rapidly progressive crescentic glomerulonephritis with a Goodpasture phenotype (see **Chapter 16**). However, the number of such cases has been extremely small.

Features common to both gold and penicillamine induced nephrotoxicity are as follows:

- ARF, haematuria, and hypertension are all rare.
- Toxicity does not seem to be dose related (gold induced toxicity much more likely if administered parenterally).
- Susceptibility is associated with HLA antigens B8 and DR3.
- Proteinuria gradually resolves over a period of months following drug withdrawal.

The pathogenesis of gold or penicillamine induced nephrotoxicity is unknown. Neither steroids nor immunosuppressive agents have been shown to be of any benefit in the treatment of these cases.

CYTOTOXIC THERAPY (see also Chapter 21)

Cisplatin

Cisplatin is a potent antineoplastic agent effective in several different types of solid tumour including small cell carcinoma of the lung, testicular, ovarian and bladder carcinoma and head and neck tumours. In early clinical trials, the incidence of nephrotoxicity was reported to be approximately 25%. Although, more recently, this incidence has fallen, the therapeutic use of cisplatin is often limited due to renal side effects.

The incidence and/or severity of cisplatin induced nephrotoxicity may be reduced by:

- **Adequate hydration** — administer intravenous fluids before, during and for at least 6 h following drug administration.
- **Maintenance of a good urine output** — by hydration alone, or with the use of diuretics if necessary.
- **For very large doses** — co-administration of sodium thiosulphate may reduce toxicity allowing the use of a more intensive therapeutic regimen.

The development of renal failure is usually dose related, often delayed and is progressive. Initial tubulointerstitial damage is characterised by tubular proteinuria and tubule casts, and is often accompanied by decreases in renal blood flow and GFR. Chronic exposure results in focal necrosis in numerous segments of the nephron. The glomerulus is rarely affected. Electrolyte disturbances, particularly magnesium, are frequent and may be persistent even after discontinuation of therapy. Increased urinary magnesium losses may be exacerbated by concurrent administration of aminoglycoside antibiotics, and may be accompanied by hypokalaemia and hypocalcaemia with symptomatic tetany.

The precise pathogenic mechanisms underlying cisplatin induced nephrotoxicity are unknown. The delay in the onset of renal dysfunction suggests that a metabolite is responsible for the toxic effects. It is quite clear, however, that toxicity is not directly related to the presence of the platinum ion *per se*, since the cis-isomer alone is nephrotoxic.

Methotrexate

Methotrexate is often used in combination therapy with other cytotoxic agents for the treatment of a wide variety of tumours ranging from acute lymphocytic leukaemia and non-Hodgkin lymphoma to choriocarcinoma and osteogenic sarcoma. It is unusual for the administration of methotrexate in conventional doses to cause renal dysfunction unless there is already some element of pre-existing renal disease. At higher doses, renal toxicity occurs in approximately 10% of patients. It is probably related, at least in part, to the intratubular precipitation of the metabolite 7-hydroxymethotrexate. Alkalinisation of the urine, adequate patient hydration and the maintenance of an adequate urine output reduce the incidence and severity of nephrotoxicity.

Mitomycin C

Mitomycin C is most commonly used in the treatment of adenocarcinoma of the breast or gastrointestinal tract. Nephrotoxicity is reported to occur in between 4 and 10% of cases, although with progressively higher cumulative doses the number of patients affected can be significantly greater. The vast majority of cases present as haemolytic uraemic syndrome (see **Chapter 15**) and non-nephrotic range proteinuria. Histological findings include fibrin thrombi in the glomeruli and small vessels, thickening of the glomerular basement membrane and fibrin exudates. Tubulointerstitial damage is thought to be secondary in origin.

Clinically, hypertension is common and, whilst the severity of renal failure varies, it is often progressive and irreversible. Therapeutically, plasma exchange and high dose steroids seem to offer the best results, although the haematological abnormalities appear to be more amenable to treatment than the renal disease. It should be noted that mitomycin C induced nephrotoxicity is associated with a significant mortality rate, with associated pulmonary and neurological manifestations being the poorest prognostic signs.

Nitrosoureas

BCNU/CCNU

These drugs can cause a slowly progressive form of renal failure that appears to be dose-dependent in nature. The onset of dysfunction is often late (median time to presentation 24 months), and frequently occurs even after the drug has been discontinued. Histological changes include tubular lesions, interstitial fibrosis and glomerulosclerosis. The mechanism of renal injury is unknown.

Streptozotocin

Streptozotocin is used for the treatment of carcinoid tumours and metastatic carcinoma of the pancreas. Its use is often limited by renal toxicity with some degree of dysfunction occurring in approximately 66% of patients. Proteinuria is most commonly seen, followed by tubular dysfunction, and histological examination usually reveals tubular atrophy with interstitial fibrosis. ARF occurs in 20 to 30% of patients. From a practical point of view, it is relevant to note that the rate of drug administration seems to be of particular importance with regard to the development of toxicity, and treatment regimens have therefore evolved to reflect this. However, in the early stages the toxic injury is usually reversible provided that the drug is withdrawn. Prolonged use of the drug, even at low dose rates, will result in permanent renal dysfunction.

HEAVY METALS

Cadmium

Approximately 50% of the cadmium in the body is found within the kidney. Cadmium causes proximal tubule dysfunction and necrosis, manifest clinically as aminoaciduria, glycosuria and renal tubular acidosis. Removal of the exposure usually leads to a stabilisation in renal function without continued deterioration. In the long-term, however, the injury may progress to a chronic and irreversible interstitial nephritis. Bony deposits of cadmium lead to severe osteopaenia and pathological fractures.

Lead

Acute lead nephropathy is predominantly seen in children who may present with gastrointestinal disturbance and neurological features, including visual abnormalities, motor dysfunction and encephalopathy. Proximal tubule dysfunction is very common, with its associated urinary findings (see **Chapter 4.2**). Adults tend to present with hypertension, proteinuria of less than 2 g/day, hyperuricaemia and a benign urinary sediment. Gouty arthritis (saturnine gout), which is rarely seen in patients with renal failure, occurs in approximately 50% of patients. Non-specific tubule atrophy is followed by interstitial inflammation ultimately leading to small contracted kidneys with an irregular surface.

An EDTA chelation test is currently the best available method for screening for lead intoxication since serum lead levels are relatively insensitive. The amount of chelatable lead found in a 24 h urine collection, following the injection of 2 g EDTA calcium disodium, correlates with bony lead stores. Intramuscular injections of EDTA calcium disodium (1 g), given once every three weeks until the chelatable lead product is normalised, is the treatment of choice and is very effective in reversing the changes of acute lead nephropathy. There is, however, no effective treatment for the more chronic interstitial renal disease.

Mercury

Whilst elemental mercury is almost completely harmless, both inorganic and organic mercuric compounds are nephrotoxic. Inorganic salts are the most nephrotoxic of all due to the relatively high degree of lipophobicity. Within a few hours of ingestion of a toxic dose, up to 50% of the mercury load may be found in the kidney, predominantly localised to the proximal tubule. Proximal tubule necrosis leads to ARF within 24 to 48 h, although with short-term exposure this is usually reversible. Early administration of 2,3-dimercaprol may improve the natural history of the disease. More chronic exposure to mercuric compounds can lead to the development of proteinuria or even nephrotic syndrome. In these situations, histological examination usually reveals the presence of a membranous nephropathy. The outcome is relatively favourable once the exposure ceases and marked changes in renal function are rare.

NON-STEROIDAL ANTI-INFLAMMATORY DRUGS (NSAIDs)

The reported incidence of NSAID induced nephrotoxicity varies widely according to the particular population studied, and is probably somewhere between 5 and 40 percent. The sheer volume of NSAID use in the UK means that, although renal complications are relatively uncommon *per se*, patients with drug induced renal side effects are seen relatively frequently. The renal syndromes associated with NSAID use include:

- Acute renal failure.
- Acute tubulointerstitial nephritis (TIN).
- Salt and water retention.
- Hypertension.
- Renal papillary necrosis.
- Hyperkalaemia.

Acute Renal Failure

Intra-renal vasodilatory prostaglandins play an important role in the control of intra-renal blood flow (see **Chapter 1**). They modulate the vasoconstrictive effects of angiotensin II and oppose vasoconstrictive actions mediated through the renal sympathetic nervous system. NSAIDs, through inhibition of cyclo-oxygenase, cause an imbalance between the vasoconstrictive and vasodilatory influences on the intra-renal vasculature, resulting in a fall in both renal blood flow and glomerular filtration rate. ARF induced in this way is usually reversible if the drug is withdrawn early on, although occasionally patients are left with some degree of chronic renal impairment. As with ACEI, risk factors for the development of this form of ARF include congestive cardiac failure, hypovolaemia or sepsis, nephrotic syndrome, cirrhosis and sodium depletion. Advanced age and pre-existing renal disease are also important predisposing factors.

Acute Tubulointerstitial Nephritis (see also **Chapter 18**)

In comparison to acute TIN secondary to other drugs, NSAID induced TIN is much more likely to present with heavy proteinuria (often nephrotic range), and is much less likely to have features of an allergic reaction, such as fever, rash, and arthralgia. Eosinophilia and eosinophiluria are much less common also. The onset of renal dysfunction is variable and abnormalities may not occur until after many months of treatment. Drug withdrawal results in improvement in renal function with a reduction in proteinuria. However, renal recovery may be incomplete and progression to chronic renal failure, with a chronic scarring TIN on biopsy, has been reported. In the acute stages, histological examination shows focal tubular damage with tubulointerstitial inflammation and a variable degree of interstitial fibrosis. Interestingly, glomerular histology is usually entirely normal even in the presence of marked proteinuria (i.e. minimal change). Possible pathogenic mechanisms include the diversion of arachidonic acid metabolites from the cyclo-oxygenase to the lipoxygenase pathways leading to an excess of pro-inflammatory leukotrienes.

Salt and Water Retention

Given that renal prostaglandins are involved in the regulation of both sodium and water excretion, it is not surprising that sodium and water retention are frequent side effects of NSAID use, occurring in up to 25% of patients. Clinically apparent peripheral and pulmonary oedema may occur, and it is important to note that the therapeutic effect of diuretics may be blunted as a consequence.

Hypertension

The use of NSAIDs may result in a mild elevation in blood pressure in the region of 5 mmHg. This is more likely to occur in patients who are already known to be hypertensive, and in those already taking anti-hypertensive medication, particularly thiazide diuretics and β-blockers. The exact mechanism by which this occurs is unknown but increased salt and water retention, and a reduction in the levels of the circulating vasodilator prostacyclin, are thought to be involved.

Renal Papillary Necrosis

Although renal papillary necrosis has traditionally been associated with the use of phenacetin, it has been described following the use of other NSAIDs such as indomethacin and phenylbutazone. It has been suggested that drug metabolism by prostaglandin H synthase leads to the formation of reactive intermediates which cause cellular damage by the covalent binding of surface macromolecules. Given that the intra-renal activity of this enzyme is at its highest in the medulla, this is a tempting hypothesis. However, at present, the exact pathogenic mechanism remains unknown.

Hyperkalaemia

NSAIDs may cause hyperkalaemia by inducing a state of hyporeninaemic hypoaldosteronism through the negative feedback effects of salt and water retention. This is more likely to occur in diabetic patients, in patients with chronic renal failure, and in patients with a pre-existing type IV renal tubular acidosis. However, it may also occur in the setting of completely normal initial renal function.

Other Clinical Syndromes

There are anecdotal reports of NSAIDs causing vasculitis and membranous GN. Chronic renal failure is most often associated with the development of either chronic tubulointerstitial nephritis or papillary necrosis. It is rarely seen with only short-term drug use.

OTHER AGENTS

Aspirin

See **Chapter 8.4**.

Chloroform

Chloroform is an example of an agent whose nephrotoxicity is dependent upon its metabolism by cytochrome P-450 in the renal proximal tubule. Subsequent reactions lead to the formation of phosgene and reactive intermediates which bind covalently to nucleophilic groups on cellular macromolecules thus causing cellular injury.

Ethylene Glycol

See **Chapter 8.4**.

Lithium

Nephrogenic diabetes insipidus, due to inhibition of vasopressin-sensitive adenylate cyclase in the distal tubule and collecting duct, is probably the most common renal abnormality seen in patients treated with lithium. In some series, polyuria and polydipsia are found in up to 40% of patients. Acutely, these changes are completely reversible, but with continued drug use, the impairment of urinary concentrating ability is progressive and often irreversible. In several studies, a correlation has been observed between the total drug dose or duration of therapy and the impairment in concentrating ability. Lithium has also been shown to cause a distal renal tubular acidosis.

Histological examination shows reversible swelling and vacuolation of cells in the distal convoluted tubule and collecting duct during the acute phase of injury. In contrast, the development of a more severe and persistent degree of renal impairment is associated with the appearance of tubule atrophy, focal tubulointerstitial fibrosis and glomerulosclerosis on renal biopsy.

Toxicity may be reduced by the careful monitoring of serum lithium levels accompanied by appropriate changes in the dosage regimen, aiming to maintain the lowest possible therapeutic serum drug level. Acute episodes of lithium intoxication should be avoided as these appear to predispose to the development of more long-term renal dysfunction.

Paracetamol

See **Chapter 25**.

RADIOCONTRAST AGENTS

Depending on the population studied, the reported incidence of radiocontrast induced nephropathy ranges from approximately 0.15% in the general population to approximately 38% in diabetic patients with a pre-existing history of renal disease. However, depending on the criteria used to establish the diagnosis, the incidence may be even higher. Radiocontrast induced nephropathy rarely occurs in patients with normal baseline renal function.

The pathogenesis is complex and involves: (i) reduced local renal blood flow secondary to contrast induced endothelin up-regulation. Endothelin mediated (calcium-dependent) vasoconstriction leads to proximal tubule cell necrosis, tubule cell detachment and lumen obstruction; and (ii) local production of reactive oxygen species.

Predisposing Factors

The two most important predisposing factors for the development of nephropathy are:

- pre-existing renal disease (serum creatinine >140 µmol/L)
- diabetes mellitus with an associated nephropathy.

  Other risk factors include:

- Heart failure and low cardiac output states.
- Concurrent administration of other nephrotoxic agents.
- Multiple myeloma.
- Advanced age.

Clinical Presentation

Clinical presentation ranges from asymptomatic biochemical abnormalities to oligoanuria requiring dialysis. The majority of cases manifest as a reversible rise in creatinine which begins within the first 24 h, peaks within two to four days, and is then followed by a spontaneous return to baseline within one week. Oliguric ARF (which is usually resistant to loop diuretics) occurs in approximately 66% of reported cases. End stage renal failure may be precipitated in those with pre-existing advanced renal disease, particularly those patients with diabetic nephropathy.

Treatment Principles

The most important management points are:

- Identify those patients at risk of radiocontrast nephropathy.
- Minimise the contrast load.
- Ensure that patients at risk are optimally hydrated using intra-venous 0.9% saline infusion.

There have been several studies examining the role of various drugs and different fluid regimens (0.45% versus 0.9% saline) in the prevention of contrast nephropathy. Administration of furosemide, mannitol, dopamine, atrial natriuretic peptide or theophylline has not been shown to be of significant benefit. In one study (Solomon *et al.*, 1994), the use of either mannitol or furosemide + intra-venous 0.45% saline resulted in a higher incidence of contrast nephropathy in patients with pre-existing renal impairment undergoing cardiac catheterisation, compared with patients receiving 0.45% saline alone. Importantly, even in this study, it was not clear as to whether or not saline hydration actually reduced the risk of nephropathy since all patients received this treatment — there has never been an adequate randomised trial of saline prophylaxis alone. The calcium dependent nature of the vasoconstrictor response has led some to advocate the use of calcium channel blocking drugs in a prophylactic role.

The use of non-ionic contrast, with its organic side chain and lower osmolality, in at-risk individuals, has also helped to reduce the incidence of toxicity. A meta-analysis of the use of non-ionic contrast, compared with standard contrast, in 25 trials revealed a pooled odds ratio for an increase in serum creatinine of more than 44 µmol/L of 0.5 (95% confidence interval, 0.4–0.7). However, subgroup analysis did not reveal any statistically significant benefit in those patients with normal baseline renal function (Barrett and Carlisle, 1993).

Recently, it has been demonstrated that prophylactic administration of the antioxidant acetylcysteine, along with hydration, prevents the reduction in renal function induced by a non-ionic, low osmolality contrast agent, in patients with chronic renal insufficiency (Tepel *et al.*, 2000). In this study, the dose of acetylcysteine used was 600 mg b.d po, on the day before and on the day of administration of the contrast agent; patients also received 0.45% saline IV at a rate of 1 mL/kg/h for 12 h before and after the contrast administration.

It is hoped that the increasing availability of newer imaging systems such as magnetic resonance angiography will reduce the incidence of radiocontrast induced nephropathy even further, as fewer numbers of at-risk patients are exposed to this nephrotoxin.

RECREATIONAL DRUGS OF ABUSE

Cocaine

The nephrotoxic effects of cocaine are usually due to the development of ARF secondary to acute rhabdomyolysis (see **Chapter 12**), although cases of cocaine induced renal artery thrombosis have been reported. There is also some evidence that maternal cocaine use may cause developmental abnormalities in the foetal urogenital tract. Rhabdomyolysis secondary to cocaine abuse carries a poor prognosis, with approximately 33% of patients developing ARF, of which 50% subsequently die. Poor prognostic features of cocaine induced rhabdomyolysis and ARF include the presence of:

- Hypotension.
- Hyperpyrexia.
- Marked elevation in creatine kinase.
- Disseminated intravascular coagulopathy.

Ecstasy

As with cocaine, the majority of cases of renal dysfunction secondary to the use of ecstasy are due to rhabdomyolysis, although ARF secondary to accelerated hypertension has been described. Again, poor prognostic features include hyperpyrexia and a disseminated intravascular coagulopathy.

Heroin

Heroin associated nephropathy is a syndrome seen almost exclusively in black heroin addicts. It presents as a nephrotic syndrome and ultimately progresses to end stage renal failure if the drug abuse continues. The underlying pathology is that of focal segmental glomerulosclerosis. Heroin can also induce rhabdomyolysis, due to direct myotoxicity or as a result of coma/muscle compression (see **Chapter 12**).

Intravenous Drug Abuse

With the widespread introduction of needle exchange programmes, the incidence of GN secondary to endocarditis has decreased significantly. When it does occur, the usual histological findings are of an acute diffuse glomerulonephritis that is indistinguishable, on light microscopy, from other types of post infectious glomerulonephritis; the most common infecting agent is *Staphylococcus aureus*. Other causes of renal dysfunction seen in intravenous drug abusers include AA amyloidosis caused by chronic suppurative infections of the skin ("skin poppers"), especially in those who inject subcutaneously, and by sequelae of Hepatitis B infection (see **Chapter 25**).

   Note that other drugs of abuse, e.g. alcohol, are associated with ARF secondary to rhabdomyolysis. These are discussed further in **Chapter 12**.

DIALYSIS AND HAEMOPERFUSION IN THE TREATMENT OF POISONING

Haemodialysis (HD) and haemoperfusion may occasionally be used in the management of drug overdose and poisoning. However, these procedures are only indicated as part of a wider management plan — **they are not a substitute for the usual management strategies associated with the treatment of such cases**. To illustrate this point, recent data from the American Association of Poison Control Centres reveal that, in a one year period, HD was used in less than 0.04% of all cases of poisoning, with haemoperfusion being used in even fewer cases.

Clinical Indications

Treatment of poisoning by HD or haemoperfusion is rarely necessary, and should only be considered if one or more of the following criteria are satisfied, **and after seeking advice from the local poisons information centre**:

- Severe intoxication and/or progressive deterioration in clinical condition in spite of appropriate therapeutic interventions.
- Intoxication with a drug known to produce metabolic and/or delayed effects.
- Impairment of the normal route of drug excretion.
- Intoxication with a drug which may be removed from the body by using either haemodialysis or haemoperfusion at a rate faster than by normal endogenous mechanisms.
- The presence of serum drug levels known to be associated with death or severe morbidity.

Choice of Modality

Haemodialysis

Haemodialysis relies upon trans-membrane drug removal down a concentration gradient, from blood into dialysate (see **Chapter 9.3**). It is therefore the treatment of choice for low molecular weight, water-soluble drugs that will rapidly diffuse across the dialysis membrane. It is also of particular benefit when the drug or its metabolite causes a metabolic acidosis, as HD simultaneously removes the drug/metabolite and corrects the acidosis.

Haemoperfusion

Haemoperfusion involves the passage of blood through a cartridge packed with an appropriate sorbent and depends upon the physical process of drug adsorption to effect drug removal. The most common sorbent used is polymer-coated activated charcoal since it effectively removes a wide variety of drugs. Both procedures may be performed via centrally placed dual-lumen vascular catheters.

Pharmacokinetic and Pharmacodynamic Considerations

Factors which may influence drug removal by HD or haemoperfusion include:

1. Drug characteristics

- Volume of distribution   } These factors have some bearing
- Degree of protein binding   } upon the blood:dialysate or
- Lipid solubility   } blood:sorbent concentration gradient.
- Intercompartmental transfer rates }
- Molecular size of the drug

2. Modality characteristics

- Blood flow rate.
- Dialysate flow rate (HD).
- Dialyser surface area (HD) or cartridge capacity (haemoperfusion).
- Membrane type (HD) or sorbent type (haemoperfusion).

Volume of distribution

The volume of distribution is the theoretical volume into which a drug is distributed following its administration. Given that HD and haemoperfusion are only able to remove drugs from the extracorporeal circuit, both procedures are considerably more efficient at removing drugs confined to the vascular compartment (low volume of distribution), compared to drugs distributed throughout, and possibly stored in, the body's tissues (large volume of distribution). However, even when the drug involved has a large volume of distribution, the use of either haemodialysis or haemoperfusion may be appropriate, in the following circumstances:

- When a transient lowering in the plasma concentration of the drug may be sufficient to prevent the development of particularly severe toxic side effects.
- When a transient lowering of the plasma concentration of the drug provides a window of opportunity for the introduction of a more specific therapeutic manoeuvre.
- Repeated treatments may be necessary for those drugs with slow intercompartmental transfer rates and large volumes of distribution.

Degree of protein binding

Independent of its effect on the volume of distribution, the degree of protein binding is an important consideration when deciding on which procedure is most appropriate. Haemoperfusion is far superior in removing highly protein bound drugs since the sorbent competes with the plasma proteins for the drug. In contrast, HD is relatively inefficient as only the free fraction of the drug in the plasma is available for removal across the dialysis membrane.

Lipid solubility

Since only the water soluble fraction of a drug is available for removal by HD, lipid soluble drugs are more readily removed by haemoperfusion, particularly if appropriate sorbents such as XAD-4, which is polystyrene based, are used.

Adverse Effects

Haemodialysis

Standard dialysate solutions are designed for use in patients suffering from acute and/or chronic renal failure with associated metabolic acidosis and hyperphosphataemia. The use of such solutions in patients without such metabolic abnormalities may result in alkalosis and hypophosphataemia respectively.

Haemoperfusion

The major adverse effect associated with haemoperfusion is thrombocytopaenia with the development of an associated bleeding tendency. The transient adsorption of calcium and glucose

Table 5. Comparison between HD & haemoperfusion in the treatment of drug overdose or poisoning

Procedure	Advantages	Disadvantages
Haemodialysis	Good for removing: — low molecular weight drugs — low volume of distribution drugs — water-soluble drugs — non-protein bound drugs Corrects metabolic acidosis	Alkalosis Hypophosphataemia
Haemoperfusion	Good for removing: — low molecular weight drugs — low volume of distribution drugs — lipid-soluble drugs — protein bound drugs	Thrombocytopaenia Hypoglycaemia Hypocalcaemia Pyrogenic reactions Cartridge saturation Does not correct metabolic acidosis

Table 6. Examples of drugs and chemicals removed by haemodialysis and haemoperfusion

Category	Haemodialysis	Haemoperfusion
Analgesics	aspirin; paracetamol	aspirin; paracetamol
Anticonvulsants	carbamazepine; paraldehyde	
Antidepressants	amphetamines; MAOI	
Barbiturates	phenobarbitone	phenobarbitone; thiopentone
Insecticides, herbicides & solvents	acetone; paraquat; toluene	carbon tetrachloride; paraquat; parathion
Other sedatives	chloral hydrate; glutethimide	chloral hydrate; chlorpromazine; diphenhydramine; glutethimide; promethazine
Miscellaneous	aminophylline/theophylline ethanol/methanol; ethylene glycol arsenic; lead lithium	aminophylline/theophylline phenol

during the procedure may also result in symptoms of hypocalcaemia and hypoglycaemia respectively, although the metabolic disturbance is usually mild. Pyrogenic reactions are relatively uncommon now following the introduction of polymer coated sorbents.

Table 5 compares the advantages and disadvantages of HD with those of haemoperfusion. **Table 6** lists drugs and chemicals, often used in poisoning and overdoses, that are removed by each of the two processes. For further information, the reader is referred to the text by Winchester, the details of which are included in the **Further Reading** section.

FURTHER READING

Bakir AA, Dunea G (1996) Drugs of abuse and renal disease. *Current Opinion in Nephrology and Hypertension*; 5: 122–126

Barrett BJ, Carlisle EJ (1993) Meta-analysis of the relative nephrotoxicity of high- and low-osmolality iodinated contrast media. *Radiology*; 188: 171–178

Cronin RE, Henrich WL (1999) Toxic nephropathy, In: Brenner BM (ed.). *Brenner & Rector's the Kidney* (6th Edition). Philadelphia: W.B. Saunders

Fillastre J-P, Godin M (1998) Drug-induced nephropathies. In: Davison AM, Cameron JS, Grünfeld J-P, *et al.* (eds.). *Oxford Textbook of Clinical Nephrology* (2nd Edition). Oxford: Oxford University Press; 2645–2658

Goldstein RS, Schnellmann RG (1996) Toxic responses of the kidney. In: Klaassen CD (ed.). *Casarett and Doull's Toxicology: The Basic Science of Poisons* (5th Edition). New York: McGraw-Hill; 417–442

Solomon R, Werner C, Mann D, *et al.* (1994) Effects of saline, mannitol and furosemide on acute decreases in renal function induced by radiocontrast agents. *The New England Journal of Medicine*; 331: 1416–1420

Tepel M, van der Giet M, Schwarzfeld C, *et al.* (2000) Prevention of radiographic-contrast-agent-induced reductions in renal function by acetylcysteine. *The New England Journal of Medicine*; 343: 180–184

Winchester JF (1990) Active methods for detoxification: Oral sorbents, forced diuresis, haemoperfusion and haemodialysis. In: Haddad LM, Winchester JF (eds.). *Clinical Management of Poisoning and Drug Overdose* (2nd Edition). Philadelphia: W.B. Saunders; 148–167

Chapter 12 _____

RHABDOMYOLYSIS

Paul Glynne and Andrew Allen

DEFINITION

Rhabdomyolysis is defined as a clinical and biochemical syndrome resulting from severe skeletal muscle cell injury and lysis, with release of cell contents (including myoglobin) into the circulation. As a consequence, acute renal failure (ARF) may develop. Rhabdomyolysis is a major cause of ARF, accounting for up to 10–15% of cases in some series. Early recognition of the syndrome is important, since prompt treatment can prevent onset of oliguric renal failure, avoiding the cost and morbidity of acute dialysis.

PATHOPHYSIOLOGY

The first clear description of rhabdomyolysis was made during World War II by Bywaters and Beall, working at Hammersmith Hospital in London during the blitz. Then termed the "crush syndrome", they presented four patients with crushed limbs who died from ARF and had pigmented casts (myoglobin-based casts) visible in renal tubules at post-mortem. Many other causes of rhabdomyolysis have subsequently been described (see below), but it is worth noting that although myoglobinaemia is relatively common (often seen in marathon runners, for example), ARF as a consequence of myoglobinuria is relatively rare. Additional factors are typically required, either genetic or environmental, before the full rhabdomyolysis syndrome develops.

Muscle Function

Muscle fibres (myocytes) function by contraction and relaxation in a calcium-dependent manner. Neural stimulation of myocytes leads to sarcolemmal (myocyte cell membrane) depolarisation and subsequent release of calcium from the sarcoplasmic reticulum (myocyte equivalent of the endoplasmic reticulum). Cytoplasmic calcium activates the actin-myosin contractile mechanism and fibre shortening occurs. To relax again, ATP-dependent calcium pumps return calcium to the sarcoplasmic reticulum and extracellular environment. In the plentiful muscle fibres of "slow" (type 1) character, this contractile cycle is highly ATP- and oxygen-dependent. Unsurprisingly, therefore, type 1 myocytes contain many mitochondria and large amounts of myoglobin, the heme-containing muscle protein which stores intracellular oxygen.

Muscle cell injury can therefore lead to loss of myocyte integrity and release of large amounts of myoglobin into the extracellular space, and hence into plasma. Of note, whole muscles are composed of multiple fibres contained within multiple sheaths of connective tissue. These collagenous sheaths optimise mechanical function of muscles, but allow little room for fibre expansion, so pressure within the sheaths can rise rapidly leading to a compartment syndrome with exacerbation of myocyte ischaemia.

Muscle Injury

Typically myocyte injury leads to ATP-depletion and cytosolic calcium overload. Free cytosolic calcium then activates degradative intracellular enzymes such as calpain and phospholipase A2, and the cell becomes necrotic. The following factors are implicated in calcium overload:

- Direct myocyte damage — can occur from prolonged exertion, muscle compression, or toxins such as snake venom, leading to a breach of cell integrity and flooding of the cytosol by extracellular calcium
- ATP-depletion — prevents normal calcium extrusion from the cytosol (into organelles or the extracellular space)
- Intracellular organelles which normally store calcium, such as mitochondria, become leaky after cellular energy-depletion

Myoglobinuria and Acute Renal Failure

The consequence of severe muscle injury, therefore, is release of myocyte contents into the circulation. As well as the hallmark hyperkalaemia, hyperphosphataemia, hyperuricaemia and elevation in plasma creatine kinase, myoglobin enters the plasma. Unlike haemoglobin (Hb), which is a large, multimeric protein (69 kDa) and binds haptoglobin after accessing the circulation, myoglobin is small (17 kDa) and has no binding protein, so immediately reaches the kidney and is freely filtered at the glomerulus. Myoglobin becomes detectable in the urine at serum concentrations ranging from 300 ng/mL to 2 g/mL, and produces visible pigmenturia ("coca-cola" coloured urine) at concentrations exceeding 100 g/mL. It has become apparent that myoglobin has several potentially nephrotoxic properties, although it should be noted that in animal studies, intravenous infusion of myoglobin (or Hb) is insufficient to precipitate ARF. In such experiments, volume depletion and/or renal hypoperfusion must also be present for induction of myoglobinuric ARF. Both in animal models of rhabdomyolysis, and in human disease, renal tissue sections typically show acute proximal tubular necrosis and distal tubular intraluminal cast formation.

These observations provide clues to the mechanisms by which myoglobin may induce ARF:

- *Renal vasoconstriction*

Nitric oxide (NO), an important renal vasodilator, is depleted by the heme proteins contained within myoglobin, and this contributes to renal ischaemia. Significantly, common causes of rhabdomyolysis are often linked with renal hypoperfusion, as in trauma (volume "third spacing") and sepsis (cytokine-induced), and inhibition of NO limits the kidney's repertoire of counter-responses. Myoglobin also directly reduces renal blood flow in hypotensive animal models, the mechanism of this effect being unclear.

- *Proximal tubular toxicity*

Renal ischaemia leads to proximal tubular cell (PTC) ATP depletion and, ultimately, necrosis. This energy depletion is facilitated by iron atoms in heme proteins. Iron, a transition metal, also catalyses free radical production, and such reactive oxygen intermediates are key mediators of PTC injury *in vivo*. In addition, normally functioning PTCs endocytose protein presented to their luminal surface, and filtered myoglobin has a direct toxic effect through excessive protein-loading of the PTC. It appears that such protein reabsorption sensitises the cell to phospholipase A_2-mediated injury.

- *Distal tubular intraluminal cast formation*

Intraluminal pigmented tubular casts are a key feature of rhabdomyolysis (detectable by urine microscopy), and are seen mostly within distal tubules. The reason for their position is that myoglobin precipitates at low concentration if Tamm-Horsfall glycoprotein (THP) is present, and THP is produced by distal tubular epithelial cells. Myoglobin precipitation is also encouraged by low urinary pH, a feature of the distal nephron. It is likely that casts cause ARF through tubular obstruction, although this is not easily demonstrable *in vivo*. The optimal therapy for rhabdomyolysis, alkaline diuresis, aims to inhibit cast formation both by reducing intraluminal myoglobin concentration and raising ambient pH.

AETIOLOGY

It is apparent from the preceding discussion that myoglobinuria plus an additional insult(s) are usually required for the development of ARF in rhabdomyolysis. It should be emphasised that multiple factors often co-exist, with alcohol, in particular, frequently playing a part in the aetiology of rhabdomyolysis. In the most comprehensive survey of the aetiology of rhabdomyolysis, studying patients presenting to a general hospital in the 1970s, Gabow *et al.* suggested that alcohol was implicated in two thirds of cases, with compression and seizures also frequently seen. Other aetiological factors are shown in **Table 1**. A list of causes, sub-divided into hereditary and acquired, is shown in **Table 2**.

In conclusion, it is clear that muscle injury and myocyte damage with myoglobin leak are a necessary but insufficient prelude to acute renal failure induced by rhabdomyolysis. The renal toxicity of myoglobin is amplified substantially by concurrent volume depletion and/or renal hypoperfusion: factors that lead to PTC ATP depletion, and a tubular fluid of sluggish flow and high myoglobin concentration. Additional derangements such as electrolyte disturbances and hyper- or hypothermia are often present, and all of these elements conspire to reduce GFR and cause PTC injury/necrosis and distal tubular myoglobin cast formation — the features of ARF seen in rhabdomyolysis.

Table 1. Aetiological factors in 87 patients with rhabdomyolysis*

Factor	Number of cases	% of cases
Alcohol	58	67
Compression	34	39
Seizures	21	24
Direct trauma	16	17
Drug abuse	13	15
Metabolic disturbance	7	8
Hypothermia	4	4
Influenza-like illness	3	3
Sepsis	2	2
Gangrene	1	1
Summary:		
No factor identified	3	3
Single factor identified	33	38
Multiple factors identified	51	59

*Adapted from Gabow *et al*. (1982) The spectrum of rhabdomyolysis. *Medicine (Baltimore)*; 61: 141–152.

Table 2. The aetiology of rhabdomyolysis

Hereditary causes	Explanation
Metabolic myopathy	Genetic predisposition towards recurrent rhabdomyolysis is found in: • myophosphorylase (McArdle's disease) deficiency: defective glycolysis leads to anaerobic type 2 muscle ATP-depletion and necrosis induced by exercise • carnitine palmitoyltransferase deficiency: defective oxidation of long-chain fatty acids depletes aerobic type 1 muscle fibres of ATP after prolonged exercise and poor nutrition
Malignant hyperpyrexia	• Induced by volatile anaesthetics in susceptible individuals • Autosomal dominant defect of the ryanodine receptor of sarcolemmal calcium release channel in some patients • Syndrome comprises fever, muscular rigidity, acidosis and rhabdomyolysis • Leads to excessive myocyte calcium release, exacerbated by anaesthetics • Cocaine and amphetamines (particularly ecstasy) can also induce MH
Neuroleptic malignant syndrome	Major tranquilisers (e.g. phenothiazines, butyrophenones) can induce this syndrome with fever, fluctuating consciousness, autonomic instability, and generalised muscular rigidity which may cause rhabdomyolysis

Table 2 (*Continued*)

Acquired causes	Explanation
Trauma	Trauma causes direct muscle injury and/or ischaemia
Compression	Compressive ischaemia of muscles may occur in comatose subjects (often alcohol or drug-induced coma), surgical patients (either through prolonged immobilisation or careless use of tourniquets) or patients who are conscious but obliged to stay in one position, such as those with certain fractures
Excessive exertion	Very severe exercise in those unaccustomed to it often leads to myoglobinaemia. This can result in myoglobinuric ARF if the ambient temperature is high, or sweating is impaired. Classic victims are new military recruits being trained in combat gear in tropical climates
Alcohol	• Alcohol is directly myotoxic • Frequently leads to compression injury • Exacerbates electrolyte abnormalities (hypokalaemia/hypophosphataemia)
Drugs	• Direct myotoxicity: heroin, HMG-CoA reductase inhibitors, fibrates • Coma/muscle compression: barbiturates, opiates, anti-psychotics • Ecstasy (see **Chapter 11**)
Toxins	• Clostridial toxin of gas gangrene, hornet/wasp sting or proteolytic snake venom can cause myonecrosis directly • Carbon monoxide poisoning causes myocyte ATP depletion by interrupting O_2 delivery
Electrolyte abnormalities	• Profound hypokalaemia or hypophosphataemia (or less commonly hypo- or hyper-natraemia) can induce muscle necrosis • Hypokalaemia can directly impair muscle glycogen synthesis and exercise-induced hyperaemia
Infection	• Viral or bacterial infections can precipitate rhabdomyolysis • Commonly implicated organisms are Influenza, HIV, Legionella, Streptococci
Status epilepticus	Prolonged seizures cause calcium-mediated muscle injury
Vascular occlusion	Macrovascular atheroma, careless use of surgical tourniquets or accidental intra-arterial injections can lead to myonecrosis
Sickle cell disease	Red cell rouleaux formation can exacerbate muscle ischaemia through microvascular occlusion, and hyposthenuria promotes a tendency towards volume depletion and renal hypoperfusion
Endocrinopathy	Diabetic hyperglycaemic crises (ketoacidosis or hyperosmolar state) or myxoedema (rarely thyrotoxicosis) can lead to rhabdomyolysis
Inflammatory myopathies	Polymyositis and dermatomyositis usually cause myoglobinuria and a high plasma creatine kinase, but ARF is very rare, illustrating that myoglobinuria alone is relatively benign
Status asthmaticus	Respiratory muscle overactivity, hypoxia, or drug-induced hypokalaemia may contribute

CLINICAL PRESENTATION

The diverse aetiology of rhabdomyolysis is reflected by the wide spectrum of clinical presentations. In some patients, with crush syndrome for example, muscle injury and its cause are apparent. However, in many patients there may be very few clinically manifest symptoms and signs. Indeed, a significant number of patients may present with an altered level of consciousness delaying early diagnosis and institution of appropriate treatment.

Specific Symptoms and Signs (seen in approximately 50% of patients)

- Cramping muscle pains: generalised or involving specific muscle groups, especially the calves and lower back
- Muscle weakness, tenderness and swelling
- Haemorrhagic discolouration of overlying skin (in 5% of patients)
- Discoloration of the urine

General Symptoms and Signs

- General malaise, tachycardia, nausea and vomiting
- Fever may be a prominent feature

Complications

The severity of complications depends on the degree of muscle injury. They arise from the local effects of muscle cell lysis and the systemic effects of the substances released. Transcellular electrolyte and solute shifts, when sarcolemmal integrity is compromised, cause significant biochemical and haemodynamic abnormalities in the hours to days following muscle injury. These are outlined below and in **Table 3**.

Hypovolaemia: commonly occurs secondary to influx of fluid into necrotic muscle. Crush injuries are usually associated with haemorrhage.

Myoglobinuric ARF: occurs in approximately 30% of patients. Established ARF secondary to rhabdomyolysis demonstrates the typical clinical and laboratory features described in **Section 2**. However, severe hyperkalaemia and hyperphosphataemia are seen much earlier in the disease. In addition, there is often an increased creatinine:urea ratio reflecting "dumping" of pre-formed creatinine from damaged muscle into the circulation.

Compartment syndrome: muscle swelling within the fascial compartment causes neurovascular compression and muscle ischaemia. Secondary oedema propagates compression and leads to muscle necrosis, scarring and Volkmann's contractures.

Disseminated intravascular coagulation: is usually present but subclinical; there are frequently abnormalities of coagulation studies with elevated fibrin degradation products but these are rarely

Table 3. Metabolic complications of rhabdomyolysis	
Cell component released	**Complications**
Potassium	Arrhythmias and cardiac arrest
	Arrythmogenic effects often exacerbated by hypocalcaemia
Phosphate	Exacerbates hypocalcaemia by binding calcium and suppressing
	1–25 dihydroxycholecalciferol production
	Increased calcium-phosphate product can cause metastatic calcification
Uric acid (following purine release)	Intra-tubular urate crystals and sludging
	Metabolic acidosis
	Encephalopathy and respiratory depression
Sulphate, lactate	Metabolic acidosis

associated with clinical haemorrhagic complications. It is probably due to coagulation cascade activation by released muscle components.

Biochemical abnormalities: following muscle injury and causing clinical disease are shown in **Table 3**.

INVESTIGATIONS

Establishing myoglobinuria confirms the diagnosis of rhabdomyolysis.

Urine

Appearance: very dark pigmented urine ("coca-cola") secondary to myoglobinuria (serum myoglobin values rarely >25 mg/L so visible pigmenturia is rare; see above).

Dipstick urine test: urine positive for blood (orthotoluidine-positive) in the presence of myoglobin (dipstick cross-reacts with haemoglobin).

Microscopy: pigmented tubular casts.

Radioimmunoassay: sensitive for detection of myoglobin. Dipstick urinalysis positive for blood in the absence of urinary erythrocytes on microscopy, is highly suggestive of rhabdomyolysis (or haemolysis).

Haematology

Sub-clinical disseminated intravascular coagulation is very common.

Biochemistry

See **Table 4**.

Table 4. Biochemical abnormalities in rhabdomyolysis

Abnormality	Comments
↑creatine phosphokinase	Hallmark of muscle damage
	CK-MM isoenzyme predominates
	Usually >5 times upper limit of normal
	Rise occurs early
	Compartment syndromes cause persistent elevation/rebound >48 hours after initial insult
↑creatinine	↑creatinine:urea ratio
↑of other muscle enzymes (aldolase, LDH, aminotransferases)	Aldolase specific for skeletal muscle injury
↑potassium	Occurs very early in disease
	Often life-threatening hyperkalaemia
↑phosphate	Occurs early in disease
	Values often markedly elevated
↑urate	Leads to hyperuricaemia and acidosis
↓calcium	Predominates during oliguric phase
↑calcium	Can complicate the diuretic phase of acute renal failure secondary to mobilisation of calcium tissue deposits and increased availability of 1–25 dihydroxycholecalciferol
↑lactate, sulphate	Contribute to acidosis

Muscle biopsy

Muscle biopsy may be indicated in patients: (i) without easily identifiable exogenous precipitants; (ii) with a history of myoglobinuria provoked by exercise (e.g. hereditary myopathies); and (iii) where the clinical picture is suggestive of an underlying inflammatory disorder such as polymyositis or dermatomyositis (e.g. associated rash, arthralgia, arthritis, dysphagia, Raynaud's phenomenon, Sjogren's syndrome). In polymyositis, the biopsy shows necrosis, swelling and disruption of myocytes with inflammation characterised by a mononuclear cell infiltrate.

Electromyography

Short polyphasic motor potentials, occasional spontaneous fibrillation and high-frequency repetitive discharges are characteristic of polymyositis.

TREATMENT PRINCIPLES

The main objectives of treatment are: (i) to treat the specific cause of the muscle damage (e.g. infection, compartment syndrome) and; (ii) to treat and prevent, where possible, the complications of rhabdomyolysis.

Table 5. Examples of the treatment of specific aetiological factors	
Aetiological factor	**Treatment/Prevention**
Hereditary causes:	
Myophosphorylase deficiency	
Carnitine palmitoyltransferase deficiency	Prevention by avoiding vigorous exercise
Malignant hyperthermia	Avoid exercise; low carbohydrate diet
	Avoid precipitating agents (see **Table 1**)
	Dantrolene is useful to control rigidity
Acquired causes:	
Compartment syndromes	Surgical expertise required
Alcohol, toxins, drugs	Conservative management where possible to reduce infection risk
	Fasciotomy if intracompartmental pressure >40 mmHg
	Withdrawal of offending agents
	Use of specific antidotes

General Considerations

Where appropriate any reversible initial insult should be treated. This clearly encompasses the vast list of conditions detailed in the AETIOLOGY section, some of which are addressed in **Table 5**; the reader is referred on to the excellent reviews listed in the final section for further information.

Treatment of the Biochemical Complications of Rhabdomyolysis

Hyperkalaemia: occurs early (within hours), is frequently very severe and is often refractory to the standard treatments, such as insulin/dextrose and sodium bicarbonate (see **Section 2**), which depend on shifting potassium intracellularly (muscle injury results in impaired ion transport and transcellular leakiness). Use ion exchange resins and consider early dialysis if dangerous hyperkalaemia develops (ECG abnormalities, arrhythmias).

Hyperphosphataemia: phosphate-binders can be administered in the awake patient. Refractory hypocalcaemia or metastatic calcification may necessitate dialysis.

Hypocalcaemia: avoid calcium infusions as they can exacerbate metastatic calcification. Calcium administration should be restricted to emergency use in patients with hyperkalaemic complications or symptomatic hypocalcaemia.

Hyperuricaemia: allopurinol may be used if severe hyperuricaemia ensues.

Prevention and Treatment of Myoglobinuric Acute Renal Failure

The aims of treatment are to: (i) aggressively correct hypovolaemia and maintain adequate renal perfusion; and (ii) enhance clearance of circulating haem proteins — see **Practice Point**.

Practice Point. Prevention of myoglobinuric ARF

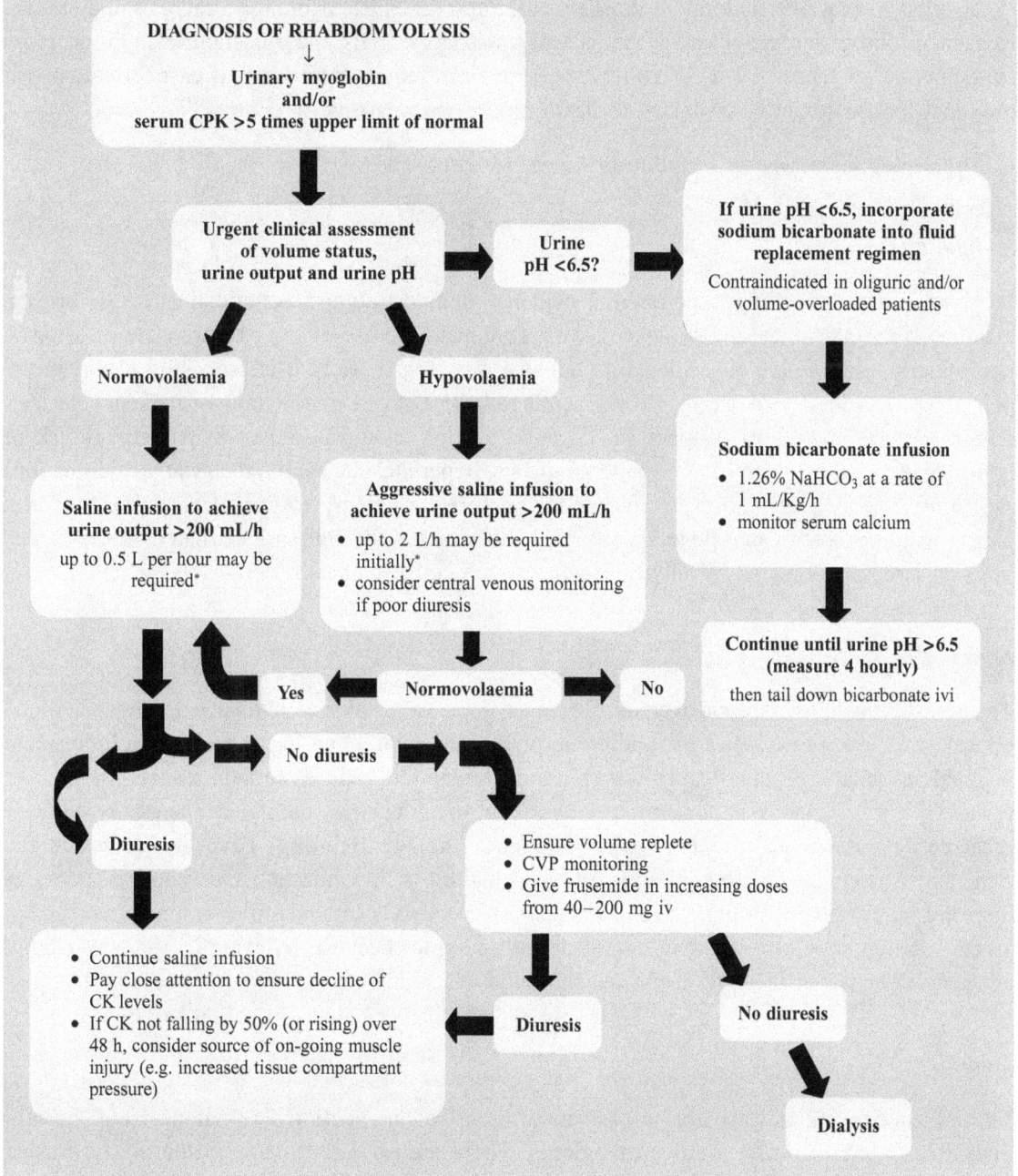

DIAGNOSIS OF RHABDOMYOLYSIS
↓
Urinary myoglobin
and/or
serum CPK >5 times upper limit of normal

Urgent clinical assessment
of volume status,
urine output and urine pH

→ Urine pH <6.5?

→ If urine pH <6.5, incorporate sodium bicarbonate into fluid replacement regimen

Contraindicated in oliguric and/or volume-overloaded patients

Normovolaemia

Hypovolaemia

Sodium bicarbonate infusion
- 1.26% NaHCO$_3$ at a rate of 1 mL/Kg/h
- monitor serum calcium

Saline infusion to achieve urine output >200 mL/h

up to 0.5 L per hour may be required*

Aggressive saline infusion to achieve urine output >200 mL/h
- up to 2 L/h may be required initially*
- consider central venous monitoring if poor diuresis

Continue until urine pH >6.5 (measure 4 hourly)

then tail down bicarbonate ivi

Yes ← Normovolaemia → No

No diuresis →

Diuresis

- Ensure volume replete
- CVP monitoring
- Give frusemide in increasing doses from 40–200 mg iv

- Continue saline infusion
- Pay close attention to ensure decline of CK levels
- If CK not falling by 50% (or rising) over 48 h, consider source of on-going muscle injury (e.g. increased tissue compartment pressure)

Diuresis

No diuresis

Dialysis

*Central venous pressure (CVP) monitoring is always required when large volumes of fluid are infused to resuscitate a hypovolaemic or shocked patient (see **Chapter 10**). An example of an appropriate fluid regimen would be to administer 1–2 mL/Kg/h crystalloid, with additional colloid challenges (e.g. gelofusine) given against the CVP and blood pressure, as described in **Chapter 8.1**.

- *Hypovolaemia*

Early and vigorous fluid replacement is undoubtedly the most important therapeutic manoeuvre in the management of rhabdomyolysis. This will improve GFR, encourage a diuresis and prevent ischaemic tubular damage. Despite the lack of prospective trials, there is significant clinical and experimental evidence that early volume repletion can reduce intra-luminal cast formation and proximal tubular toxicity secondary to haem protein endocytosis.

- *Enhancing clearance of circulating haem proteins*

Sodium bicarbonate

In view of the compelling experimental evidence demonstrating a beneficial effect of urinary alkalinisation (but no clinical evidence), we recommend the use of early bicarbonate infusion in non-oliguric, volume replete patients, to achieve a urine pH >6.5. It is especially useful in the patient who has developed severe hyperkalaemia following severe muscle injury (markedly elevated CPK), acidosis and renal dysfunction. Extreme caution should be taken in patients at risk of hypocalcaemia (those with severe rhabdomyolysis, hyperphosphataemia, metastatic calcification) as the bicarbonate may cause precipitous fall in serum calcium; a hypocalcaemic seizure in a patient with pre-existing muscle injury is highly undesirable! The high sodium load of a bicarbonate infusion is contraindicated in oliguric, volume-overloaded patients.

Mannitol

The role of mannitol is controversial. There is good experimental evidence for its beneficial effects most likely as a result of its diuretic properties (facilitating haem protein excretion) and its renal vasodilatory properties. However, although mannitol reduces sodium reabsorption, it can paradoxically increase ATP consumption which, in the context of tubular damage may increase renal cortical ischaemia. Better *et al.* (1990; see **Further Reading**) advocate its use in the treatment of traumatic rhabdomyolysis in combination with saline and bicarbonate. However, there are no prospective trial data to prove that mannitol adds any benefit to volume replacement alone. Caution should be used in administering mannitol because an osmotic diuresis without adequate volume replacement might worsen hypovolaemia.

Dialysis

The indications for dialysis are as previously described in **Section 2**. Peritoneal and haemo-dialysis do not adequately remove myoglobin. There are no data to support the use of plasma exchange.

OUTCOME

Typically the muscle disorder is self-limiting and resolves within days to weeks, due to the regenerative capacity of muscle. Independent renal function returns in the vast majority of patients with dialysis-dependent renal failure.

HAEMOGLOBINURIC RENAL FAILURE

Although much rarer than ARF from rhabdomyolysis, haemoglobinuric renal failure (HRF) is well described in disorders associated with massive intravascular haemolysis. These include:

- Incompatible blood transfusions
- Falciparum malaria (blackwater fever)
- Red cell enzyme defects (e.g. G6PD deficiency)
- Autoimmune or drug-induced haemolytic anaemias (e.g. chloroquine, aspirin, chloramphenicol)
- Infection (mycoplasma)
- Favism
- Eclampsia
- Absorption of large volumes of hypotonic solution into the circulation (as may occur in endoscopic prostate surgery where large volumes of glycine are instilled into the bladder, some absorbed, and the glycine metabolised, leading to effective free-water absorption and consequent hypotonic red cell lysis)
- Poisoning with copper sulphate, arsine, quinine sulphate, naphthalene, or snake and insect bites
- Paroxysmal nocturnal haemoglobinuria (ARF may occur during an acute haemoglobinuric crisis)

Extravascular haemolysis leads to production of bile pigments and urobilinogen, but does not cause ARF. In contrast to myoglobin, there is a specific plasma protein which binds Hb, haptoglobin, which must first be saturated (occurring at a free Hb concentration of 100 mg/dL) before there is free plasma Hb to render the serum dark in colour. Even then, because of its large size (tetramer is 69 kDa), Hb enters the urinary filtrate poorly (unlike the small, freely filtered myoglobin molecule) and this may account for the relative rarity of HRF. These physical differences underlie the classic test to distinguish between HRF and rhabdomyolysis in a patient with ARF and a positive urine dipstick test for blood without visible urinary red cells: if the plasma is dark, then haemoglobinuria is probable, whereas myoglobin released from myocytes is very rapidly filtered into the urine such that the plasma concentration is invisibly low and the plasma remains clear. It is generally assumed that the pathophysiology of HRF is similar to that of myoglobinuric ARF, developing through a combination of intratubular Hb cast formation and obstruction, tubular toxicity and coincident renal ischaemia.

The laboratory features of ARF include:

- Anaemia
- Low plasma haptoglobin
- Elevated free plasma haemoglobin
- Hyperbilirubinaemia
- Elevated LDH
- Hyperkalaemia

Unsurprisingly, given similar pathophysiology, treatment principles of HRF are similar to those of myoglobinuria, and consist of volume repletion with intensive efforts to establish a diuresis, often using mannitol and loop diuretics. The importance of urinary alkalinisation is not defined, and firm recommendations cannot be made. Prognosis for the renal disease is generally good, with recovery of renal function expected even if there is a period of dialysis-dependence. Significantly though, other consequences of the anaemia and its inciting factors may carry mortality greater than that of ARF.

FURTHER READING

Better OS, Stein JH (1990) Early management of shock and prophylaxis of acute renal failure in traumatic rhabdomyolysis. *New England Journal of Medicine*; 322: 825–829

Gabow PA, Kaehny WD, Kelleher SP (1982) The spectrum of rhabdomyolysis. *Medicine (Baltimore)*; 61: 141–152

Kakulas BA, Mastaglia FL (1992) Drug-induced, toxic and nutritional myopathies. In: Mastaglia FL and Walton J (eds.). *Skeletal Muscle Pathology* (2nd Edition). New York: Churchill Livingstone; pp. 511–540

Poels PJE, Gabreëls FJM (1993) Rhabdomyolysis: A review of the literature. *Clinical Neurology and Neurosurgery*; 95: 175–192

Singh U, Scheld WM (1996) Infectious aetiologies of rhabdomyolysis: Three case reports and review. *Clinical Infectious Diseases*; 22: 642–649

Zager RA (1996) Rhabdomyolysis and acute renal failure. *Kidney International*; 49: 314–326

Chapter 13 _____

RENOVASCULAR DISEASE AND CHOLESTEROL EMBOLI
Graham Lord

DEFINITION

Renovascular disease or ischaemic nephropathy may be either acute or chronic. This chapter will concern itself with acute forms of this syndrome, as the management of chronic renovascular disease and renovascular hypertension is beyond the scope of this text. Acute ischaemic nephropathy (AIN) may be defined as a reduction in glomerular filtration rate (GFR) as a consequence of arterial obstruction to renal blood flow (RBF). The commonest clinical scenario is that of an acute deterioration in GFR upon a background of a chronic impairment of RBF. An acute rise in serum creatinine from baseline will of course only occur in the presence of a single functioning kidney or in the context of bilateral renovascular disease.

Cholesterol embolism or atheroembolic disease occurs in the context of systemic embolisation, usually as a consequence of an iatrogenic vascular procedure, where the kidney is subjected to showers of emboli causing an acute reduction in microvascular renal blood flow. There are also other systemic effects caused by distal emboli.

PATHOPHYSIOLOGY

A detailed review of renal haemodynamics is provided in **Chapter 1** and will not be repeated here. Given what we know about the anatomy of the renal blood supply, it is of note that acute occlusion of the renal artery does not necessarily cause infarction. Analogous to the coronary circulation, collateral vessels can develop, particularly where the kidney has previously been subject to chronic ischaemia. However, chronic ischaemia itself may cause significant renal damage, despite providing a degree of protection against infarction following acute occlusion. The pathophysiological basis of AIN is complex. Animal models demonstrate that experimental stenosis induces marked interstitial damage with relative glomerular preservation, which is mirrored by the histological appearances seen in human renal ischaemia. Other models show that renal artery stenosis can induce fibrotic interstitial changes which are significantly worsened by the concomitant administration of angiotensin converting enzyme inhibitors (ACEI). The clinical link between ACEI and AIN will be discussed later in the chapter. It is clear from animal models that the damage caused by renal ischaemia can be reversible. However, in certain circumstances, the ischaemic changes are progressive, leading to irreversible structural changes. The cellular mechanisms whereby hypoxia and altered renal haemodynamics cause renal damage are complex and include Fas-mediated apoptosis, alterations in nitric oxide pathways and disturbance of the synthesis of prostaglandins and other vasoactive mediators.

Obstruction to RBF can occur in the context of either normal or abnormal renal arteries. By far the commonest situation is occlusion of the renal artery in the presence of atherosclerotic renovascular disease. Rarely, occlusion may occur in previously normal renal arteries.

Cholesterol emboli commonly cause lesions in the kidney, spleen, muscle and skin, although almost any distal site can be affected. In the kidney, histology reveals characteristic clefts that are left after the cholesterol has been dissolved during fixation of the tissue sample (see **Chapter 7**). These clefts are seen in the arcuate and interlobular arteries and the deposition of cholesterol at these sites incites a giant cell foreign body inflammatory reaction in the subsequent 48 hours. Over the next few weeks, endothelial cell proliferation and luminal obliteration are observed leading eventually to wedge-shaped scarring. Rarely, cholesterol emboli have been reported to cause crescentic and membranoproliferative glomerulonephritis. The most typical pattern however, is widespread fibrosis and the typical cholesterol cleft may be difficult to find.

AETIOLOGY

The aetiology of AIN differs depending on whether the renal arteries are normal or diseased (**Table 1**). Cholesterol embolism shows many features similar to macrovascular renal pathology, except that it occurs both in the presence of normal and abnormal renal arteries. However, its occurrence is much more likely in the context of widespread atheromatous changes, given that the source of the emboli is often either a spontaneously or iatrogenically ruptured proximal atheromatous plaque.

Table 1. Causes of acute ischaemic nephropathy	
Previously abnormal renal arteries	Thrombosis at a site of atherosclerotic stenosis
	Thrombosis at a site of stenosis caused by fibromuscular dysplasia
	ACEI treatment in the presence of bilateral renal artery stenosis
	Thrombosis in a renal artery aneurysm
	Angioplasty damage to a stenosed renal artery
Previously normal renal arteries	Aortic dissection
	Traumatic rupture of renal artery
	Trauma induced thrombosis of renal artery
	Thrombosis caused by a pro-coagulant state
	Embolus from a central source
	Takayasu's aortitis
	Idiopathic
Cholesterol embolism	Angiographic procedures on arteries proximal to renal artery
	Anticoagulation
	Vascular surgery
	Thrombolysis
	Idiopathic

AIN in the Presence of Abnormal Renal Arteries

The main abnormality predisposing to acute renal ischaemia is stenosis of the renal arteries. The most common situation in which this occurs is acute renal artery occlusion in the presence of chronic renal artery stenosis due to atherosclerosis. Atheromatous plaques occur most commonly in the proximal third of the renal artery. Often, aortic plaques may encroach on the ostia of the renal arteries. It is important to differentiate between these two situations, since their response to angioplasty is not the same (see **Treatment Principles**). The natural history of these plaques is progression to complete occlusion, which is often unrecognised. The prevalence of renovascular disease is high, being up to 50% in patients requiring investigation for peripheral vascular disease and 30% of patients undergoing coronary angiography. Renovascular disease causes 15% of all cases of end-stage renal failure and is a causative factor in up to 15% of all cases of acute renal failure. When an acute presentation is observed, it is usually on a background of a more subacute or chronic process.

To a certain extent, it is possible to predict which patients are at risk of acute renal artery occlusion in the context of a background of atherosclerotic renal disease. In patients with a renal artery stenosis of less than 60% as assessed by doppler ultrasound, no progression to complete occlusion was seen within two years. However if the stenosis was greater than 60%, then the rate of complete occlusion was 5% at one year and 11% at two years. It is important to remember that progression to occlusion usually only causes a slight elevation of plasma creatinine, due to the presence of a functional contralateral kidney and the development of a relatively efficient collateral circulation. However, in the presence of a single functioning kidney, occlusion will lead to an acute decline in GFR. Such a scenario is made more likely due to the fact that atherosclerotic renovascular disease is commonly bilateral.

Fibromuscular dysplasia of the renal arteries may cause renal artery stenosis and occlusion. Although much less common than atherosclerotic disease, it is more likely to occur in young patients with hypertension. Total occlusion in this situation is very rare, and therefore this condition is unlikely to present acutely.

Glomerular filtration pressures in the face of a reduced renal blood flow are maintained by angiotensin II-mediated vasoconstriction of the efferent arteriole (**Chapter 1**). Patients with pre-existing bilateral renal artery stenosis are at risk of an acute deterioration in renal function following the institution of angiotensin converting enzyme inhibitors (ACEI) for the treatment of either hypertension or cardiac failure. Any blockade of conversion to angiotensin II will reduce efferent arteriolar constriction and hence lower renal artery pressure and GFR.

Renal artery aneurysms are a rare but important cause of acute occlusion since they are amenable to surgical treatment and can cause haemorrhage as well as thrombose. Finally, acute occlusion of a renal artery may occur during or after angioplasty to an atherosclerotic renal artery, either due to induced thrombosis following plaque fracture or due to renal artery dissection.

AIN in the Presence of Normal Renal Arteries

Acute renal ischaemia occurs much less commonly in the presence of previously normal renal arteries. Given that there is no background of chronic ischaemia, it is much more likely that acute renal artery occlusion will produce renal infarction and a more dramatic presentation. Aortic dissection extending to and including the renal arteries can obviously cause an acute reduction in renal blood flow, as can traumatic rupture or trauma-induced thrombosis of the renal artery.

Procoagulant states can induce *de novo* renal artery thrombosis and include protein C and S deficiency, the nephrotic syndrome and the antiphospholipid syndrome. Takayasu's arteritis can induce renal artery narrowing and renal ischaemia. Spontaneous occlusion has also been rarely reported.

A rare, but important cause of renal ischaemia is a clot embolus from a central source. This differs from cholesterol embolism, in that a clot embolus can cause complete occlusion and renal infarction, whereas cholesterol emboli tend to cause incomplete vascular occlusion and distal ischaemia rather than infarction. A clot embolus usually originates from a mural thrombus in the heart in patients with atrial arrhythmias, prior myocardial infarction or a ventricular aneurysm. Occasionally, a central thrombus can originate from valvular vegetations in endocarditis or from a necrosing tumour. Even more rarely, a fat embolism may be the cause of acute renal artery occlusion.

Cholesterol Emboli

Patients who have diffuse atherosclerosis are at risk of plaque fragments breaking off and embolising to the kidneys and other distal sites. It can occur in the presence of normal renal arteries but given that atheroma is usually multifocal, it is more commonly seen on a background of renal artery stenosis. Embolisation may be spontaneous but often arises in the context of instrumentation to proximal vascular beds. It has been estimated that 48% of cases could be attributed to angiography, 13% to anticoagulation and 5% to vascular surgery. Thrombolysis for myocardial infarction has been reported as a cause of cholesterol embolism. In a proportion of cases, there is no clear precipitating factor.

CLINICAL PRESENTATION

Acute Ischaemic Nephropathy

Specific symptoms and signs are rare in AIN. The patient may experience acute loin pain and haematuria and occasionally have a pyrexia. However, on a background of chronic ischaemia, which allows an effective collateral circulation to develop, renal infarction and hence flank pain are absent. A renal bruit may be present on examination, but its absence does not exclude the diagnosis. Indeed, if the artery is totally occluded, then a bruit will be absent. Acute renal failure (ARF) due to AIN shares most of the clinical features associated with other aetiologies of ARF, with the caveat that a rapid onset of pulmonary oedema is more common (so called "flash" pulmonary oedema). Indeed, bilateral renal artery stenosis should be considered in any patient who presents with hypertension and pulmonary oedema and is clinically euvolaemic with normal left ventricular function. There may be evidence of macrovascular disease at other sites, such as lower limb ischaemia, cardiovascular and/or cerebrovascular disease. Signs of end-organ damage due to prior hypertension caused by pre-existing renal artery stenosis may be present, such as hypertensive retinopathy and left ventricular hypertrophy. Central embolism from a cardiac thrombus to the renal artery often causes renal infarction, since chronic ischaemia and hence a collateral circulation is not present. In this situation, the patient will complain of an acute onset of vomiting, flank pain and fever.

Cholesterol Emboli

Occasionally renovascular disease can present with symptoms and signs suggesting an embolic aetiology, on the background of worsening renal function. Patients are often hypertensive and have evidence of atheroma at other sites. Distal gangrene and so called "trash feet" may occur and livedo reticularis and myalgia are not uncommon. The features of cholesterol emboli often suggest a multisystem disease and can be misdiagnosed as vasculitis. Focal neurological defects, such as transient ischaemic attacks (TIAs), seizures, retinal emboli and strokes may be observed. Occasionally, gut haemorrhage or infarction may be a presenting feature.

A unique clinical feature of cholesterol emboli is that they can be observed directly in the retina on fundoscopy. A retinal embolus is an important prognostic and diagnostic marker in this condition and should be specifically looked for. **Table 2** summarises the clinical features seen in this condition and includes rarer findings.

Table 2. Clinical features of cholesterol emboli

Distal gangrene
Myalgia/myositis
Livedo reticularis
Worsening hypertension
Retinal emboli
Focal neurological signs — TIAs, seizures, stroke
Neuropathy
Abdominal pain due to gut infarction or haemorrhage
Addisonian crisis
Features of crescentic glomerulonephritis
Occasionally asymptomatic

INVESTIGATIONS

Acute Ischaemic Nephropathy

Clinical suspicion of acute ischaemic nephropathy should be high where an elderly patient presents with rapidly deteriorating renal function in the context of atheromatous disease elsewhere, as previously described.

The urinary sediment is typically inactive with a 24-hour protein excretion of less than 1 g. There is rarely evidence of an acute phase response, in contrast with cholesterol embolism (see later). There may be laboratory evidence of a procoagulant state.

In the case of renal infarction, gross or microscopic haematuria is seen in about 30% of patients. Additionally, a markedly raised lactate dehydrogenase (LDH) in the presence of normal transaminase levels strongly suggest infarction.

Ultrasound scanning may show asymmetrical renal size which is highly suggestive of previous renal artery stenosis in the smaller kidney, which may then be prone to complete occlusion. In the presence of symmetrical disease, however, there will be no size disparity. Conversely, in the setting of an acutely deteriorating creatinine and asymmetrical renal size on ultrasound, it may be that the blood supply to the normal sized kidney has occluded acutely, with the smaller kidney having silently occluded previously.

If the renal outline is normal on ultrasound, and renovascular disease is suspected, lack of function on a DTPA or a MAG3 scan indicates a high probability of renal artery occlusion. Further information about renal blood flow may be gained by the use of duplex doppler ultrasonography. However, this is a difficult and time-consuming technique which is very operator dependent.

The gold standard for the diagnosis of renal artery stenosis and occlusion is intra-arterial renal artery angiography. However, this may exacerbate the disease process by dislodging showers of emboli or causing dissection of the renal artery. There is also the risk of a contrast load in the context of an already impaired renal blood flow. Due to these concerns and the relatively invasive nature of renal angiography, other investigations are currently being assessed as screening tools and are even being used as a first line in some centres, depending on local expertise and availability.

Spiral CT scanning and gadolinium-enhanced magnetic resonance angiography (MRA) have both been used to image the renal arteries in the situation of impaired renal function and a strong clinical suspicion of renovascular disease. The advantage of these investigations is that they are non-invasive and so do not carry the risk of embolisation and dissection. Their sensitivity and specificity for detection of significant disease is high, but unlike conventional angiography, they do not offer the opportunity for intervention (i.e. angioplasty or stent placement) should the need arise. Spiral CT is less accurate in the face of a raised creatinine, reducing its usefulness in acute occlusion. Furthermore, MRA is currently not sensitive enough for detecting stenoses in branch or accessory renal arteries and stenoses can be underestimated due to blood flow turbulence. If surgical intervention is required, then the definition provided by a standard angiogram is usually needed.

Cholesterol Emboli

Urinalysis is typically benign and proteinuria is mild (although nephrotic range proteinuria has been reported). Some patients may have an active sediment with red cells and red cell casts leading to a suspicion of acute glomerulonephritis. Eosinophiluria may be observed with Hansel's stain.

Blood testing often reveals a raised ESR and hypocomplementaemia, particularly if measured in the acute phase of the disease. This is thought to be due to immunological activation at the surface of exposed atheroemboli. These findings resolve or normalise within a week and therefore recurrence suggests continuation of the atheroembolic process.

Given that angiography is a frequent cause of cholesterol emboli, its use in diagnosis is contraindicated. In the appropriate clinical circumstances, the diagnosis is reached by biopsy of a skin lesion if present or a renal biopsy. Renal biopsy is generally the diagnostic procedure of choice.

An algorithm for the clinical diagnosis of AIN and cholesterol emboli is given in the **Practice Point** at the end of this chapter.

TREATMENT PRINCIPLES

Acute Ischaemic Nephropathy

The management principles will depend on the clinical situation and the specific causative factor(s). Clearly, in certain situations such as aortic dissection, other management issues will take priority and treatment of renal dysfunction will be supportive replacement therapy. There are several specific clinical situations that need to be considered separately.

1. *Suspected renal infarction due to clot embolus*

If renal infarction is diagnosed, it will usually have occurred unilaterally, and plasma creatinine will not rise. In this situation, the priority is to prevent embolic occlusion of the contralateral kidney. This will generally involve medical treatment such as anticoagulation or thrombolysis. Surgery is better able to restore vascular patency than medical treatment, but has a higher mortality with no improvement in functional renal recovery. The one exception to this is in the case of traumatic renal artery thrombosis, where early surgical intervention is the preferred management option.

Medical therapy will be of use with a partial occlusion or if a degree of patency can be restored by thrombolysis within 2 to 3 hours. This is the "warm ischaemic time" of a kidney, which is the time a kidney can survive when deprived of its blood supply at 37C. If an early diagnosis is made, then consideration should be given to thrombolysis, which can be given by local intraarterial infusion in order to reduce systemic bleeding problems.

2. *Pharmacologically-induced renal failure*

Any patient who presents with acute renal failure and is taking an ACEI should probably have the drug discontinued until the aetiology of the renal failure is diagnosed. This is certainly true if the patient has any signs or symptoms of systemic or renal atheroma. Patients are particularly sensitive to the effects of ACEI in the context of sodium depletion, where the GFR is dependent on angiotensin II. Therefore ACEI can be most deleterious if the patient is concomitantly taking diuretics or has excessive extrarenal losses such as vomiting or diarrhoea. Cessation of therapy may produce a dramatic improvement in renal function, particularly if a patient who has been hypovolaemic is simultaneously rehydrated. The speed and extent of renal recovery will depend on several factors such as the degree of tubular necrosis caused by the hypoperfusion, the amount of prior chronic ischaemic damage to the kidney and whether the reduction in renal blood flow has caused renal artery thrombosis and subsequent infarction (in a single functional kidney). Indeed, the renal failure induced by ACEI may be permanent.

Other classes of antihypertensive agents can cause a reduction in GFR and RBF when prescribed in the presence of bilateral renal artery disease. Therefore, one should consider stopping any such therapy in the acute situation if a diagnosis of acute ischaemic nephropathy is entertained.

3. *Renal failure due to renal artery thrombosis*

Medical revascularisation should be considered as for renal infarction due to a clot embolus (see above). If the clinical history suggests a recent event, or the thrombosis has occurred during or soon after renal artery angioplasty, then the initial treatment of choice is probably direct intra-arterial fibrinolysis with either streptokinase or recombinant tissue plasminogen activator. Placing a catheter with its tip in close proximity to a renal artery thrombus is a relatively safe procedure especially if the thrombus has occurred as a result of an angioplasty during the procedure. Some reports demonstrate that renal function can be restored up to 25% of patients with this treatment.

Revascularisation can also be brought about by angioplasty (percutaneous transluminal renal angioplasty — PTRA) or surgery, particularly in the cases of failed medical therapy. It is cogent to note that the survival of patients with renovascular disease on long-term dialysis is poor. The degree of atherosclerotic renal artery disease can predict survival on dialysis, such that there is probably less than a 50% 5-year survival rate in dialysis patients with severe renovascular disease. However, no study has convincingly shown that revascularising kidneys improves long-term survival, as the mortality may be a reflection of widespread atheroma, particularly in the coronary circulation. Long-term dialysis is known to be associated with accelerated atheroma formation, so intuitively it would seem logical to attempt to delay end-stage renal failure as long as possible. Prior to either PTRA or surgical revascularisation, it is probably advisable to perform a DMSA scan and a renal biopsy. The renal biopsy will ensure that the kidney is not severely damaged by cholesterol emboli or end-stage ischaemic nephropathy, in which case attempted revascularisation is not an option.

PTRA may be useful in bringing about a return of renal function in patients presenting with AIN. After aggressive fluid management and the withdrawal of ACEI and other antihypertensive medication, which are often precipitating factors, PTRA is a useful treatment option. Some authors, however, have reported a high incidence of complications, so the decision of whether to proceed with interventional revascularisation is often not clear-cut. The most amenable lesions to PTRA are those producing incomplete occlusion in the main renal artery. Ostial lesions and complete occlusions are not suitable for standard PTRA. Ostial lesions can sometimes be treated by placement of a renal artery stent, whereas complete occlusion is usually dealt with surgically. No randomised trial has yet proven the benefit of renal artery stents, although their use in difficult cases and to prevent re-stenosis is increasing. There are several series of cases that demonstrate the ability of PTRA to improve renal function in the setting of AIN. Overall, approximately 45% of patients have an improvement in renal function, 35% are stabilised and 20% are made worse. Complications include renal artery dissection, cholesterol emboli and contrast nephropathy.

Surgical revascularisation is often considered if the patient has unsuitable angiographic findings for PTRA. Again, no randomised trials exist in the setting of AIN to decide when surgery is better than PTRA. Given that many patients will have coronary and cerebral vascular disease, PTRA has the advantage of avoiding general anaesthesia and its attendant risks. There are reports of success with surgical approaches even after prolonged occlusion and anuria. The operative intervention can either be embolectomy/thrombectomy or a bypass procedure such as an aortorenal shunt. If there is a complete occlusion of the renal artery, surgery is probably the preferred option. Indeed, there are some studies which seem to show a better outcome in terms of renal function with surgery. However, with stenting procedures being improved and radiological teams gaining more experience in their use, it may be that PTRA with stent placement will become the treatment of choice. In the absence of randomised controlled trials, local expertise will often decide the appropriate treatment modality.

Cholesterol Emboli

Unfortunately, no intervention has been demonstrated to be effective in the treatment of cholesterol emboli. It has been suggested that peritoneal dialysis should be used in preference to haemodialysis as it avoids the need for further anticoagulation. Certainly, angiography or any vascular manipulation must be avoided, as this will only aggravate the situation. Despite the lack of available treatment, the diagnosis is important to make because it avoids confusion with other systemic diseases. The commonest mistaken diagnosis is systemic vasculitis and a correct diagnosis avoids unnecessary immunosuppression. Anticoagulation is best avoided, as it may further destabilise an unstable plaque. A recent report suggests that prostacyclin therapy may improve distal extremity lesions and renal function in patients with cholesterol emboli (Elinav *et al.*, 2002)

OUTCOME

Outcome is determined to some extent by making or suspecting the diagnosis of acute ischaemic nephropathy. If the diagnosis is made early, then the prospects for revascularisation are good, as described above. If renal function is not stabilised or improved and the patient requires long-term dialysis, then the outlook is poor, with a 5-year survival rate less than 50%.

In situations such as aortic dissection, factors other than renal function will have a greater influence on outcome. It must also be remembered that the vast majority of patients are elderly with widespread atheromatous disease, which will often be the main determinant of long-term prognosis.

Patients with clot emboli tend to do badly despite effective medical treatment, due to extrarenal emboli (especially brain and gut) and underlying disease which is usually ischaemic heart disease.

The prognosis in patients with cholesterol emboli is poor. Approximately 50% of patients die during the follow up period of studies, which range from 1 to 3 years, commonly from coronary artery disease.

FURTHER READING

Elinav E, Chajek-Shaul T, Stern M (2002) Improvement in cholesterol emboli syndrome after iloprost therapy. *BMJ*; 324: 268–269

Pickering TG, Blumenfeld JD, Laragh JH (1998) Renovascular hypertension and ischemic nephropathy. In: Saunders, Brenner, Rector (eds.). *The Kidney* (5th Edition). pp. 2106-2125

Robson MG, Scoble JE (1996) Atheroembolic disease. *British Journal of Hospital Medicine*; 55: 648–651

Rose BD (1998) UpToDate© Version 6.3 (CD ROM)

Scoble JE (1998) Ischaemic renal disease. In: Davison, Cameron, Grünfeld, *et al.* (eds.). *The Oxford Textbook of Clinical Nephrology* (2nd Edition). Oxford University Press; 1679–1688

Vidt DG (1997) Cholesterol emboli: A common cause of renal failure. *Annual Review of Medicine*; 48: 375–385

Practice Point. Clinical diagnosis of acute ischaemic nephropathy and cholesterol emboli

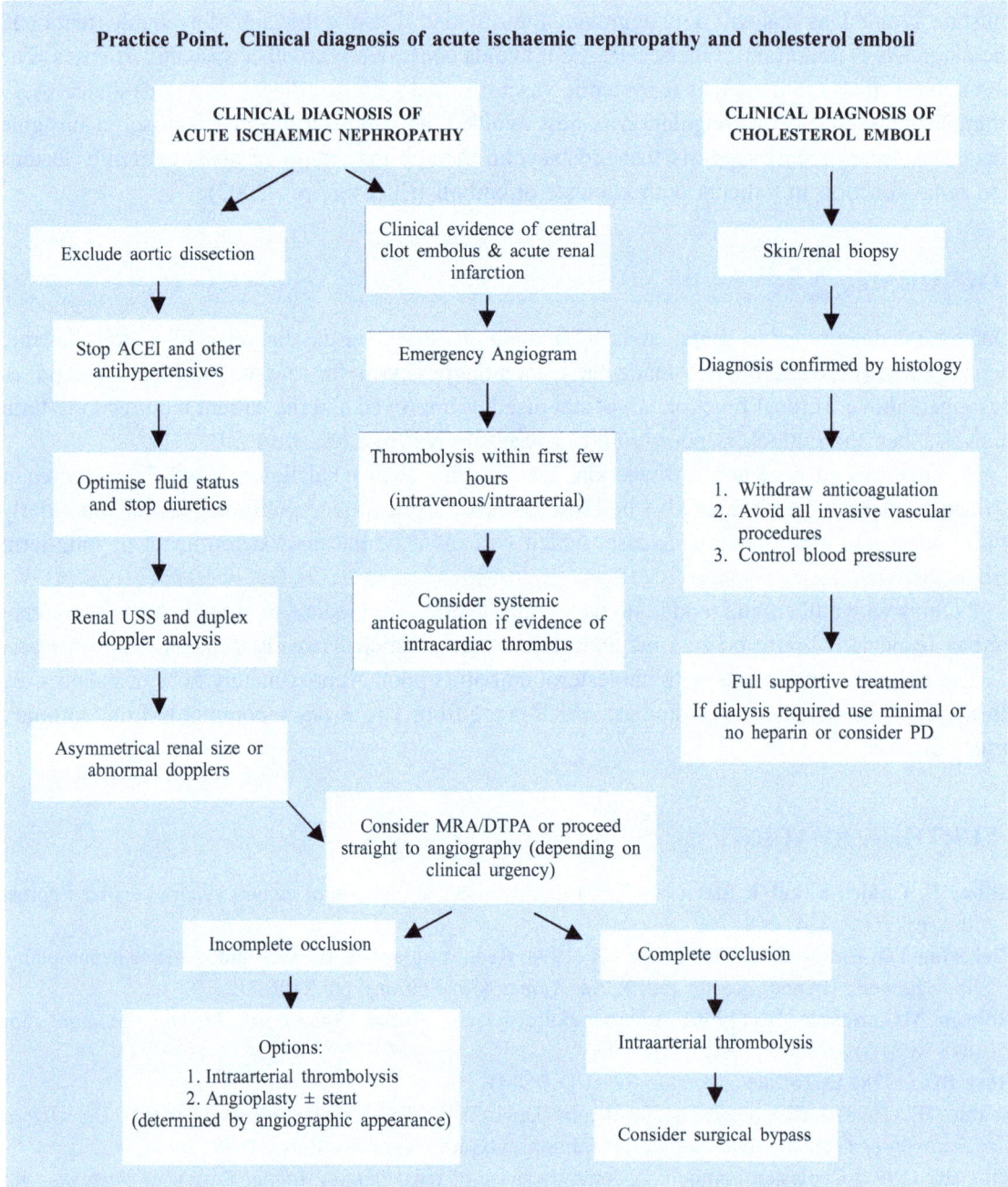

CLINICAL DIAGNOSIS OF
ACUTE ISCHAEMIC NEPHROPATHY

CLINICAL DIAGNOSIS OF
CHOLESTEROL EMBOLI

Exclude aortic dissection

Clinical evidence of central
clot embolus & acute renal
infarction

Skin/renal biopsy

Stop ACEI and other
antihypertensives

Emergency Angiogram

Diagnosis confirmed by histology

Optimise fluid status
and stop diuretics

Thrombolysis within first few
hours
(intravenous/intraarterial)

1. Withdraw anticoagulation
2. Avoid all invasive vascular
   procedures
3. Control blood pressure

Renal USS and duplex
doppler analysis

Consider systemic
anticoagulation if evidence of
intracardiac thrombus

Full supportive treatment
If dialysis required use minimal or
no heparin or consider PD

Asymmetrical renal size or
abnormal dopplers

Consider MRA/DTPA or proceed
straight to angiography (depending on
clinical urgency)

Incomplete occlusion

Complete occlusion

Options:
1. Intraarterial thrombolysis
2. Angioplasty ± stent
(determined by angiographic appearance)

Intraarterial thrombolysis

Consider surgical bypass

Chapter 14 _____

MALIGNANT HYPERTENSION
Raj Thuraisingham

DEFINITION

Severe hypertension can be associated with retinal damage, manifested as haemorrhages and exudates (grade III hypertensive retinopathy) or papilloedema (grade IV). Prior to the advent of effective anti-hypertensive therapy, such changes were associated with dismal survival, and the phrase "malignant hypertension" was thus coined. The term accelerated hypertension has been used to describe patients with grade III hypertensive retinopathy, but this distinction is an artificial one as the aetiology, pathophysiology, treatment and prognosis are similar in patients with grades III and IV retinal changes. Grade I ("silver wiring") and grade II (arteriovenous nipping) hypertensive retinopathy are secondary to atherosclerotic retinal disease, and are not associated with the characteristic end-organ damage seen in malignant hypertension. Early studies suggested malignant hypertension affected 1–7% of the hypertensive population, with men twice as likely to be affected as women. Recent data estimate the annual incidence of malignant hypertension to be 1–2 per 100,000 of the general population.

PATHOPHYSIOLOGY

Blood Pressure

The critical factor for the development of malignant hypertension is the degree and rapidity of the rise in blood pressure as opposed to absolute blood pressure levels. Patients with chronic hypertension will tolerate blood pressures far higher than previously normotensive patients. Hence, absolute blood pressure recordings do not play an important part in the diagnosis of this condition. Typically, however, malignant hypertension is associated with blood pressure readings above 200/120 mmHg.

Malignant hypertension occurs when there is loss of vascular autoregulation. In vascular beds a rise in blood pressure causes distal vasoconstriction at arteriolar level, thus protecting end-organs from the effects of hypertension. This mechanism also ensures relatively constant blood flow under normal conditions and modulates minor alterations in blood pressure. In severe hypertension, however, the vasoconstrictor response fails, resulting in transmission of the hypertension to the microvasculature. Endothelial injury ensues as a result of mechanical trauma. Damage to the endothelium leads to enhanced vascular permeability with leakage, allowing plasma proteins such as fibrinogen to enter the vessel wall. In the brain, failure of autoregulation leads to cerebral oedema.

Endocrine Factors

There may be an initial pressure-induced natriuresis as a result of the rise in blood pressure. This causes activation of the renin-angiotensin-aldosterone-system (RAAS), hence patients often have elevated plasma renin activity. In fact, some cases of malignant hypertension have been precipitated by the use of diuretics in severe hypertension, causing volume depletion and thus activating the RAAS. Patients with severe volume depletion at presentation may respond to volume loading alone, by reducing plasma renin activity and reversing the "malignant" process. Increased circulating concentrations of endothelin, cortisol, catecholamines and vasopressin have all been detected in malignant hypertension, but their specific pathophysiological roles have not been defined. Severe volume depletion may also result in non-osmotic release of antidiuretic hormone, resulting in pure water retention and hyponatraemia.

Paracrine Factors

Local tissue production of angiotensin II (AII) may be very important in the pathogenesis of malignant hypertension. When angiotensin converting enzyme inhibitors (ACEIs) with high tissue binding were administered to an animal model of malignant hypertension, end-organ damage was prevented. This protective effect was seen despite similar blood pressure recordings in control and treated animals, as non- hypotensive doses were used. This suggested that local AII may play an important role in the end-organ damage that occurs in this condition. Recent work has highlighted the importance of other endothelium-derived vasoactive mediators in the pathogenesis of malignant hypertension. An imbalance in the production of the potent vasodilator nitric oxide, and vasoconstricting peptides such as endothelin, may lead to the characteristic loss of vascular autoregulation seen in this condition.

There is also local activation of the coagulation cascade and platelets, resulting in a vicious cycle of fibrin deposition and tissue ischaemia leading to fibrinoid necrosis. Abnormal circulating concentrations of fibrinogen, factor VIIIc and beta-thromboglobulin have been documented in malignant hypertension. Their importance, however, is questionable as similar levels are also found in essential hypertension, which may suggest that these factors are the result rather than the cause of endothelial damage.

Sympathetic Activation

There is evidence for activation of the sympathetic nervous system in malignant hypertension. Recordings from tibial nerves in patients showed increased activity compared to patients with benign hypertension. This increase in sympathetic tone correlated with activity of the RAAS, as administration of ACEIs resulted in a reduction of RAAS activity and sympathetic outflow. This is consistent with the known phenomenon of AII-mediated facilitation of sympathetic neurotransmission.

A summary of the pathophysiology of malignant hypertension is outlined in **Figure 1**.

Figure 1. Summary of the pathophysiology of malignant hypertension

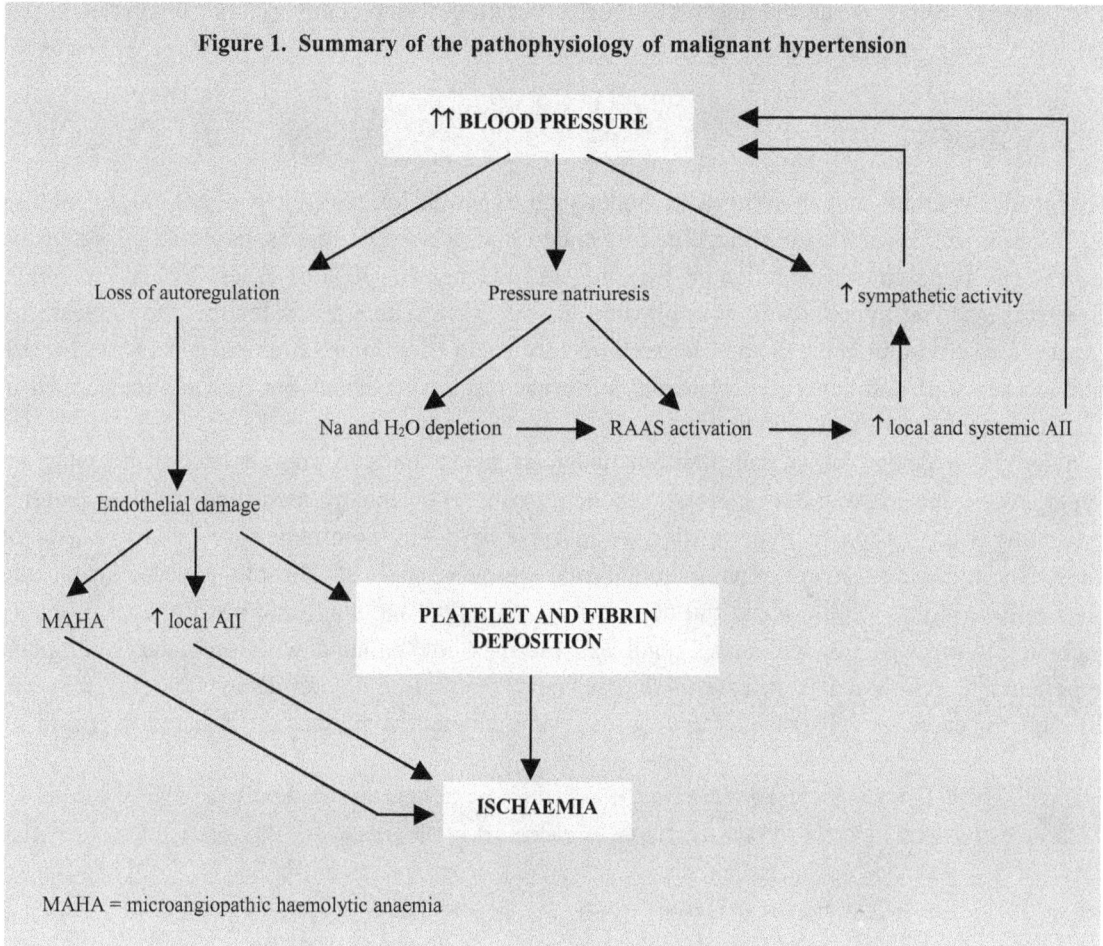

MAHA = microangiopathic haemolytic anaemia

HISTOLOGY

The characteristic histological changes of malignant hypertension are the consequence of endothelial injury. These changes are particularly well demonstrated in the kidney. Macroscopically, the kidneys are usually of normal size, often with cortical and subcapsular haemorrhages and hyperaemia of the medulla. Microscopic abnormalities include proliferative endarteritis of small arteries and arterioles, arteriolar necrosis and mucoid material in small and medium size arteries. Arterioles typically show fibrinoid necrosis with subendothelial lipid deposits and hyaline thrombi (see **Chapter 7**). Interlobular arteries demonstrate intimal fibrin deposition. This occurs in the presence of intimal hyperplasia, with concentric layers of collagen resulting in the characteristic "onion skin" appearance. Fibrinoid necrosis is seen in the vascular pole of the glomerulus. Focal mesangial proliferation and crescent formation are sometimes present. There are frequently signs of glomerular ischaemia such as basement membrane wrinkling and tuft shrinkage. Features of an underlying glomerulonephritis may be evident. Hypertrophy of the juxtaglomerular apparatus with increased renin-secreting granules is seen. Acute tubular necrosis (ATN) occurs commonly, as does chronic tubular atrophy. On immunohistochemistry, fibrin is usually demonstrable in glomeruli, arterioles and small arteries, with non-specific IgM and C3 in the mesangium.

The vascular lesions described are not unique to the kidney, and occur in other organs including the heart, brain, adrenal glands, liver, pancreas and intestine.

AETIOLOGY

Malignant hypertension can complicate underlying hypertension regardless of aetiology, but also occurs *de novo*. Several studies have demonstrated that, in white subjects, essential hypertension is the underlying cause of malignant hypertension in only 20–30% of cases. In black patients, however, essential hypertension is implicated in over 80%. The reasons for this are unclear, but genetic and environmental factors, as well as low socio-economic status have been suggested. The incidence of malignant hypertension is decreasing in Caucasians but remains unchanged in the Black and Indo-Asian populations.

Essential hypertension causing malignant hypertension tends to present later than malignant hypertension due to secondary causes. Secondary causes are mostly identified in white patients presenting with malignant hypertension at an early age. The commonest secondary causes of malignant hypertension are renal parenchymal diseases such as chronic pyelonephritis and glomerulonephritis. Tubulointerstitial nephritis due to reflux and analgesic nephropathy probably account for most of the remaining renal causes. In white patients with secondary malignant hypertension, renovascular disease is increasingly recognised to be responsible for between 20–50% of cases. A full list of known causes of malignant hypertension is listed in **Table 1**.

Table 1. Causes of malignant hypertension

Essential hypertension

Renal parenchymal disease
chronic pyelonephritis
glomerulonephritis
tubulointerstitial nephritis

Systemic diseases
systemic sclerosis
HUS/TTP
diabetes mellitus
SLE
vasculitides
familial homocysteinuria
antiphospholipid syndrome

Renovascular disease
atheroma
fibromuscular hyperplasia
Takayasu's arteritis
acute occlusion
polyarteritis nodosa

Congenital disorders
renal aplasia/dysplasia
polycystic kidney disease

Endocrine
Cushing's syndrome
Conn's syndrome
phaeochromocytoma

Drugs
cocaine
amphetamines
ecstasy
clonidine withdrawal
MAOI interactions
erythropoeitin
cyclosporin
FK 506

Tumour-related
renal cell carcinoma
Wilm's tumour
lymphoma

Coarctation of the aorta

Pre-eclampsia/eclampsia

CLINICAL PRESENTATION

Symptoms

There are no pathognomonic symptoms to suggest a diagnosis of malignant hypertension. Patients may present with non-specific general manifestations such as weakness, weight loss, malaise and fatigue. More specific symptoms and signs are listed in **Table 2**.

Symptom/sign	Comments
Eyes	impaired vision, 35–60% of cases
	grade III or IV hypertensive retinopathy
Blood pressure	although there is no specific threshold for making the diagnosis most patients at presentation have blood pressures >160/100 mmHg
Headaches	60% of cases
Dizziness	30% of cases
Shortness of breath	left ventricular failure, 11% of cases
Chest pain	angina, 4% of cases
	myocardial infarction, 3–4% of cases
Hemiparesis	stroke, 7% of cases
Encephalopathy	fits
Cortical blindness	
Reduced conscious level and confusion	

Table 2. Symptoms and signs associated with malignant hypertension

Complications

Renal

ARF occurs in 30% at presentation. This may be due to intrinsic renal damage as described above or to volume depletion or ischaemia. It is important to recognise that an intrinsic renal lesion may compound renal impairment.

Cardiovascular

Heart failure is the presenting complication in 11% of cases. However underlying left ventricular hypertrophy is present in 75%. Angina and myocardial infarction (MI) may also occur, as may aortic dissection, although these are rarer complications.

Neurological

Hypertensive encephalopathy is now relatively rare but non-specific symptoms such as dizziness and drowsiness are common. Encephalopathy is caused by cerebral oedema due to failure of cerebral autoregulation. Other neurological complications include cerebrovascular accidents, subarachnoid haemorrhage and transient ischaemic attacks. Visual impairment due to hypertensive retinopathy is well described, as is cortical blindness.

Haematological

Anaemia is often present and may reflect the degree of renal impairment. More commonly, there is evidence of a microangiopathic haemolytic anaemia (MAHA).

Miscellaneous

Pancreatitis may occur due to haemorrhagic infarction. Ischaemia of the adrenal cortex may also lead to adrenal insufficiency.

INVESTIGATIONS

Important investigations to be performed in the patient with malignant hypertension are given in **Table 3**.

Table 3. Investigations in malignant hypertension

Urine	
Dipstick	blood, protein
Microscopy	red cells, granular casts
Chemistry	proteinuria, occasionally nephrotic range, impaired creatinine clearance
Blood	
Urea and creatinine	↑2° to ARF or acute on chronic renal failure
pH	↑2° to activation of RAS and hence hypokalaemic alkalosis or ↓2° to ARF
K$^+$	↓2° to activation of RAS or ↑2° to ARF
Na$^+$	may be ↓ due to non-osmotic activation of ADH secretion 2° to volume depletion
Haematology	features of MAHA may be present, i.e. ↓Hb, ↓plt, ↑presence of red cell fragments, ↓haptoglobins
	anaemia 2° to renal impairment or MAHA
	↑ESR
ECG	LVH, ischaemia, MI
ECHO	LVH, aortic dissection
Renal biopsy	features as described above

TREATMENT PRINCIPLES

The ideal rate of blood pressure reduction is determined by the complications at presentation. Under most circumstances a gradual reduction in blood pressure to ~160/100 mmHg over 24–36 hours is required in order to minimise the chance of ischaemic complications such as cerebral infarction or worsening of renal failure. Should the patient present with hypertensive encephalopathy, severe hypertensive heart failure or aortic dissection, a more rapid blood pressure reduction is required.

- *Hypertensive encephalopathy*

Rapid reduction in blood pressure to ~160/100 mmHg over 3–4 hours. IV therapy may be required as patients' conscious level may be impaired.

- *Hypertensive heart failure*

Rapid reduction with the use of vasodilators IV over 3–4 hours.

- *Aortic dissection*

Rapid reduction of blood pressure to prevent extension of dissection. β-blockers are particularly useful (e.g. esmolol).

- *Acute renal failure*

Gradual reduction in blood pressure. There is often a decline in renal function initially but this is usually temporary.

- *Eye disease*

Gradual reduction in blood pressure.

Drugs

Oral therapy should be used where possible as it results in a gradual and steady fall in blood pressure. IV therapy should only be used when rapid reduction in blood pressure is required (see above). For details of drugs see **Table 4** and **Appendix A**.

Supportive Measures

Volume depletion if severe should be treated with normal saline. If renal failure is severe, dialysis may be required. Fluid removal should be carried out cautiously as this may result in a rapid fall in blood pressure.

OUTCOME

It was initially thought that patients presenting with grade IV retinopathy had a poorer prognosis than those with grade III. More recent data, however, do not support this and suggest similar outcomes. In early studies, before ready access to dialysis and effective antihypertensive therapy

Table 4. Drugs used in the treatment of malignant hypertension

Drug	Route of administration/dose	Comments
Labetalol	**IV** 2 mg/min until satisfactory response; usual total dose 50–200 mg **Oral** 100 mg b.d. (Max. of 2.4 g/day)	1st line intravenous therapy as it can be administered on the ward and dose titrated according to blood pressure. Patients can then be transferred onto oral labetalol. Safe in pregnancy so can be used in eclampsia (see **Chapter 27**)
Esmolol	**IV** 50–200 µg/kg/min	Particularly useful for aortic dissection. Very short half-life (2 min). No dose adjustment in renal failure. For immediate BP control can give initial 80 mg bolus (~1 mg/kg) over 1 min
Nitrates (GTN)	**IV** 10–200 µg/min	IV GTN is useful in the treatment of severe heart failure and can be administered on the ward
Sodium nitroprusside	**IV** Start 0.3–1.5 µg/kg/min (↑ by 0.5 µg/kg/min every 5 min until satisfactory response) Range 0.3–8 µg/kg/min	Potent vasodilator. Requires intensive blood pressure monitoring on ITU. Cyanide toxicity not usually a problem if used for less than 72 hours
Hydralazine	**IV** Start 200–300 µg/min Maintenance dose 50–150 µg/min	
	ORAL THERAPY	
Calcium channel blockers	Start with nifedipine (modified release) 10 mg **oral** 12 hourly; Max. 40 mg 12 hourly	Oral nifedipine in small doses is often used as first line therapy. Doses are then gradually increased. Safe in pregnancy. Nimodipine is the drug of choice if malignant hypertension complicated by subarachnoid haemorrhage Immediate release capsules and sublingual nifedipine NOT recommended
ACE inhibitors	Start at small doses and increase as required. Those with high tissue binding have theoretical benefits e.g. Quinapril, Ramipril	Very effective drugs and in scleroderma crisis are 1st line therapy. For other causes of malignant hypertension ACEIs probably should not be used on admission as volume depletion may be present. Also, underlying renal artery disease should be excluded first
Oral β blockers	Start with atenolol 50 mg	Not usually used 1st line but useful additional oral therapy

Table 4 (*Continued*)

Drug	Route of administration/dose	Comments
Diuretics	Depends on degree of renal failure	Should be used with extreme caution as can cause deterioration in condition. However useful if severe fluid overload or as an adjunct to other oral therapy
Minoxidil	5 mg o.d. increasing to 50 mg	Useful additional agent but not used 1st line. Causes fluid retention therefore requires coadministration of diuretics
Doxazosin	2 mg b.d. increasing to 16 mg/day	Useful 2nd line agent

were available, survival with malignant hypertension was 10–20% at 1 year. Renal failure was the cause of death in 60–70% of cases. Now the outlook is much improved with 5 year survival of around 70%.

A peculiar feature of the renal failure that occurs as a result of malignant hypertension is the late recovery of renal function. A series by Yaqoob *et al.* demonstrated that patients requiring dialysis may recover independent renal function up to a year later. Despite late recovery, the renal function of patients with underlying renal disease was more likely to deteriorate eventually.

Kidney survival depends on the degree of renal impairment at presentation. In one study, 90% of patients with serum creatinine <300 μmol/L remained dialysis free whereas 90% of those with serum creatinine >300 μmol/L progressed to end stage renal failure. The underlying disease process also affects the prognosis. Patients with malignant hypertension due to essential hypertension have a better prognosis than those with a primary renal disease.

FURTHER READING

Kincaid-Smith P, McMichael J, Murphy EA (1958) The clinical course and pathology of hypertension with papilloedema (malignant hypertension). *Quarterly Journal of Medicine*; 37: 117–153

Kitiyakara C, Guzman NJ (1998) Malignant hypertension and hypertensive emergencies. *Journal of the American Society of Nephrology*; 9: 133–142

McGregor E, Isles CG, Jay JL, et al. (1986) Retinal changes in malignant hypertension. *British Medical Journal*; 292: 233–234

Montgomery HE, Kiernan LA, Whitworth CE, et al. (1998) Inhibition of tissue angiotensin converting enzyme activity prevents malignant hypertension in TGR(mREN2)27. *Journal of Hypertension*; 16: 635

Raine AEG, Ritz E (1998) Accelerated hypertension. In: Davidson AM, Cameron JS, Grunfeld, J-P, et al. (eds.). *Oxford Textbook of Clinical Nephrology* (2nd Edition). Oxford: Oxford University Press; 1488–1503

Yaqoob M, McClelland P, Ahmad R (1991) Delayed recovery of renal function in patients with ARF due to accelerated hypertension. *Postgraduate Medical Journal*; 67: 829–832

Chapter 15 _____

HAEMOLYTIC URAEMIC SYNDROME AND THROMBOTIC THROMBOCYTOPAENIC PURPURA

Alan Salama

DEFINITION

Thrombotic Thrombocytopaenic Purpura (TTP) and Haemolytic Uraemic Syndrome (HUS) are examples of thrombotic microangiopathies — vasculopathies in which tissue injury is secondary to microvascular occlusion and ischaemia.

TTP was first described in 1924 by Moschowitz in a sixteen year old girl with fever, purpura, anaemia, paralysis and coma. Her post mortem examination revealed arteriolar and capillary thrombi, consisting predominantly of platelets. Subsequently, Symmers and others described the histopathological features of the condition as thrombotic microangiopathy (TMA). The term Haemolytic Uraemic Syndrome was first coined by Gasser in 1955, reporting on a group of children with haemolytic anaemia, thrombocytopaenia, renal cortical necrosis and ARF. He differentiated it from TTP on the basis of the severe and isolated renal disease. Habib later described the histologic features in this condition and noted their similarity to those found in TTP.

As noted, there is extensive overlap between these syndromes which are now often considered as one, HUS/TTP, the clinical features being dictated by the affected vascular beds. The histological feature which is common to both, thrombotic microangiopathy, also occurs in a number of other vasculopathies (see under differential diagnosis). Due to the similarities in pathology it has been proposed that the terms HUS and TTP be replaced by TMA, then further classified based on the aetiological agent, e.g. TMA secondary to verotoxin. This classification however has not yet gained widespread usage. In some cases, HUS is used to refer to children with diarrhoea related disease and TTP to adults with relapsing disease. Confusion over nomenclature has made investigation of pathogenesis and trials of treatment difficult.

In HUS, there is a triad of microangiopathic haemolytic anaemia, renal impairment and thrombocytopaenia. It occurs in two forms, the "typical" form, associated with bloody diarrhoea (D+), which is a common cause of acute renal failure (ARF) in children. The second form is not associated with diarrhoea (D−) and is termed "atypical", occurring more in adults, with a much poorer prognosis and resembling the clinical course of TTP more closely. TTP consists of a pentad of central nervous system disorders, thrombocytopaenia, renal impairment, fever, and microangiopathic haemolytic anaemia. Examples of overlapping features are the occurrence of neurological symptoms in HUS, the absence of a diarrhoeal prodrome in some cases of typical

HUS and the occurrence of TTP following haemorrhagic colitis. It is still useful to differentiate typical (D+) HUS from the others, because of prognostic and therapeutic implications.

PATHOPHYSIOLOGY

The underlying abnormality in all cases of HUS/TTP is widespread microvascular thrombosis consisting of a platelet-rich thrombus. Depending on the endothelial bed affected, differing end organ damage results with varied clinical features. Platelet thrombus production is caused by a breakdown in the natural anticoagulant mechanisms which normally operate. This is thought to be due to primary endothelial cell (EC) injury, with loss of its anticoagulant surface, and/or due to a pro-coagulant platelet aggregating factor(s). There is evidence from patients that both of these abnormalities occur; however the exact mechanism by which the disease is initiated remains to be elucidated.

Aggregation of platelets within the thrombus leads to their continual consumption with resultant thrombocytopaenia. Passage of red cells through obstructed microvasculature, and oxidant injury to the cells, is responsible for the microangiopathic haemolysis.

Endothelial Cells and Coagulation

Resting, unactivated endothelial cells (EC) provide an effective anticoagulant surface allowing the free passage of blood over them. They employ a number of mechanisms to achieve this:

- Inhibiting the coagulation pathway
- Inducing fibrinolysis
- Preventing platelet aggregation

The production of heparan sulphate, catalysing the anti-thrombin III pathway, and thrombomodulin, catalysing the activated protein C pathway, effectively inhibit the coagulation cascade. Release of plasminogen activators (t-PA and u-PA) allow fibrinolysis to occur. The production of prostacyclin (PGI$_2$) and the conversion of adenosine diphosphate to adenosine serve to inhibit platelet aggregation.

Following activation or damage, EC change from an anti-coagulant to a pro-coagulant surface. Expression of tissue factor, which binds factor VIIa and initiates the extrinsic clotting pathway, and loss of thrombomodulin and heparan sulphate from the EC surface serve to promote coagulation. Reduced plasminogen activators and increased production of the plasminogen activator inhibitors I and II shift the balance to promote fibrin deposition. Platelet aggregation is achieved by release of von Willebrand factor (vWF), normally stored in EC Weibel-Palade bodies (along with P-selectin), which binds platelet glycoprotein Ib as well as IIb/IIIa complexes, in the presence of calcium and ADP. Von Willebrand factor also serves to promote factor VIII activation by thrombin. Furthermore, reduced production of PGI$_2$ and nitric oxide by the EC encourages platelet aggregation. There is therefore a critical balance between preventing and promoting thrombosis, and any injurious event to EC can tip the balance in favour of thrombus formation at the site of damage.

Endothelial Cell Damage

A number of different aetiological agents associated with HUS/TTP can injure EC and may therefore play a role in initiating disease. Damage to particular vascular beds explains the predominant clinical manifestations of the syndromes.

The verocytotoxin (VT) of *E. coli* and *Shigella* species, causative agents of the D+ HUS, is toxic to EC and some epithelial cells. It is made up of two subunits. The A subunit which is biologically active, inhibits intracellular protein synthesis leading to cell death and the B subunit binds disaccharides found in globotriosyl ceramide (Gb3), a surface receptor on some endothelial cells. The distribution and density of these VT receptors dictate which vascular bed is involved in disease. VT receptors are found in the kidney, within the glomeruli of children but not adults, the brain and colon. Lipopolysaccharide appears to enhance the cytotoxic effect of verotoxin, in part by upregulating the Gb3 receptors, as do certain cytokines (IL-1 and TNFα).

Even in cases of HUS/TTP not caused by VT, certain EC seem more susceptible to damage than others. Plasma from patients with HUS/TTP induces apoptosis in EC from cerebral, renal and dermal microvasculature, but not from pulmonary or hepatic beds. This is paralleled by an upregulation of the pro-apoptotic molecule Fas. It has become apparent that there are many differences in behaviour and expression of key molecules on EC from different vascular beds; however which molecules determine the susceptibility to damage and apoptosis have not yet been elucidated. Interestingly, the increased apoptosis did not occur when using sera from patients with D+ HUS, possibly explaining some of the differences between the two syndromes.

Certain drugs are directly toxic to EC, such as mitomycin C and cyclosporin. Other cancer chemotherapy agents have been associated with the development of anti-EC antibodies; these antibodies may bind to EC, leading to cell activation and rendering the EC pro-coagulant and susceptible to apoptosis. In some cases, these antibodies may be capable of fixing complement and inducing EC lysis. Some antibodies only bind and activate EC in the presence of certain cofactors, as is the case in quinine induced HUS. Anti-EC antibodies are also present in certain autoimmune diseases, e.g. SLE and PAN.

A number of the anticoagulant properties of the EC have been reported to be affected in HUS/TTP. PGI_2 can be found in diminished levels in blood and its metabolites in urine are also diminished during acute disease, returning to normal in remission. There has been a suggestion that a PGI_2 stimulating factor is missing in patients, and can be corrected by the therapeutic use of antioxidants such as vitamin E. Unusually large Von Willebrand factor multimers (UL-vWFm), which are normally stored within EC Weibel-Palade bodies, are found in the circulation suggesting EC damage. They are also found within the microthrombi in patients with HUS/TTP. A number of different changes in the levels of UL-vWFm have been reported, with differing explanations. Levels were found to be raised in acute disease and returned to normal in remission, possibly reflecting the degree of EC damage. Similarly, levels of P-selectin were raised in patients' serum compared to controls. In other studies, levels of UL-vWF were found to be lower in disease and returned to normal in remission, possibly due to its binding of activated platelets in acute disease, causing its consumption. It is apparent that collection artefacts may explain some of the vagaries in vWF measurement, since vWF may be broken down *in vitro* by proteases. *In vivo* differences in the fragmentation of vWF may also occur in disease, with a decrease in the 225 kDa subunit and a relative increase in a 176 kDa fragment. The latter may be a more potent platelet aggregator. These changes normalise in remission.

Platelet Aggregators

Normal platelets may aggregate in the presence of serum from HUS/TTP patients, suggesting that an endogenous aggregator is present. It has been proposed that this may be UL-vWF multimers, which bind platelets and cause their aggregation. These are normally degraded in the circulation by proteases, but may escape this degradation if the appropriate protease is lacking in disease. Cryosupernatant (the plasma fraction left after removal of cryoprecipitate) retains the ability to degrade UL-vWf multimers to the size of those found in normal plasma. Low levels of a vWF-cleaving protease were found in some patients with TTP during acute disease, which normalised in remission. An inhibitory factor was found in the sera from non-familial cases but not from familial ones. This was identified as an IgG molecule. The conclusion from these studies was that inherited deficiencies of a vWF-cleaving protease would explain the familial syndromes whereas an acquired autoimmune process could lead to production of a protease inhibitor.

Alteration in autoantibody production may explain the relapsing-remitting form of the syndrome. Further support for these theories comes from the response to treatment with plasma infusions, containing normal levels of the proteases, as well as plasmapheresis and splenectomy allowing removal of the autoantibody. Interestingly the use of immunosuppressants (steroids and azathioprine) has been associated with the loss of UL-vWf multimers from the circulation. No explanation as to why temporary aberrations of the immune system should occur and why temporary treatments should have long-lasting effects on the disease, have been made. These abnormalities were only found in patients with clinical TTP and not HUS, suggesting a possible pathophysiological difference between the syndromes.

Alternative suggestions for the platelet aggregator is plasminogen-activator type 1, found at higher levels in children with D+ HUS, or a cystine protease called calpain. This is a cytosolic protease whose normal function is to hydrolyse cytoplasmic proteins, including vWF.

There is evidence for each of these mechanisms occurring in certain patients. It may be that one or more abnormalities can lead to the common final pathway resulting in platelet microthrombi. The heterogeneity in aetiology would suggest that this may be the case.

Neutrophils and Oxygen Free Radicals

There is evidence for neutrophil activation with production of oxygen free radicals and lipid peroxidation, which is injurious to EC. Neutrophils from patients damage EC *in vitro*, verotoxin increases neutrophil adhesion to EC and a high neutrophil count is a predictor of poor outcome in patients.

Vitamin E levels have been found to be reduced in patients and in animal models of HUS, in association with increased lipid peroxidation and reduced PGI_2 levels. Furthermore there is some evidence in children with HUS that therapy with vitamin E may be beneficial.

Complement Regulatory Proteins

Reduced levels of the complement component C3 have been described in both familial and sporadic HUS/TTP. In the sporadic forms it reflects consumption of C3 in the microvasculature during acute disease. Release of complement cleavage products such as C3a and C5a could further contribute to the pathogenesis by allowing neutrophil recruitment and activation, or direct EC damage through the membrane attack complex (C5-9). A number of studies have found genetic deficiencies in factor H, a regulatory protein of the alternative pathway of complement, which leads to low C3 levels. Further analysis of some families with HUS/TTP has shown linkage with a region of chromosome 1 in which factor H (as well as other complement regulatory proteins) resides. Mutations in the factor H gene have also been described although correlation with altered protein activity was not shown. There is therefore a possible role for complement C3 and factor H in familial and relapsing HUS/TTP, which requires further investigation. This also raises the possibility that there is some genetic predisposition to developing HUS following exposure to an environmental agent, such as verotoxin. Recent multivariate analysis has shown that low C3 levels are strongly associated with development of HUS/TTP, and factor H abnormalities are correlated with low C3 levels in patients. Factor H deficiency may allow uncontrolled complement deposition in vessels, which is normally regulated by its inhibition of the C3bBb convertase.

Other Genetic Factors

An increased prevalence of HLA B40 has been reported in a series of children with HUS. This may be in linkage disequilibrium with other susceptibility genes, which have not yet been identified.

CLINICAL PRESENTATION AND INVESTIGATIONS

Patients with HUS/TTP present with microangiopathic haemolytic anaemia, renal failure and thrombocytopaenia. Fever and neurological features such as seizures, focal signs and altered levels of consciousness may also occur. Symptoms and signs relating to uraemia, and bleeding secondary to the thrombocytopaenia dominate the picture. In addition, gastrointestinal symptoms prevail in the D+ form. Hypertension is common.

Haemoglobin in the range of 8–10 g/dL is typical, with evidence of haemolysis, increased bilirubin and LDH, and reduced haptoglobins. Blood films show fragmented red cells, burr and helmet cells. Platelet counts of $30–100 \times 10^9$/L are usual with reduced platelet survival time. Elevated white cell counts ($>20 \times 10^9$/L) are predictors of poorer outcome in D+ HUS. Levels of the complement component C3 are reduced in a third of the patients (see **Table 1**).Urinalysis generally reveals proteinuria, in the non-nephrotic range (1–2 g/day), as well as red cells, but rarely red cell casts.

D+ HUS/TTP

- Occurs in epidemics
- Has a seasonal incidence, higher in summer months
- Typically affects females more than males

Reported cases of the disease in children have increased over recent years. Most patients have a prodromal gastrointestinal illness with bloody diarrhoea leading to their presentation, or they

Table 1. Investigations in HUS/TTP

Haematology	Biochemistry
⇩ haemoglobin	⇧ LDH
⇩ platelets	⇧ bilirubin
⇧ or ⇨ neutrophils	⇩ haptoglobins
normal clotting times	⇧ urea/creatinine
normal fibrinogen and FDP's	⇩ sodium
Coomb's test negative*	⇧ urate
⇧ reticulocytes	

Blood film
- red cell fragments
- burr cells
- helmet cells

*Except in association with pneumococcal disease.

may present later with renal symptoms (oedema, oligo-or poly-uria), hypertension, cardiac symptoms, or neurological dysfunction. Convulsions, irritability, and restlessness are frequent neurological features, as a result of cerebral microangiopathy and hyponatraemia. Young children are commonly affected, with mean peak incidence between 1 and 2 years. Epidemic outbreaks in adults, especially affecting the elderly, have also been reported, and traced to food products such as contaminated meats and apple cider.

Renal failure requiring dialysis occurs in about half the patients, but recovery is the general rule (see **Outcome**).

In over half the cases VT-producing *E. coli*, generally of the 0157:H7 serotype, can be isolated in the stool. Anti-VT antibodies may be found and VT can be isolated in faecal filtrates. Other *E. coli* serotypes, as well as *Shigella dysenteriae* type 1, can also produce disease. Only 10–30% of children with *E. coli* 0157H diarrhoea will develop D+ HUS, suggesting that other susceptibility factors, environmental or inherited, are required.

D− HUS/TTP

- Has no seasonal incidence
- Accounts for about 10% of all cases
- Generally exhibits no gastrointestinal prodrome, although upper respiratory tract infections may precede presentation

Clinical features for D− disease are as for the D+ form, except proteinuria which may be in the nephrotic range and hypertension which is generally more severe. The disease may have a remitting-relapsing nature and familial cases are well recognised with autosomal recessive or dominant inheritance (see above).

Aetiological factors for HUS/TTP are shown in **Table 2**.

Table 2. Aetiology of HUS/TTP

Agent/insult	Explanation
Infectious agents	
Escherichia coli O157:H7 *Shigella dysenteriae*	Verocytotoxin (VT) induced direct EC damage, with inhibition of cellular protein synthesis. VT receptor distribution determines the vascular beds affected.
Streptococcus pneumoniae	Neuraminidase producing organisms cleave sialic acid from surface of EC, erythrocytes and platelets, exposing Thomsen-Friedenreich antigen. Binding of IgM to this antigen induces platelet and erythrocyte agglutination. Associated with positive Coombs test.
HIV, CMV/HSV	AIDS defining illness often present. Certain viral tropism for EC.
Drugs	
Mitomycin	*In vitro* drug induced reduction of PGI_2 levels in human umbilical vein endothelial cell cultures. Risk increases with cumulative drug dose >60 mg.
Vincristine	Used in regimens to treat refractory cases of HUS/TTP. Presumed to act by inhibition of platelet aggregation. Mechanism of disease induction unknown.
Cisplatin	Increased plasma levels of vWF found on treatment.
5 Flurouracil	Implicated because frequently used with mitomycin. Little direct evidence.
Tamoxifen	Possible interaction with other anti-cancer drugs. Mechanism unknown.
Quinine	Quinine dependent antibodies react with glycoproteins on EC, platelets, leucocytes and erythrocytes, inducing platelet aggregation, neutrophil and EC activation.
Ticlopidine	Suggestion that drug or its metabolites may induce or act as an inhibitor of vWF-cleaving protease.
Cyclosporin A	Direct toxic effect of CsA on EC; reduced PGI_2 and endothelin levels. Improves on drug withdrawal and plasma exchange.
Oral contraceptive pill (oestrogen containing)	Reports of disease in patients with familial HUS/TTP.
Hereditary	
Familial HUS/TTP	Diminished C3 levels and associated abnormalities in factor H found in some families. Complete factor H deficiency in some, and mutations in factor H gene in others. Linkage to chromosome 1q32, in HUS. Diminished levels of UL-vWF multimer cleaving protease in familial TTP.
Others	
Bone marrow transplantation	EC damage caused by radiation or cytotoxic drug induction regimens, or cyclosporin.
Pregnancy	HUS generally occurs postpartum. TTP occurs during the first two trimesters and in the early post-partum period, differentiating it from pre-eclampsia and HELLP. The procoagulant state of pregnancy may provoke disease.

Table 2 (*Continued*)	
Agent/insult	**Explanation**
Others	
Malignancy (adenocarcinoma of GI tract, pancreas and prostate, squamous carcinomas, thymomas and lymphomas)	Increased levels of immune complexes and decreased complement components in patients, which normalise following immunoadsorption.
Accelerated hypertension	Multiple endothelial alterations, including increased vasoconstrictors, adhesion molecule expression, reduced prostacyclin and increased oxygen free radical production.

HUS/TTP may be associated with pregnancy, in the context of pre-eclampsia, the HELLP syndrome (see also **Chapter 27**), acute fatty liver of pregnancy and up to three months post-partum. This may explain the female predominance. Differentiating these pregnancy related conditions can be difficult, the best clues coming from their timing during gestation. TTP occurs within the first 24 weeks, but can occur up to three months post-partum, when the syndrome of HUS is commoner. Pre-eclampsia and the HELLP syndrome occur in the third trimester and unlike HUS/TTP improve rapidly after foetal delivery. Pregnancy or oral contraceptives may provoke disease in familial cases of HUS/TTP, possibly due to the generalised pro-coagulant state induced. Interestingly, although cyclosporin is known to cause disease, some reports of benefit from using cyclosporin as treatment in refractory cases have also been made. Similarly, the antiplatelet agent ticlopidine, which acts by inhibiting ADP binding to platelets, has been implicated in causing HUS/TTP.

Recently an increasing number of cases have been reported in association with HIV infection (see also **Chapter 20**). Renal failure is less common in HIV associated disease, and patients generally present with haematological abnormalities and neurological dysfunction. Most have co-existing AIDS defining illnesses.

Many cases are associated with cancer or cancer chemotherapy. It is not always easy to differentiate whether the underlying tumour or its treatment is responsible. In cases of HUS/TTP where patients are being treated for cancer and true tumour remission exists, the chemotherapy may be held responsible.

Differential diagnosis of HUS/TTP is detailed in **Tables 3** and **4**.

Histology

There are differences in the biopsy findings between younger children (<2 years) with predominant D+ disease, and older children and adults. In the former group, the glomeruli are mainly involved, with thickening of the glomerular capillary wall, EC swelling, narrowing or occlusion of the capillary lumina and widening of the subendothelial space. This may be filled with electron dense material, producing a double contour or tram track appearance. Arteriolar damage is rare. By

Table 3. Other causes of thrombotic microangiopathy

Condition	Associated features
Scleroderma	Serology, clinical features
Malignant hypertension	HTN, retinopathy
Pre-eclampsia	Proteinuria in last trimester, HTN, clotting abnormalities
HELLP syndrome	⇧ liver enzymes, pre-eclampsia, clotting abnormalities
Renal vascular rejection	Anti-donor antibodies, graft dysfunction
Primary antiphospholipid syndrome	Serology, clinical features

HTN = hypertension.

Table 4. Causes of renal failure in association with thrombocytopaenia and haemolytic anaemia

Condition	Associated features
SLE	Serology, clinical features
Acute bacterial endocarditis	Blood cultures, clinical features
DIC	Coagulopathy, ⇩ fibrinogen, rash
PNH	Haematuria, cryoglobulins

PNH = Paroxysmal Nocturnal Haemoglobinuria; DIC = Disseminated intravascular coagulation.

contrast, the latter group has a more heterogeneous appearance on biopsy with ischaemic glomerular changes, arteriolar and arterial involvement with intimal swelling, proliferation and necrosis of the vessel wall. Microaneurysms may also occur. Mesangial matrix oedema and reticulation can occur (termed mesangiolysis) (see **Chapter 7**).

TREATMENT PRINCIPLES

Due to the rarity of these conditions, their heterogeneity and difficulties with classification, few prospective clinical trials have been carried out. Anecdotal reports and retrospective analyses of treatment strategies are numerous.

D+ HUS/TTP

Supportive therapy with transfusion and renal replacement is the mainstay of management. Aggressive treatment of hypertension is required. Prophylactic anti-epileptics in cases with neurological irritability may be useful. Anti-motility agents can aggravate the condition by increasing exposure of the gut mucosa to verotoxin. Antibiotics are not of benefit (possibly with the exception of fluoroquinolones) and have been shown to increase release of verotoxin from the verotoxin producing bacteria *in vitro*. There are reports that the outcome of patients treated with antibiotics, following certain epidemics, was worse than those without treatment. Very recent convincing prospective cohort data also supports the contention that antibiotics are contra-indicated in D+ HUS/TTP. Antibiotic treatment of children with *E. coli* O157:H7 infection has recently been shown to increase the risk of developing HUS (Wong *et al.*, 2000). There is no benefit from anti-coagulant or thrombolytic therapy; nor from intravenous prostacyclin, steroids or gammaglobulin. Use of plasma infusions may reduce the incidence of cortical necrosis in follow up biopsies, but have not been shown to alter long term renal function. Plasma exchange may be used in patients who fail with supportive treatment but there is little evidence to support any benefit. Some benefit from vitamin E was reported in one uncontrolled trial.

D− HUS/TTP

Changes in management have reduced the appalling mortality of this condition from 90% to about 10%. The introduction of plasma exchange and plasma infusion has mainly been responsible and remains the mainstay of treatment. Since infusion of plasma provides therapeutic benefit, and plasma exchange with albumin or saline is not beneficial, it was concluded that replacement of a missing substance found in plasma was the mode of action. Prompt initiation of therapy is required since delay increases the risk of treatment failure. Prospective comparison of plasma infusion and exchange in TTP found plasma exchange to be superior, with more rapid haematological improvement and better patient survival. However the plasma exchange allowed greater quantities of plasma to be infused. Other studies in which equal volumes of plasma were used showed equal benefit of the two treatments.

Patients should undergo exchanges of between 1 and 1.5 times their plasma volume (40–80 mL/kg) with fresh-frozen plasma (FFP) using citrate anticoagulation, or plasma infusion with FFP at the maximally tolerated dose, dictated by fluid status, until clinical/haematological improvement occurs. Solvent detergent treated plasma (used to inactivate viral particles) is still effective. Albumin, however, should not be used for exchange. Sensitivity reactions to plasma may be treated with steroids, antihistamines and ephedrine.

Patients with severe disease, or those who fail to respond to treatment with plasma exchange, may benefit from increased doses of FFP (80 mL/kg) or substitution of FFP with cryosupernatant. This may be related to its ability to degrade the UL-vWF multimers more effectively (see Pathophysiology section). Refractory disease has also been treated with combinations of steroids, azathioprine, vincristine, splenectomy or gammaglobulin, all with varying levels of success. In milder forms of HUS/TTP (without neurological or renal features) treatment with high dose steroids (200 mg prednisolone/day, with rapid reduction to 60 mg on remission induction) was sufficient, and it is reasonable to include steroids in a therapeutic regimen in all cases lacking contraindications. Aspirin and dipyridamole, used as adjunctive measures, do not seem to be of benefit. Prostacyclin has not been shown to help in trial settings, but there are some anecdotes of benefit. To date there are no reports of the use of monoclonal antibodies directed against glycoprotein IIb/IIIa being used in patients with HUS/TTP, although they are beneficial in experimental models. A recent early report of the use of retinoic acid in relapsing TTP was hopeful, and further trials are needed. Retinoic acid abrogates pro-coagulant factors on endothelial cells and promotes fibrinolytic and anticoagulant factors.

Platelet infusions are contraindicated unless life threatening haemorrhage occurs, because of reports of clinical deterioration following platelet transfusions. This is thought to be due to promotion of further microvascular thrombosis.

An algorithm for the management of HUS/TTP is given in the **Practice Point** at the end of this chapter.

Special Treatment Cases

In HIV associated TMA there is a role for anti-retroviral therapy, in view of the evidence for HIV mediated EC damage. No systematic study has been undertaken, but there is an example of a patient with relapsing disease who responded to treatment with AZT. Conventional treatment with plasma exchange has been shown to be effective in HIV associated TMA.

In cancer associated HUS/TTP, as well as other refractory cases, immunoadsorption using a protein A column has been helpful.

Pregnancy associated HUS/TTP, unlike pre-eclampsia or HELLP, does not seem to improve following delivery of the foetus.

In pneumococcal disease, plasma should be avoided since it may contain IgM antibodies against the Thomsen-Friedenreich antigen, inducing further intravascular agglutination and thrombosis.

OUTCOME

Familial cases of HUS/TTP, whether related to verotoxin or not, are associated with a poorer outcome than sporadic disease and respond less well to plasma therapy.

D+ HUS/TTP

The mortality rate is low at 0–8%. The condition generally resolves within 1–2 weeks and has a lower incidence of chronic sequelae, with up to 30% suffering from proteinuria, hypertension or renal impairment. Relapse is uncommon. Up to 16% of patients reach end stage renal failure and require renal replacement therapy.

D– HUS/TTP

Is associated with a significantly higher mortality rate and a high incidence of chronic sequelae. With treatment, mortality is now of the order of 5–10%. Recovery of the haematological features occurs first, with renal recovery generally being slower. Up to 50% of patients may have chronic renal failure. Relapse is reported in TTP in approximately 10–70% of patients in different series. It generally occurs within one to four weeks, although it may be as late as five years. There are no good predictors of relapse. In pregnancy related HUS/TTP, the prognosis is generally poor with mortality rates approaching 50%. In the survivors, approximately 12% required renal replacement therapy. No cases of foetal involvement have been reported in HUS/TTP, suggesting that the factor responsible does not cross the placenta. Foetal survival is generally poor in TTP as a result of placental infarction. Recurrence is rare in HUS, but commoner in pregnant patients with a history of TTP. The outcome in pregnant patients with familial disease is uncertain.

Table 5. Poor prognostic indicators in sporadic HUS/TTP	
D+ HUS	**D− HUS**
Neutrophilia $>20 \times 10^9/mm^3$	Failure to respond to initial plasmapheresis treatment
Age >3 years at presentation	Haemoglobin <6 g/L at presentation
Anuria >8 days or oliguria >15 days	Preglomerular arteriolar lesions on biopsy
Glomerular microangiopathy with >50% glomeruli affected, arterial microangiopathy or cortical necrosis	

TRANSPLANTATION

D+ HUS/TTP

Recurrence of HUS in the allograft is rare. Graft outcome is improved if an interval of about a year is allowed prior to transplantation. Cyclosporin is often withheld in this group. However, there is little evidence that this is necessary.

D− HUS/TTP

Recurrence following renal transplantation in those patients reaching end stage is well described and complicated by the use of cyclosporin and FK506. In some series up to 46% of patients experience recurrence in their allografts. This generally manifests within two months of transplantation, although late recurrences also occur. Risk factors for recurrence include older age, shorter time between disease and transplantation, hereditary form of HUS/TTP and live related donation. Reports of recurrence following treatment with anti-lymphocyte globulin (ALG) and OKT3 have also been made. Graft outcome is worse in patients with HUS/TTP compared to other causes of renal disease. In the event of recurrence in the graft, cyclosporin should be reduced or stopped altogether and plasma exchange instituted. FK506 may subsequently be used without adverse effect. *De novo* HUS-TTP in a transplant is rare.

FURTHER READING

Brandt JR, Avner ED (1996) Haemolytic uraemic syndrome and thrombotic thrombocytopaenic purpura. In: Neilson EG and Couser WG (eds.). *Immunologic Renal Diseases Lippincott-Raven*; pp. 1161–1179

Moake JL (1997) Studies on the pathophysiology of thrombotic thrombocytopaenic purpura. *Seminars in Haematology*; 34: 83–89

Remuzzi G, Ruggeneti P (1995) The haemolytic uraemic syndrome. *Kidney International*; 47: 2–19

Wong CS, Jelaic S, Habeeb RL (2000) The risk of the hemolytic uremic syndrome after antibiotic treatment of *Escherichia coli* O157:H7 infections. *The New England Journal of Medicine*; 342: 1930–1936

Practice Point. Treatment of HUS/TTP

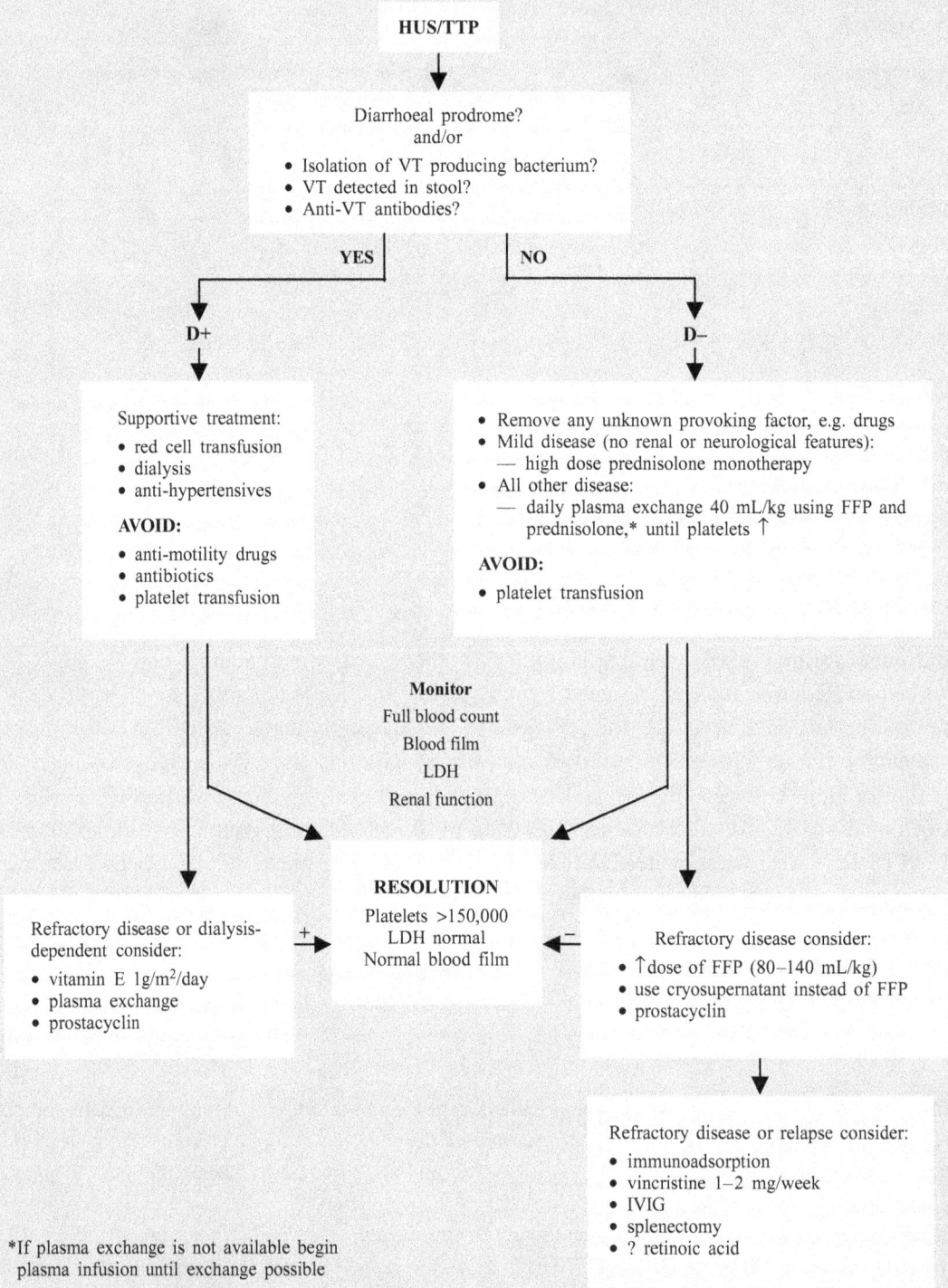

HUS/TTP

↓

Diarrhoeal prodrome?
and/or
- Isolation of VT producing bacterium?
- VT detected in stool?
- Anti-VT antibodies?

YES   **NO**

D+   **D–**

Supportive treatment:
- red cell transfusion
- dialysis
- anti-hypertensives

AVOID:
- anti-motility drugs
- antibiotics
- platelet transfusion

- Remove any unknown provoking factor, e.g. drugs
- Mild disease (no renal or neurological features):
  — high dose prednisolone monotherapy
- All other disease:
  — daily plasma exchange 40 mL/kg using FFP and prednisolone,* until platelets ↑

AVOID:
- platelet transfusion

Monitor
Full blood count
Blood film
LDH
Renal function

RESOLUTION
Platelets >150,000
LDH normal
Normal blood film

Refractory disease or dialysis-dependent consider:
- vitamin E 1g/m^2/day
- plasma exchange
- prostacyclin

Refractory disease consider:
- ↑ dose of FFP (80–140 mL/kg)
- use cryosupernatant instead of FFP
- prostacyclin

Refractory disease or relapse consider:
- immunoadsorption
- vincristine 1–2 mg/week
- IVIG
- splenectomy
- ? retinoic acid

*If plasma exchange is not available begin plasma infusion until exchange possible

Chapter 16 _____

RAPIDLY PROGRESSIVE GLOMERULONEPHRITIS
Gill Gaskin

DEFINITION

Rapidly progressive glomerulonephritis (RPGN) is a clinically-defined syndrome, in which glomerular disease — indicated by microscopic haematuria and proteinuria — leads to the loss of renal function in a matter of weeks (see **Figure 1**). It is an important cause of acute renal failure (ARF) developing outside hospital, and should always be considered when features of systemic inflammation are present. Early recognition is important as treatment may prevent the development of end-stage renal failure.

Figure 1. Typical course of untreated rapidly progressive glomerulonephritis in ANCA-associated vasculitis

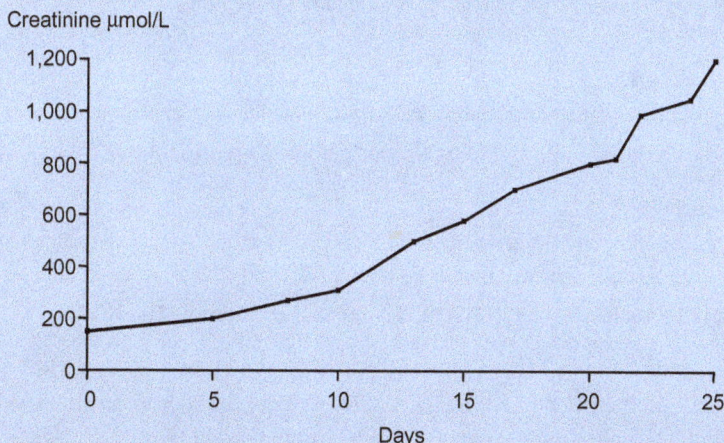

PATHOLOGY AND AETIOLOGY

The characteristic renal pathology in RPGN is a crescentic glomerulonephritis, in which inflammatory cells in Bowman's space surround a damaged glomerular tuft (see **Chapter 7**). Historically, crescentic glomerulonephritis was classified according to the findings on staining of renal tissue for immunoglobulin deposition, and this technique remains useful in making a specific diagnosis. Three categories of RPGN were identified using this approach.

The first category was crescentic glomerulonephritis with deposition of immunoglobulin in a linear pattern on the glomerular basement membrane. This corresponds to anti-glomerular basement membrane antibody-mediated (anti-GBM) or Goodpasture's disease, a rare syndrome associated with circulating antibodies directed against the non-collagenous domain of the $\alpha 3$ chain of type IV collagen, a component of selected basement membranes. In anti-GBM disease, which can lead to renal failure in a matter of days, it is common to find all the glomeruli in a biopsy specimen affected by crescents of similar ages.

The second historical category was crescentic glomerulonephritis with scanty or absent immune deposits: "pauci-immune" crescentic glomerulonephritis. This is now recognised as the renal lesion of primary, small vessel vasculitis. The earliest lesion is necrosis of the capillary loop in a segment of the glomerulus but, as the nephritis progresses, the lesions become more extensive and crescents form. It is usual to identify lesions of different ages in a biopsy specimen. Primary small vessel vasculitis is associated with circulating anti-neutrophil cytoplasm autoantibodies (ANCA), specific for one of two granule enzymes: proteinase 3 and myeloperoxidase, which are found in both neutrophils and monocytes. Pauci-immune crescentic glomerulonephritis without extrarenal vasculitis is also considered part of the ANCA-associated vasculitis (AASV) spectrum. The ANCA-associated syndromes are listed in **Table 1**. In a minority of cases, the illness appears to be provoked by exposure to certain drugs; Hydralazine, Propylthiouracil and Penicillamine are the most commonly reported. Occupational exposure to silica also confers an increased risk of developing ANCA-associated RPGN.

Table 1. ANCA-associated syndromes

Wegener's granulomatosis
Necrotising vasculitis affecting small-to-medium sized vessels; granulomatous inflammation in the respiratory tract.
Associated with proteinase 3-specific C-ANCA > myeloperoxidase-specific P-ANCA.

Churg-Strauss syndrome
Necrotising vasculitis affecting small and medium-sized vessels; eosinophil-rich and granulomatous inflammation in the respiratory tract; asthma and eosinophilia ($>1.5 \times 10^9$/L).
Associated with myeloperoxidase-specific P-ANCA > proteinase 3-specific C-ANCA.

Microscopic polyangiitis
Necrotising vasculitis affecting small vessels. (Distinguished from cryoglobulinaemic vasculitis and Henoch-Schönlein purpura by the paucity of immune deposits.)
Associated with myeloperoxidase-specific P-ANCA or proteinase 3-specific C-ANCA.

Renal-limited vasculitis
Isolated pauci-immune necrotising and crescentic glomerulonephritis.
Associated with myeloperoxidase-specific P-ANCA > proteinase 3-specific C-ANCA.

RPGN, with few immune deposits on biopsy, may occur in all the ANCA-associated small vessel vasculitis syndromes. Note that Polyarteritis Nodosa is a vasculitis affecting medium size muscular arteries, which does not cause RPGN, and which is only rarely associated with ANCA.

ANCA have a variety of activating effects *in vitro* on neutrophils and monocytes; ANCA-activated neutrophils can kill cultured endothelial cells, and this interaction occurring *in vivo* could contribute to the pathological features of vasculitis. The evidence that this actually occurs is not watertight, however, since ANCA may persist during remission of vasculitis, and some patients with clinically typical disease are ANCA negative. Current rodent models of anti-myeloperoxidase immunity do not faithfully imitate the human disease, and rodents do not have a neutrophil enzyme which cross-reacts with human proteinase 3.

The third historical category of crescentic glomerulonephritis was crescentic glomerulonephritis with prominent granular immune deposits. This is a heterogeneous group which includes nephritis associated with systemic illnesses such as Henoch-Schönlein purpura, mixed essential cryoglobulinaemia and systemic lupus, nephritis associated with or following infection, and crescentic change occurring in a primary glomerular disease such as IgA nephropathy or mesangiocapillary glomerulonephritis.

ANCA-associated vasculitis is the most common cause of RPGN. Anti-GBM disease affects only 0.5–1/million of the population/year in the United Kingdom, while the incidence of AASV is nearer 20/million/year and appears to be increasing. Most cases of RPGN are considered to have an autoimmune basis; circulating autoantibodies (ANCA, anti-GBM, or antinuclear and anti-double-stranded DNA antibodies) are detectable, and they respond to immunosuppressive drugs.

CLINICAL PRESENTATION AND DIFFERENTIAL DIAGNOSIS

The overall clinical picture is determined by a number of factors, including the severity and consequences of the renal failure (see **Section 2**), and the extra-renal features of the underlying disease.

Features of Crescentic Glomerulonephritis

The crescentic glomerulonephritis is associated with proteinuria and microscopic, and occasionally macroscopic, haematuria (typically the colour of coca-cola). The amount of blood and protein in the urine varies, and does not correlate directly with the severity of glomerular injury. Hypoalbuminaemia, if present, is often due to the acute phase response, or a prolonged prodromal illness, rather than due to heavy urinary losses. Red cell casts (see **Chapter 4.2**) are an important urinary finding, indicating bleeding from the damaged glomerular tuft into the urinary space and distinguishing glomerular bleeding from bleeding due to structural lesions of the lower urinary tract. Granular casts are not specific for glomerulonephritis and are common in acute tubular necrosis. Hypertension may occur (perhaps least commonly in AASV) and may sometimes be treated by correction of fluid overload. Occasionally, the patient has loin pain and tenderness, due to renal swelling and capsular distension in a severely destructive glomerulonephritis.

Extra-Renal Features of the Underlying Disease

Up to two-thirds of patients with **anti-GBM disease** have alveolar haemorrhage, since the anti-GBM immune response also targets the alveolar basement membrane; the haemorrhage may be sufficient to cause significant anaemia. However, access of antibodies and other immune reactants to the alveolar basement membrane may require a degree of lung injury, for example from exposure to industrial or environmental toxins (including cigarette smoke), or perhaps as a result of certain cytokines during infection. Lung haemorrhage is therefore not an invariable occurrence.

Patients with **AASV** may have a range of extra-renal features, including constitutional features mimicking "prolonged Flu"; **Table 2** lists typical clinical features. It is worth noting that AASV is not only the most common cause of crescentic glomerulonephritis, but also the most common cause of pulmonary haemorrhage. Thus, while "Goodpasture's syndrome", comprising RPGN and lung haemorrhage, is classically associated with anti-GBM disease, it is actually more commonly due to vasculitis. The common causes of the "pulmonary-renal syndrome" — the combination of acute renal and respiratory failure — are set out in **Table 3**. Clinic features of alveolar haemorrhage include dyspnoea, haemoptysis, and anaemia, though not all are present in every case. Investigations usually reveal hypoxaemia, diffuse alveolar shadowing on the chest radiograph, and a raised transfer factor for carbon monoxide (KCO) since the gas is taken up by red cells in the alveolar space. Bronchoscopy and bronchoalveolar lavage may be performed to exclude pulmonary infection, and will demonstrate fresh blood in the presence of active bleeding, and haemosiderin-laden macrophages subsequently.

A small subgroup of patients has features of both anti-GBM disease (linear IgG on biopsy, circulating anti-GBM antibodies) and vasculitis with detectable ANCA.

Table 2. Clinical features of ANCA-associated vasculitis

Constitutional
Fever, night sweats, weight loss, malaise, arthralgia, myalgia

Organ-specific

Kidney	necrotising and crescentic glomerulonephritis
Lung	alveolar capillaritis causing diffuse alveolar haemorrhage
	granulomas* **
	asthma**
ENT	epistaxis, nasal bridge collapse, deafness, subglottic stenosis*
	nasal polyps**
Eye	episcleritis, scleritis, retinal vasculitis
	orbital granuloma*
Skin	purpura, nail-fold infarcts, splinter haemorrhages
Nervous system	mononeuritis multiplex, cerebral vasculitis causing focal signs, fits, haemorrhage
Gut	abdominal pain, bleeding, perforation
Heart (rare)	cardiac failure (especially**), valve lesions,* pericarditis

*Denotes features of Wegener's granulomatosis; **denotes features of Churg-Strauss syndrome.
The most common features are noted here; the list is not exhaustive.

Table 3. Differential diagnosis of the "pulmonary-renal syndrome"
Lung haemorrhage and glomerulonephritis
ANCA-associated vasculitis
Anti-GBM disease
Systemic lupus erythematosus
Cryoglobulinaemic vasculitis
Henoch-Schönlein purpura
Pulmonary infections with renal failure
Any severe pneumonia with ATN
Legionella
Hantavirus
Severe pulmonary oedema associated with renal failure of any cause
Pulmonary emboli with IVC thrombosis
Paraquat poisoning

Vasculitic features do not guarantee a diagnosis of AASV. In **Henoch-Schönlein purpura** there is classically a purpuric rash on extensor surfaces, and arthralgias and gut vasculitis complete the picture. In **cryoglobulinaemia** a vasculitic rash affects the extremities, and other features of vasculitic organ injury include mononeuritis multiplex and pulmonary haemorrhage. However, both conditions are less common in adults than AASV. One important differential diagnosis, which requires a different line of treatment, is **infective endocarditis** with vasculitic features in the skin and nails, and an associated nephritis. Another syndrome which can occasionally cause diagnostic confusion is **cholesterol embolisation** (see **Chapter 13**), leading to purpuric lesions in the skin, and progressive renal failure. However, the clinical context of severe generalised vascular disease, with recent intervention or anticoagulation, often points to the diagnosis before confirmation is gained from further investigations.

Systemic lupus erythematosus (SLE) may cause a variety of glomerular lesions, including a severe proliferative nephritis with crescent formation (see **Chapters 7** and **17**). When compared with AASV, the extrarenal features have some similarities (joint pains, occasional cutaneous vasculitis, and CNS disturbances) and some differences (polyserositis, cytopaenias, photosensitivity). SLE typically affects young females, and is more common in non-Caucasian groups; in contrast, ANCA-associated vasculitis is most common in the 6th and 7th decades, and in Caucasians. However, the distinction is not absolute.

Rapidly progressive renal failure without evidence of extrarenal inflammation may occur in **renal-limited AASV**, **anti-GBM disease**, and in **crescentic transformation of primary glomerulonephritis**. ARF due to **tubulo-interstitial nephritis** (which is often associated with haematuria, and occasionally with red cell casts) and **myeloma kidney** may also present a similar picture. A firm diagnosis cannot therefore be made on clinical grounds alone, and serological tests (serum and urinary immunoglobulins, autoantibodies and complement) and renal biopsy are required urgently.

INVESTIGATIONS

RPGN is a nephrological emergency and prompt treatment is required if maximum recovery of renal function is to be achieved. This is especially true in anti-GBM disease, where the pace of the disease is particularly rapid, and renal failure usually permanent once oliguria has developed. Treatment may be required before the results of all investigations are available.

The aims of the investigations are:

- To identify any immediate action required (e.g. treatment of hyperkalaemia, fluid overload)
- To confirm that RPGN is the likely cause of the renal failure
- To eliminate any other diagnoses which would respond unfavourably to immunosuppressive treatment
- To make a specific diagnosis to guide short-term and longer-term management

The plan of investigation is illustrated in **Figure 2**.

There are a number of non-specific laboratory findings which support a diagnosis of AASV, including anaemia (normochromic normocytic, or hypochromic microcytic due to lung or gut bleeding), neutrophil leucocytosis, thrombocythaemia, and an acute phase response (raised C-reactive protein, hyperglobulinaemia, low albumin, raised alkaline phosphatase). Importantly, complement levels are normal or even raised.

Screening tests for ANCA commonly employ an indirect immunofluorescence (IIF) assay on ethanol-fixed neutrophils. This method distinguishes two patterns of positivity: the cytoplasmic or C-ANCA pattern and the perinuclear or P-ANCA pattern. Antibodies to Proteinase 3, found most commonly in Wegener's granulomatosis, produce the C-ANCA pattern, while antibodies to Myeloperoxidase, found most commonly in microscopic polyangiitis and renal-limited vasculitis, produce the P-ANCA pattern. Unfortunately, autoantibodies of other specificity, in rheumatoid, SLE and inflammatory bowel disease, may mimic the P-ANCA pattern and, in isolation, finding of P-ANCA has a low specificity for vasculitis. ANCA testing is therefore most reliable when IIF is combined with ELISA assays detecting antibody binding to purified antigens. In a large European study using a combination of standardised IIF and ELISA assays for ANCA, the likelihood of a false positive result was no more than 1%. The false negative result in vasculitis was higher, at 15–20% (reflecting the assay cut-off needed to minimise the rate of false positive results). There are case-reports of false positive ANCA results in endocarditis and cholesterol emboli, when specific immunoassays to detect antibodies against the vasculitis-associated ANCA antigens Proteinase 3 and Myeloperoxidase were not used.

TREATMENT PRINCIPLES

Treatment in RPGN has three main strands:

- Management of the resulting renal failure.
- Therapy directed against the immune response and glomerular inflammation.
- Measures to prevent complications of treatment.

Management of the renal failure follows the same principles as management of renal failure in other settings: modification of diet and fluid input, and renal replacement therapy (see **Chapters 8**

Figure 2. Approach to investigation of rapidly progressive glomerulonephritis

Consider RPGN
- in renal impairment with systemic symptoms or
- in renal impairment progressing over days/weeks

Without factors predisposing to "acute tubular necrosis"

Check urinalysis and microscopy for blood, protein ± red cell casts
- Negative: consider vascular causes, myeloma, obstruction
- Positive: suggestive of RPGN

Send blood for immunoassays
- ANCA, anti-GBM, complement, ANA, dsDNA
- Analysis for cryoglobulin (blood kept at 37°C until serum separated) if distal purpura or hepatitis C present and there are no other features characteristic of other diagnoses

Arrange renal ultrasound
- Proceed to renal biopsy if 2, normal-sized, non-obstructed kidneys
- Samples for light microscopy, immunohistology, electron microscopy

Meanwhile, consider likely clinical diagnosis
- Consider age, gender, ethnicity
- Look for presence and distribution of extrarenal vasculitis and for pulmonary haemorrhage
- Look for serositis and cytopaenias which would favour diagnosis of SLE
- Look for risk factors and stigmata of endocarditis
- If no extrarenal organ involvement apparent, check drug history (?allergic interstitial nephritis)

Start immunosuppressive treatment while awaiting results if
- Pulmonary haemorrhage is present *or* anti-GBM disease is a significant possibility *or* renal deterioration is rapid
  and
- Endocarditis is unlikely

and **9**). In general, patients are haemodynamically stable and can be treated with intermittent haemodialysis. Anticoagulation should be minimised in the presence of alveolar haemorrhage, or gastrointestinal bleeding from vasculitic injury, and following renal biopsy.

Specific therapy typically consists of corticosteroids with cyclophosphamide, with addition of plasma exchange in anti-GBM disease, and sometimes in ANCA-associated vasculitis (plasma exchange is discussed in greater detail below). Typical drug regimens are listed in **Table 4**. Treatment may be commenced before the diagnosis is confirmed by renal biopsy, when the clinical picture is highly suggestive, and if the probability of a diagnosis in which the treatment would be harmful (e.g. endocarditis) is low. The confidence to commence immunosuppression is greatly enhanced when positive immunoassay results can be obtained urgently.

Complications of therapy are common. A high proportion of patients experience **infection**, and causative agents include bacterial infections in damaged tissues, related to dialysis lines and urine catheters, opportunist organisms in patients inadvertently rendered neutropaenic, lymphopaenic or maintained on high dose therapy, and reactivated tuberculosis. Consideration should therefore be given to low dose cotrimoxazole for pneumocystis prophylaxis, isoniazid to prevent TB reactivation, and antifungal agents to prevent mucosal candida infection. The leucocyte

Table 4. Oral steroid/cyclophosphamide regimens for treatment of anti-GBM disease and ANCA-associated vasculitis

	Anti-GBM disease	ANCA-associated vasculitis
Induction therapy	Prednisolone 1 mg/kg/day (60 mg/day for average sized patients) Cyclophosphamide 2–3 mg/kg/day	Prednisolone 1 mg/kg/day (60 mg/day for average sized patients) Cyclophosphamide 2–2.5 mg/kg/day (to maximum of 150 mg/day in patients <60, 100 mg/day in patients >60)
Adjunctive treatment	Daily plasma exchange for 14 days, or until anti-GBM antibody level within normal range	For severe renal impairment: 7–10 plasma exchanges in first 14 days *or* i.v. Methylprednisolone 0.5 g–1 g on days 1–3
Steroid taper	1–2 weekly to a dose of 20 mg/day by 6 weeks; 2–4 weekly thereafter, stopping by 3–6 months	1–2 weekly to a dose of 20 mg/day by 6 weeks, then more slowly to 10 mg/day by 6 months, and 5–7.5 mg/day by 12 months
Maintenance therapy	None required	Substitute Azathioprine dose-for-dose for Cyclophosphamide at 3 months, provided in remission

Prophylaxis against complications — consider:

Proton pump inhibitor, Cotrimoxazole 960 mg 3x/week, Isoniazid + Pyridoxine if previous TB, oral antifungal agent (e.g. Amphotericin lozenges), Calcium/Vitamin D.

Readers are advised to consult original publications (e.g. Adu *et al.* 1998) for details of pulsed/intravenous cyclophosphamide regimens, which are complex.

count must be monitored carefully in Cyclophosphamide-treated patients, and the drug withdrawn temporarily if the level falls to an unacceptable level ($<4 \times 10^9$/L in our protocol) or is falling rapidly. The drug can be introduced at a lower dose when the white cell count has recovered. Patients on high dose immunosuppression should be advised to report symptoms of infection immediately.

Other complications include **peptic ulceration** (consider proton pump inhibitor), **osteoporosis** due to steroids (consider early documentation of bone density, calcium/vitamin D, and bisphosphonates once severe renal impairment has been reversed) and **haemorrhagic cystitis** due to Cyclophosphamide (give mesna when Cyclophosphamide is used in high-dose pulses). Some complications do not have specific preventive measures, but are dose-related (**infertility** and **risk of malignancy** due to Cyclophosphamide, and **cataracts**, **avascular necrosis** and **diabetes** due to steroids). It is therefore imperative that the risks and benefits of therapy are constantly assessed, particularly where the presentation is isolated renal disease, and there appears to be no response to initial therapy. Ideally, cyclophosphamide therapy in young males should be preceded by semen banking, but in the setting of RPGN, this is often precluded by the urgency of the treatment and by how ill the patient feels.

Controversies in Immunosuppressive Treatment of PRGN

Regimens for anti-GBM disease have developed empirically, and the disease is sufficiently rare that randomised controlled trials to identify the crucial components of existing therapies are unlikely to take place.

Treatment regimens for proliferative nephritis in SLE have received considerable attention at the US National Institutes of Health and elsewhere, and combined regimens have been shown to be superior to steroids alone. Pulse administration of cyclophosphamide is now widely preferred over oral therapy. However, it is worth noting that a rapidly progressive course is not the norm in SLE: ARF occurs in only 1–2% of cases. One should therefore apply the general messages about treatment with a little caution.

The controversies in initial treatment of RPGN mainly apply to the most common underlying cause, AASV, and are as follows:

- The place of pulses of methylprednisolone
- The place of plasma exchange
- The route of administration of cyclophosphamide

Methylprednisolone and plasma exchange are generally considered to be adjunctive therapies to be reserved for the more severe cases of AASV, including those with severe renal impairment due to RPGN. Methylprednisolone is typically given as 3 pulses of 0.5 g–1 g on consecutive days (although both less and more intensive regimens have been published). The value of adjunctive pulsed steroid in milder disease has not been subjected to randomised controlled trial but the known dose-related toxicity of steroids and the known efficacy of regimens without pulsed steroids should mitigate against its routine use. Published controlled trials suggest that there is no benefit to the addition of plasma exchange in milder disease.

There is considerable debate as to which of these adjunctive approaches should be preferred in RPGN with ARF. A head-to-head comparison (for efficacy and toxicity) has not yet been completed, and the decision must presently rest on local practice and availability, and whether an alternative diagnosis of anti-GBM disease, or the presence of co-existing anti-GBM antibodies, has been excluded.

Plasma Exchange

The indications for plasma exchange in RPGN are outlined above. In general, it is employed when circulating factors are considered or suspected to be pathogenic (e.g. anti-GBM antibodies). Whole blood is separated into plasma and blood cells in a pumped extracorporeal circuit, the cells are returned to the patient, and the plasma is discarded and replaced by an albumin solution to which physiological concentrations of potassium and calcium are added. Blood can also be transfused, but the procedure is sometimes poorly tolerated in severely anaemic patients and prior transfusion (on dialysis if necessary) is to be preferred. The separation of plasma and cells is achieved using either a cytocentrifuge (the haematologist's usual method) or a highly permeable plasma filter (the nephrologist's usual method). A number of machines exist, with varying degrees of automation of the fluid replacement. The usual aim is to deplete one plasma volume in a treatment session, and allowing for the decreasing efficiency as the treatment proceeds (the same plasma is "re-treated"), a typical exchange volume is 60 ml/kg (with a practical maximum of 4 litres). In anti-GBM disease, the treatment is performed more or less daily for two weeks, or until the circulating antibody is undetectable. In vasculitis, a typical protocol consists of 7–10 exchanges during the first two weeks of treatment. In these settings, vascular access for the procedure is usually a "Vascath" dual-lumen venous line.

Plasma exchange removes normal plasma proteins. Fresh frozen plasma may be added into the replacement regimen at the end of the exchange when the removal of clotting factors poses a particular risk, e.g. after an invasive procedure or in the presence of alveolar haemorrhage, but should not be used routinely or as the sole replacement solution; past experience suggests that severe allergic reactions to plasma constitute the greatest potential danger of the treatment. Bleeding, complications of fluid shifts, and problems related to vascular access are the other major problems.

Route of Cyclophosphamide Administration

Conventional treatment for AASV involves daily oral Cyclophosphamide, a treatment which is effective in inducing remission, if toxic. Pulsed Cyclophosphamide offers the potential advantage of a lower monthly dose, and ease of concurrent administration of mesna to protect the bladder, and its efficacy in lupus nephritis has led to a number of clinical trials in vasculitis. The regimens used have varied considerably, in dose size and interval, in treatment duration, and in modifications for age and renal function. The results, unsurprisingly, are also heterogeneous, but taken together they suggest that pulsed therapy is effective at inducing remission and associated with fewer infections than daily dosing. However, the rate of escape of disease is high, and the experience in severe renal impairment is limited. In view of this, a dose regimen is not recommended in this chapter and the reader is advised to consult individual research reports for further details.

Maintenance Therapy and Long-Term Management

Anti-GBM disease relapses infrequently, and it is usual to discontinue Cyclophosphamide at around three months, and to taper the Prednisolone over three to six months. Treatment may be curtailed sooner if there is no recovery of renal function and pulmonary haemorrhage has not occurred. Vasculitis requires more prolonged therapy, and it is usual to continue therapy for at least a year after the induction of remission, with progressive reduction in the corticosteroid dose. We substitute Azathioprine for Cyclophosphamide at three months; this strategy has recently been shown to be as effective as continuing Cyclophosphamide in a randomised European trial, and avoids the cumulative risks of prolonged therapy with an alkylating agent. Even with such therapy, a relapse rate of 10–15% can be expected in the first year.

There is no consensus on the optimum duration of maintenance immunosuppression in vasculitis. Fifty per cent of patients will relapse eventually. The pattern of organ involvement does not always mimic the initial presentation, the severity varies, and the consequences are influenced by any irreversible damage already inflicted by the disease. Long-term follow-up is desirable. Prolonged maintenance treatment probably reduces the relapse rate, but carries the risk of cumulative toxicity, and should ideally be reserved for those at highest risk of relapse. Risk factors for relapse include persisting ANCA, ANCA specificity for Proteinase 3, and nasal carriage of *Staphylococcus aureus* in Wegener's granulomatosis. A rise in the ANCA concentration precedes relapse in some cases but the relationship is not strong enough to dictate changes in treatment. Rather, it suggests that increased vigilance is required.

Treatment of Relapse in Vasculitis

Treatment depends on the drug doses at the time of relapse, and the severity of the clinical picture. Mild relapses can often be managed with moderate doses of Prednisolone (20–30 mg/day), while more severe relapses will require the reinstitution of Cyclophosphamide, and in life-threatening cases, adjunctive therapies as used in the presenting illness. Anti T-lymphocyte antibodies, both polyclonal and humanised monoclonal, have been used in specialist centres to treat refractory disease.

Alternative Treatments in Vasculitis

A number of other drugs may prove useful in long-term management, either to improve remission maintenance following relapse, or in the event of adverse reactions to first-line agents. **Methotrexate** (using an escalating weekly dose regimen, as employed in rheumatoid arthritis) is useful in the treatment of Wegener's granulomatosis, but cannot be used if there is significant residual renal impairment. **Intravenous immunoglobulin** has been used to treat mild vasculitis relapses or to improve long-term disease control. A typical regimen is 2 g/kg (in four divided doses) for initial treatment and 0.5–1 g/kg 1–3 monthly in maintenance regimens. The main disadvantages are cost, only modest efficacy, and the risk of nephrotoxicity in patients with pre-existing renal impairment. **Cotrimoxazole** (960 mg b.d) has been shown to reduce the rate of respiratory relapses in patients with Wegener's granulomatosis, although up to 20% of patients fail to tolerate the drug. Newer immunosuppressive drugs, including **Mycophenolate mofetil** and

Deoxyspergualin (developed as anti-rejection drugs for transplantation) and **Leflunomide** (recently licensed for treatment of rheumatoid) are promising, and are being studied.

Treatment of RPGN in Association with Infection

Here the priority is to treat the underlying infection, whether streptococcal or endocarditis, and this may be sufficient to reverse the renal failure. Where crescentic nephritis persists after adequate treatment of the infection, anecdotal successes have been reported with high dose steroid therapy, but this is not an option to be undertaken lightly, or outside specialist centres.

Treatment of Crescentic Phase of Primary GN

The treatment of crescentic transformation in primary glomerulonephritis has not been subjected to rigorous study, and evidence-based recommendations cannot be made. Some have elected to treat crescentic IgA nephropathy with a similar immunosuppressive regimen to RPGN in AASV, and there are anecdotal reports of both success and failure. The small literature in mesangiocapillary glomerulonephritis is similarly mixed. In any patient in this category, the risks of therapy must be balanced against the chance of deferring or preventing need for dialysis.

OUTCOME

Survival

Historically, Goodpasture's syndrome was often fatal, either as a result of overwhelming pulmonary haemorrhage or renal failure, though with hindsight not all cases were attributable to anti-GBM disease. With current therapeutic regimens containing plasma exchange and cytotoxic drugs, and as a result of improvements in supportive care for renal and respiratory failure, one year mortality has reduced to 10–20%.

In vasculitis, outcome depends on the severity of the illness at presentation. The highest mortality is seen in patients requiring ventilation for pulmonary haemorrhage, at approximately 50%. Patients with severe renal impairment due to RPGN have a one year mortality of 25–30%, with a significant number of deaths due to the complications of therapy; older patients are particularly susceptible. Late deaths include a small number due to relapse and a proportion due to the adverse effects of therapy, including haematological malignancies in patients with prolonged exposure to cyclophosphamide. The remainder are attributable to unrelated causes. Prognosis appears to have improved, with better recognition of relapse and the more judicious use of immunosuppression.

Renal Recovery

Renal outcome in anti-GBM disease remains unsatisfactory, largely because renal impairment is often advanced at presentation. Few patients presenting with a creatinine higher than 500 or 600 µmol/l avoid long-term dialysis, though occasional patients recover renal function after an initial requirement for dialysis. Early referral is therefore critical, but rarely achieved, perhaps because the renal injury progresses so rapidly.

In vasculitis, the rate of recovery of renal function following treatment for RPGN varies substantially between series, perhaps reflecting the variation of treatment policies between, and even within, centres. In our experience, over 70% of patients are alive with independent renal function at two months and recovery from dialysis-dependence occurs frequently. Patients who make a good response to initial therapy and then remain in remission generally maintain stable renal function long-term. Some features of the renal biopsy correlate with outcome when large groups of patients are studied; the proportion of normal glomeruli and the extent of tubulo-interstitial scarring are predictive but the crescent score is not. However, the prediction for individual patients is unreliable, and the biopsy appearances should not be used to decide whether to withhold immunosuppressive therapy.

Long-Term Dialysis and Transplantation

In patients who fail to recover renal function after initial therapy, or who later progress to endstage renal failure, a long-term plan for renal replacement therapy is required. Listing for transplantation should usually be deferred until the patient has been in clinical remission for at least six months. Anti-GBM antibodies have the potential to cause nephritis in the transplanted kidney, and levels should be consistently undetectable prior to transplantation; under such circumstances the risk of recurrent anti-GBM disease in the graft is low. In vasculitis, current data suggest that ANCA positivity should not preclude transplantation, but there remains a small risk of disease relapse, and necrotising glomerulonephritis may recur in the graft.

The optimal dialysis modality for immunosuppressed patients is debated; one vasculitis series did not identify particular problems with either haemodialysis or peritoneal dialysis, while data from Guys' Hospital, London suggested that immunosuppressed patients on Continuous Ambulatory Peritoneal Dialysis, including patients with vasculitis, had a higher incidence of infectious complications than non-immunosuppressed patients. Other reports suggest that infections of haemodialysis vascular access may be problematic. Overall, the prognosis for vasculitis patients on renal replacement therapy is comparable to UK Registry patients as a whole.

Long-Term Complications

Patients with RPGN, especially those with vasculitis — a relapsing multisystem disease requiring prolonged treatment — are at risk of damage from both their disease and their treatment. Renal impairment has already been discussed. Non-renal disease damage includes pulmonary fibrosis in a small proportion of patients presenting with alveolar haemorrhage due to vasculitis, residual neurological deficits after mononeuritis multiplex, and deafness, chronic nasal deformities and sinus drainage problems in Wegener's granulomatosis. Treatment-related damage is common; nearly half of the patients in a large series from the National Institutes of Health suffered adverse effects from their treatment for Wegener's granulomatosis. Significant infections occurred during follow-up in 46 per cent, especially in the early stages of treatment. The range of infectious organisms is wide, reflecting the diverse precipitating factors: drug effects on humoral and cell-mediated immunity, disease-induced organ damage, hospitalisation and invasive procedures.

Common opportunist infections include Pneumocystis (particularly in the presence of drug-induced lymphopaenia) and Herpes Zoster; Nocardia and Aspergillus have also been reported. Fatal infections are most common in the first year of treatment, and elderly patients appear to be particularly susceptible. Infection can progress rapidly in immunocompromised patients, particularly in the presence of drug-induced leucopaenia, and empirical treatment is often warranted. The differential diagnosis may also include manifestations of vasculitis, and a two-pronged approach to investigation, and even to treatment, may be required. Long-term use of cytotoxic agents increases the risk of malignancy. Cyclophosphamide is associated with haematological malignancies and bladder cancer, while prolonged Azathioprine (and combined regimens in general) add to the skin cancer risk. Infertility is another important adverse effect of Cyclophosphamide.

ARF IN OTHER GLOMERULAR DISEASES

ARF in Severe Nephrotic Syndrome

ARF is a well-recognised, if infrequent, complication of severe nephrotic syndrome. Contributory factors can include intravenous contrast agents (rare now that ultrasound is the standard imaging modality), allergic interstitial nephritis due to diuretics, renal vein thrombosis and superimposed sepsis, but many cases are "idiopathic". ARF typically occurs in older patients with minimal change nephrotic syndrome, very heavy proteinuria and marked hypoalbuminaemia, and usually precedes therapy. The clinical differential includes a variety of other causes of ARF, and the diagnosis is made on biopsy, which shows acute tubular necrosis, often with considerable interstitial oedema, in addition to the characteristic foot process effacement. Not all patients are clinically hypovolaemic, and the pathophysiology is unclear. Indeed, it is a rare complication in nephrotic children, even though they are frequently more overtly volume depleted. Management requires judicious fluid removal by ultrafiltration, together with specific therapy for the nephrotic syndrome if the patient's general condition permits. Attention to nutrition and good general nursing care are also crucial. Recovery can be slow and incomplete, and there is a significant mortality in the oldest patients.

RPGN: Practice Points

- Think of the diagnosis — look for the evidence — start treatment if there is strong suspicion
- Confirm the diagnosis with specific investigations
- Be aware of the risks of therapy and ensure that the patient is informed appropriately of the risks and benefits of treatment
- Plan long-term follow-up

FURTHER READING

Adu D, Pall A, Luqmani RA, *et al.* (1997) Controlled trial of pulse versus continuous prednisolone and cyclophosphamide in the treatment of systemic vasculitis. *Quarterly Journal of Medicine*; 90(6): 401–409

A controlled trial report which gives the details of a pulsed cyclophosphamide regimen for vasculitis

Gaskin G, Pusey CD (1998) Systemic vasculitis. In: Davison AM, Cameron JS, Grunfeld J-P, *et al.* (eds.). *Oxford Textbook of Clinical Nephrology* (2nd Edition). Oxford: Oxford University Press

A comprehensive account of ANCA-associated systemic vasculitis

Hewins P, Cohen Tervaert JW, Savage COS, Kallenberg CGM (2000) Is Wegener's granulomatosis an auto-immune disease? *Current Opinion Rheumatology*; 12: 3–10

A recent discussion of the evidence that Wegener's granulomatosis is an autoimmune disease

Hoffman GS, Kerr GS, Leavitt RY, *et al.* (1992) Wegener granulomatosis: An analysis of 158 patients. *Annals of Internal Medicine*; 116: 488–498

An important paper which describes the disease and treatment-related morbidity in a large cohort of patients with Wegener's granulomatosis

Jennette JC, Falk RJ, Andrassy K, *et al.* (1994) Nomenclature of systemic vasculitides. Proposal of an international consensus conference. *Arthritis and Rheumatism*; 37: 187–192

Current approach to nomenclature of ANCA-associated vasculitis

Specks U (2000) Are animal models of vasculitis suitable tools? *Current Opinion Rheumatology*; 12: 11–19

A discussion of current animal models of vasculitis and their applicability to human disease

Turner AN, Rees AJ (1998) Antiglomerular basement membrane disease. In: Davison AM, Cameron JS, Grunfeld J-P, *et al.* (eds.). *Oxford Textbook of Clinical Nephrology* (2nd Edition). Oxford: Oxford University Press

A comprehensive account of anti-GBM disease

Chapter 17 _____

CONNECTIVE TISSUE DISEASES AND ACUTE RENAL FAILURE

Aine Burns

DEFINITION

Connective tissue diseases encompass a group of systemic disorders all of which may be associated with acute renal failure (ARF). The cause of the ARF varies according to which of these disorders is present in the individual patient. There is some overlap between these conditions and many patients demonstrate features of more than one connective tissue disease; in 25%, a phenotypic evolution occurs from one category to another over time. Such patients are said to have overlap syndrome. Current classifications recognize five major diffuse connective tissue diseases:

- SLE.
- Scleroderma.
- Polymyositis.
- Dermatomyositis.
- Rheumatoid arthritis.

Sjogren's syndrome is commonly associated with each of these disorders, but can also occur in isolation when it is referred to as primary Sjogren's syndrome. The most common connective tissue disease to affect renal function is systemic lupus erythematosus (SLE), which can be associated with ARF either because of lupus nephritis or occasionally because of haemolytic uraemic syndrome (HUS) (see **Chapter 15**). Scleroderma or systemic sclerosis (SSC) is a disorder in which 4–10% of affected patients develop devastating ARF, and which prior to the 1970s was almost universally fatal. Other connective tissue disorders such as rheumatoid arthritis, mixed connective tissue disease and anti-phospholipid syndrome can also cause both acute and chronic renal failure. Early recognition and correct diagnosis of renal involvement in these disorders is important as the progression of the ARF can be arrested and mortality reduced by appropriated intervention. This chapter focuses on SLE and SSC.

SLE NEPHRITIS

Some renal involvement on renal biopsy is almost universal in SLE, as even patients without clinical signs of renal disease are often found to have evidence of mesangial or diffuse proliferation on renal biopsy. However, only 50% of patients have abnormal urinalysis or impaired renal function at diagnosis and this rises to 75% over the entire course of the disease. Although most of these abnormalities develop in the first few years of disease, renal failure is uncommon and is usually the result of long-standing disease. Exceptions to this general rule occur when SLE is associated with intra-vascular volume depletion and the nephrotic syndrome, or when anti-phospholipid antibodies are present, which predisposes to ARF related to thrombotic microangiopathy (discussed below). Approximately one third of SLE patients have progressive renal impairment over the course of their disease, with 25% developing end stage renal failure within 10 years of diagnosis.

PATHOPHYSIOLOGY OF SLE NEPHRITIS

Glomerulonephritis in SLE

Most lupus-related renal disease is immune complex-mediated. Standard WHO classification is given in **Table 1**, and the prevalence, clinical findings, prognosis, and treatment of SLE nephritis according to histological classification are given in **Table 2**. Although helpful, this classification is imperfect as many patients have findings suggesting more than one type of nephritis on a single biopsy specimen, and further renal biopsies often demonstrate evolution from one type to another. The location of the immune complex deposition is important in determining the severity of injury and likelihood of ARF. Subendothelial and mesangial deposits are associated with neutrophil and monocyte infiltrates, giving rise to the proliferative types of GN. This response may be partly driven by Fc receptor-mediated pro-inflammatory pathways. Like all proliferative glomerular lesions, an active urine sediment is demonstrable and renal function may decline acutely. It is generally believed that the culprit immune complexes in this type of lesion are derived from the circulation rather than fashioned *in situ*. A growing body of evidence from animal models and clinical studies supports the concept that impaired clearance of immune complexes predisposes to SLE. A good example is the massively increased risk of SLE occurring in families in which complement components are genetically defective — such patients have been shown to dispose of circulating immune complexes poorly *in vivo*. The immune deposits contain DNA-anti-DNA complexes, but chromatin, laminin, Ro, ubiquitin, ribosomal material, and C1q may also be found. Occasionally crescentic glomerulonephritis (GN) ensues to cause ARF (see **Chapter 16**).

Table 1. Classification of SLE glomerulonephritis	
No abnormality detected	Type I
Mesangial proliferation	Type II
Focal proliferative*	Type III
Diffuse proliferative	Type IV
Membranous	Type V
Sclerosing	Type VI

*<50% of glomeruli affected on light microscopy.

Table 2. Prevalence, clinical findings, prognosis, and treatment of SLE nephritis according to histological classification

Classification & prevalence in SLE nephritis patients	Complement and autoantibody levels	Main clinical findings	Prognosis and recommended treatment
Type II Mesangial proliferation (10–20%)	Minimal complement reduction and low anti-DNA Ab titres	Microscopic haematuria/ proteinuria usually detectable HT, NS, ARF almost never seen	Prognosis excellent, no treatment necessary (unless for other features of SLE)
Type III Focal proliferative (10–20%)	Moderate complement reduction and elevated anti-DNA Ab titres	Haematuria/proteinuria almost always present HT, NS, renal impairment may all be present	Prognosis variable, <25% of glomeruli involved usually benign: no treatment required 25–40% of glomeruli involved treat depending on severity of lesions, NS or renal impairment 40–50% of glomeruli involved treat as for diffuse disease
Type IV Diffuse proliferative (40–70%)	Significant hypocomplementaemia and elevated anti-DNA levels especially during active disease	Haematuria, proteinuria and active urine sediment almost always seen HT, NS, renal impairment common	Focal necrosis and crescents may be seen and changes involve more than 50% of glomeruli sampled Immunosuppressive therapy generally required
Type V Membranous (10–20%)	May be no serological markers of SLE	Present with signs of NS May have haematuria and HT, renal impairment uncommon	Prognosis good in general Treat only if patient has severe NS or progressive renal impairment as for diffuse proliferative disease BP control and cholesterol lowering likely to be beneficial Value of proteinuria reduction with ACEI/AII blockers unproven but likely to be beneficial

Table 2 (*Continued*)

Classification & prevalence in SLE nephritis patients	Complement and autoantibody levels	Main clinical findings	Prognosis and recommended treatment
Type VI Sclerosing (2%)	Markers of SLE activity usually low	Bland urine sediment, proteinuria and HT often present, slow progressive renal impairment	Treat as for chronic renal disease with excellent BP control; ACEI/AII blockers likely to be beneficial Special attention should be paid to cardiovascular risk factors such as cholesterol

HT = hypertension; NS = nephrotic syndrome; BP = blood pressure.

In the non-proliferative types of GN associated with SLE, antibodies are believed to be directed against planted antigens which have already crossed the basement membrane or are part of the epithelial cell. In these situations there is little or no inflammatory cell infiltrate and hence the disease phenotype is less acute, with proteinuria and nephrotic syndrome being the usual presentation. In addition, the IgG subclass of the anti-DNA antibody may be important in determining the severity of inflammation in the glomeruli, as IgG1 and IgG3 are more powerful activators of complement than either IgG2 or IgG4. Immune complexes themselves can also induce adhesion molecule expression on vascular endothelial cells which, together with cytokine production by both infiltrating macrophages and T-cells and the injured glomerular cells, recruits further inflammatory cells. These cytokines include tumour necrosis factor alpha (TNF-α), interleukin-6 (IL-6), platelet derived growth factor (PDGF) and interferon-gamma (IFN-γ).

Non-glomerulonephritic renal lesions in SLE

The presence of inflammatory cell infiltration and scarring in the interstitium has important prognostic significance and is commonly seen when there is active glomerular disease. Immune deposits may be present along the tubular basement membrane. The severity of these changes correlates well with the presence of hypertension and likelihood of progressive renal impairment. Occasionally, interstitial changes can occur in the absence of glomerulonephritis. The consequences of this process can be severe with the development of tubular dysfunction. This may present as renal tubular acidosis, hyperkalaemia due to impaired distal potassium secretion, or salt wasting with hypokalaemia resulting from intra-vascular volume depletion and hyperaldosteronism. Some patients may have antibodies directed against acid secreting cells of the collecting tubule. Drugs such as non-steroidal anti-inflammatory agents may also cause acute tubulointerstitial nephritis, and this possibility should be borne in mind as discontinuation of the offending drug may lead to resolution of the inflammation. Very occasionally, immune complexes are deposited under the vascular endothelium in lupus patients leading to an aggressive vasculitic process with features of thrombotic thrombocytopaenic purpura (TTP). Interestingly, the immune deposits do not usually induce inflammation and the patients are often severely hypertensive, which may contribute to the vascular injury. SLE patients with anti-phospholipid auto-antibodies are at increased risk of malignant hypertension and ARF; this is discussed separately in the next section. Drug-induced lupus rarely affects the kidneys but nephrotic syndrome and diffuse proliferative GN have both been described.

Treatment Options in SLE Nephritis

Treatment of lupus nephritis is a vast and difficult subject marred by lack of controlled clinical trials and too many anecdotes. Nevertheless, immunosuppression is effective in treating progressive renal disease and is widely used. The weight of evidence supports the use of cytotoxic agents in all patients with class IV nephritis, as well as some with types III and V disease. An extensive review of this topic is beyond the scope of this chapter. Chemotherapeutic strategies which have been used in human lupus nephritis include the use of cyclophosphamide, administered either orally or as intravenous pulses, azathioprine, cyclosporin A, tacrolimus (FK-506), chlorambucil and steroids (as oral agents or as intra-venous pulses). Other agents directed against lymphocytes, cytokines or their receptors have been tried, as have plasma exchange, intravenous immunoglobulin and occasionally oestrogen antagonists. Total lymphoid irradiation and even bone marrow transplantation have been used in animal models, and occasionally in humans with very aggressive disease.

There is convincing evidence, much of it from classic National Institutes of Health (NIH) sponsored trials over the last 30 years, that azathioprine, cyclophosphamide, ATG, steroids and cyclosporin are beneficial in therapy of SLE nephritis. However, controversy still surrounds when and how these agents are best used. When treating aggressive diffuse proliferative glomerulonephritis, most specialists would agree that monthly pulses of intravenous cyclophosphamide are warranted according to the NIH regimen (monthly at 5–10 mg/kg followed by quarterly pulses for two years). How frequently to administer the cyclophosphamide, and for how long, remains controversial and many units switch to azathioprine after 6 or 9 pulses of cyclophosphamide. There is some evidence that prolonged pulsed cyclophosphamide treatment decreases the risk of relapse, doubling creatinine or reaching end stage renal failure, when patients are followed up for up to ten years. However, the cost of such aggressive treatment in terms of infection, fertility and risk of cancer, particularly bladder cancer, is difficult to determine. Most units would now recommend the use of bisphosphonates to ameliorate osteoporosis in those patients likely to require prolonged steroid treatment. Others use the oral contraceptive pill to try to reduce the chances of infertility, which reach 100% in the over 31 age group who have received prolonged courses of intra-venous cyclophosphamide.

My own preference is to use pulsed intra-venous cyclophosphamide monthly for 6 months then alternate months for a further 6 months followed by conversion to azathioprine. More recently we have had considerable success in some patients using mycophenolate mofetil. A pilot study is currently underway to evaluate its efficacy and safety in treating lupus nephritis. Proteinuria of >2 g per 24 hours, and a serum creatinine of greater than 200 µmol/L at the start of treatment are thought to be poor prognostic signs. The extent of interstitial scarring on renal biopsy, together with the presence of crescents, are also likely to predict a poor long-term outcome but this is not always true.

SCLERODERMA

Scleroderma or systemic sclerosis (SSC) is a relatively uncommon disorder (incidence = 2/100,000, prevalence = 1/8,000 in UK) which affects women predominantly, but approximately 18% of patients are male. The disease may occur in a diffuse (33%) or limited (67%) form. The main pathology lies in the skin dermis, where there is excessive deposition of collagenous material. There is, however, increasing evidence that SSC is an inflammatory vasculopathy. The characteristic skin thickening is commonly preceded by Raynaud's phenomenon (72%) which may either be of recent onset or longstanding. Early in the course of the disease there is clear evidence of elongation and increased tortuosity of nail fold capillaries. Raynaud's phenomenon often progresses to irreversible digital arteriolar narrowing with loss of finger-tip pulp, painful ulceration and gangrene. Angiography demonstrates pruning and irregularity of digital blood vessels. Prolonged and exaggerated vasoconstriction in response to cold stimuli can be demonstrated by thermography. Systemic involvement causing pulmonary fibrosis (40% diffuse disease, 25% limited disease, 30% overall), hypertension (17% diffuse disease, 21% limited disease, 20% overall), restrictive cardiomyopathy, oesophageal dysmotility (59% diffuse disease, 56% limited disease, 57% overall), gut involvement and diverticulosis occur commonly and complicate patient management. The characteristic skin telangiectasia are further evidence of abnormal vasculature in this condition and can also be found in the GI tract, where they can be responsible for significant haemorrhage.

SCLERODERMA RENAL CRISIS

Renal involvement in SSC was first described by Sir William Osler more than one hundred years ago. Many subsequent authors have described renal vascular pathology in scleroderma patients dying with normal renal function. Proteinuria and/or hypertension are frequent findings in scleroderma patients. Further, Kovalchik et al. found vascular abnormalities in 6 of 9 renal biopsies from scleroderma patients who were normotensive with no evidence of renal dysfunction. Thus, it appears that large numbers of patients with SSC have sub-clinical or minor evidence of renal disease. However, since the 1970s it has been recognised that a significant subgroup of SSC patients (4–10%) develop ARF which is characterised by accelerated hypertension. These patients develop what is now termed a **scleroderma renal crisis** (SRC).

DEFINITION

The definition of SRC is controversial but the major and minor criteria, as defined by Traub et al. based on 68 patients with SRC, are listed (**Table 3**). These combine evidence of an abrupt rise or aggravation of BP(>160/90 mmHg) with evidence of grade III or IV hypertensive retinopathy, a plasma renin activity of more than twice normal, and ARF for which no other cause can be found. Evidence of encephalopathy, microangiopathic haemolytic anaemia (MAHA — see also

Table 3. Diagnostic criteria for SRC

In a patient with known SSC two major or one major plus two minor criteria should be present

Major

Evidence of an abrupt rise or aggravation of BP(>160/90 mmHg)
Grade III or IV hypertensive retinopathy
Plasma renin activity of more than twice normal
ARF for which no other cause can be found

Minor

Encephalopathy
Microangiopathic haemolytic anaemia (MAHA)
Characteristic changes on renal biopsy

Chapter 15) or characteristic changes on renal biopsy support the diagnosis. A small number of patients develop the renal hypertensive crisis before they develop the skin abnormalities or when the changes are subtle and undiagnosed. ARF without hypertension can occur and carries a particularly poor prognosis, perhaps because left ventricular failure has already resulted from the massive systemic vascular resistance (SVR) characteristic of a renal crisis. The cardinal feature of SRC is a steady increase in SVR. ARF rapidly ensues if diagnosis and treatment is not commenced. The renal failure may be accompanied by evidence of intravascular haemolysis. Falling haemoglobin and platelet counts together with increased LDH, AST and ALT, and modest elevation in bilirubin levels, are usually accompanied by evidence of RBC fragments on blood film and decreased haptoglobin levels. Clotting studies are characteristically normal.

Epidemiology

The average age of onset of scleroderma is 45 ± 3 years. SRC typically occurs early in the course of aggressive disease. Mean duration of scleroderma prior to development of a renal crisis in our patient group was 22.6 months, with a range of 3–144 months, excluding one patient who had no evidence of scleroderma at the time of SRC. The average skin score (based on severity and extent of skin involvement) in our series of patients increased from 22.3 one year prior to SRC to 35.5 at presentation with crisis ($P < 0.06$). In this series, the average age of onset of SRC was 47.9 years. Forty-one percent of patients had been categorised as having limited disease and 59% diffuse. Worldwide, SRC is more common in black patients than Caucasians; however, in our series of 33 UK residents, 29 were Caucasian, one black West Indian, one Asian, one Ugandan, and one Japanese. There is a slight increase in incidence during the winter months, which may be more pronounced in more severe climates than the UK.

PATHOPHYSIOLOGY

The elevated blood pressure (BP) which is the primary manifestation of SRC is generated within the kidney. Renin and angiotensin levels are raised and bilateral nephrectomy is known to normalise

BP. The hypotensive effect of angiotensin converting enzyme inhibitors (ACEI) is further evidence that the angiotensin generated within renal tissue is a key player in the development of hypertension in SRC. However, to analyse this further, we need to examine the physiology of BP generation: BP is the product of cardiac output (stroke volume times heart rate) and peripheral resistance, which is determined by the product of vascular tone and effective arterial blood volume (see also **Chapter 5**). During SRC, heart rate is often increased but stroke volume may be diminished, either because of restrictive cardiomyopathy or pulmonary hypertension, or more likely because the left ventricle is pumping against extraordinarily elevated systemic vascular resistance (SVR). Systemic vascular resistances of up to three times the upper limit of normal have been recorded in these circumstances. Effective arterial blood volume is likely to play a minor role when compared with the effect of SVR.

Sokoloff *et al.* put forward the theory in 1952 that SRC was triggered by Raynaud's phenomenon of the kidney, with consequent renal cortical ischaemia and massive renin and angiotensin generation leading to intense vasoconstriction and aldosterone-induced salt and water retention. Certainly, renal angiography performed during SRC demonstrates profound pruning of vessels in the renal cortex (**Figure 1B**), although **Figure 1A** shows that there was considerable vascular abnormality when the patient was not undergoing SRC. Others have claimed that angiography performed at post-mortem fails to demonstrate the renal vascular spasm, supporting the idea that there is reversible spasm of renal vessels during SRC. Although cold may be one of the triggers for vascular spasm, and patients with SSC show an exaggerated renin response to a remotely applied cold stimulus (cold pack applied to side of neck), most patients with SRC do not give a history of cold exposure prior to SRC and there is only a modest increased incidence in the winter months. Steroids are known to provoke crises as are drugs which can cause vascular injury; e.g. cyclosporin A precipitated SRC in several patients in the 1980s.

Figure 1. Renal angiography (A) prior to and (B) during a scleroderma renal crisis

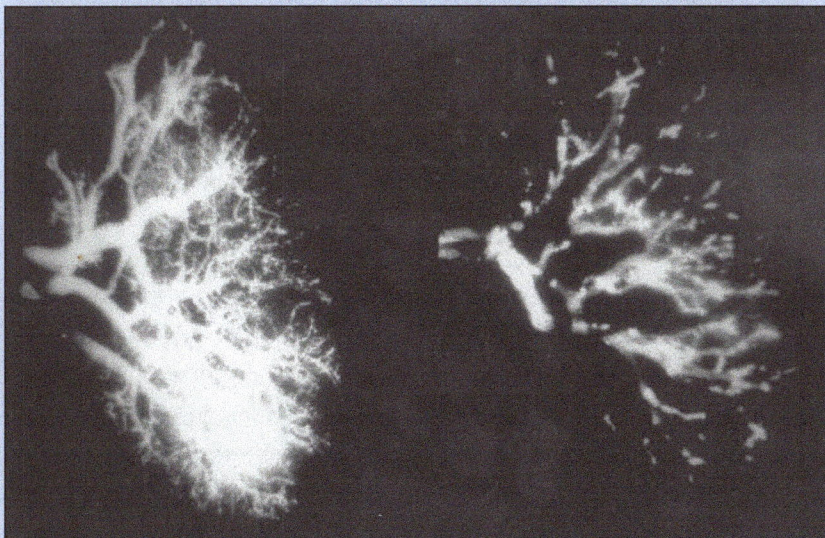

(A)   (B)

What is clear, is that the ability of SSC patients to tolerate shifts in effective intra-vascular blood volume is very limited. Their vascular compartment behaves in an inflexible or stiff manner. Shear stresses caused by changes in intra-vascular volume may contribute to the onset of a renal crisis by the local release of endothelin and ultra-large von-Willebrand factor multimers from vascular endothelial cells. This inability to accommodate changes in intra-vascular volume makes management of SRC difficult, as a single unit of packed cells can precipitate pulmonary oedema. Similarly, reduction of peripheral vascular resistance may cause effective intra-vascular volume depletion. It is our experience that the exquisite sensitivity to intra-vascular volume lasts for some weeks after a crisis, and patients often need to return to ICU several times to manage these "after shocks". These exaggerated responses are not seen in other patients with malignant hypertension, who are in general much easier to manage.

Whether or not renal blood vessels in this condition are more susceptible to shear stresses caused by hypertension is not known, but high circulating levels of endothelin (ET) have been measured during SRC. The endothelins are a homogenous group of vasoconstrictors which also play a role in mitogenesis and angiogenesis. Endothelin-1 causes reduced renal blood flow and GFR. They are synthesised by the vascular endothelium in response to numerous stimuli: injury, ischaemia, endotoxin, inflammatory mediators, thrombin, transforming growth factor β, turbulent blood flow, stretch and shear stress. Plasma ET levels are increased in SRC as are mediators such as PGI_2 (vasodilator) and TxA_2 (vasoconstrictor). Increased renin activity as a consequence of renal under-perfusion, and increased angiotensin II which has smooth muscle proliferative activity, may be partly responsible for the intimal proliferation which is so characteristic of this condition. However, renin and angiotensin levels are elevated in other conditions of renal underperfusion such as hepatorenal syndrome, where no such vascular changes are seen (see **Chapter 25**). It is likely that the additional effect of vascular shear stresses and stretch, perhaps together with fibrin deposition, activation of the clotting cascade and endothelial injury, are required for initiation and perpetuation of the intimal proliferation characteristic of SRC — but common also to ARF associated with malignant hypertension and HUS (see **Chapters 14** and **15**).

Vasodilator and vasoconstrictor prostanoids are also likely to play an important role in SRC. The most important renal vasodilator PGE_2 may be reduced, and treatment with Iloprost, a synthetic equivalent, may improve outcome in this condition. Stratton *et al*. have shown that there are increasing levels of circulating ICAM, VCAM and E-selectin in patients with Raynaud's, limited and diffuse scleroderma, reaching maximum levels in those suffering SRC. Patients in whom sequential measurements were obtained showed incremental rises in these markers of endothelial injury as their disease progressed to SRC.

HISTOPATHOLOGY

It is generally unsafe to perform a renal biopsy during an acute SRC, and biopsies are usually performed when the crisis has abated and BP and platelet counts are back to normal. The renal biopsy findings in SRC are characteristic though not exclusive to SRC. The major changes are seen within the small muscular arteries, which show massive intimal proliferation, often occluding the vessel lumen (**Figure 2A**). These changes are referred to as onion skinning, and fibrinoid necrosis can often be found within the vessel wall. **Figure 2A** (silver stain) clearly shows the internal elastic lamina, which is intact, with massive intimal proliferation obliterating the vascular

Figure 2. (A) Muscular artery showing an intact internal elastic lamina (arrow) with profound intimal proliferation ("onion skinning") obliterating the vascular lumen (silver stain); (B) Collapsed glomerulus with wrinkled basement membrane from a patient recovering from SRC (silver stain)

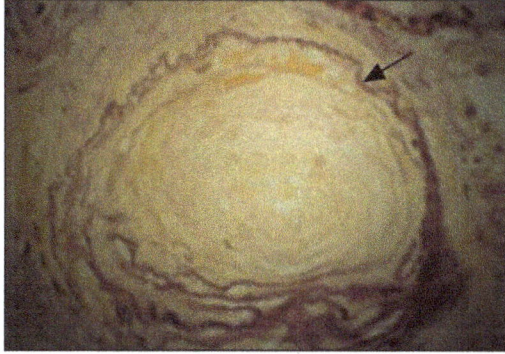 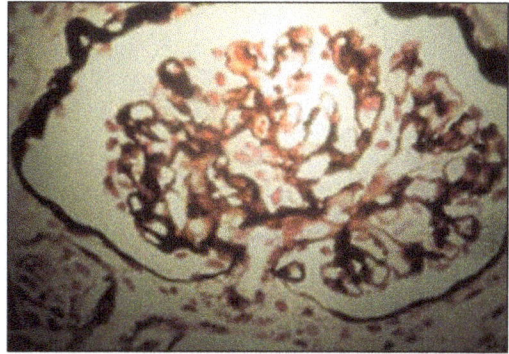

(A)   (B)

lumen. The glomeruli are frequently collapsed or ischaemic with wrinkled basement membranes (**Figure 2B**). Fibrin thrombi can be seen within the afferent arterioles and occasionally within the glomerular capillaries, especially in patients with predominant intravascular haemolysis. Juxta-glomerular hyperplasia has been noted and probably reflects excess renin production. Immunofluorescence staining is usually negative except for complement deposition within the vessel walls. If cortical necrosis has occurred there may be extensive infarction and haemorrhage.

CLINICAL FEATURES AND DIAGNOSIS

• *Symptoms*

Patients undergoing SRC present with a wide range of symptoms which generally reflect the duration and severity of the crisis. Patients whose BP is monitored regularly, and whose crisis is therefore recognised early, often have few if any symptoms. More commonly, however, patients present with headache, vomiting, blurred vision, severe dyspnoea or fitting. Occasional patients present with cerebral haemorrhage. Symptoms related to ARF and intravascular haemolysis may complicate the picture further. Haemorrhage secondary to platelet consumption associated with MAHA is rare but very difficult to manage, although platelet counts are often reduced and of prognostic significance. One characteristic feature of full-blown SRC is profound peripheral vasoconstriction causing the patient's extremities to feel like marble.

• *Clinical signs*

Clinical examination of these patients often reveals a tachycardia with gallop rhythm, and evidence of left and right heart failure. Skin changes are usually diffuse and severe but may be minimal, localised or absent. Hypertensive retinopathy is usually present. The patient may be pale and sweating with a mottled livido-like appearance of the skin. Pericardial effusions may be seen on echocardiography and are occasionally clinically obvious. Mentation may be poor and consequently the patient may be unable to give a clear history.

INVESTIGATIONS

Important investigations are listed in **Table 4**. Certain investigations deserve special mention:

- *Haematological investigations*

It is important to establish whether there is ongoing intra-vascular haemolysis as this carries a particularly poor prognosis. Haemoglobin estimates need to be repeated frequently in the initial stages of management. Platelet counts reflect the severity of MAHA. A film to look for fragmented RBCs is mandatory (a few RBC fragments is normal on film examination; an experienced observer makes this investigation more reliable). Flow cytometric examination of RBCs to estimate the percentage of hyperchromic microcytic cells may become a useful tool, but is still being evaluated as a marker of ongoing haemolysis. LDH levels are also a useful measure of ongoing haemolysis, together with AST, ALT and less reliably bilirubin and haemoglobin. Serum haptoglobin levels are seldom available during an acute illness and are therefore of little use in monitoring haemolysis, but can be helpful in confirming its presence.

Table 4. Investigations during SRC

Haematology/biochemistry	Radiology	Histopathology	Immunology
FBC (Hb*, platelet counts*)	CXR*	Renal biopsy (when BP controlled and platelet count normal)	ANA
U&E (creatinine*/clearance)	US kidneys (size/rule out obstruction)		ENA (Scl 70, RNA polymerase, U1 RNP)
LDH*	Cardiac ECHO		Anti-DNA antibodies
Haptoglobins	CT lungs		C_3/C_4
Bilirubin	DTPA scan of lungs[1]		
AST*	Lung function tests		
ALT*			
RBC film (fragmented RBCs*)			
Arterial blood gases			
SaO_2**			
Renin levels (academic interest only)			

*Useful in monitoring progress; **Use ear lobe as fingers may be inaccurate due to very poor perfusion of digits.
[1]Used to assess degree of pulmonary fibrosis.

- *Immunological investigations*

Autoantibody profiles may help to confirm the diagnosis of SSC and anti-topoisomerase (Scl 70) antibodies in particular are more likely to be present in patients undergoing SRC than in other SSC patients. Anti-RNA polymerase autoantibodies were present in 9/14 (65%) of our SRC patient group compared with 7.3% of the general scleroderma population ($P < 0.0001$). Anti-Scl 70 antibodies were found in 5/24 (21%) of patients with SRC and in 17/50 (34%) of control SSC patients. Clearly, the presence of these auto-antibodies is seldom of use during the acute illness but may identify patients with SSC who are at particular risk of SRC.

- *Physiological investigations*

Blood gases are required to assess respiratory function. CXR may reveal an enlarged heart with a distinct globular outline, suggesting a pericardial effusion. There may be changes of pulmonary oedema or fibrosis, although the latter is more easily demonstrated by fine cut CT scanning or DTPA lung scans.

An ECG usually confirms the tachycardia and may show evidence of left heart strain or RV hypertrophy in patients with known pulmonary hypertension. Voltage may be diminished in patients with pericardial effusions.

During the acute crisis, patient monitoring is greatly facilitated by insertion of a central line with measurement of central venous pressures. In the case of patients who are severely unwell, Swan-Ganz monitoring, which facilitates measurement of peripheral vascular resistance (PVR) and cardiac output (CO), is very valuable (see **Chapter 5**).

MANAGEMENT OF SCLERODERMA RENAL CRISIS

The management of SRC is directed at controlling the severe hypertension; however, unlike other causes of malignant hypertension, the extreme rigidity of the vasculature and frequent co-existence of restrictive cardiomyopathy and pulmonary hypertension makes this a difficult task. The key issues are:

- How quickly to reduce the blood pressure?
- Which are the best agents to achieve this?
- How best to maintain this reduction?

If possible, rapid reduction of BP should be avoided. However, if the patient has severe left heart failure or evidence of cerebral haemorrhage or ongoing intra-vascular haemolysis then a more rapid correction of BP is desirable. Under these circumstances Swan-Ganz monitoring is advisable in order to optimise right and left ventricular filling pressures while BP is being reduced.

Oral Therapy

Very fast acting agents such as sub-lingual nifedipine and β-blockers should be avoided, the latter because tachycardia may be appropriate for the patient undergoing SRC and β blockade may cause an abrupt decrease in CO.

The use of ACEI has heralded a dramatic improvement in outcome in this condition, which as recently as 1970s was universally fatal. It is sensible to use a low-dose short acting agent, such as captopril 6.25 mg t.d.s, initially during a crisis in order to facilitate adjustments in accordance with the patient's response. Later, when the patient's condition stabilizes, longer acting ACEI which have preferential binding to renal tissues may be more appropriate. This is a personal preference not supported by evidence, as there is none available to guide management. Patients whose crises are identified early may require nothing more than the introduction of an ACEI to gently reduce BP; however, patients undergoing severe crises require intravenous agents to assist BP reduction. Very often these patients are vomiting and therefore cannot tolerate oral agents.

Intravenous Therapy

The choice of intravenous agent is important. Agents such as GTN and hydralazine have been used successfully, but the vasodilator PGE_2 analogue iloprost offers many advantages over its older rivals. Firstly, dosage can be titrated accurately to achieve targeted BP lowering. Secondly, its anti-platelet activity may be beneficial in breaking the cycle of platelet aggregation and fibrin deposition. In addition, in our series of patients, renal function was more likely to be preserved in those treated with iloprost, and in those who required dialysis, recovery was more likely to occur if iloprost had been used in the initial management.

Recommended Treatment Regimen

Commence an iloprost infusion at low dose (5 ng/kg/min) increasing every 10 min in order to achieve a 10–15 mmHg BP reduction over the first 24 h of treatment. At the same time the ACEI can be commenced. Once the BP target is achieved, the iloprost infusion can be maintained at a constant dose. Further daily target BP reductions of 10 mmHg can be achieved by incremental increases in the iloprost dose. At the same time it is usually possible to increase the ACEI until a dose of captopril 25 mg t.d.s is achieved. A short acting α-blocker (prazosin) can also be introduced gradually to allow reduction and eventual cessation of the iloprost infusion within 3–7 days. After 2–3 weeks, when the patient's condition is stable, longer acting agents can be substituted instead of captopril and prazosin.

In a retrospective examination of our 33 patients' outcome, BP was restored to pre-crisis levels over an average of nine days in patients who recovered without requiring dialysis, whereas those patients who required dialysis had their BP lowered to pre-crisis levels in three days. Clearly, these data are subject to bias as patients undergoing a full blown crisis, with severe cardiac decompensation, were more likely to have their BP lowered aggressively. Nevertheless, maintaining perfusion through renal blood vessels narrowed by intimal proliferation is likely to enhance renal survival.

In the months following a renal crisis, patients frequently demonstrate a reduced requirement for anti-hypertensive medication. It would seem sensible that a low dose of a long-acting ACEI be maintained if possible in these patients as repeated renal crises can occur.

Figure 3. (A) CXR of a patient prior to developing SRC; (B) CXR during SRC demonstrating severe pulmonary oedema. Note the presence of an endotracheal tube and Swan-Ganz catheter, the tip of which can be seen in the right pulmonary artery; (C) CXR taken when the patient's PVR had been lowered and the pulmonary oedema resolved. Note the right sided subclavian catheter which was used for dialysis

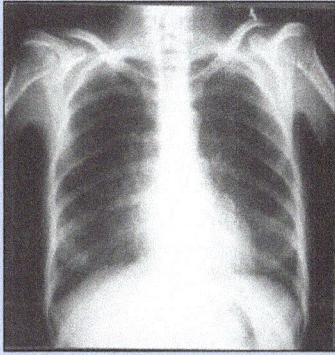 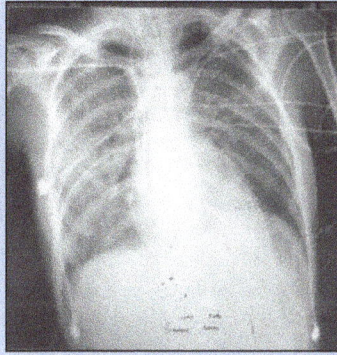 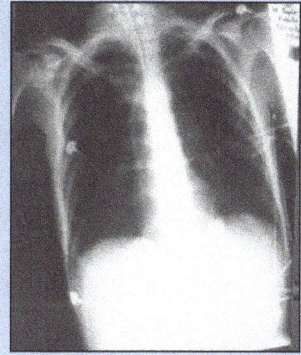

| (A) | (B) | (C) |

Supportive Therapy

Full supportive care with ventilation and intensive care may be necessary. Fitting should be controlled with diazepam, sodium valproate or phenytoin. Pain relief may be required in those patients with painful ulceration of fingers. Nephrotoxic agents, NSAIDs, contrast, and aggravating agents such as steroids, the oral contraceptive pill and cyclosporin A, should be stopped. If intravascular haemolysis is a significant feature, plasma exchange for fresh frozen plasma should be considered. In patients not requiring dialysis a further rise in creatinine is usually seen for 7–10 days after initiation of treatment. The usual pattern then is for creatinine to stabilise before falling gradually. Continued improvements in renal function have been recorded in patients following renal crises for up to 10 years. **Figures 3A**, **3B** and **3C** demonstrate the CXR changes in one patient who was treated on ICU during a renal crisis. The improved appearances coincided with reduction of PVR with intravenous iloprost, which improved CO and facilitated resolution of pulmonary oedema.

Dialysis in SRC

Both haemodialysis (HD) and peritoneal dialysis (PD) can be undertaken in patients who develop renal failure secondary to a renal crisis. During the acute illness, when management of intravascular volume is critical, continuous methods of renal replacement therapy, e.g. CVVH, may be easier to manage (see **Chapter 9**). If intermittent HD is used, daily dialysis may be necessary to avoid large fluctuations in intra-vascular volume, especially as temperature reduction is not advisable to assist with the ultrafiltration process. PD can, however, provide an acceptable alternative as the warmed PD fluid may be beneficial; during the acute phase of the crisis ultrafiltration volumes can be unpredictable and may therefore complicate management. CAPD and intermittent

HD have both been used to maintain stable scleroderma patients whose renal function has not yet recovered. No reliable information is available to suggest which modality enhances the chances of renal recovery. We have encountered patients whose renal function has recovered while maintained on both methods of treatment.

OUTCOME OF SCLERODERMA RENAL CRISIS

- Early 1970s: universally fatal within one year of onset (Medsger *et al.*).
- Late 1970s: anecdotal survivors with ACEI.
- 11/62 (18%) survivors (Traub *et al.*).
- Post ACEI analysis — patient survival 73%, kidney survival 50% (Stein *et al.*).
- Maintained on ACEI after starting dialysis — 11/20 recovered renal function versus 0/15 not maintained on ACEI (Stein *et al.*).

RENAL TRANSPLANTATION FOLLOWING SCLERODERMA RENAL CRISIS

Based on recent data from the American United Network for Organ Sharing (UNOS) Renal Transplant Registry, and from the European renal registry, renal transplantation appears to be an effective method of treatment for scleroderma patients who do not regain renal function within 1–2 years of their renal crisis. Special consideration needs to be given to co-morbid factors, such as restrictive cardiomyopathy and pulmonary hypertension. Chang *et al.* have reported the results of transplanting 86 such patients over a ten year period. The overall mortality was 24% and 44% of the grafts failed over the ten year period. One year graft survival was 62%. Two patients had a recurrence of SRC which caused the transplanted kidney to be lost. Interestingly, 60% of patients were treated with cyclosporin, in addition to prednisolone and azathioprine, without apparent triggering of SRC.

ANTI-PHOSPHOLIPID SYNDROME

In the early 1980s, a clinical syndrome of widespread arterial and venous thrombosis associated with antibodies directed against phospholipids was described. Though initially termed anti-cardiolipin syndrome, it is now agreed that the condition is more appropriately called the anti-phospholipid syndrome (APS). Features include stroke, transient ischaemic attacks, hypertension, recurrent abortions, migraine, livido reticularis, pulmonary hypertension, thrombocytopenia, ocular ischaemia and heart valve abnormalities. Up to one third of patients with SLE also have anti-phospholipid antibodies, but in long-term follow-up, patients with anti-phospholipid antibodies alone do not develop SLE. This has led to the term primary anti-phospholipid syndrome (PAPS). It is now recognised that anti-phospholipid antibodies are in fact a diverse group of antibodies which require a plasma protein co-factor, β_2-glycoprotein 1 (β_2-GPI), to bind to their negatively charged phospholipid antigen targets. Patients with this condition may develop ARF associated with thrombotic microangiopathies, which are particularly likely to occur during pregnancy.

Bilateral renal vein thrombosis has been reported in this condition. Catastrophic APS is also recognised, where patients develop acute collapse with multi-organ failure, including ARF, associated with widespread thrombosis, thrombocytopaenia and acute respiratory distress syndrome. Management of the ARF is by anti-coagulation and supportive treatment. Renal biopsies taken from such patients resemble those of SRC, although some observers have noted increased numbers of glomerular thrombi. Pregnancy carries an increased risk of pre-eclamptic toxaemia and ARF (see **Chapter 27**). In these circumstances, the pathogenesis is likely to be placental thrombosis and ischaemia.

MIXED CONNECTIVE TISSUE DISEASE

Mixed connective tissue disease (MCTD) is a controversial subject and many clinical investigators do not view it as a separate clinical entity. Nevertheless, it defines a group of patients with distinct clinical features, autoantibody profiles and prognosis. The characteristic antibodies, usually found in high titres, are directed against U1 RNP (a ribonuclease-sensitive extractable nuclear antigen). Most patients have Raynaud's phenomenon, hand oedema, or puffy fingers and many develop pulmonary hypertension, but rarely have seizures or psychosis. Patients with MCTD seldom develop the diffuse proliferative glomerulonephritis often seen in SLE; therefore ARF is uncommon unless the patient develops a scleroderma like vasculopathy. The characteristic antigen U1 RNP is now known to consist of RNA plus three proteins A, C and a 68 kDa protein. The clinical disease is most closely associated with antibodies directed against the A and 68 kDa proteins; however, as yet these specific antibodies cannot be measured routinely. Further, some of these patients also demonstrate IgM antibodies against another extractable nuclear antigen, Sm (a 28 kDa protein complex), and switching of these antibodies to an IgG class can herald a phenotypic change in disease from MCTD to more classical SLE.

FURTHER READING

Balow JE, Boumpas DT, Fessler BJ, Austin HA (1996) Management of lupus nephritis. *Kidney International*; 49(suppl. 53): 88–92

Bennett RM (1990) Scleroderma overlap syndromes. *Rheumatic Diseases and Clinics of North America*; 16: 185–198

Black C, Isenberg DA (1992) Mixed connective tissue disease-goodbye to all that. *British Journal of Rheumatology*; 31: 695

Hughes G (1993) The antiphospholipid antibody syndrome: Ten years on. *Lancet*; 342: 341

Medsger TA Jr., Masi AT, Rodnan GP, et al. (1971) Survival with systemic sclerosis (scleroderma). A life-table analysis of clinical and demographic factors in 309 patients. *Annals of Internal Medicine*; 75: 369–376

Steen VD, Medsger TA (1984) Factors predicting development of renal involvement in progressive systemic sclerosis. *American Journal of Medicine*; 76: 779

Steen VD, Medsger TA (2000) Long-term outcomes of scleroderma renal crisis. *Annals of Internal Medicine*; 133: 600–603

Steinberg AD (1995) Insights into the basis of systemic Lupus. *Journal of Autoimmunity*; 8: 771–775

Stratton RJ, Coghlan JG, Pearson JD, et al. (1998) Different patterns of endothelial cell activation in renal and pulmonary vascular disease in scleroderma. *Quarterly Journal of Medicine*; 91: 561–566

Traub YM, Shapiro AP, Rodnan GP, *et al.* (1983) Hypertension and renal failure (scleroderma renal crisis) in progressive systemic sclerosis. Review of a 25-year experience with 68 cases. *Medicine (Baltimore)*; 62: 335–352

Tuffanelli DL, Winkelman RK (1961) Systemic scleroderma: A clinical study of 727 cases. *Archives of Dermatology*; 84: 359

Uramoto KM, Michet CJ, Thumboo J (1999) Trends in the incidence and mortality of systemic lupus erythematosus 1950–1992. *Arthritis and Rheumatism*; 42: 46–50

Chapter 18 _____

ACUTE TUBULOINTERSTITIAL NEPHRITIS
Richard Baker

DEFINITION

Acute tubulointerstitial nephritis (ATIN) encompasses the clinical syndrome of acute renal impairment and florid tubulointerstitial inflammation, with absent or minimal glomerular abnormalities, on renal biopsy. Notably this definition excludes ARF secondary to glomerular or vascular disease, both of which may have prominent interstitial infiltrates, and also pyelonephritis due to direct bacterial invasion. The exact incidence of ATIN is hard to gauge, partly due to the different indications for renal biopsy in different series. In a series of 109 patients from a large centre, biopsied for unexplained renal impairment with normal sized kidneys, ATIN accounted for 27% of cases. Recognition of this disease is therefore important as it represents a significant cause of ARF, particularly when no obvious cause of acute tubular necrosis exists. In addition, amelioration of renal function usually follows the identification and cessation of any inciting agent. There is also some evidence that treatment with corticosteroids leads to both more rapid and more complete renal recovery.

PATHOPHYSIOLOGY

Acute interstitial nephritis (ATIN) was first described by Councilman in 1898, at Harvard Medical School, Boston. He described a series of forty-two autopsies, all of whom had characteristic, "cellular and fluid exudation in the interstitial tissue..." These cases were largely caused by diphtheria and scarlet fever. He noted that the exudate was not purulent and that the kidneys were themselves sterile. He speculated that the cells might accumulate because "soluble substances may exert a positive chemotaxis". Crucially, he had made the observation that the tissue damage was not due to direct microbial invasion but due to "allergic-type" immunopathology. In 1946, a series of patients with ATIN was described in which all the patients had been treated with sulphonamides, but it was not entirely clear whether the inciting agent was the drug itself or the underlying infection. However, in the ensuing years, links between phenindione, and then methicillin, and ATIN were established, confirming drug allergy as a cause of ATIN. With the widespread use of percutaneous biopsies throughout the 1950s and 1960s, ATIN became increasingly recognised as a cause of acute renal impairment.

The exact pathophysiology remains far from clear but there are a number of observations, predominantly derived from series of drug-related ATIN, that suggest the renal damage is immune mediated.

Evidence for Immune Aetiology

- Clinical features suggestive of an allergic phenomenon — rash, fever, arthralgia and eosinophilia.
- Histopathology — biopsies reveal intense interstitial infiltrates of lymphocytes and other immune effector cells, which stain for markers of activation.
- Delayed-type hypersensitivity (DTH) response to intradermal injection of the offending drug in some patients.
- Positive *in vitro* lymphocyte stimulation tests — incubation of patients' T lymphocytes with the offending drug, *in vitro*, causes them to proliferate.
- Memory response — inadvertent rechallenge with the offending drug has led to accelerated recrudescence of disease in some cases.
- Animal models — two murine models of tubulointerstitial inflammation, the *kd/kd* mouse and the *anti-TBM* model, have been clearly shown to be caused by nephritogenic T cells and antibodies respectively.

Immunopathogenesis

Despite the circumstantial evidence linking an aberrant immune response to the tissue damage in ATIN, surprisingly little is known about the disease process in man. Putative immunopathological mechanisms are derived largely from animal models and are illustrated in **Figure 1**. It is helpful to divide the T cell response into an afferent phase, whereby CD4+ T cells become activated by nephritogenic antigens, and an efferent phase in which effector cells bring about renal inflammation.

- *Afferent phase*

The afferent part of the immune response to a renal antigen is likely to be mediated by migratory antigen presenting cells (APCs), such as macrophages and dendritic cells, which carry immunogenic peptides from the kidney into regional lymph nodes. In the lymph node, APCs can prime CD4+ T cells which in turn orchestrate the efferent phase of the response. The identity of these immunogenic peptides is unknown as none of the antigens in human ATIN have been characterised, unlike in animal models of TIN, where a 30 kDa tubular protein, 3-M1, has been shown to be the target antigen in the murine anti-tubular basement membrane (TBM) model . In humans, putative nephritogenic antigens might be derived from a number of sources:

- They might be intrinsic renal antigens or exogenous antigens that become deposited in the kidney.
- In the case of drug related ATIN, it is possible that the drug acts as a hapten, whereby it binds to intrinsic renal structures, such as the GBM, and facilitates the recognition of a new conformational antigen by T cells. In this context, the discovery of a metabolite of methicillin, dimethoxyphenylpenicilloyl, along the TBM in methicillin-related ATIN was encouraging but it was soon offset by the demonstration of similar deposits in patients who did not develop ATIN.
- In theory, drugs might directly damage renal structures, rendering them immunogenic.

Figure 1. Possible mechanisms for immunopathogenesis of ATIN

Nephritogenic antigens, which may be either planted antigens or parts of intrinsic renal structures, are processed by antigen presenting cells (APCs) and presented to CD4$^+$ T cells in association with class II MHC molecules. This causes CD4$^+$ T cell activation and proliferation. Once activated, these CD4$^+$ T cells are able to orchestrate three main immune effector mechanisms. Firstly they can assist B cells to produce nephritogenic antibodies against renal structures. Secondly they can help to activate cytotoxic CD8$^+$ T cells with receptors specific for renal tubular cells. Finally CD4$^+$ T cells may recirculate to the kidney themselves and initiate delayed-type hypersensitivity (DTH) reactions. These effector mechanisms collectively bring about renal inflammation with eventual resolution or fibrosis and chronic renal impairment. Alternatively CD4$^+$ T cells may be activated directly by antigens on the renal tubular cells themselves. Finally, other proteins may share antigenic sequences with renal tubular epithelial cells (RTEC), and an immune response to the unrelated antigen could lead to renal damage as a result of "molecular mimicry".

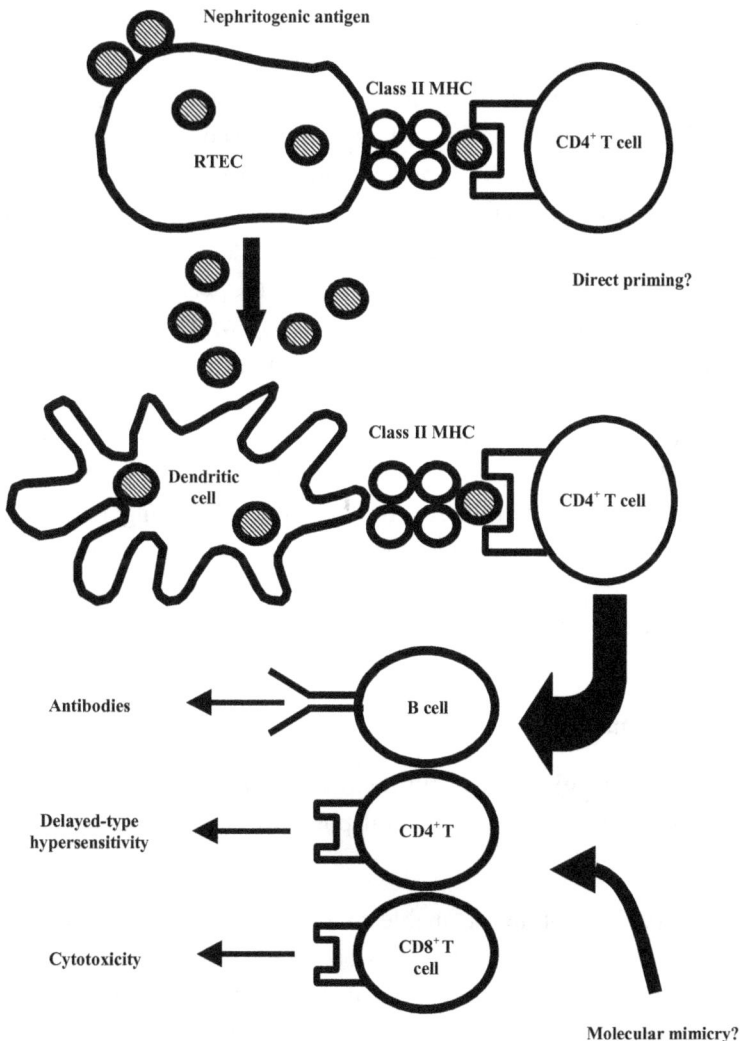

- Cross-reaction or "molecular mimicry", such that the T cells would be primed elsewhere in the body, by non-renal antigens, and the effector cells would then cross-react with renal tubular antigens. Indeed it has been shown that there are antibodies to nephritogenic streptococci that cross-react with type IV collagen, and antibodies to *Escherichia coli* that cross-react with Tamm-Horsfall protein.

The afferent part of the response might also be brought about by CD4$^+$ T cells primed directly on renal tubular epithelial cells, by any of the first three mechanisms above. These cells express the necessary MHC class II antigens, but there is uncertainty as to whether they possess the other requisite molecules to function as APCs.

- *Efferent phase*

Once CD4$^+$ T cells are activated they are then equipped to unleash the effector arm of the immune response. They can cooperate with B cells to produce antibodies, activate cytotoxic CD8$^+$ T cells, or travel to the kidney themselves to set up a delayed-type hypersensitivity (DTH) reaction, releasing cytokines that attract and activate macrophages to augment the inflammation. Amplification is further facilitated by the increased expression of adhesion molecules (e.g. VLA-4/VCAM-1 and LFA-1/ICAM-1) and chemokines (e.g. MCP-1) within the mononuclear infiltrates in ATIN . In different animal models each of the above three effector mechanisms can be shown to predominate, but in human ATIN it would appear that DTH is the main protagonist, as evidenced by the presence of granulomas on biopsy and positive skin-prick testing in some patients. Immunofluorescence is usually negative on biopsy which mitigates against a prominent humoral mechanism, except in the extremely rare cases of anti-TBM disease. CD8$^+$ cytotoxic T cells may be important in tubulitis leading to tubular atrophy.

The conclusion of the immune response is either resolution, with near complete recovery of function, or fibrosis, tubular atrophy and chronic renal failure. Interestingly, in animal models, fibrogenesis can be demonstrated within seven days of the initiating insult. In addition, renal tubular epithelial cells can alter their phenotype, synthesising collagen and contributing to this process. Fibrosis is mediated by a number of cytokines amongst which transforming growth factor-β (TGF-β) and platelet derived growth factor (PDGF) are prominent.

Mechanism of Acute Renal Failure

ATIN leads to a reduction in glomerular filtration rate (GFR) despite there being little or no morphological changes in the glomeruli. Several possible explanations have been advanced to explain this:

- "Clogged drain theory" — filtrate is unable to flow from glomeruli into tubules that have become blocked by a combination of distortion secondary to profound interstitial cellular infiltrates, and the shedding and aggregation of damaged tubular cells.
- The hydrostatic pressure within the oedematous interstitium rises leading to increased resistance in both glomerular arterioles, and therefore a decline in renal blood flow with a consequent reduction in GFR.

- Interstitial inflammation and tubular damage reduce the amount of sodium reabsorbed in the proximal tubule and thick ascending limb. This leads to an increased tubular flow rate which is detected by cells in the *macula densa* of the juxtaglomerular apparatus. Tubuloglomerular feedback counteracts this effect by reducing GFR, predominantly via vasoconstriction of the afferent arteriole.
- Decreased GFR might be mediated by an alteration in the balance of vasoactive hormones and cytokines produced not only by intrinsic renal cells but also by the infiltrating inflammatory cells.

In general, the magnitude of the reduction in GFR correlates with the extent of interstitial cellular infiltrates on the biopsy.

HISTOPATHOLOGY

Grossly the kidneys appear swollen and grey with occasional petechial haemorrhages. Light microscopy reveals the following notable features (see also **Chapter 7**):

- Increased interstitial volume, mainly due to oedema.
- Focal mononuclear cell infiltrates within the interstitium, especially at the corticomedullary junction. These infiltrates predominantly consist of CD4$^+$ and CD8$^+$ T lymphocytes.
- Monocytes/macrophages are also abundant.
- Plasma cells may be present to a lesser degree.
- Eosinophils may be prominent, especially in drug-related ATIN.
- Granulomas, particularly in drug-induced ATIN, infection-related ATIN and sarcoidosis.
- Varying degrees of damage to tubular cells with tubulitis, i.e. lymphocytic invasion of tubular epithelium across the TBM.
- Minimal change disease may be present in association with NSAID-induced ATIN.
- Sparing of glomerular and vascular structures.
- Phenotypic analysis of infiltrating T lymphocytes reveals a variable CD4$^+$/CD8$^+$ ratio and increased expression of activation markers, e.g. MHC class II, LFA-1 and CD25.
- Phenotypic analysis of tubular cells shows increased expression of MHC class II antigens and adhesion molecules such as ICAM-1 and VCAM-1.
- Immunofluorescence studies are usually negative except in rare cases of anti-TBM disease.
- Electron micrographs show non-specific, chaotic interstitial hypercellularity and tubular damage.

AETIOLOGY

There are four broad categories of ATIN (see **Table 1** and **Table 2**):

1. Drug-Related

Many drugs have been implicated in the aetiology of ATIN and it is important to be vigilant for new associations. Drug-related cases seem to form an increasing percentage of more recent series, although it is often unclear whether the ATIN is causally related to the antecedent infection or to the drug itself. In many cases the only clinical manifestation is ARF which improves with

Table 1. The aetiology of ATIN

Causes	Common specific examples
1. Drug-related	
β-Lactam antibiotics	Methicillin, ampicillin, cephalosporins
Macrolides	Erythromycin
Sulphonamides	Cotrimoxazole
Quinolones	Ciprofloxacin
Aminoglycosides	Gentamicin
Tetracyclines	Minocycline
Anti-mycobacterial	Rifampicin
Antiviral	Aciclovir
H_2-antagonists	Cimetidine, ranitidine
Diuretics	Thiazides, triamterene, furosemide
NSAIDs	Fenoprofen, mefenamic acid
Anticonvulsants	Carbamazepine, phenytoin
5-aminosalicylates	Mesalazine
Analgesics	Paracetamol, 5-ASA, aspirin
Herbal medicines	Aristolochic acid
Anticoagulants	Phenindione
Other	Allopurinol, phenytoin, clofibrate, α-methyldopa
2. Infection-related	
Bacterial	Streptococci, Staphylococci, Corynebacteria, Brucella, Legionella, Campylobacter
Viral	CMV, HIV, EBV, Hantavirus
Other	Toxoplasma, Mycoplasma, Leishmania, Rickettsia, Leptospira
3. Associated with multisystem disease	
Sarcoidosis	
Systemic lupus erythematosus	
Sjögren's syndrome	
Cryoglobulinaemia	
Primary systemic vasculitis	
4. Idiopathic	
Unassociated idiopathic	
With uveitis (TINU)	
Anti-TBM disease	
With anti-neutrophil cytoplasmic antibodies (ANCAs)	

Table 2. Accumulated aetiological data from four recent series

	Buysen et al. (1990)	Hammersmith (1986–1997)	Shibasaki et al. (1991)	Laberke et al. (1980)	OVERALL	%
β-lactams	3	7	8	7	25	22.5
Sulphonamides	1	3		2	6	5.4
Rifampicin	1	3		1	5	4.5
Macrolides		3			3	2.7
Aminoglycosides		2		1	3	2.7
Chloramphenicol				1	1	0.9
Quinolones			2		2	1.8
Tetracyclines	1	1	1	5	8	7.2
Diuretics		2			2	1.8
NSAIDs	3	2	2	1	8	7.2
H$_2$ antagonists	3	1			4	3.6
Anticonvulsants	2			2	4	3.6
Allopurinol		1			1	0.9
Analgesics	1	1	1	2	5	4.5
Drug-related	**15**	**26**	**14**	**22**	**77**	**69.4**
Pneumococci	1				1	0.9
Streptococci	2			1	3	2.7
Mycobacteria	1	4			5	4.5
Leptospira	3				3	2.7
Legionella	1				1	0.9
Syphilis	1				1	0.9
Infection-related	**9**	**4**	**0**	**1**	**14**	**12.6**
Idiopathic	3	3		11	17	15.3
TINU		2			2	1.8
Sarcoid		1			1	0.9
Other	**3**	**6**	**0**	**11**	**20**	**18.0**
TOTAL	**27**	**36**	**14**	**34**	**111**	**100.0**

the cessation of multiple drugs. In this case, there is a tendency to incriminate the drug that is most commonly associated with ATIN. Thus, it is often difficult to establish a definite culprit. The published series of patients with ATIN should be considered with this in mind.

2. Infection-Related

Despite the original description of ATIN in patients with infectious diseases, this cause is becoming increasingly uncommon in the antibiotic era. Infection-related disease may be either due to direct

Table 3. Infection-related ATIN

Mechanism	Common specific examples
1. Allergic-type	
Bacteria	Streptococci, Staphylococci, Corynebacteria, Brucella, Legionella, Salmonella, Mycoplasma, Pneumococci
Viruses	EBV, HIV, Rubeola, Kawasaki disease, Hepatitis A
Parasites	Leishmania, Toxoplasma
2. Direct invasion	
Bacterial	Pyelonephritis (multiple species), Mycobacteria, Leptospira
Fungi	Pyelonephritis (multiple species), Histoplasma
Rickettsia	Rickettsia rickettsii, Mediterranean spotted fever
Viruses	CMV, Hantaviruses, Polyoma viruses (BK and JC), Adenovirus, Enterovirus

invasion or by indirect allergic-type reactions to a systemic infection. Direct infection is distinguished from acute pyelonephritis by a number of features.

- Pyelonephritis is associated by characteristic local and systemic clinical features.
- Pyelonephritis is focal, with sharp demarcation from the surrounding parenchyma, and it is usually limited to one individual pyramid.
- The pyelonephritic infiltrate is dominated by neutrophils.

The distinction between directly invasive ATIN and reactive disease is illustrated in **Table 3**; however in some infections the differentiation between these two entities is not entirely clear-cut. Leptospira, for example, can only be demonstrated in about two-thirds of biopsy samples from patients with leptospirosis.

3. Associated with Multisystem Disease

ATIN may be the predominant histological finding in SLE although it is far more common to have significant accompanying glomerular lesions. Similarly, ATIN is occasionally the predominant feature in primary systemic vasculitis. Histological evidence of tubulointerstitial nephritis is probably common in sarcoidosis although usually it is clinically silent. Occasionally, however, patients may present with an acute TIN, i.e. with acute renal impairment.

4. Idiopathic

Some of these cases have an association with uveitis, anti-TBM antibodies or even anti-neutrophil cytoplasmic antibodies (ANCA). However their pathogenesis remains obscure.

CLINICAL PRESENTATION

Although the evolution is highly variable, ATIN commonly presents with ARF which may be slower in onset than rapidly progressive glomerular disease. When there is no obvious precipitant for acute tubular necrosis and an ultrasound examination reveals normal sized kidneys then there is a high likelihood that ATIN is the cause of renal failure (10–25% of cases in different series). However, the clinical findings are inconsistent and this is reflected in some series where biopsy-proven ATIN has been mistaken clinically for other forms of ARF. With this qualification in mind, there are some features to look for during the clinical assessment:

History

- Prior history of infection or drug exposure may be obtained.
- Details should be sought of over the counter medications such as NSAID creams and herbal remedies.
- The patient may already be suffering from an associated multisystem disease.
- Non-specific features such as malaise, anorexia and fatigue are common.
- Typically a low-grade fever and arthralgia are present.
- There may have been a fleeting skin rash.
- Non-specific symptoms of uraemia may be evident.
- Gross haematuria is unusual.
- Urinary output is variable.
- Rarely, flank pain may be described, presumably due to renal capsular stretching.

Examination

- Pyrexia.
- There may be a rash, which is usually an erythematous maculopapular eruption.
- Joint movement may be uncomfortable.
- Hypertension and signs of fluid retention are unusual except in the case of NSAID-induced ATIN.
- Uveitis.
- Evidence of a multisystem disease.

  With regard to drug exposure the following points should be borne in mind:

- ATIN is an idiosyncratic reaction and *not* dose related.
- It may occur at any time after starting drug therapy, i.e. not necessarily 2–3 weeks.
- The triad of fever, rash and eosinophilia is present in only a minority of cases.
- Prior tolerance to a medication does not preclude its involvement in ATIN.

INVESTIGATIONS

Certain Diagnosis of ATIN is only Possible by Renal Biopsy

Despite this, a number of other tests are usually carried out and they may have characteristic results. It is a fact, however, that none of them is either specific or sensitive enough to ensure the diagnosis:

- *Biochemistry*

A rise in both urea and creatinine is observed and increasingly often this occurs in a hospitalised patient undergoing treatment for an unrelated condition. Immunoglobulin levels and liver function tests are sometimes elevated.

- *Haematology*

Eosinophilia is sometimes seen, particularly in drug-related ATIN.

- *Autoantibodies*

Positive tests for P-ANCA have been observed in some cases of drug-related ATIN (omeprazole and ciprofloxacin) while C-ANCAs have been described in the TINU syndrome. ANA and anti-dsDNA levels may be raised in lupus-related ATIN.

- *Urinalysis*

Eosinophiluria is commonly seen with Hansel's stain. The urinary sediment usually contains red cells, white cells and white cell casts. Red cell casts have been described only exceptionally and suggest glomerular disease. Proteinuria is almost universal but is only moderate (<1 g/24 h). Nephrotic range proteinuria may occur in association with NSAID-related ATIN.

- *Functional tubular abnormalities*

Salt-wasting, magnesium-wasting, Fanconi's syndrome and renal tubular acidosis have all been reported and are probably common if sought.

- *Ultrasonography*

Ultrasound usually shows normal-sized or sometimes enlarged kidneys.

- *67-Gallium scanning*

Typically diffuse, bilateral and intense renal uptake is observed, corresponding with the dense interstitial cellular infiltrates. However these findings are not universal and may be seen in other renal disorders.

TREATMENT PRINCIPLES (see **Practice Point**)

1. General Considerations

- Withdraw any drug that might be implicated. Where the patient is on multiple drugs then any non-essential agents should be withdrawn immediately. Essential drugs can then either be substituted with an alternative or withdrawn serially allowing seven days for a response to occur.
- Treat any possible underlying infection.
- General supportive treatment of renal failure, including the provision of dialysis.

2. Specific Treatment

Corticosteroids

There have been no large-scale prospective randomised trials of corticosteroid therapy in ATIN. However there is considerable evidence from small retrospective case-controlled studies suggesting that treatment with corticosteroids hastens the improvement in renal function and ensures a more complete recovery. Once the diagnosis is made, treatment should begin with prednisolone 1 mg/kg/day (Maximum 60 kg/day). This dose should be maintained for two weeks and then tapered off over two to three months. If no response occurs after a month then the drug can be stopped. An alternative is to give three pulses of i/v methylprednisolone (0.5–1.0 g) on three consecutive days at the outset.

Plasma exchange

May be justified in the exceptional case of anti-TBM disease.

Cyclophosphamide and cyclosporin

Though both these agents have been shown to be efficacious in animal models, there is only anecdotal evidence to support their use in refractory cases of human ATIN.

3. Prevention

- It is important that clinicians are aware of the drugs that commonly cause ATIN. Through regular reporting of adverse reactions, certain drugs have been withdrawn, e.g. methicillin, phenacetin and glafenin.
- Any offending drug should be clearly marked in the patients' notes to prevent inadvertent rechallenge.

OUTCOME

Renal function usually improves rapidly within the first 6 to 8 weeks. It may continue to improve slowly over the ensuing year. However, a significant minority of patients (<10%) may recover only partially or even remain dialysis-dependent. The limited data available suggest that the following are associated with poor prognosis:

1. Biopsy

- Diffuse disease.
- Atrophic tubules and advanced interstitial fibrosis.
- Prominent neutrophils.
- Granulomas.

The focal nature of the disease and the highly selective sampling of core biopsies should be borne in mind.

2. Clinical features

- Increasing age.
- Renal failure of greater than three weeks duration.

DISTINCT CLINICAL SUBGROUPS

Methicillin

This drug, which has now been discontinued, was associated with the highest incidence of ATIN. It caused a distinctive and florid type of ATIN with a number of characteristic features:

- Mean duration of drug treatment was 15 days (range 10–45 days).
- Overall 2% of patients exposed to methicillin developed ATIN, rising to 15% if courses were over 2 weeks.
- An accelerated recrudescence of disease was observed in those who were re-exposed.
- Fever, skin rashes, arthralgia, fevers and eosinophilia were common.
- Renal failure was non-oliguric in two-thirds of cases.
- Recovery was usually rapid and complete.

Rifampicin

Many cases of ATIN associated with rifampicin have been described and the clinical picture is often characteristic:

- ATIN may occur many months after the initiation of treatment.
- It was previously more common with intermittent administration, i.e. two doses weekly.
- Circulating antibodies to rifampicin are often detected.
- Clinically the onset is abrupt with fever, chills, vomiting, diarrhoea, abdominal pain and myalgias.
- Abnormal liver function tests, haemolysis and thrombocytopaenia may occur.
- Rapid and severe recrudescence upon re-exposure.

Non-Steroidal Anti-Inflammatory Drugs (NSAIDs)

These drugs are amongst the most widely prescribed, particularly amongst an ageing population. Moreover they are available without prescription in a number of different preparations, including topical creams. It is therefore crucial to enquire quite specifically about their use during the clinical history. ATIN is one of the rarer renal side effects of these drugs but it has a number of distinctive clinical features:

- Pre-morbid exposure may range from 2 weeks to many years.
- Propionic acid derivatives, fenoprofen, ibuprofen and naproxen account for 75% of cases.
- Reactivation of ATIN has been noted with other groups of NSAIDs.
- ATIN is accompanied in up to 85% of cases by nephrotic syndrome, secondary to minimal change disease.
- The nephrotic syndrome is usually insidious in onset and can occur without ATIN (10% of cases).
- Flank pain may be prominent.
- Systemic allergic-type clinical features are usually absent.
- The biopsy often reveals prominent B cell infiltrates and eosinophils.
- An occasional association with vasculitis.
- Response to drug withdrawal is usually prompt though abnormalities of urine sediment may persist.

Chinese Herb Nephropathy

This distinct clinical entity was first described in 1993 after an epidemic in Belgium associated with Chinese herbal preparations used in slimming treatments. More recently similar syndromes have been associated with other herbal remedies, e.g. for eczema. Distinctive clinical features include:

- Rapidly progressive renal failure.
- Poor prognosis — a high proportion of cases result in permanent renal failure.
- Extensive interstitial fibrosis on biopsy.
- Severe anaemia.
- Hypertension.
- Aortic regurgitation is common.
- Glycosuria.
- Asymmetrical kidneys on ultrasound.
- Linkage to urothelial tumours.
- Identification of Aristolochic acid as nephrotoxin.

Leptospirosis (see also **Chapter 20**)

This spirochaetal infection is rare with approximately 60 cases per year in the United Kingdom. The development of leptospirosis is linked with environmental exposure to contaminated water in rivers or canals. ATIN usually develops during the second week of the infection, during the icteric phase, after the septicaemic phase. Clinical features include:

- Myalgia, conjunctival injection and jaundice.
- Intravascular haemolysis.
- Hyperuricaemia.
- The development of ARF in about half of all cases.
- Diagnosis by serology.

Practice Point. Management of acute tubulointerstitial nephritis

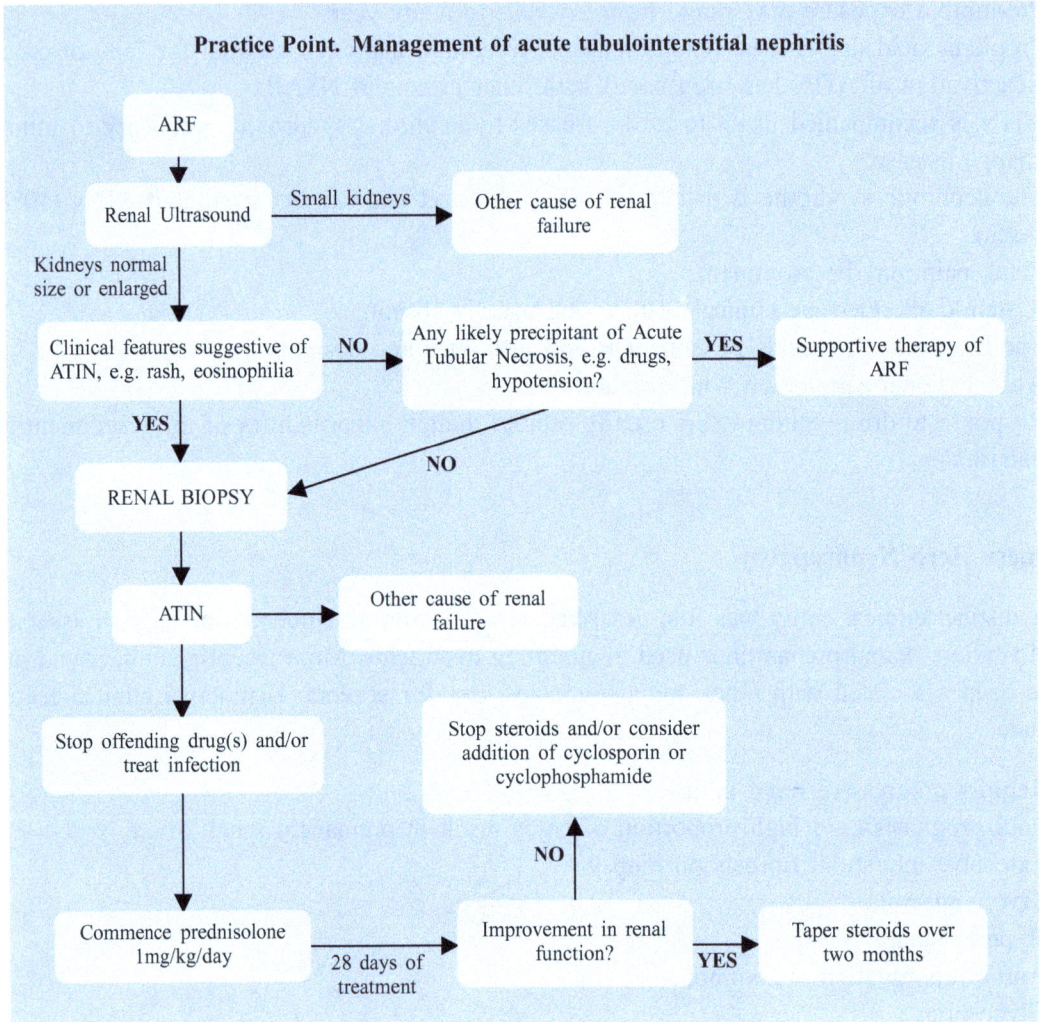

- Visible Leptospira in the urine by dark field microscopy.
- Intravenous penicillin or erythromycin is the treatment of choice in renal failure.

Hantavirus Infection (see also **Chapter 20**)

Infection with this virus is associated with the development of ATIN throughout Asia and also continental Europe. The European variety is usually milder and is associated with an animal reservoir in the bank vole. It is endemic in Scandinavia, the Balkans and Western Europe. Clinical features include:

- A preponderance for young men (M/F 4:1) working in rural areas in contact with rodents.
- Incubation lasting between 10 and 30 days.
- Presentation with high fever, headaches, myalgia and conjunctival injection.
- Later loin pain.
- A second phase of disease with ARF.

- Thrombocytopaenia, leucocytosis and a raised ESR.
- Vascular congestion and medullary interstitial haemorrhages on biopsy.
- Diagnosis by serologic tests for antibodies.
- Good prognosis with spontaneous recovery.

Acute Tubulointerstitial Nephritis with Uveitis (TINU)

This syndrome was first described in 1975 as the association of ATIN with anterior uveitis in adolescent females. Since that time many further cases have been described in adults, including some males. There are a number of common clinical features:

- Bone marrow and lymph node granulomas.
- Fever, weight loss, myalgias and anaemia are common.
- An association with C-ANCA.
- An elevated ESR.
- Eosinophilia, both in peripheral blood and on renal biopsy.
- Possible association with chlamydial or mycoplasma infection.
- Good response of both uveitis and ATIN to steroids.

FURTHER READING

Buysen JG, Houthoff HJ, Krediet RT, Arisz L (1990) Acute interstitial nephritis: A clinical and morphological study in 27 patients. *Nephrology Dialysis and Transplantation*; 5: 94–99

Farrington K, Levison DA, Greenwood RN, et al. (1989) Renal biopsy in patients with unexplained renal impairment and normal kidney size. *Quarterly Journal of Medicine*; 70: 221–233

Laberke HG, Bohle A (1980) Acute interstitial nephritis: Correlations between clinical and morphological findings. *Clinical-Nephrology*; 14: 263–273

Michel DM, Kelly CJ (1998) Acute interstitial nephritis. *Journal of the American Society of Nephrology*; 9: 506–515

Neilson EG (1989) Pathogenesis and therapy of interstitial nephritis [clinical conference]. *Kidney International*; 35: 1257–1270

Pusey CD, Saltissi D, Bloodworth L, et al. (1983) Drug associated acute interstitial nephritis: Clinical and pathological features and the response to high dose steroid therapy. *Quarterly Journal of Medicine*; 52: 194–211

Rastegar A, Kashgarian M (1998) The clinical spectrum of tubulointerstitial nephritis. *Kidney International*; 54: 313–327

Shibasaki T, Ishimoto F, Sakai O, et al. (1991) Clinical characterization of drug-induced allergic nephritis. *American Journal of Nephrology*; 11: 174–180

Chapter 19 _____

SEVERE SEPSIS AND ACUTE RENAL FAILURE

Paul Glynne and Nicholas Price

DEFINITION

Severe sepsis comprises a syndrome of vascular collapse and multi-organ dysfunction secondary to bacterial infection, of which there are 30–50,000 cases per annum in the United Kingdom. Sepsis is a major risk factor for the development of acute renal failure (ARF), associated with approximately 50% of cases in the intensive care unit. In one prospective study, the incidence of ARF was 19% in sepsis, 23% in severe sepsis and 51% in septic shock.

Table 1. **Definitions of sepsis and septic shock** (adapted from Bone *et al.* 1992)	
Bacteraemia	Bacterial growth in blood cultures (clinical features of sepsis not necessarily present)
Sepsis	Clinical infection* plus systemic response to infection indicated by 2 or more of the following: • Temperature >38°C or <36°C • Pulse rate >90 beats/minute • Respiratory rate >20 breaths/minute or $PaCO_2$ <32 mmHg (<4.3 kPa) • White cell count >12 × 10^9/mL or <4 × 10^9/mL, or >10% immature (band) forms **Note** that the systemic inflammatory response syndrome (SIRS) describes a similar systemic response to that in sepsis, but it is unrelated to infection
Severe sepsis	Sepsis plus organ dysfunction (e.g. hypotension, oliguria, lactic acidosis, confusion, hypoxia, disseminated intravascular coagulation)
Septic shock	Sepsis-induced hypotension or the requirement for inotropes despite adequate intravascular volume fluid resuscitation

*Infection describes the presence of organisms in a normally sterile site ± inflammatory host response.

PATHOPHYSIOLOGY

Sepsis

Following bacterial infection, microbial products (e.g. lipopolysaccharide (LPS) or endotoxin) interact with components of the host innate immune system leading to an extensive pro-inflammatory response mediated by a complex pathway of cellular, cytokine and plasma protein

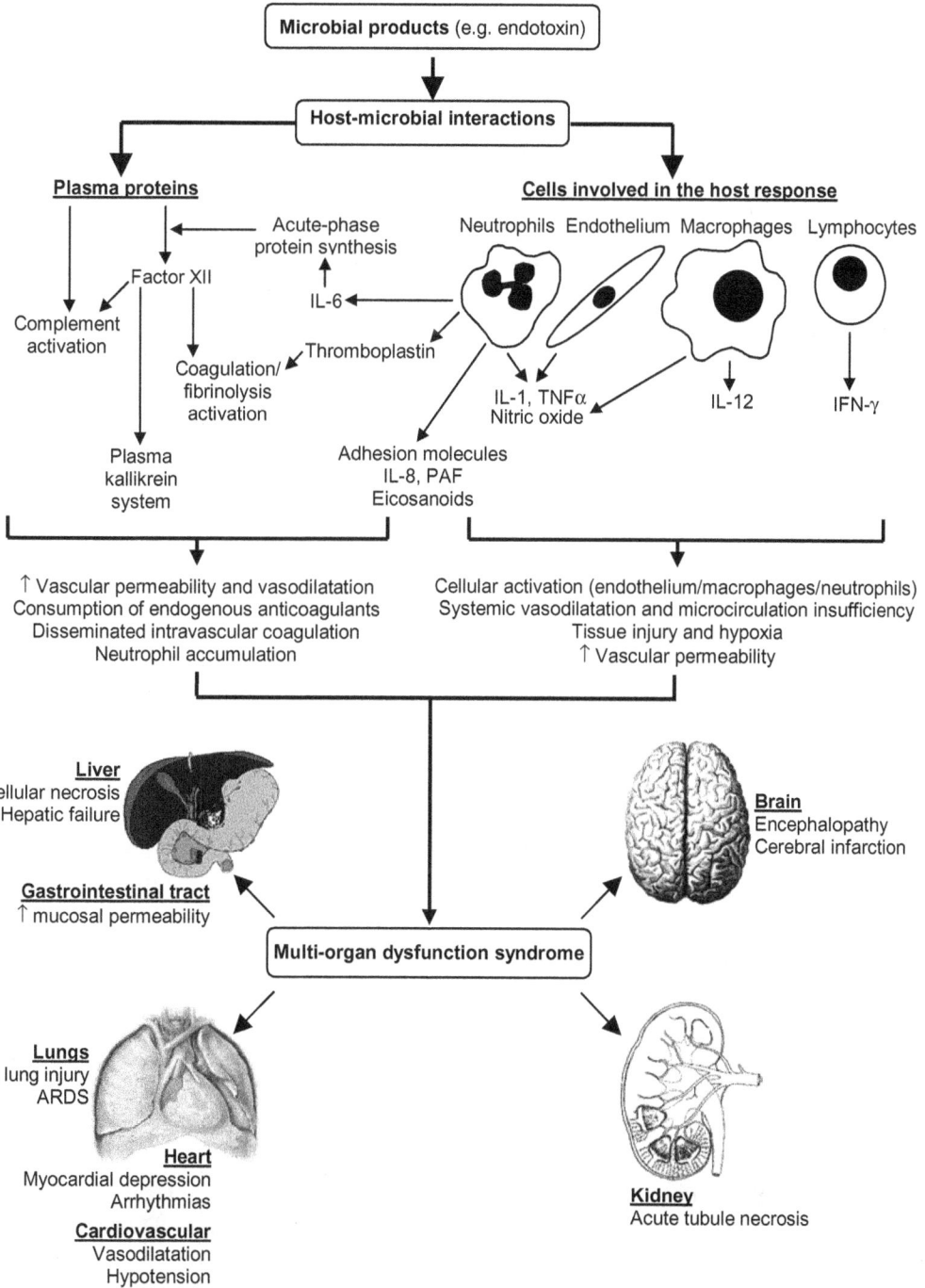

Figure 1. The pathogenesis of sepsis

IL = interleukin; IFN = interferon; PAF = platelet activating factor; ARDS = acute respiratory distress syndrome

cascades (see **Figure 1**). This severe inflammation plays a major role in the pathogenesis of the circulatory failure and multi-organ dysfunction that characterises severe sepsis and septic shock.

Pathophysiology of Acute Renal Failure in Sepsis

The main histopathological changes in ARF during sepsis are confined to the proximal renal tubule. Most morphological data comes from work performed in experimental models of sepsis and endotoxaemia, as there is limited availability of human renal tissue for histological examination (few biopsies are performed on patients with severe sepsis!). In addition, post-mortem specimens from cases of sepsis are subject to severe autolysis, making morphological examination difficult. In contrast to non-septic shock, widespread acute tubule necrosis (ATN) is uncommon; indeed, in endotoxin shock models, tubule epithelial cells often appear microscopically normal although peritubular capillaries demonstrate endothelial oedema and neutrophil sequestration. In animals challenged with live bacteria, proximal tubule damage is more pronounced, characterised by tubule cell apoptosis and necrosis, similar to that described for ischaemic ATN in **Chapter 8.2**.

A variety of humoral and cellular factors contribute to renal tubule damage through: (i) alterations in renal blood flow and glomerular filtration; and (ii) direct tubule cell injury.

(i) *Altered renal blood flow and glomerular filtration*

In patients with sepsis, and in experimental models of sepsis or endotoxaemia, ARF is caused by a reduction in glomerular filtration. Prolonged renal hypoperfusion secondary to a reduction of renal blood flow (RBF) plays a major pathogenic role, leading to ischaemic renal injury and ATN. However, there are marked variations in RBF between patients and between different experimental models. In some series, fluid replete patients with severe sepsis and high cardiac output demonstrate a decline in RBF, suggesting regional vasoconstriction and redistribution of blood flow away from the kidneys. In other cases, the renal vasculature participates in systemic vasodilatation, so that ARF develops despite normal RBF. These differences may reflect varying renal vascular compensatory mechanisms, whether or not patients were ventilated (which lowers RBF, as discussed in **Chapter 28**), variations between animal models, and differences in techniques used to measure RBF. A fall in glomerular filtration, despite normal global RBF, may occur as a result of intrarenal redistribution of blood flow to the corticomedullary junction away from outer cortical nephron regions.

Taken together, renal function may deteriorate without a significant decline in RBF. Therefore, although haemodynamic changes are important in the pathogenesis of ARF during sepsis, non-haemodynamic factors are also involved.

• *Vasoactive mediators*

Pro-inflammatory cytokines, e.g. tumour necrosis factor-alpha (TNF-α), interleukin-1 (IL-1) and platelet activating factor (PAF), are released into the circulation at high levels early in the sepsis cascade (see **Figure 1**). These cytokines induce haemodynamic changes of sepsis when infused directly in animal models, and activate complement, coagulation and fibrinolysis cascades leading to endothelial dysfunction. Endothelial dysfunction is associated with abnormal production of vasoactive mediators, including both vasoconstrictors (e.g. endothelin, thromboxane, angiotensin and catecholamines) and vasodilators (e.g. nitric oxide and prostaglandins). Increased production of endothelial nitric oxide (NO) induces the systemic vasodilatation characteristic of severe sepsis, and NO output correlates with the degree of renal failure. *In vivo* studies of endotoxaemia have demonstrated that non-specific NO inhibition leads to deteriorating renal function and intrarenal thrombosis, whereas specific inhibition of the inducible isoform of NO synthase (iNOS) prevents the fall in glomerular filtration.

(ii) *Direct tubule cell injury*

• *Pro-inflammatory cytokines and endotoxin*

In vitro studies have shown that pro-inflammatory cytokines induce alterations of specific tubule cell actin cytoskeletal functions. These include loss of cell polarity, increased epithelial permeability, altered solute transport and dissolution of integrin-mediated cell-matrix adhesion (see **Figure 2**). Consequently, tubule cells detach from the basement membrane into the lumen leading to tubule obstruction, increased intra-tubular pressure, and back-leak of glomerular filtrate out of the tubule into the interstitium and renal venous blood. Endotoxin infused into experimental animals induces intrarenal vasoconstriction, production of pro-inflammatory cytokines, and activation of complement and coagulation systems, often leading to widespread intravascular coagulation.

• *Nitric oxide*

The effects of NO in the kidney during sepsis are complex. As a vasodilator, constitutive low level production of NO, produced by endothelial NO synthase within the renal vascular

Figure 2. Schematic diagram of tubule injury in sepsis

Acute tubule injury in sepsis results from altered blood flow (ischaemia) and direct tubule cell injury. Damaged tubule cells lose their polarity and apical brush border, and demonstrate apical redistribution of basolateral Na^+/K^+-ATPase (causing cell swelling) and β_1 integrins (causing cell detachment). Tubule cells undergo apoptotic and necrotic cell death, and are shed into to the lumen leading to tubule obstruction. Pro-inflammatory cytokines and nitric oxide are key mediators in these pathogenic effects.

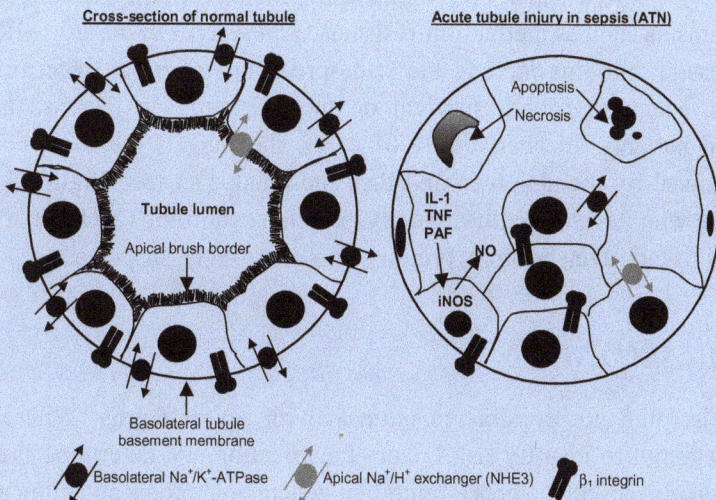

Cross-section of normal tubule

Acute tubule injury in sepsis (ATN)

Apoptosis

Necrosis

Tubule lumen

Apical brush border

IL-1
TNF
PAF

NO

iNOS

Basolateral tubule
basement membrane

Basolateral Na^+/K^+-ATPase   Apical Na^+/H^+ exchanger (NHE3) β_1 integrin

endothelium, is essential for continued renal perfusion (see above). However, a variety of cells within the kidney can be induced to produce high levels of NO following pro-inflammatory cytokine and/or LPS induction of iNOS. These include proximal renal tubule epithelial cells, mesangial cells and infiltrating tissue macrophages. In murine models of sepsis, using live bacteria, iNOS is induced within renal tubule cells in both Gram-negative and Gram-positive infections. Infiltrating neutrophils may also be an important source of NO in the kidney in sepsis, since they too produce iNOS and NO following cytokine-activation.

The effects of high output NO in the kidney (from iNOS) during sepsis remain unclear, and both cytotoxic (e.g. tubule cell shedding and apoptosis) and cytoprotective roles (e.g. maintenance of organ perfusion, regulation of solute transport) have been demonstrated. NO can also react with superoxide ions leaking from the mitochondrial electron transport chain, to give the highly toxic product, peroxynitrite. There is evidence that peroxynitrite is produced in the kidney during sepsis and may induce cellular damage and tubule cell apoptosis.

- *Infiltrating leucocytes*

Activated neutrophils, that have accumulated within peritubular capillaries, interact with the renal vascular endothelium leading to endothelial dysfunction, coagulation activation and tubule cell injury. The release of reactive oxygen species from neutrophils can also directly induce tubule cell damage. Endotoxin-primed neutrophils are thought to play a major role in renal ischaemia-reperfusion injury (perfusion after a period of renal hypoperfusion) through production of oxygen free radicals.

A striking feature of ATN is that, following tubule injury, renal tubule epithelia have a remarkable capacity for repair and regeneration. Indeed, patients who survive the underlying sepsis syndrome usually regain significant renal function (see Outcome).

AETIOLOGY

Historically, Gram-negative infections have been regarded as the major cause of septic shock, but over the past few decades the importance of Gram-positive organisms has become increasingly recognised (**Table 2**). There has also been an alarming increase in the incidence of infection with drug-resistant organisms such as methicillin-resistant *Staphylococcus aureus* (MRSA), enterococci and fungi. The reasons for this include the widespread use of broad-spectrum antibiotics and intra-venous lines, extended patient survival on the ICU, and an increase in the number of immunosuppressed patients. In nearly 50% of cases, the lung is the most common source of severe sepsis, followed by the abdomen and then the renal tract (see **Figure 3**). Importantly, in 20–30% of patients who develop multi-organ dysfunction syndrome (MODS), a definite infective source is not established, even when a primary site is strongly suspected.

CLINICAL PRESENTATION

Taking a history is often not possible in patients with severe sepsis. Wherever possible, the physician should attempt to identify risk factors for infection and determine the infection source (and therefore the likely causative agent). Important general symptoms and clinical signs associated with sepsis are detailed in **Figure 4**. More specific symptoms aid localisation of the infective

Table 2. Spectrum of aetiological agents in community-acquired and nosocomial infection

Microbiology	Community acquired (%)	In-hospital bacteraemia (%)	ICU bacteraemia (EPIC)* (%)	Anti-TNF mAb in sepsis study (%)
Gram positive	51	39	76	36.3
Gram negative	45	35	31	38.9
Mixed	NS	21	NS	11.1
Fungi	NS	NS	9.7	5.4

*Total >100% as mixed infections are included. EPIC = European Prevalence of Infection in Intensive Care Study; ICU = Intensive Care Unit; TNF = tumour necrosis factor; mAb = monoclonal antibody; NS = not stated.

Adapted from Green & Lynn (2000).

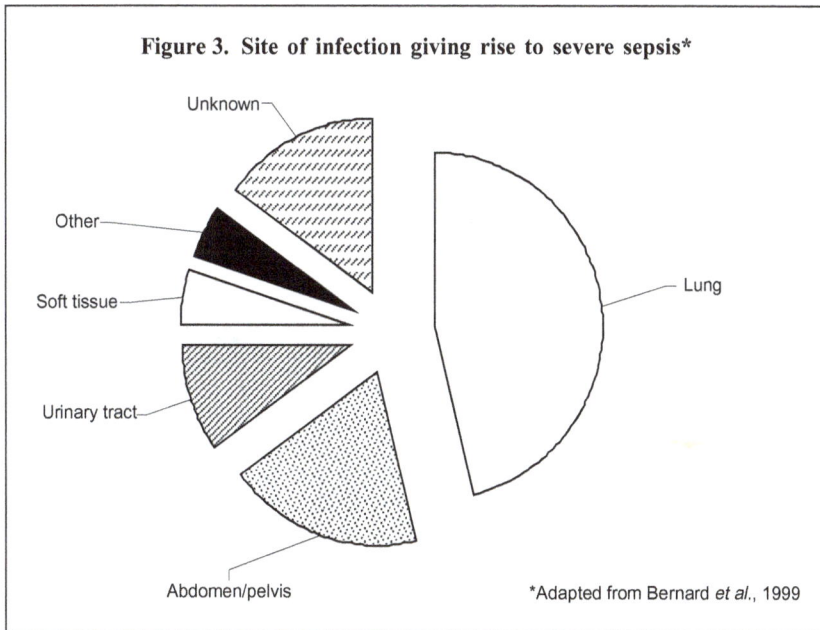

Figure 3. Site of infection giving rise to severe sepsis*

*Adapted from Bernard et al., 1999

source, e.g. productive cough. Acute renal failure during sepsis typically presents with oliguria, elevated serum creatinine and a reduction in creatinine clearance.

Contributory factors predisposing to infection include:

- Increasing age.
- Concurrent illness (including poor nutrition).
- Immunosuppression (chemotherapy, risk factors for HIV).
- Surgery (wounds, prostheses).
- Instrumentation (catheters, cannulae).
- Prolonged hospital admission (ICU versus non-ICU, local flora and resistance patterns).
- Recent travel abroad (malaria, viral haemorrhagic fever and rickettsial infections should be considered where there is an appropriate history of foreign travel).

Figure 4. Clinical signs of sepsis

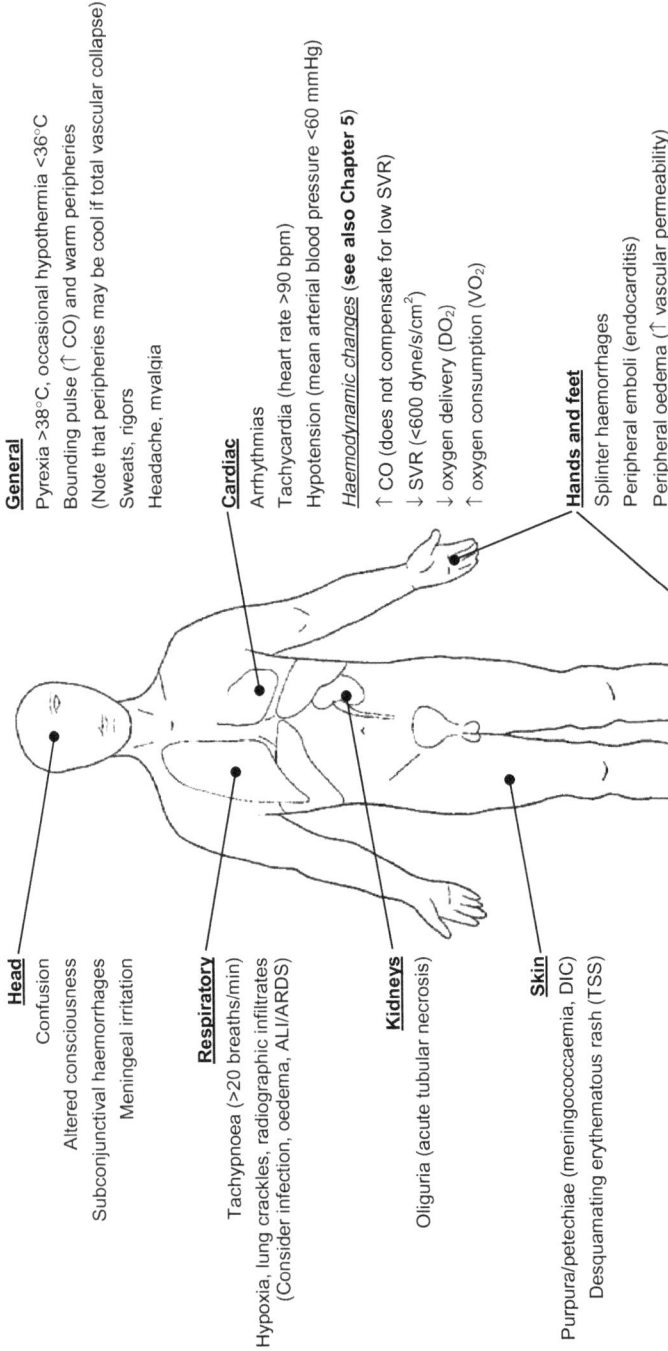

Head
Confusion
Altered consciousness
Subconjunctival haemorrhages
Meningeal irritation

Respiratory
Tachypnoea (>20 breaths/min)
Hypoxia, lung crackles, radiographic infiltrates
(Consider infection, oedema, ALI/ARDS)

Kidneys
Oliguria (acute tubular necrosis)

Skin
Purpura/petechiae (meningococcaemia, DIC)
Desquamating erythematous rash (TSS)

General
Pyrexia >38°C, occasional hypothermia <36°C
Bounding pulse (↑ CO) and warm peripheries
(Note that peripheries may be cool if total vascular collapse)
Sweats, rigors
Headache, myalgia

Cardiac
Arrhythmias
Tachycardia (heart rate >90 bpm)
Hypotension (mean arterial blood pressure <60 mmHg)
Haemodynamic changes (**see also Chapter 5**)
↑ CO (does not compensate for low SVR)
↓ SVR (<600 dyne/s/cm^2)
→ oxygen delivery (DO$_2$)
↑ oxygen consumption (VO$_2$)

Hands and feet
Splinter haemorrhages
Peripheral emboli (endocarditis)
Peripheral oedema (↑ vascular permeability)

TSS = toxic shock syndrome
DIC = disseminated intravascular coagulation
SVR = systemic vascular resistance; CO = cardiac output
ALI = acute lung injury (PaO$_2$/FiO$_2$ <300 mmHg, bilateral infiltrates, no ↑ left atrial pressure)
ARDS = acute respiratory distress syndrome (PaO$_2$/FiO$_2$ <200 mmHg, bilateral infiltrates, no ↑ left atrial pressure)

INVESTIGATIONS

Table 3. Investigations in the patient with severe sepsis

Investigation	Specific comments
Haematology	
Full blood count	White cell count (WCC) $>12 \times 10^9$/mL or $<4 \times 10^9$/mL; blood film shows "left shift"
Coagulation, fibrinogen and fibrin degradation products	$\downarrow$ fibrinogen, $\downarrow$ platelets, $\uparrow$ APTT/PT suggests disseminated intravascular coagulation
Biochemistry	
C-reactive protein	Perform baseline measurement as may help assess response to treatment
Electrolytes	Falling albumin suggests "capillary leak" (or $\downarrow$ hepatic synthesis) Liver function test abnormalities common but hepatic failure rare Hypoglycaemia and hypocalcaemia may occur
Arterial blood gases	Plasma lactate often increased up to 5-fold Respiratory alkalosis early to compensate for hyperlactataemia Metabolic acidosis late (lactic acidosis) Hypoxia suggests pulmonary oedema, pneumonia or ALI/ARDS
Microbiology	
Blood cultures	Take 3 sets from different sites. Take set from IV line if catheter-related sepsis suspected
Urine specimens	10^5 organisms/mL indicates significant infection Send urine for Legionella or pneumococcal antigen if indicated
Intra-vascular catheter tips	Send for Gram stain and culture
Pus/swabs from wounds, drains & catheter sites	Send for Gram stain and culture
Aspirates (naso-tracheal, pleural, ascitic fluid)	Send for Gram stain and culture Send pleural & ascitic fluid for WCC & differential, glucose & protein concentration
Lumbar puncture if meningitis suspected	Send for Gram stain, culture, WCC & differential, protein and glucose concentration Consider pneumococcal latex agglutination test or meningococcal PCR on CSF Send skin lesion aspirates in suspected meningococcaemia for Gram stain & culture
Bronchoscopy	Consider if patient immunosuppressed (suspected fungal or viral pneumonia) or deteriorates despite treatment
Serology	Antibody titres for Legionella, Weil's disease if indicated; save serum
Invasive monitoring	**Figure 3** details the haemodynamic changes associated with severe sepsis
Imaging	
Chest X-ray	Infiltrates may indicate pulmonary oedema, pneumonia or ARDS
CT and ultrasound scanning	Consider if collection suspected (e.g. intra-abdominal); CT brain if impaired consciousness
Echocardiography	If endocarditis suspected; consider trans-oesophageal echo if trans-thoracic echo negative

PCR = polymerase chain reaction; CSF = cerebrospinal fluid.

TREATMENT PRINCIPLES

The most important aspect of clinical management is early recognition of the "at-risk" patient, aiming to intervene rapidly and prevent progression to septic shock and the multi-organ dysfunction syndrome, conditions that carry extremely high mortality. Unfortunately, many patients continue to deteriorate despite early therapeutic intervention. All patients with severe sepsis should be managed on an intensive care unit.

The key treatment principles are:

(1) Treatment of the underlying infection.
(2) Provision of general supportive care and prevention of further complications.
(3) Provision of "organ-specific" supportive management.

1. Treatment of the Underlying Infection

Treatment of infection involves early surgical drainage of pus and debridement of necrotic tissue. Antibiotic treatment covering the likely causative organisms should commence without delay, after specimens for culture have been collected, and until definitive microbiological results are available. Antibiotic doses should be adjusted to the level of renal and hepatic function and mode of renal support. The toxic effects of some of these agents are increased in ARF and, where applicable, drug levels should be monitored closely (see **Appendix A**). In addition, to minimise the risk of drug-resistance and treatment-related adverse effects, it is imperative that initial antibiotic therapy is modified once subsequent positive culture results are known. The infectious diseases team should be closely involved, especially in cases of hospital-acquired sepsis, when the choice of antibiotic therapy is guided by knowledge of local bacterial flora, patterns of drug-resistance and the hospital prescribing policy. Some examples of empirical regimens are suggested in **Table 4**, which depend on the suspected primary site of infection. Note that Candida species are common isolates from clinical specimens taken from patients receiving broad-spectrum antibiotic therapy, and usually represent colonisation or contamination rather than true infection. Rational reduction of antibiotic therapy and removal/replacement of catheters from affected sites is usually sufficient in these cases. However, true infection should be considered if there is growth from more than one peripheral site. Candida grown from blood cultures should always be taken seriously and treated with antifungal therapy.

2. General Supportive Care and Prevention of Further Complications

Recent improvements in outcome in certain subgroups of patients with severe sepsis, in the absence of any novel beneficial therapies, are most likely associated with improved basic supportive care. This includes: provision of enteral nutrition; skin care; physiotherapy; prevention of superadded nosocomial infection; blood product replacement; stress ulcer prophylaxis. These general supportive measures are discussed in detail in **Chapter 28**.

Table 4. Possible empirical antibiotic therapy for the treatment of severe sepsis

Suspected origin of sepsis	Causative organisms	Antibiotic treatment
Pneumonia		
Community-acquired	*S. pneumoniae, H. influenzae, Legionella pneumophila*	Cefotaxime + erythromycin
Hospital-acquired	GN rods (e.g. *P. aeruginosa*, coliforms), *S. aureus*	Vancomycin* + ciprofloxacin **or** piperacillin + gentamicin **or** piperacillin-tazobactam **or** imipenem
Renal tract		
Community-acquired	Enteric GN organisms (*E. coli* most likely) + enterococci	Cefotaxime **or** co-amoxiclav + gentamicin
Hospital-acquired		Ciprofloxacin alone **or** piperacillin + gentamicin
Skin and soft tissue		
Community-acquired	*S. aureus*, Group A streptococci most commonly	Benzyl-penicillin + flucloxacillin
Hospital-acquired	GN organisms & anaerobes (including *Clostridium* spp), especially if "dirty" wound or diabetic patient	Cefotaxime + vancomycin* (need benzyl-penicillin if "gas gangrene")
Intra-abdominal		
Suspected gut source (e.g. bowel-perforation, post-operative infection)	Enteric GN organisms, enterococci + *Bacteroides fragilis* & other anaerobic cocci (plus *S. pneumoniae* in primary peritonitis)	Cefotaxime + metronidazole
Biliary tract	Above + clostridia, *fusobacterium*	Piperacillin + gentamicin **or** imipenem
Vascular access devices	*S. aureus, S. epidermidis*, enterococci, diptheroids, rarely GN organisms	Vancomycin* + ciprofloxacin/ gentamicin
Meningitis		
Immunocompetent adults	*N. meningitidis, S. pneumoniae, H. influenzae, Listeria monocytogenes* (if pregnant, immunosuppressed or >50 years old)	Cefotaxime **or** ceftriaxone (add ampicillin if suspect Listeria)
Endocarditis	Viridans streptococci, *S. aureus, S. epidermidis*, enterococci	Benzylpenicillin + gentamicin + flucloxacillin*
Neutropaenic sepsis§ (neutrophil count <500/mm³)	*P. aeruginosa* & other enteric GN rods, *S. aureus*, viridans streptococci	Piperacillin + gentamicin **or** vancomycin* + ciprofloxacin **or** teicoplanin + gentamicin **or** imipenem

*Use vancomycin if infection with MRSA suspected; §Consult unit policy; GN = Gram negative.

3. "Organ-Specific" Supportive Management

Circulatory support

Provision of adequate circulatory support aims to maintain organ perfusion and tissue oxygenation. Early and aggressive intravascular fluid resuscitation is critically important to improve cardiac output and renal blood flow. Patients with severe sepsis are typically hyperdynamic, vasodilated and hypotensive (see **Figure 4**), and usually require intravenous infusion with large volumes of colloid or crystalloid. The assessment of intravascular volume status can be guided by measurement of central venous pressure (CVP) and cardiac output (obtained from a pulmonary artery catheter or oesophageal Doppler monitor) prior to, and after colloid challenges. For example, following a 200 mL colloid bolus, if there is no significant change in CVP and/or a rise in stroke volume of >10%, then the patient requires further fluid resuscitation. Conversely, a sustained rise in CVP of >3 mmHg and the absence of any change in stroke volume, following colloid filling, suggests that the patient is intravascularly volume replete. If clinically important hypotension persists with evidence of impaired tissue perfusion (e.g. oliguria), despite adequate intravascular volume resuscitation, then the patient has by definition, septic shock, and requires vasopressor therapy. In general, high cardiac output states, such as septic shock, are managed using the vasopressor norepinephrine, which has been shown to increase urine output and GFR in patients with hyperdynamic septic shock. A more detailed discussion of haemodynamic, inotropic and vasopressor support in critically ill patients is provided in **Chapter 28**.

Respiratory support

Respiratory failure occurs commonly in association with severe sepsis and septic shock. Indeed, a primary pulmonary focus of infection accounts for almost 50% of cases of severe sepsis (see **Figure 3**). Acute lung injury and the acute respiratory distress syndrome (see **Figure 4**) occur as part of the multi-organ dysfunction syndrome that may follow severe sepsis. Patients frequently require intubation and mechanical ventilation. Ventilation strategies in critically ill patients are discussed further in **Chapter 28**.

Renal support

The prevention and management of ARF have been described extensively elsewhere in this book (see **Chapters 8** and **9**). Other than optimising renal perfusion through adequate circulatory support, there is no evidence that any other specific therapies (e.g. dopamine, furosemide) are of benefit in the prevention or treatment of ARF in sepsis. The generally accepted treatment for established ARF, in patients with severe sepsis on the intensive care unit, is continuous renal replacement therapy, discussed further in **Chapter 9**. In addition, renal replacement therapies have the potential to remove mediators from the blood that have been implicated in the pathogenesis of sepsis and SIRS (systemic inflammatory response syndrome). Cytokines (pro-inflammatory and anti-inflammatory) and other mediators are removed by filtration or adsorption onto the filter. Despite promising results from animal experiments there are no data from randomised clinical trials to support the use of renal replacement therapies as specific treatment for sepsis.

OUTCOME AND FUTURE PROSPECTS

Despite improvements in supportive care and increased use of continuous renal replacement techniques, mortality in patients with severe sepsis is high (~40–50%), and is dependent on co-morbid conditions and the number of organ system failures. Although ARF in sepsis usually occurs as part of a multi-organ dysfunction syndrome, it independently adversely affects the prognosis of patients in intensive care units, and the outcome of renal failure associated with sepsis is worse than in non-septic cases. Renal function recovers in most patients with ATN who survive the underlying sepsis syndrome, and only a small proportion (~5%) require long term renal replacement therapy. Mixed bacterial infections and infection with *P. aeruginosa* or fungi are associated with a poorer outcome.

Recent trials of experimental agents in the prevention of ARF have been disappointing (see **Chapter 8**), although these have generally been undertaken in the context of ischaemic ATN rather than sepsis-related ARF *per se*. Experimental therapies for the treatment of severe sepsis and septic shock have predominantly been designed to intervene in the host inflammatory response that results in organ failure. Monoclonal anti-TNF and anti-endotoxin antibodies, and NO synthase inhibition, have failed to reduce mortality in randomised controlled trials. The anti-endotoxin agent, recombinant bactericidal/permeability increasing protein (rBPI) is under evaluation. Exciting recent developments have stemmed from strategies aimed at replacing endogenous anticoagulants, which are consumed in severe sepsis (see **Figure 1**). A randomised, double-blind, placebo-controlled multi-centre trial evaluating recombinant activated protein C demonstrated a significant beneficial effect on mortality and morbidity of the drug over placebo.

It seems unlikely that any of these novel agents will directly influence the pathogenesis of renal injury in sepsis. However, attempts to increase our understanding of the mechanisms underlying renal dysfunction in sepsis will undoubtedly lead to more promising treatments in the future.

FURTHER READING

Bernard GR, Vincent JL, Laterre PF, et al. (2001) Efficacy and safety of recombinant human activated protein C for severe sepsis. *N Engl J Med*; 344: 699–709

Bone RC, Balk RA, Cerra FB, Dellinger RP, et al. (1992) Definitions for sepsis and organ failure and guidelines for the use of innovative therapies in sepsis. *Chest*; 101: 1644–1655

Glynne PA, Picot J, Evans TJ (2001) Coexpressed nitric oxide synthase and apical beta(1) integrins influence tubule cell adhesion after cytokine-induced injury. *J Am Soc Nephrol*; 12: 2370–2383

Green J, Lynn WA (2000) Septicaemia. *Journal of the Royal College of Physicians*; 34: 418–423

Groeneveld ABJ (1994) Pathogenesis of acute renal failure during sepsis. *Nephrology Dialysis and Transplantation*; 9(S4): 47–51

Groeveneld ABJ, Tran DD, van der Meulen J, et al. (1991) Acute renal failure in the medical intensive care unit: Predisposing, complicating factors and outcome. *Nephron*; 59: 602–610

Lynn WA (1999) Sepsis. In: Armstrong D and Cohen J (eds.). *Infectious Diseases* (1st Edition). London: Mosby

Neveu H, Kleinknecht D, Brivet F, Loirat P, Landais P and The French Study Group on Acute renal failure (1996) Prognostic factors in acute renal failure due to sepsis. Results of a prospective multicentre study. *Nephrology Dialysis and Transplantation*; 11: 293–299

Rangel-Frausto MS, Pittet D, Costigan M, *et al.* (1995) The natural history of the systemic inflammatory response syndrome (SIRS). A prospective study. *Journal of the American Medical Association*; 273: 117–123

Wheeler AP, Bernard GR (1999) Treating patients with severe sepsis. *The New England Journal of Medicine*; 340: 207–214

Chapter 20

INFECTIOUS DISEASES AND ACUTE RENAL FAILURE
Thomas Evans

INTRODUCTION

A variety of microbiological agents cause acute renal failure (ARF; see **Table 1**). Some of these have been described in detail in other chapters. Here, I will describe those infections that have a particular ability to produce ARF. As the pathophysiology, clinical features and treatment of each of these infections is quite specific, each will be described in turn. This will make the chapter a little more fragmented than others, but will allow easy access to specific management of ARF associated with a particular infection.

Table 1. Microbiological causes of acute renal failure	
1. General	
Syndrome	**Causative agent**
Sepsis	Gram-negative and Gram-positive bacteria + fungi; see **Chapter 19**
Rhabdomyolysis	Diverse organisms; see **Chapter 12**
Haemolytic uraemic syndrome	*E. coli* O157/Shigella; see **Chapter 15**
Post-infectious glomerulonephritis	*Streptococcus pyogenes*; see **Chapter 16**
Tubulointerstitial nephritis	Diverse organisms; see **Chapter 18**
2. Specific	
Syndrome	**Causative agent**
Viral	HIV
	Hantavirus
Bacterial	Leptospirosis
Parasitic	Malaria

SPECIFIC INFECTIONS

HIV

Human immunodeficiency virus (HIV) infection may be associated with ARF through a wide spectrum of different disease processes. These may be specifically related to the HIV virus, they may be due to coincidental opportunistic infection, or they may be secondary to drug therapy. Since many patients with HIV disease present with complex clinical problems, it is often very difficult to be certain from the clinical presentation which of these processes is responsible for ARF. I have chosen one study of ARF in the course of HIV infection, from France, to illustrate the diversity of disease processes involved (**Table 2**).

This study was a retrospective analysis of 92 HIV-infected patients, 60 of whom underwent renal biopsy. The inclusion criteria required that serum creatinine increase from <110 µM to >180 µM within 20 days, and that kidney size was not reduced on ultrasonography. The separate aetiological factors will be considered below.

Table 2. Aetiology of HIV associated acute renal failure (data from Peraldi et al. 1999)

Cause	Number of cases		% of cases		Renal biopsies	Number died	
Haemolytic uraemic syndrome	32		35		26	7	
Acute tubular necrosis	24		26.1		7	8	
— *rhabdomyolysis*		6		6.5	4		0
— *ischaemic/toxic*		18		19.6	3		8
Obstruction	16		18.2		8	3	
— *drug-induced tubule obstruction*		13		15	7		0
— *lymphoma*		2		2.1	0		2
— *paraproteinaemia*		1		1.1	1		1
HIV-associated nephropathy	14		15		13	0	
Glomerulonephritis	4		4.3		4	0	
Acute tubulointerstitial nephritis	2		2.1		2	0	
TOTAL	92		100		60	18	

AETIOLOGY

- The commonest cause of ARF in this cohort was haemolytic uraemic syndrome (HUS; see **Chapter 15**), in 35% of patients. Although this probably reflects the particular unit's interest in this condition, other studies have also found that HUS is a common cause of ARF in HIV. Extrarenal manifestations, including neurological impairment, suggest an overlap with thrombotic thrombocytopaenic purpura. Men were affected far more than women. The pathophysiology of HUS in HUV infection is obscure. Shiga-like toxin producing bacteria were only found in one of the patients in this study; a direct role of the HIV virus is postulated.

- Acute tubular necrosis (ATN) was the cause of ARF in 26% of cases. The underlying processes were rhabdomyolysis (see **Chapter 12**), shock (**Chapter 10**) or drugs (**Chapter 11**).
- Obstruction was the cause of ARF in 18% of the cases. Most of these were due to drug-induced tubular obstruction (see **Chapter 11**). The drugs involved were sulfadiazine, foscarnet and indinavir.
- HIV-associated nephropathy (HIVAN) caused ARF in 15% of the cases, This is a condition peculiar to HIV infection, considered in more detail below. It is a cause of acute or rapidly progressive renal failure, so leads to both acute and chronic renal failure in HIV.
- The remaining conditions were individually uncommon. Membranoproliferative glomerulonephritis occurred in 2 cases associated with hepatitis B and C. Two cases of a lupus-like syndrome were found.

HIV-ASSOCIATED NEPHROPATHY (HIVAN)

This is a syndrome of massive proteinuria, haematuria, renal failure and unusual pathological features that occurs in patients infected with HIV, usually at a late stage of disease. The most common histopathological finding is that of focal and segmental glomerulosclerosis. Visceral epithelial cells are enlarged with coarse cytoplasmic vacuoles, and underlying capillary walls show collapse. Renal tubules dilate, the lumen filling with casts. As the disease progresses, renal tissue shows increasing sclerosis, but with no vascular changes. IgM and C3 are deposited in the mesangium and sclerotic areas. Electron microscopic studies show fusion of glomerular foot processes and detachment of epithelial cells. Tubuloreticular inclusion bodies are visible in capillary endothelial cells. Although direct cytopathic effects of HIV on renal tissue are thought to be important in the pathogenesis, it is not clear how this disease is caused.

HIVAN commonly presents as the nephrotic syndrome with accompanying renal impairment. As discussed above, this can be of sufficiently rapid onset to produce ARF. There is usually haematuria, occasionally gross. Patients are typically normotensive, with enlarged and highly echogenic kidneys. Most patients are young African-American men, suggesting a genetic component in disease pathogenesis. The syndrome progresses very rapidly, with onset of end-stage renal disease in 3–4 months.

Controlled studies analysing specific treatment of this condition are not available. Available data suggest that suppression of HIV replication by the most effective drug combination available should be commenced. Small studies suggest that corticosteroids may have some effect, but no long term benefits are evident. Angiotensin-converting enzyme inhibitors in small studies have been shown to slow progression, despite lack of hypertension.

INVESTIGATIONS

- Diagnosis of HIV is by detection of anti-HIV specific antibodies after careful counselling of patients. Results are available in hours. In most cases, ARF will not be the presenting feature of HIV disease. HIVAN, however, can be the first evidence of HIV infection. Patients with features of this condition, especially of African-American origin, should be carefully evaluated for the presence of risk factors for HIV infection and tested accordingly.

- Given the diverse causes of ARF evident in **Table 2**, renal biopsy should be performed in all patients, unless prognosis is judged so poor that further intervention is unwarranted. Given more effective treatment for HIV, outlook is now not nearly so bleak, making accurate diagnosis by biopsy more important (see below).
- HUS should be specifically sought (**Chapter 12**). A blood film will show the changes of microangiopathic haemolytic anaemia, in association with thrombocytopenia and normal clotting. Because of marrow impairment produced by HIV, there is little elevation of the reticulocyte count.

TREATMENT PRINCIPLES

1. Determine the aetiology of ARF from clinical features and renal biopsy.
2. Correct any reversible cause found.
3. Dialysis in most cases is appropriate, as many causes of ARF are reversible and outcome is good.
4. In most cases, antiretroviral therapy will not alter the course of ARF in HIV. An important exception is HIVAN, where there is some evidence that institution of therapy to reduce HIV replication will alleviate the renal failure (see above). This should be planned and initiated with an infectious disease specialist. An angiotensin converting enzyme inhibitor should be started. I do not feel there is strong enough evidence to commence steroids in this disease.

OUTCOME

Prognosis is better than might be expected. The mortality rate of the patients shown in **Table 2** was 18% at 2 months after presentation. With more effective antiretroviral therapy, long-term survival of patients with HIV disease will become normal. Apart from tumour related causes of ARF, most of the causes detailed in **Table 2** are potentially reversible. Thus, dialysis should not be withheld from this group of patients, although provision should be made for dedicated machinery to provide renal replacement for HIV infected individuals.

HANTAVIRUS

Hantaviruses are membrane-bound negative-sense RNA viruses belonging to the family Bunyaviridae. They are endemic in specific rodent reservoirs, from which transmission to man occurs by inhalation of infectious aerosols of rodent excreta. They cause a number of clinical syndromes. In Europe, the main disease pattern is that of Haemorrhagic Fever with Renal Syndrome (HFRS). Related viruses in the Americas cause a disease referred to as Hantavirus Pulmonary Syndrome. I will discuss here HFRS only.

PATHOPHYSIOLOGY

The exact distribution and incidence of human hantaviral infections in Europe are not well characterised. There are a variety of different viral strains with particular distributions and differing rodent vectors. Dobrava, found in the Balkans, is transmitted by the yellow-necked field mouse and causes a relatively severe form of the disease. A milder form, Puumala, is transmitted by bank voles and is prevalent in Northern and Western Europe. Other strains include Seoul, carried by the Norwegian rat, and Hantaan, carried by the striped field mouse. Data on infection rates are limited, but in Germany the seroprevalence rate is 1–2%, rising to 3–4% in known endemic areas and higher in those whose occupations lead to exposure to the rodent vector, e.g. forestry workers. There was an outbreak in Belgium between 1995–1996 when there were 217 documented cases of HFRS, caused almost entirely by the Puumala strain. Data from the UK are scant, but one survey of farmers in England and Wales found a seroprevalence rate of 4.7%, with a further 4.8% seroconverting in the subsequent year. In Nothern Ireland, a seroprevalence rate of 2.1% was found amongst those presenting with features of HFRS; the predominant strain identified was the rat-borne Seoul virus. Isolated case reports of HFRS in England and Scotland have been made; undoubtedly, the disease is underdiagnosed.

Hantavirus infects endothelial cells preferentially, and it is assumed that an increase in capillary permeability leads to the majority of the clinical features of disease. Why the European forms of Hantavirus preferentially target the kidney and how the virus produces ARF are not known.

CLINICAL FEATURES

The incubation period is estimated to be 2–3 weeks. The disease is divided into 4 stages:

1. A febrile stage, lasting between 3–7 days, with associated thirst, nausea and vomiting, flushing of the face and anterior chest, conjunctival suffusion, blurred vision and periorbital oedema. Lumbar back pain is prominent, reflecting retroperitoneal oedema. Petechiae may appear and proteinuria becomes increasingly evident.
2. A hypotensive phase, which may last a few hours to 2 days. Haemorrhages are more obvious and ecchymoses appear. Although in many cases the hypotension is very mild, in severe illness it can be fatal.
3. The oliguric phase, which may last between 3–14 days. Renal function progressively deteriorates. Most deaths from the disease occur in this period.
4. A polyuric phase then supervenes, lasting days to several weeks, as renal function returns to normal.

INVESTIGATIONS

- The mainstay of specific diagnosis is serology. IgM antibodies to Hantavirus appear between 8–15 days after disease onset. Reference laboratories should be able to provide more specific speciation. Rising titres during the course of the illness confirm the infection. PCR based diagnostic methods may prove more sensitive in the future.
- Thrombocytopenia is virtually universal in the early stages of infection, but not sufficiently profound to account for the bleeding tendency observed. Disseminated intravascular coagulation may occur.

TREATMENT PRINCIPLES

- **Treatment of the Infection**

One trial of intravenous ribavirin in China found some evidence of benefit, reducing the incidence of renal failure and decreasing bleeding complications. The dosages used were:

- loading dose of 33 mg/kg;
- then a dose of 16 mg/kg every 6 h for 4 days;
- then 8 mg/kg every 8 h for 3 days.

Since the only side effect of this therapy was reversible anaemia, this drug should be administered if the disease is confirmed. About one-third of drug elimination is renal, so dosage adjustment in renal failure is probably not necessary, although studies are lacking. The drug is not removed to any great extent by haemodialysis.

- **Dialysis**

Dialysis required in severe renal failure. Volume adjustment is critical because of the endothelial leak and, as the disease recovers, management of the polyuric phase requires close monitoring of salt and water balance.

OUTCOME

If the patient survives, complete recovery of normal renal function is the rule.

LEPTOSPIROSIS

Leptospirosis is a generalized disease caused by infection with spirochetes of the genus *Leptospira*. It is a zoonosis found worldwide, affecting many different mammalian species. Humans are accidental hosts of the organism, and human–human spread is virtually unknown. The main animal vectors are rats, dogs, livestock, and other wild mammals. A single species, *L. interrogans*, is responsible for human disease, of which there a number of different serotypes — these include *icterohaemorrhagiae*, *hebdomidis* and *canicola*.

PATHOPHYSIOLOGY

Leptospires can persist in the renal tubules of infected animals for long periods and are shed into their urine. The spirochetes penetrate abraded skin or mucous membranes of humans and are carried by the blood to all parts of the body. Renal damage is chiefly in tubule cells, with functional impairment worse than histological findings, which usually show mild tubular degeneration. The cause of the tubular lesions is not clear. Leptospires can directly invade renal tubule cells, suggesting a direct toxic effect. In addition, acute tubulointerstitial nephritis has been associated with *Leptospira*. Hypovolaemia from endothelial leakage caused by the infection may exacerbate the renal damage. Glomerular damage is not common, although there are case reports of histological findings suggestive of immune-complex mediated glomerulonephritis. Hepatocellular damage without necrosis can occur in severe disease, leading to jaundice (Weil's disease). Haemorrhage is secondary to capillary vasculitis.

CLINICAL FEATURES

The source of infection is usually contaminated water containing leptospires. The disease is commonest in those who are exposed through occupation, such as farmers, sewage workers and veterinarians, or leisure activity, such as fisherman and canoeists. After an incubation period of 7–12 days, a septicaemic phase begins, characterized by a "flu-like" illness with fever, headache, myalgia, nausea and vomiting. Leptospires can be isolated from blood and CSF. This persists for about 4–7 days. Fever then abates, and in a small number of cases the disease progresses no further. However, most patients then enter the second "immune" stage of the illness, with severe headache, myalgia, photophobia, neck-stiffness, nausea and vomiting. Clinical findings in this phase include conjunctival suffusion and haemorrhage, splenomegaly in about 20% of cases, and lymphadenopathy. Pulmonary involvement can occur, with cough, chest pain and bloodstained sputum. A generalized rash can be found in a small minority of cases. Aseptic meningitis is common in this phase of the illness (see below). Leptospires are shed into the urine during this stage of the infection. This phase may last up to 1 month, or longer, with complete resolution. However, in severe disease, a third icteric phase begins. Leptospires return in blood, CSF and urine. Jaundice, with mild elevation of transaminases occurs, associated with renal failure, petechial haemorrhages, thrombocytopenia (50%) and myocarditis (50%). The estimated mortality of severe leptospirosis is 5–10%, with death usually occurring in this stage of the illness.

INVESTIGATIONS

- Definitive diagnosis depends on laboratory evidence of infection, either from isolation of the organism or demonstration of a serological response. Leptospires can be isolated from blood and CSF during the first 10 days of the illness, although growth of the organism may take some days. Leptospires appear in the urine during the second week of the illness, and they may be visualized by dark field illumination. Organisms in the CSF may also be visualized by this technique. Serology is the mainstay of diagnosis. Specific antibody appears after about 6–12 days of illness and will peak in the third or fourth week of illness. This leptospiral IgM can be detected by a variety of ELISA techniques. A rising titre during the course of infection is diagnostic. Low level titres of antibody will persist for many years after infection has resolved.
- CSF examination in the second "immune" phase of the illness is often performed because of the intense headache, photophobia and neck-stiffness. 80–90% of patients will have a CSF pleocytosis during the second week of illness, usually with fewer than 500 cells per mm^3, predominantly mononuclear. CSF protein may show mild elevation, and sugar is normal. The CSF is usually sterile, unless lumbar puncture is performed in the first week of illness, when polymorphs may predominate.
- Creatinine phosphokinase is usually elevated, although true rhabdomyolysis is rare.

- Pulmonary involvement may produce diffuse infiltrates on chest X-ray.
- Myocarditis may be detected by ECG changes and echocardiography.

TREATMENT PRINCIPLES

Treatment of the Infection

Antibiotics should be administered in patients with leptospirosis and renal failure. **The treatment of choice remains intravenous Penicillin G at a dose of 1.5 MU given four times a day**; given the safety profile of penicillin, this dose does not need to be altered in renal failure. Penicillin can precipitate a Jarish-Herxheimer reaction, although this is rare and rarely requires more than symptomatic relief. If oral therapy can be tolerated, an alternative is doxycycline 100 mg b.d. In severe illness with penicillin allergy, there is no clear best second-line systemic antibiotic. Third generation cephalosporins such as cefotaxime are effective *in vitro*, and erythromycin may also be used.

OUTCOME

In surviving patients, complete renal recovery is to be expected.

MALARIA

Infection with the human malarial protozoan parasite *Plasmodium falciparum* can result in ARF; other human malarial species do not cause ARF.

PATHOPHYSIOLOGY

P. falciparum is transmitted by the bite of an infected anopheline mosquito. There are a number of different stages in the life cycle of the parasite, which are important in understanding the pathophysiology and clinical features of the infection. The insect transmits malarial sporozoites, usually about 10 per bite, which then invade hepatocytes and mature to become tissue schizonts. These then rupture to release a total of about 10^5–10^6 merozoites. Merozoites infect erythrocytes, where they undergo an asexual cycle of replication in the next 48–72 h period. Each infected erythrocyte then lyses to release 24–32 merozoites, which can go on to infect yet more red cells. In this fashion, there is an exponential increase in the numbers of parasites, which can proceed largely unchecked in *P. falciparum* infection, to reach parasitaemias in excess of 50% with a parasite burden of greater than 10^{14} organisms. Some of the merozoites will develop into long-lived motile gametocytes, which can then be passed to a biting female anopheline mosquito, where the remainder of the life-cycle is completed.

The key pathophysiological feature of infection with *P. falciparum* is its ability to induce adherence of parasitised erythrocytes to the microvascular endothelium. This sequestration occurs during the latter part of the protozoon's asexual life cycle in the red cell, and thus these more mature stages of the parasite are never seen on peripheral blood films. This also has the extremely

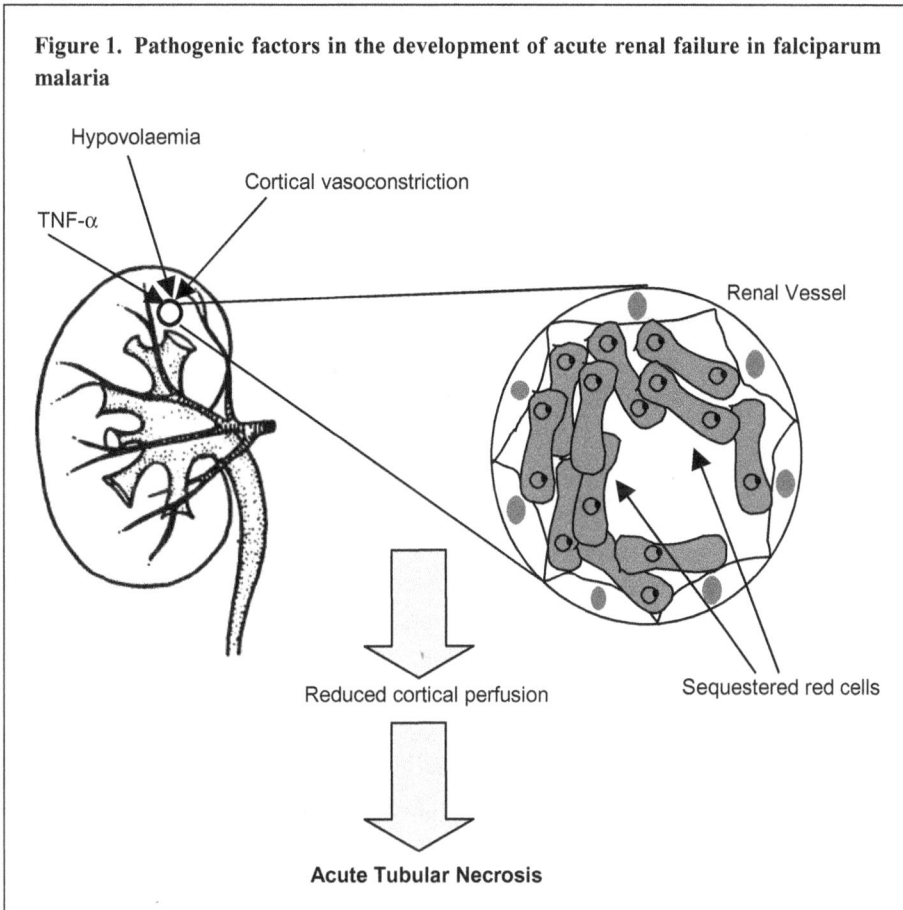

Figure 1. Pathogenic factors in the development of acute renal failure in falciparum malaria

important corollary that the parasite count in the peripheral blood of a patient with falciparum malaria does not necessarily reflect the severity of disease, since towards the end of its life cycle an increasing proportion of parasitised erythrocytes are sequestered. In addition, parasite load can increase following treatment as sequestered red cells lyse, releasing fresh merozoites into the circulation, which infect more red blood cells.

Sequestration is greatest in the cerebral vasculature, but also is evident in other organs including the kidneys. Occlusion of the renal vasculature by sequestered red cells leads to anoxic damage, principally to the proximal tubule cells, resulting in acute tubular necrosis (**Figure 1**). This process is exacerbated by renal cortical vasoconstriction, of uncertain aetiology, and by dehydration consequent to high fever and patient debility. There is little evidence of significant glomerular damage. In addition to direct occlusion of the renal microvasculature, the host releases large amounts of pro-inflammatory cytokines, which may contribute to tubular damage. Raised TNF-α levels have been specifically linked to the development of ARF in falciparum malaria.

Rarely, falciparum malaria can precipitate massive intravascular haemolysis and consequent haemoglobinuria, so-called "blackwater fever". The precise aetiology is unclear, but it most commonly results from associated quinine ingestion and glucose-6-phosphate dehydrogenase deficiency. Aciduria converts filtered haemoglobin to methaemoglobin, which can precipitate in the tubules leading to obstruction and tubular cell necrosis. Surprisingly, ARF in blackwater fever is unusual; in 50 cases reported from Southern Vietnam, only 3 required dialysis.

CLINICAL PRESENTATION

The clinical features of malaria are dependent on the immune status of the patient. In the Tropics, where malaria is endemic, severe malaria usually occurs in children between the ages of 6 months and 3 years of age. In this group, hypoglycaemia, acidosis and cerebral malaria are common, but multi-organ failure and renal involvement rare. Surviving children develop progressively more effective immunity, so that the indigenous adult population of malarious areas of the world typically only experience mild symptoms on infection. Non-immune adults who acquire malaria show a quite different pattern of disease, in which renal involvement and multi-organ failure are common. Travellers to the Tropics are at high risk of acquiring malaria, and it is this group that comprises the majority of cases of severe malaria seen in Western Europe and North America. Malaria should be suspected in *any* patient with fever returning from a malaria endemic region. Classic cyclical fever with a 48 h periodicity is very rarely seen; more commonly, the fever is continuous with irregular peaks. The mean incubation period between infection with *P. falciparum* and symptoms is 13 days in experimental infection, but can be prolonged in patients who have taken some chemoprophylaxis, in those with partial immunity and those with co-infection by *P. vivax*. Malaria can be transmitted in blood, and this has rarely given rise to infections in patients who were inadvertently inoculated with blood from an infected individual, causing much diagnostic confusion. It is also vital to appreciate that immunity to malaria is species specific and wanes once constant exposure to the parasite is removed. Thus, a patient who grew up in the Tropics but is now resident in Northern Europe will have the same risk of acquiring severe malaria on revisiting a malarial region as a native of a non-malarious zone.

ARF in severe malaria can present in the acute phase of the disease or it may be delayed until the recovery phase. Usually, when ARF develops in the acute phase of the disease, it is oliguric or anuric and associated with other features of severe disease, such as coma, acidosis and jaundice. Patients with severe malaria are usually dehydrated due to fever and debility. However, pulmonary oedema can develop in falciparum malaria even with normal left atrial pressures. ARF developing in the recovery phase is more likely to be non-oliguric. Hypertension and oedema are not features of malaria-induced ARF, and proteinuria is usually mild. In common with other causes of ATN, there may be a polyuric phase as renal function returns to normal. Blackwater fever is very obvious, with gross dark discolouration of the urine.

INVESTIGATIONS

- **Detecting the Parasite**

The diagnosis is established by detecting the parasite in blood. Thick films are more sensitive for detecting the parasite, but precise speciation is best achieved with a thin film. In the context of renal failure, absence of malarial parasites makes the diagnosis very unlikely, but it is always worth repeating the films on two further occasions. A little-used, but probably slightly more sensitive technique, is to analyse smears made from intradermal blood. This is obtained by making half a dozen punctures with a 25G needle into the dermis of the volar surface of the upper forearm. These should not bleed spontaneously, but will produce serosanguineous fluid when squeezed. This material can then be directly smeared onto a glass slide for analysis. A number of ELISA-based kits are also available for diagnosis. They are probably of most use where laboratory facilities are limited or there is no experienced person able to read a blood film. Although parasite load can be misleading, because of sequestration, there is some correlation between parasite load and outcome.

- **Urinary Sediment**

The urinary sediment may contain granular casts and leukocytes. There may be dip-stick positivity to blood and protein. In blackwater fever, the urine will be uniformly dark.

- **Haematology**

Anaemia and thrombocytopenia are very common. DIC can be a complication of severe infection, giving rise to prolonged clotting times with reduced fibrinogen and presence of fibrinogen breakdown products. Neutrophils and monocytes may contain parasite pigment. If more than 5% of neutrophils contain pigment, this is associated with an adverse prognosis.

- **Biochemistry**

Low sodium is common. In severe disease, acidosis with an elevated lactate may be present. Biochemical changes of ARF will be apparent. Conjugated bilirubin, creatinine phosphokinase and transaminases may all be elevated. Low blood glucose can be a severe complication and must be monitored closely.

TREATMENT PRINCIPLES

1. Treatment of the Infection

In most parts of the world, chloroquine-sensitive *P. falciparum* is uncommon, so therapy should be initiated with quinine. Most patients with ARF in association with malaria will require parenteral therapy with quinine dihydrochloride. The patient should be weighed and the drug administered as follows. Infusions can be in saline or dextrose.

- *Loading dose*

7 mg salt/kg infused over 30 min by infusion pump followed by 10 mg salt/kg over 4 h

The loading dose should *not* be altered in renal impairment, but should be withheld if the patient has received more than 15 mg salt/kg quinine in the preceding 24 h prior to in-patient care. There is a theoretical risk of toxic interaction with mefloquine (which may have been given for prophylaxis), but in practice this has not been reported, so the loading dose should still be given even if mefloquine has been administered.

- *Maintenance dose*

10 mg salt/kg infused over 2 h given every 8 h

Renal failure produces little change in quinine plasma levels, as only about 20% of the dose is eliminated unchanged by the kidney. After 48 h of treatment, it is usual to reduce the dose by 1/3 to avoid accumulation. Levels of the drug can be measured, but results are unlikely to be available acutely. The drug is not removed by dialysis, so no adjustment to this regimen is required in patients requiring dialysis. Once the patient has recovered sufficiently to take oral medication, quinine can be continued orally at 10 mg salt/kg every 8 h. Treatment should continue for 7 days, or until blood films have shown no parasites on 3 consecutive days.

Quinine stimulates β-cell release of insulin, so close monitoring of blood sugar is required during intravenous therapy. The drug predictably increases the QT_c interval, but iatrogenic dysrhythmias are exceptionally rare. There is thus no need specially to monitor the ECG during therapy, although in practice on intensive care units this will be done in any event. Rapid bolus injection must be avoided, as this produces hypotension. Cinchonism — tinnitus, high-tone hearing loss, nausea and vomiting — is reasonably common.

- *Artemesinin derivatives*

Partial and complete resistance to quinine (and other antimalarials), initially noted on the Thai/Myanmar/Cambodia borders, has now been reported in many areas of the world. Imported malaria in the UK with quinine resistance remains uncommon. However, if parasitemia does not fall by >75% in the 48 h following quinine treatment, this indicates high-grade resistance. Under these circumstances, artemesinin derivatives such as artemether or artesunate should be used. They are only available on a named patient basis at present, and advice concerning their use should be obtained from the nearest specialist centre in Tropical Medicine. They also have the advantage of producing a more rapid clearance of parasites than quinine, and in a sick patient with parasitemia in excess of 30% at presentation, advice concerning their possible use should be sought as above.

Because of the possibility of some degree of resistance to quinine, once a parasitological cure has been achieved a course of a different drug is given, to eliminate the possibility of late recrudescence. Doxycycline 200 mg o.d. should be given for 7 days. An alternative in pregnancy is clindamycin 900 mg t.d.s. for 5 days.

2. Treatment of Renal Failure

Dialysis reduces the mortality of malaria-associated renal failure. Although peritoneal dialysis is effective, continuous veno-venous haemofiltration is preferable. Severe acidosis, hyperkalaemia, fluid overload and signs or symptoms of uraemia are all indications for dialysis. However, disease can progress very rapidly, and in fulminant infection severe acidosis can occur before creatinine levels have risen, in which case dialysis should be started early.

3. General Supportive Measures

As malarial-induced ARF usually arises in the context of multi-organ failure, patients are best managed on an intensive care unit, with the treatment principles as outlined in **Section 2** of this volume. Falciparum malaria can precipitate non-cardiac pulmonary oedema, so great care must be taken with fluid balance. A CVP line should be inserted and the level kept between 0 to 5 cm H_2O. Blood glucose should be monitored frequently and glucose infusions given as required.

4. Exchange Transfusion

Considerable controversy exists concerning the role of exchange transfusion or erythrocytapharesis (removal of red cells by cell separator) in the management of patients with severe falciparum malaria. Removal of parasitised red cells and malarial "toxins" seems an attractive idea, but the fact that many parasitised red cells are sequestered in the circulation (and thus not removed by these procedures) militates against the potential benefit. In addition, exchange transfusion is not without risk; complications include cerebral haemorrhage, fluid overload, transfusion reactions and metabolic disturbance. Many patients with high (>10%) parasitaemias have survived with drug therapy alone. On the other hand, many case reports have argued that institution of exchange transfusion has been associated with clinical benefit. There is no trial that has evaluated exchange transfusion, so the strict adherent of evidence-based medicine could not recommend its use. If the facilities are available, it can be used in very ill patients with parasitaemias in excess of 30% who are failing to respond rapidly to conventional therapy. However, with the more widespread use of artemesinin derivatives (see above), these circumstances may arise less commonly.

FURTHER READING

Day NPJ, Phu NH, Loc PP (1997) Malaria and ARF. *Journal of the Royal College of Physicians of London*; 31: 146–148

Faulde M, Sobe D, Kimmig P, Scharninghausen J (2000) Renal failure and Hantavirus infection in Europe. *Nephrology Dialysis and Transplantation*; 15: 751–753

Peraldi MN, Maslo C, Akposso K, Mougenot B, Rondeau E, Sraer JD (1999) ARF in the course of HIV infection: A single-institution retrospective study of ninety-two patients and sixty renal biopsies. *Nephrology Dialysis and Transplantation*; 14: 1578–1585

Peters CJ, Simpson GL, Levy H (1999) Spectrum of Hantavirus infection: Hemorrhagic fever with renal syndrome and Hantavirus pulmonary syndrome. *Annual Reviews of Medicine*; 50: 531–545

Rao TKS (1996) Renal complications in HIV disease. *Medical Clinics of North America*; 80: 1437–1451

Winearls CG, Chan L, Coghlan JD, Ledingham JGG, Oliver DO (1984) ARF Due to Leptospirosis: Clinical features and outcome in six cases. *Quarterly Journal of Medicine*; 212: 487–495

Chapter 21

MALIGNANT DISEASES
Peter Choi

INTRODUCTION

The management of ARF in the patient with malignant disease represents a significant challenge. The incidence of ARF in patients with cancer exceeds that in many other patient groups. Between 20–30% of patients with acute leukaemia will experience an episode of acute renal impairment at some time during treatment and up to 50% of patients receiving unrelated bone marrow transplants will develop ARF. Similar statistics exist for patients receiving chemotherapy for metastatic carcinoma. ARF directly confers significant morbidity and mortality upon the patient, who is likely to be in the midst of a prolonged illness, and additionally may delay or prevent definitive anti-cancer therapy. For these reasons, the development of ARF in the patient with cancer is invariably associated with a worsening of prognosis.

Patients with cancer may develop ARF arising from many possible aetiologies. It should be emphasised that, as in many cases of ARF, multiple renal insults may co-exist. The principle causes of ARF in the context of malignancy are listed in **Table 1**. The relative incidence of these pathologies will be dependent upon on the workload bias of referring units, but most surveys have indicated the importance of acute tubular necrosis (ATN) as the predominant renal insult in these patients. One 10 year review of ARF in patients with haematological malignancy, excluding

Table 1. Causes of ARF in patients with malignant disease

Acute tubular necrosis (secondary to ischaemia)

Drugs
Cytotoxic drugs
Other nephrotoxic drugs
e.g. NSAIDs, aminoglycosides, amphotericin

Acute interstitial nephritis

Urinary obstruction

Tumour lysis syndrome

Tumour infiltration

Paraneoplastic syndromes
Haemolytic uraemic syndrome
Crescentic glomerulonephritis
Renal vein thrombosis

Bone marrow transplantation complications
Bone marrow infusion syndrome
Hepatorenal syndrome

myeloma, identified ATN in 83% of patients (Harris *et al.*). This key observation would imply that many cases of ARF in patients with cancer are potentially preventable.

Some of the pathologies listed are discussed in detail elsewhere and, in this chapter, will only be further mentioned in the context of the general management principles. This chapter highlights the pathophysiology and management of tumour-lysis syndrome and renal tumour infiltration, and reviews those cytotoxic drugs and paraneoplastic syndromes that may lead to ARF.

1. TUMOUR LYSIS SYNDROME

DEFINITION

Tumour lysis syndrome (TLS) results from the toxicity of free cellular breakdown products which are synchronously released from malignant tissue, usually due to induced cell lysis following chemotherapy, but rarely due to spontaneous cell lysis resulting from ischaemic necrosis. Renal dysfunction in TLS results principally from acute uric acid accumulation. Hyperkalaemia, hyperphosphataemia and hypocalcaemia, each of which may be associated with its own specific complications, are also characteristic of TLS.

PATHOPHYSIOLOGY

Acute Urate Nephropathy

Uric acid is the end product of purine metabolism. The purines adenine and guanine are constituents of DNA and RNA and are components of many essential intracellular cofactors and regulatory molecules. The normal turnover of purines involves reuse of some breakdown products to resynthesise fresh purine nucleotides, and the oxidation of the excess to uric acid, via hypoxanthine and xanthine. Humans and higher primates excrete uric acid as they lack the enzyme uricase, which other mammals utilise to convert uric acid into allantoin, which is more water-soluble than uric acid.

Approximately 0.8 g of urate is formed each day, of which one-third is eliminated via the gut and two-thirds excreted via the kidneys. Urate is freely filtered at the glomerulus and undergoes a complex pattern of renal handling. Complete active proximal tubular reabsorption is followed by tubular secretion and post-secretory reabsorption.

Cell lysis is associated with a rapid increase in nucleotide metabolites and saturation of the purine salvage pathways, such that urate production is increased. When urate delivery to the distal tubule exceeds re-absorptive capacity, excess urinary urate may precipitate out. Crystallisation of urate occurs preferentially in the distal tubule due to the progressive reabsorption of water, and because urate becomes less soluble in the acidic conditions that predominate in the distal tubule. This pathological urate crystallisation, which results in intraluminal tubular obstruction, is the basis of acute urate nephropathy. Urate crystals may also precipitate in the renal pelvis or ureters and contribute to ARF due to outflow obstruction.

It follows that the development of TLS is dependent on the balance of uric acid release and renal uric acid excretion. Therefore the likelihood of TLS increases in situations where malignant tissue is highly sensitive to cytolytic treatment and where tumour bulk is high. Indeed, an elevated pre-treatment LDH or uric acid is predictive of TLS for haematological and solid malignancies. Similarly, TLS becomes more likely in the face of pre-existing renal impairment by virtue of reduced uric acid excretion. One review of patients with high grade Hodgkin's lymphoma found that those with a pre-treatment serum creatinine over 132 µmol/L were 18 times more likely to develop TLS than those with normal renal function (Hande and Garrow).

Hyperkalaemia (see also **Chapter 8.3**)

Potassium, the major intracellular cation, is maintained in the intracellular compartment by an active ATP-requiring process. Derangements to cellular metabolism and depletion of ATP are induced in malignant cells by chemo- and radio-therapy prior to the onset of complete cell lysis. Consequent dysfunction of ion pumps results in early loss of the potassium gradient, 12–24 hours after initiation of therapy. Therefore, potentially life-threatening hyperkalaemia can precede the onset of hyperuricaemia or hyperphosphataemia. Hyperkalaemia is more likely to develop in patients with pre-existing renal impairment.

Hyperphosphataemia and Hypocalcaemia (see also **Chapter 8.5**)

Phosphate is the most abundant intracellular anion and is a vital component of many co-enzymes and second messengers. Serum phosphate is freely filtered at the glomerulus and approximately 60–70% is actively reabsorbed in the proximal tubule under the influence of PTH, with an additional 5–10% being reabsorbed more distally. However, a reabsorptive threshold does exist, such that delivery of excess phosphate will result in its excretion.

Synchronous cell death in response to chemotherapy is associated with massive release of intracellular phosphate into the blood. If glomerular filtration is maintained, phosphate in excess of renal reabsorptive capacity will be excreted. However, the concomitant development of acute urate nephropathy tends to favour the progressive onset of hyperphosphataemia, which is usually maximal 48–96 h after the initiation of therapy. Hyperphosphataemia affects the kidney in two ways. Firstly, it is known to directly exacerbate experimental ARF by an unknown mechanism and, secondly, may result in renal calcium phosphate deposition which is tubulotoxic.

Hyperphosphataemia leads to a reciprocal depression of serum calcium levels by precipitation of calcium phosphate and depression of calcitriol production.

CLINICAL PRESENTATION

Tumour lysis syndrome is characterised by the onset of hyperkalaemia, hyperuricaemia, hyperphosphataemia and hypocalcaemia, often associated with loin pain and oliguric renal failure. The syndrome develops within four days of commencing chemotherapy. Considerable variability exists in the clinical presentation, and subclinical metabolic abnormalities frequently follow chemotherapy without development of the full-blown syndrome. A key observation is that, amongst patients who go on to develop ARF, hyperphosphataemia is the most consistent biochemical abnormality seen. In cases where diagnosis is not clear, a urinary uric acid: creatinine ratio

Table 2. Tumour types associated with acute tumour lysis syndrome	
Those underlined are more commonly associated. Those indicated in italics are case reports	
Haematological malignancies associated with TLS	**Solid tumours associated with TLS**
<u>Burkitt's lymphoma</u>	Breast carcinoma
<u>Acute lymphocytic leukaemia</u>	Small cell lung carcinoma
<u>Other non-Hodgkin's lymphomas</u>	Neuroblastoma
Acute leukaemias	*Medulloblastoma*
Chronic lymphocytic leukaemia	*Rhabdomyosarcoma*
Chronic myeloid leukaemia — in blast crisis	*Ovarian carcinoma*
	Seminoma
	Hepatoblastoma
	Melanoma

>1 is highly suggestive of acute urate nephropathy. Examination of urinary sediment is rarely diagnostic, and usually shows amorphous debris or is normal, but may reveal uric acid crystals which are rhomboidal in shape (see **Chapter 4.2**).

TLS has traditionally been associated with a number of chemosensitive haematological malignancies. It is likely that the future development of more aggressive treatment strategies will result in an increased incidence of TLS in malignancies not usually associated with TLS. **Table 2** lists those malignancies which have been associated with TLS to date.

TREATMENT PRINCIPLES

The key to management of TLS is identification of at-risk patients prior to the initiation of chemotherapy. With appropriate prophylaxis, most cases of oliguria can be avoided. The prevention of TLS is especially important as, by definition, the syndrome occurs in patients who have responded to treatment (**Table 3**). Rare patients, such as those with Burkitt's lymphoma or those with impaired renal function, may develop oliguria with severe metabolic abnormalities despite prophylactic measures. An algorithm describing prophylaxis of TLS is shown in **Practice Point 1**.

If oliguric TLS does develop, the principle aim of management then becomes to control life-threatening hyperkalaemia and the sequelae of ARF (see **Section 2**), whilst encouraging dissolution of uric acid crystals and renal recovery (**Table 4**). Use of intravenous urate oxidase (Uricozyme®, Sanofi Winthrop Ltd., UK) to render uric acid more soluble for urinary excretion may be effective in limiting the progression of and hastening recovery from TLS. A number of studies have demonstrated a rapid fall in serum urate levels and increase in urine output following administration of urate oxidase at a dose of 100 units/kg/day over 3–5 days. Presently, this drug must be prescribed on a named-patient basis.

Table 3. Prevention of acute tumour lysis syndrome	
Treatment aim	**Rationale**
Hyperhydration (with invasive pressure monitoring if necessary)	Urate and phosphate in excess of reabsorption threshold can be excreted if glomerular filtration is maintained. Animal data support the pre-eminent role of diuresis in preventing acute urate nephropathy
Loop diuretic	Aids high urine flow rate if not achieved by hydration alone. Additional phosphaturic effect
Alkalinisation of urine with bicarbonate	Uric acid is 13 times more soluble at pH 7.0 than pH 5.0
Allopurinol	Inhibits xanthine oxidase mediated production of uric acid from xanthine and hypoxanthine
	NB. In exceptional cases, allopurinol may cause xanthine to exceed its solubility product and precipitate in distal tubule

Table 4. Treatment of established TLS	
Treatment aim	**Comments**
Control hyperkalaemia	Insulin and dextrose may prove ineffectual as potassium transport mechanisms are damaged. Early dialysis may be indicated
Control hyperphosphataemia	Dialysis may be necessary to prevent metastatic calcification. Limit oral phosphate
Consider continuing hydration	Only if urine output allows, and in conjunction with invasive pressure monitoring/strict fluid balance in order to prevent pulmonary oedema. Fluid overload may develop quickly in acute TLS
Consider continuing urinary alkalinisation	Stop if Ca^{2+}/PO^{2-}_4 product rising, as increases likelihood of metastatic calcification
Consider IV Uricozyme	Converts uric acid into allantoin, which is ten-fold more soluble at urinary pH

Dialysis has two roles in the treatment of acute TLS. Firstly, haemodialysis is conventionally indicated for treatment of:

- Hyperkalaemia.
- Hyperphosphataemia and metastatic calcification.
- Fluid overload.
- ARF.

Practice Point 1. Prevention of TLS

Consider risk factors
- High tumour load
- Chemosensitivity
- Renal impairment
- Elevated LDH
- Elevated uric acid

If any one factor present, commence prophylaxis

Hyperhydrate

Allopurinol
300–600 mg/day. Start at least 3 days before treatment

Urinary alkalinisation

Saline infusion to achieve UO >200 mL/hour
Commence 24 hours prior to onset of therapy

Check urinary pH once diuresis established

Diuresis achieved

Diuresis not achieved

pH >7.0

pH <7.0

IV frusemide 50–250 mg to achieve UO >200 mL/h

Sodium bicarbonate: 75–100 mmol per litre

e.g. alternate 500 mL 1.26% NaHCO$_3$ with 500 mL dextrose

Diuresis achieved

Diuresis not achieved

Recheck pH

pH >7.0

pH <7.0

Continue fluids until biochemistry becomes normal, or for 2 days after therapy

Tail down input to match output + insensible losses

No alkali
Recheck urinary pH daily

Recommence alkali if pH falls below 7.0

Continue alkali therapy

Secondly, haemodialysis should be considered as definitive therapy for hyperuricaemia and as such greatly speeds recovery from acute urate nephropathy, particularly as the return of renal function mirrors serum urate levels. Haemodialysis is highly efficient at removal of uric acid as well as phosphate, and may induce a brisk diuresis after relatively few treatment sessions. Haemodialysis may therefore be considered in acute TLS, even in the absence of conventional indications.

There is no role for acute peritoneal dialysis in treatment of TLS.

OUTCOME

The release of toxic cellular breakdown products is self-limiting and renal prognosis is good if the patient can be managed through the acute phase. However , the development of TLS should have implications for the planning of subsequent chemotherapy. Prophylactic uric acid oxidase may be considered.

2. TUMOUR INFILTRATION

Bilateral infiltration of the renal parenchyma by malignant cells is a post-mortem finding in up to 30–50% of patients who die from leukaemia or lymphoma. Such renal infiltration is usually clinically silent, but may result in acute or chronic renal failure. Conversely, tumour infiltration by metastatic solid tumours usually results in ARF by involvement of lymph nodes, causing ureteric obstruction or vascular occlusion, and few cases of bilateral parenchymal infiltration from solid tumours have been described.

PATHOPHYSIOLOGY

ARF due to renal infiltration may arise from any histological variant of acute or chronic leukaemia, or lymphoma. Spread to the kidney may be haematogenous, lymphatic or by direct invasion through Geronta's fascia from the adrenals or extra-renal lymph nodes. The malignant cells accumulate in the interstitium of the cortex, resulting in compression of the tubules and increased glomerular back-pressure. Renal impairment ensues. Histologically, glomeruli appear normal. Renal infiltration may be nodular or diffuse in pattern. Diffuse infiltration is more often associated with renal failure.

CLINICAL PRESENTATION

Tumour infiltration may result in silent chronic renal failure. ARF due to tumour infiltration presents with oliguria and loin pain, in association with constitutional upset. Physical examination often reveals bilateral loin masses, which are confirmed as enlarged kidneys by ultrasonography or CT scanning. It is important to exclude co-existent obstruction. Urine examination shows proteinuria, microscopic haematuria but rarely malignant cells.

TREATMENT PRINICIPLES

Definitive management requires chemotherapy for the infiltrating tumour. However, in the face of renal impairment, this carries a high likelihood of precipitating tumour lysis syndrome and dosing of cytotoxic drugs may be difficult. Therefore, prior local irradiation of the kidneys should be considered to allow some recovery of renal function, before commencing definitive therapy.

OUTCOME

In most cases, recovery of renal function is rapid following radiotherapy or chemotherapy, unless TLS supervenes. Improvement is associated with a decrease in renal size. Overall prognosis is dependent on the underlying malignancy.

3. ANTI-CANCER DRUGS AND ARF

The use of cytotoxic agents at high dose and in combinations that potentiate nephrotoxicity is increasingly associated with ARF in patients with malignant disease (**Table 5**). In addition to their ability to induce tumour lysis syndrome, anti-cancer drugs may cause direct nephrotoxicity in one of two ways. Some drugs, notably cisplatin, methotrexate, mithramycin, streptozotocin, and interleukin-2, induce a predictable, dose-dependent fall in GFR, often after the first dose. Other drugs, such as mitomycin and CCNU, result in a less predictable, but often irreversible, nephrotoxicity after multiple exposures.

The nephrotoxicity of anti-cancer drugs is discussed further in **Chapter 11**. Note that in **Table 5**, where doses are given, these are intended to serve as a clinical guide in assessing the contribution of a given drug to ARF, and are not intended to define safe dosages for treatment. It should be remembered that other drugs commonly given to cancer patients, such as aminoglycosides, NSAIDs and amphotericin, have the potential to enhance the nephrotoxic effects of cytotoxic therapy, and should be avoided.

The cornerstone of prophylaxis is adequate hydration, with intravenous fluids for 24 h prior to onset of therapy in situations where renal dysfunction is common. The use of correct drug dosages and administration in split doses may also lessen the risk of nephrotoxicity. Many specific prophylactics have been advocated, particularly with the use of cisplatin, but none has been of proven benefit.

4. PARANEOPLASTIC SYNDROMES

A paraneoplastic syndrome is a syndrome arising from the activity of a protein directly produced by cancerous cells or induced from other cell-types by cancerous cells. Renal paraneoplastic syndromes may rarely contribute to ARF in one of three ways, as outlined in **Table 1**. In the majority of cases, the nature of the causative bioactive agent is unknown.

Haemolytic uraemic syndrome (HUS), which is characterised by ARF in association with a microangiopathic anaemia, results from abnormal endothelial activation in response to a circulating factor. HUS in the context of malignancy usually arises as a complication of cytotoxic drugs, but

Table 5. Anti-cancer drugs and ARF

Drug	Comments
1. Alkylating agents	
Cisplatin	Intracellular toxin which accumulates in tubular cells. Gradual onset non-oliguric renal failure 3–5 days after therapy. Also associated with urinary Na^+, Ca^{2+}, Mg^{2+} and PO^{2-}_4 wasting
	>100 mg/m^2 associated with ARF
	50–75 mg/m^2 may cause delayed renal impairment
Carboplatin	Less nephrotoxic than cisplatin
BCNU	Nephrotoxicity not often seen as pulmonary toxicity is limiting
CCNU	Progressive renal failure after multiple doses
Methyl CCNU	Progressive, irreversible renal failure after doses >1500 mg/m^2
Streptozotocin	Dose dependent renal failure with Fanconi's syndrome
	>4 g/m^2 total dose associated with nephrotoxicity
Ifosfamide	Dose dependent renal failure and tubular dysfunction, especially when used with cisplatin
2. Antimetabolites	
Methotrexate	Non-oliguric ARF at doses >1 g/m^2. Poorly removed by dialysis
Cytosine arabinoside	50% incidence of renal failure when used in multi-drug regimens
3. Antitumour antibiotics	
Mitomycin-C	Dose dependent ARF, most pronounced in combination with other drugs. Also associated with HUS, which is unresponsive to plasma exchange
Mithramycin	Renal failure after multiple doses
4. Cytokines	
Interferon-α	Minimal change nephropathy. Occasionally ARF
Interferon-γ	Associated with ARF and ATN
Interleukin 2	Dose dependent oliguric ARF with vascular leak syndrome. May be prevented by low-dose dopamine. Rarely associated with crescentic nephritis

has also been associated with specific malignancies (acute promyelomonocytic leukaemia, prostate carcinoma, gastric carcinoma and pancreatic carcinoma) and vascular tumours (giant haemangiomas and haemangioendotheliomas). The pathophysiology and treatment of HUS are described in detail in **Chapter 15**.

A number of glomerulonephritides are associated with malignancy, and there exists strong circumstantial evidence for a causal relationship: successful treatment of malignant disease is often accompanied by a remission of nephropathy; recurrence of tumour may be associated with a recurrence of nephropathy; and, in rare cases such as melanoma, cancer antigen and anti-cancer antibodies have been demonstrated in affected glomeruli.

The most common histological appearances associated with malignancy are membranous nephropathy (accounting for 60–70% of cases), mesangiocapillary nephritis, IgA nephropathy and amyloid nephropathy. In general, the clinical presentation is nephrotic syndrome or asymptomatic proteinuria/haematuria, and impairment of renal function is unusual. The exception is crescentic nephritis, which may be associated with lymphoma or carcinoma, and presents with acute renal failure. Although this pathology is rarely associated with malignancy, two separate reviews of patients with crescentic nephritis revealed that 7–9% of these patients had a co-existent cancer. Crescentic nephritis was usually diagnosed after the diagnosis of cancer, and tumour removal was sometimes associated with complete remission of the renal condition. The management of rapidly progressive glomerulonephritis is discussed in **Chapter 16**.

Severe nephrotic syndrome, particularly when due to membranous nephropathy, may be complicated by bilateral renal vein thrombosis, presenting as oligo-anuric ARF with loin pain and macroscopic haematuria. The diagnosis may be confirmed by venous Doppler studies, though these are technically difficult and venography or MRI scanning may be required. Aggressive anticoagulation with heparin and warfarin according to a pulmonary embolus protocol may preserve renal function. The use of fibrinolytics or surgical thrombectomy does not confer greater benefit. However, renal prognosis may be poor, especially as thrombosis is often precipitated by underlying venous tumour invasion.

MANAGEMENT OF ARF IN THE CONTEXT OF MALIGNANCY

Management of patients with cancer who develop ARF is fraught by many conflicting influences. It is vital throughout the process of care that a clear goal is defined, including the limits of treatment in the event of failure to respond. These goals should be clearly agreed between all medical and nursing teams involved. In many cases, it is appropriate to communicate this to the patient and relatives, but this should not remove the primary responsibility from medical staff.

DIAGNOSIS OF ARF IN THE CONTEXT OF MALIGNANCY

This section will provide a general overview of the diagnosis of ARF in patients with cancer. Details of the diagnostic investigations for specific disorders are provided in the relevant chapters and will not be restated here.

Early diagnosis of the cause of ARF is necessary for successful treatment of patients with cancer. Progression to dialysis-dependency or multiple organ failure is often associated with a poor outcome. The following general principles apply to the algorithm in **Practice Point 2**.

- Consider the high likelihood of ATN as the cause of ARF, as revealed by clinical studies.
- Correct assessment of volume status is vital. Where clinical doubt exists, it is short-sighted to avoid early invasive monitoring, unless the overall management of the patient is clearly palliative.
- Consider the possibility of multiple renal insults co-existing and therefore complete the algorithm for all patients.
- Diagnosis is urgent and important investigations should not be delayed. In particular, ultrasound scanning should be performed immediately.
- Consider the underlying malignant diagnosis and its association with specific renal pathologies.

Practice Point 2. Guidelines for diagnosis of ARF in malignancy

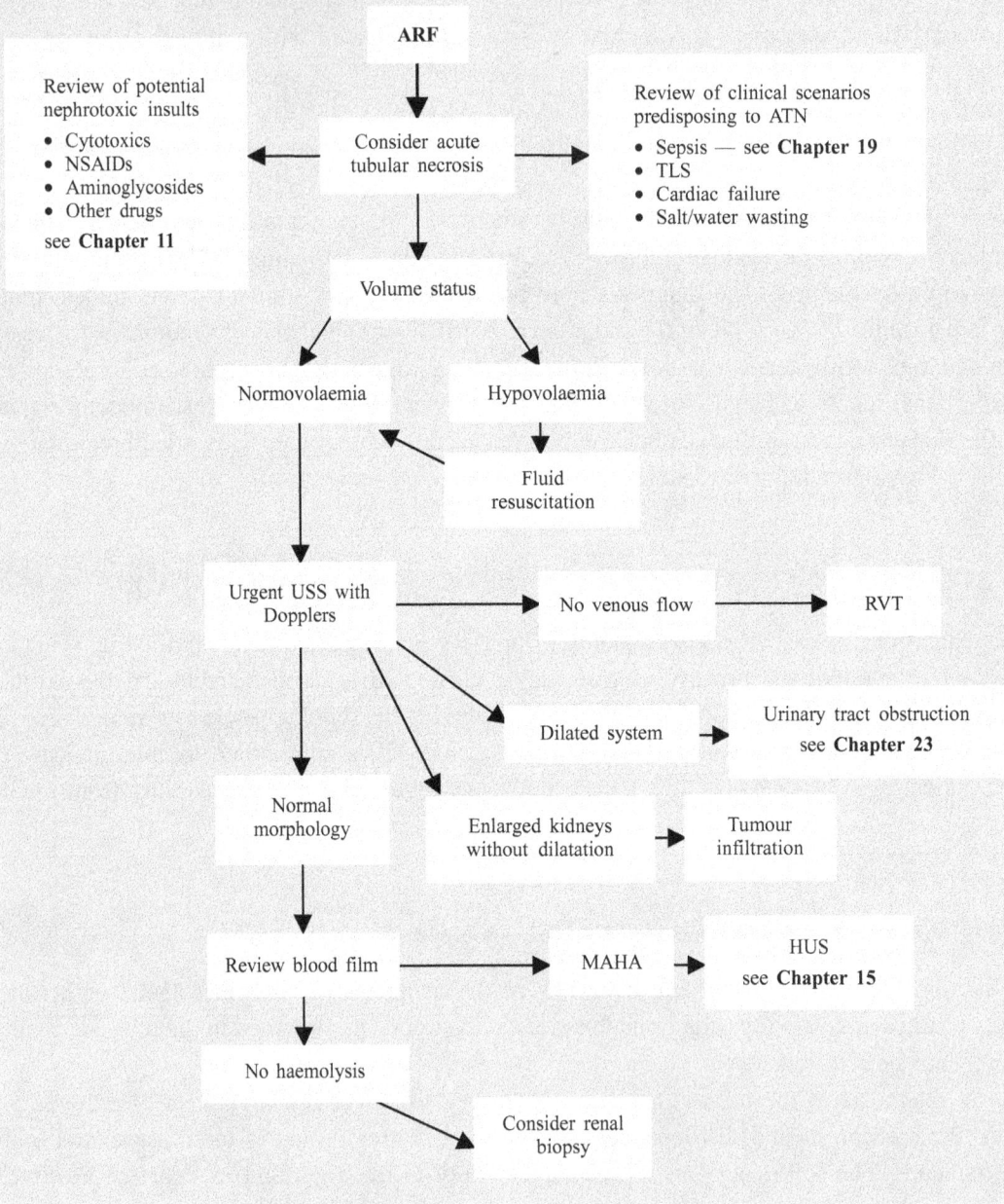

ARF

Review of potential
nephrotoxic insults
- Cytotoxics
- NSAIDs
- Aminoglycosides
- Other drugs
see **Chapter 11**

Consider acute
tubular necrosis

Review of clinical scenarios
predisposing to ATN
- Sepsis — see **Chapter 19**
- TLS
- Cardiac failure
- Salt/water wasting

Volume status

Normovolaemia

Hypovolaemia

Fluid
resuscitation

Urgent USS with
Dopplers

No venous flow

RVT

Dilated system

Urinary tract obstruction
see **Chapter 23**

Normal
morphology

Enlarged kidneys
without dilatation

Tumour
infiltration

Review blood film

MAHA

HUS
see **Chapter 15**

No haemolysis

Consider renal
biopsy

TREATMENT OF ARF IN THE CONTEXT OF MALIGNANCY

Following diagnosis, the treatment of ARF in patients with cancer may not differ significantly from the treatment of ARF in patients who do not have cancer. This is particularly the case where attention to fluid balance and removal of nephrotoxic drugs is sufficient to rescue incipient ATN. The principle factor imposed by the co-existence of malignancy is the need to consider the appropriateness of more invasive manoeuvres with respect to the overall prognosis of the patient's cancer. However, the existence of malignancy should not itself constitute reason to pursue a sub-optimal management plan.

The reader is referred to the relevant sections for specific management protocols.

OUTCOME

Amongst patients with cancer, the occurrence of ARF confers a poor prognosis. One survey found that only 28% of patients with cancer who developed ARF which required dialysis were discharged from intensive care. Cancer patients who developed ARF in the context of sepsis or who required ventilatory support were especially vulnerable and had greater than 90% short-term mortality. However, most surveys have concentrated on patients requiring intensive care and the prognosis of patients with lesser degrees of acute renal impairment may be substantially less gloomy. One review of the mortality of bone marrow transplant recipients in relation to the severity of their renal failure showed that dialysis requiring patients had an 84% mortality, falling to 37% in patients with acute renal impairment not requiring dialysis, and 17% in patients with preserved renal function.

FURTHER READING

Hande KR, Garrow GC (1993) Acute tumor lysis syndrome in patients with high-grade non-Hodgkins lymphoma. *American Journal of Medicine*; 94: 133–139

Harris KPG, Hattersley JM, Feehally J, Walls J (1991) Acute renal failure associated with haematological malignancies: A review of 10 years experience. *European Journal of Haematology*; 47: 119–122

Leach M, Parsons RM, Reilly JT, Winfield DA (1998) Efficacy of urate oxidase (uricozyme) in tumour lysis induced urate nephropathy. *Clinical Laboratory Haematology*; 20: 169–172

Maesaka JK, Mittal SK, Fishbane S (1997) Paraneoplastic syndromes of the kidney. *Seminars in Oncology*; 24: 373–381

Safirstein RL (1997) Renal diseases induced by antineoplastic agents. In: Schrier RW and Gottschalk CW (eds.). *Diseases of the Kidney*. Boston. Little Brown

Zager RA (1994) Acute renal failure in the setting of bone marrow transplantation. *Kidney International*; 46: 1443–1458

Chapter 22 _____

MYELOMA AND ACUTE RENAL FAILURE
Jeremy Levy

DEFINITION

Myeloma is one of a number of plasma cell dyscrasias characterised by the uncontrolled proliferation of a single B cell clone. The incidence of myeloma is approximately 40 new cases per million population per year, and 10% of patients will have severe acute renal failure (ARF). Other related diseases include AL amyloidosis, Waldenstrom's macroglobulinaemia, monoclonal immunoglobulin deposition diseases and monoclonal gammopathy of uncertain significance (MGUS). In all these cases, an aberrant B lymphocyte population secretes a paraprotein: either an intact monoclonal immunoglobulin, or a derived fragment (usually a light chain alone). Clinical features may be caused by the B cells themselves, by the secreted immunoglobulin molecule, by the suppression of normal antibody synthesis or by metabolic effects. ARF is a common and important complication of myeloma. Up to 50% of all patients with myeloma will have renal dysfunction, of whom 20% will have severe renal failure. Historically, renal failure was thought to be a poor prognostic feature of myeloma; however, more recently it has been recognised that renal failure occurs in patients with increased tumour loads, and that renal failure *per se* may not be an independent marker of poor outcome. Furthermore, renal failure may be reversible in a significant proportion of patients. Other important causes of renal failure in plasma cell dyscrasias include cryoglobulinaemia, light chain deposition disease and AL amyloidosis.

PATHOPHYSIOLOGY

The most important cause of ARF in myeloma is the production of a nephrotoxic paraprotein by the abnormal B cells. However, there are a number of other causes for renal dysfunction in myeloma, and frequently a precipitating event is required before patients with myeloma develop renal failure. Furthermore, many patients with myeloma have water, electrolyte and acid-base disturbances, all of which may require nephrological input (**Table 1**).

Henry Bence Jones and William McIntyre first described the unusual thermal stability properties of urinary proteins in patients with bone pain and oedema in 1845. Hence, light chain proteinuria is also referred to as Bence Jones proteinuria. Excess urinary light chains (normally found together with heavy chains in the immunoglobulin molecule) are the most important underlying cause of renal failure in myeloma, since they directly contribute to cast nephropathy, which in turn is the commonest cause of renal failure. Renal failure predates the diagnosis of myeloma in 50% of patients in whom it will occur, and develops in most of the remainder within one month of the diagnosis of myeloma.

Table 1. Causes of renal dysfunction in myeloma

Renal disease	Precipitants	Electrolyte and fluid disturbances
Light chain proteinuria	Volume depletion	Hypercalcaemia
Light chain cast nephropathy	Non-steroidal anti-inflammatory drugs	Dehydration
Light chain deposition disease	Hypercalcaemia	Pseudohyponatraemia
Hypercalcaemic nephropathy	Radiocontrast media	Hyperviscosity
AL amyloidosis	Furosemide	Hyperuricaemia
Acute urate nephropathy	Septicaemia	Hyperkalaemia
Obstructive uropathy	Urinary tract infection	
Pyelonephritis		
Acute interstitial nephritis		
Cryoglobulinaemia		
End stage renal disease		

Table 2. The incidence of renal manifestations (light chain proteinuria and renal failure) in myeloma patients with different immunoglobulin class paraproteins

	All myeloma (%)	Light chain proteinuria (%)	Renal failure (%)
IgG	55	50–70	25–50
IgA	25	50–70	30–60
IgD	1	90	90–100
Light chains only	20	100	50–90

Why only some light chains are nephrotoxic, and why different light chains cause different patterns of renal disease, is unclear. There is no good association between the isoelectric point or isotype of individual light chains and their nephrotoxicity. Some nephrotoxic light chains are relatively resistant to proteolysis, and some are able to self aggregate into multimers under physiologic conditions. There is certainly a difference in the incidence of renal failure according to the class of immunoglobulin present in excess, being highest in patients with IgD myeloma and pure light chain myeloma (**Table 2**).

The risk of developing renal failure is twice as high in patients with pure light chain myeloma than in the commonest IgG myeloma, and increases with increasing light chain excretion. There is no real difference in the incidence of renal failure in patients with λ or κ light chains.

There are two main mechanisms for the nephrotoxicity of renally excreted light chains. Firstly, free light chains are directly nephrotoxic: renal failure is rare in myeloma patients without Bence-Jones proteinuria; identical light chain crystals are found in plasma cells, casts and proximal tubule cells; and mice injected intra-peritoneally with purified light chains from patients with myeloma develop similar renal lesions to those of the patients from whom the light chains were obtained. Furthermore, in these studies, light chains from patients with myeloma but no renal failure rarely deposited in the kidneys of mice. In a microperfusion model some (but not all) light chains injected into proximal tubules caused loss of the microvillus border, cellular shedding and fragmentation, and subsequent obstruction of the distal tubule. Light chains from a patient without renal failure did not cause such tubular damage and obstruction.

The second major mechanism of renal damage by light chains is the formation of casts in distal tubules. Although nephrotoxic light chains are necessary for the development of cast nephropathy, there are usually concomitant factors which precipitate the renal failure. Free light chains produced during normal immunoglobulin synthesis are filtered through the glomerulus and reabsorbed in the proximal tubule by a low affinity endocytotic receptor. As noted, an excess of tubular light chains directly causes morphological changes in proximal tubule cells, and overwhelms the normal mechanisms for disposal of filtered light chains. Dehydration, NSAIDs, or other causes for a reduced GFR, will increase the concentration of light chains in the tubular fluid, increasing the extent of proximal tubule damage, and thus increasing the delivery of light chains to the distal tubule. Proximal tubule damage itself causes salt and water loss, and further exacerbates a reduction in GFR, initiating a vicious circle leading to rapidly rising distal tubule concentration of light chains. Under these conditions light chains readily precipitate in the distal tubules as obstructing casts.

Myeloma casts are composed principally of monoclonal light chains and Tamm-Horsfall glycoprotein (THP), a major constituent of normal urine synthesised exclusively by cells of the thick ascending limb of the loop of Henle. THP is able to form high molecular weight aggregates at high (but physiologic) concentrations of sodium and calcium, and at low urinary pH. Light chains are able to bind specifically to THP along its peptide core, a process which can be inhibited by anti-peptide antibodies. The aggregation of light chains and THP can be encouraged experimentally by reducing extracellular volume or by furosemide. Pre-treatment of animals with colchicine completely prevents tubular obstruction and cast formation, possibly by altering the sialic acid content of the THP, even though binding is not thought to be to carbohydrate residues. THP from normal human volunteers given colchicine also has diminished aggregation *in vitro* in the presence of pathogenic light chains. Not all tubular casts in myeloma kidney contain THP, however, and in some patients light chains can undergo homotypic precipitation alone. Distal tubular cast formation of any type subsequently causes back leak of tubular fluid into the interstitium, and disruption of tubular basement membranes and tubular integrity. This leads to the presence of THP and light chains within the interstitial regions of the kidney, where they can elicit an intense inflammatory reaction. Immunomorphological studies have clearly demonstrated THP in Bowman's space within glomeruli in patients with myeloma renal failure, indicating intratubular urinary backflow. Some (but not all) clinical studies have shown a correlation between the extent of cast formation and the degree of renal failure.

Thus, light chains can cause tubular damage by a number of mechanisms which may vary from one light chain to another. However, renal failure often evolves rapidly, implicating extrinsic factors as a major precipitant. Dehydration, diuretics, NSAIDs, hypercalcaemia, contrast media and antibiotics may all play a role by decreasing GFR, and thus increasing the intratubular concentration of light chains. Drugs and contrast media may also act as tubular epithelial cell toxins and decrease proximal tubular absorption of light chains. Hypercalcaemia causes vasoconstriction and reduced GFR, and impairs renal concentrating and sodium reabsorption mechanisms, leading to polyuria and dehydration. NSAIDs decrease renal blood flow and decrease sodium reabsorption. Increased distal tubular sodium and calcium concentration both exacerbate THP aggregation with light chains.

CLINICAL PRESENTATION

Renal failure antedates the diagnosis of myeloma in 50% of patients in whom it will occur, and is thus frequently the presenting feature. Myeloma is also a common cause for ARF of undetermined origin prior to biopsy. The mean age at presentation is 65 years, and there is a slight excess of men. The presence of renal failure is strongly associated with advanced disease.

Clinical Features

- Signs and symptoms are usually those of myeloma, including bone pain, weight loss, weakness and infections. 75% of patients have osteolytic lesions on radiography.
- Patients usually have an acute precipitating event for their renal failure, e.g. infection, hypercalcaemia, dehydration or the use of NSAIDs (**Table 3**). A careful drug history is important.
- Over 70% of patients will have urinary light chains (not detectable with urine dipsticks).
- Albuminuria is rarely >1g/day — in these cases the renal lesion is much more likely to be amyloid or light chain deposition disease (see later).
- Tumour mass is usually large — most patients (>70%) will have Durie and Salmon grade IIIB disease.
- Most patients present with severe renal failure — the mean creatinine at presentation is >800 μmol/L, and >50% of patients require immediate dialysis.

Contrast media represent only a small risk in patients with myeloma, the prevalence of renal failure increasing from 0.15% of the general population given radiocontrast to 0.6–1.25% in patients with myeloma.

Table 3. Incidence of precipitating factors in the development of renal failure in patients with myeloma

Precipitating events	Overall incidence
Dehydration	10–65%
Hypercalcaemia	19–57%
Infection	10–44%
NSAIDs	0–26%
Contrast medium	0–11%

INVESTIGATIONS

Investigations should focus on confirming the diagnosis of myeloma itself, the extent of disease, and establishing a cause for the renal failure (**Table 4**).

Table 4. Important investigations in the patient with suspected myeloma and ARF

FBC	↑platelets may be associated with worse outcome, though pancytopaenia common
ESR/plasma viscosity	May be normal in light chain disease Particularly ↑ in Waldenstrom's macroglobulinaemia
Biochemical profile	Pseudohyponatraemia can occur as increased protein reduces plasma sodium concentration Alkaline phosphatase usually normal
Serum calcium	30–50% of patients have ↑ calcium. Even moderate ↑ in calcium may precipitate cast nephropathy
Uric acid	Frequently ↑, but urate nephropathy rare
Anion gap (from serum chloride & bicarbonate)	Usually low in the presence of paraproteinaemia, except IgA myeloma. Normal anion gap may mask a true (raised anion gap) metabolic acidosis
Serum immunoglobulins	Immune-paresis common
Immunoelectrophoresis (serum & urine)	Up to 50% of patients will not have a serum M band (intact paraprotein), but only light chains
Serum paraprotein concentration	May be indicative of tumour load
Cryoglobulins	Type I cryoglobulins particularly may occur in myeloma
β_2 microglobulin (serum)	Elevation denotes a poor prognosis (reflection of tumour mass)
24 h urine protein	Nephrotic syndrome rare in pure myeloma kidney May indicate light chain deposition disease or AL amyloid
Urine glucose, phosphate & amino acids	Adult Fanconi syndrome can occur but is rare
Bone marrow aspiration and trephine	Mean plasma cell infiltrate ~40% in patients with renal failure
Blood and urine culture	Infection is an important precipitant of renal failure and the commonest cause of death in patients with myeloma
Renal biopsy	See below
Imaging	Renal U/S for obstruction Plain X Rays for lytic lesions

Renal Biopsy

The characteristic findings in myeloma kidney are the presence of tubular casts associated with alterations in the tubule epithelium, and an associated inflammatory response. The casts are usually present in distal tubules and collecting ducts, and often have a fractured or laminated appearance. Both casts and tubular cells frequently contain crystals of light chains. Immunostaining confirms that casts are composed of monoclonal light chains and Tamm-Horsfall protein, though up to 25% stain with both anti-λ and anti-κ antibodies. Casts are surrounded by denuded epithelial cells, mononuclear cells and by multinucleated giant cells. Tubular damage is a consistent finding, involving proximal and distal tubules, with epithelial degeneration and tubular necrosis. Interstitial infiltrates, interstitial fibrosis, oedema and tubular atrophy are also very common. Granuloma-like lesions can be found close to myeloma casts. In contrast to these interstitial changes, the glomeruli are usually normal. Glomerular changes are very rare and should raise the possibility of monoclonal immunoglobulin deposition disease (MIDD) rather than myeloma kidney (cast nephropathy).

Is a Renal Biopsy Needed in a Patient with Confirmed Myeloma and Renal Failure?

A renal biopsy is not without risk in a patient with acute uraemia, prolonged bleeding time, functional platelet deficiencies, etc. However, renal failure can have many causes in patients with myeloma, and cast nephropathy, LCDD, AL amyloidosis, ATN and interstitial nephritis have very different outcomes. Furthermore, in some patients the renal injury is chronic with marked interstitial fibrosis and glomerulosclerosis. Thus, a biopsy will often provide prognostic information about renal recovery, and may guide therapy (e.g. the use of plasma exchange).

TREATMENT (see **Practice Point**)

Prevention of renal failure is paramount in patients with myeloma. Potential precipitants of renal failure should be avoided and renal function monitored closely. Serum calcium should be maintained in the normal physiologic range and dehydration aggressively prevented.

For patients with myeloma and established renal failure, treatment must focus on the renal failure itself, its underlying cause, and on the plasma cell dyscrasia. Thus, precipitants must be reversed or removed, light chain concentrations reduced and plasma cell secretion of further light chains inhibited. Hydration is the most crucial aspect of management (see below).

Precipitants

- NSAIDs, nephrotoxic antibiotics and diuretics should be stopped if possible, or alternatives substituted.
- Volume replete rapidly with intravenous normal saline and oral fluids. Fluid intake should be >3 L/day.
- Identify and treat infections, especially urinary sepsis.
- Correct hypercalcaemia, initially by rehydration. Prednisolone (or dexamethasone) will lower serum calcium and is usually part of a chemotherapeutic regimen for myeloma (see below). If severe hypercalcaemia occurs, consider bisphosphonates (pamidronate 60–90 mg IV over 4–24 hours).
- Prevent hyperuricaemia with allopurinol (reduce dose in renal failure).

Active Management of Renal Failure

- Maintaining urine flow rates of >3 L/day in patients who can tolerate volume expansion will improve renal function in most patients with renal failure and myeloma (good evidence from MRC trials). For most patients this will be sufficient therapy.
- Alkalinisation of urine is sometimes used, without substantive evidence. *In vitro*, some light chains can be prevented from precipitating with Tamm-Horsfall protein at high urine pH, but there is no evidence in humans that bicarbonate improves the outcome. In the MRC trial of the treatment of myeloma and renal failure, rehydration alone was successful in reversing renal dysfunction in most patients.
- Furosemide is calciuric and may help maintain urine output during aggressive fluid management, but may also increase light chain nephrotoxicity (by increasing distal tubule calcium concentration) and worsen hypovolaemia. Furosemide should therefore be used cautiously, if at all.

Plasma Exchange

There are a large number of case reports of the benefits of plasma exchange in patients with myeloma and renal failure, but only two small controlled trials. The aim of plasma exchange in myeloma is to reduce the concentration of circulating light chains as rapidly as possible, and thus limit their continued toxicity within tubules and the renal interstitium. However the volume of distribution of light chains is large, and plasma exchange is not a very efficient way of removing them. Despite this theoretical objection, plasma exchange has been used in patients with myeloma cast nephropathy and myeloma interstitial nephritis. There is no role for plasma exchange in treating ATN, dehydration, obstruction or hypercalcaemic nephropathy. Simultaneous or sequential inhibition of light chain production by plasma cells must be attempted by chemotherapy (see below).

   Uncontrolled studies have shown increased rates of renal recovery (from 20% up to 60%) in patients treated with plasma exchange in addition to chemotherapy. In the first controlled trial of plasma exchange, Zuchelli *et al.* randomised 29 patients with myeloma and renal failure to receive either plasma exchange and chemotherapy (prednisolone and cyclophosphamide) or chemotherapy alone, after initial treatment with intravenous fluids, furosemide and sodium bicarbonate. Plasma exchange was performed on five consecutive days by plasmafiltration (3–4 L) for saline, albumin and fresh frozen plasma. To complicate the study, all patients receiving plasma exchange were treated with haemodialysis, whilst those in the control group received intermittent peritoneal dialysis. All patients had >1 g/day light chain proteinuria, and in 19 patients the renal failure was the first presentation of their myeloma. Renal failure was defined by a rise in creatinine >440 µmol/L, not reversible by rehydration. Twenty-four of the 29 patients required dialysis, and 16 were oliguric. Renal biopsy in 17 patients showed cast nephropathy in 16. The results showed a clear benefit for plasma exchange: 11 of 13 dialysis dependent patients receiving plasma exchange recovered renal function compared with only two of 11 receiving IPD and chemotherapy. One year survival was 66% versus 28% in favour of those patients treated with plasma exchange. Interpretation of this study should be tempered by the difference in dialysis modality employed in the two groups, and by the high mortality in the control group despite apparently good matching for extent of disease.

The second trial of plasma exchange, by Johnson *et al.* 1990, randomised 21 patients after initial treatment with forced diuresis (intravenous fluids, sodium bicarbonate and furosemide), melphalan and prednisolone. Renal disease was less severe in this trial, with only five of the 24 patients being oliguric, and 13 requiring dialysis. Renal failure was defined as a rising creatinine despite fluid therapy or a creatinine >270 µmol/L. Patients with the most rapid deterioration in renal function were excluded. The biopsies from seven of 16 patients had cast nephropathy, and nine had a predominant severe interstitial nephritis. Plasma exchange (for albumin) was performed only three times per week for one to four weeks. Overall recovery of renal function was associated with response to chemotherapy and with the extent of cast formation in the biopsy, but not with plasma exchange. However of the five patients who were oliguric, three who received plasma exchange recovered renal function. Similarly three of seven dialysis dependent patients receiving plasma exchange recovered renal function, compared with none of five dialysis dependent patients in the control group.

The precise place for plasma exchange thus remains poorly defined. Certainly, aggressive hydration should be the first approach to the renal failure of myeloma, and a biopsy considered in all patients not recovering renal function. Patients with cast nephropathy or interstitial nephritis and circulating light chains should be considered for plasma exchange, especially if they are oliguric and dialysis dependent. If plasma exchange is to be performed it should be done frequently (daily for five to seven days) to maximise the clearance of light chains, and combined with chemotherapy. There is undoubtedly a need for a properly controlled trial of plasma exchange in myeloma renal failure.

Dialysis

The overall prognosis of patients with myeloma and renal failure is similar to patients with equivalent tumour burdens and normal renal function (see below), and thus dialysis should be considered in all patients with renal failure having chemotherapy for myeloma. Dialysis should begin early to avoid prolonged uraemia in patients who already have an immune paresis and dysfunctional bone marrow. Peritoneal dialysis and haemodialysis have both been used. The major complication in myeloma patients on dialysis is infection: peritonitis in peritoneal dialysis and line-related sepsis in haemodialysis. Infection is the commonest cause of death. Haemodialysis is probably the preferred method for renal replacement therapy, since peritonitis is almost universal as patients become neutropaenic and are receiving steroids. Line sepsis is easier to treat and the incidence can be reduced by using tunnelled catheters from an early stage. Residual renal function should be monitored closely in patients on dialysis since renal recovery can occur several months after treatment has begun.

Chemotherapy of Myeloma

Aggressive treatment of myeloma is justified in most patients. The presence of renal failure *per se* is indicative of tumour burden and is probably not itself an independent risk factor for poor outcome. The regimens most commonly used are melphalan and prednisolone, or vincristine, doxorubicin (adriamycin) and dexamethasone (VAD). VAD acts faster in reducing light chain secretion, and the drugs are hepatically metabolised, but the regimen has not been shown to improve survival over the older regimens. Melphalan and prednisolone stabilise or improve renal function in two thirds of patients, but melphalan is excreted renally; dosing is thus difficult, and there is a high incidence of leucopaenia or thrombocytopenia in patients with renal failure. Both autologous and allogeneic bone marrow transplantation after myeloablation have been used to treat patients with myeloma, but are not in common practice. Relapse is common after autologous transplantation, and allogeneic transplants have a very high morbidity and mortality.

OUTCOME

Overall survival of patients with myeloma and renal failure varies widely in different series, from medians of 4 months to 28 months (mean 17 months). Twenty percent of patients will die within one month of presentation, but one third of patients will survive for more than one year, and of these a significant number will survive 3–5 years. Survival is significantly worse in patients with renal failure compared to all patients with myeloma, but not to stage matched patients. Early studies did suggest that an increased creatinine at presentation was associated with an adverse outcome, but more recent studies have shown that extent of disease is the crucial element rather than renal failure itself. Response to chemotherapy is the major factor determining overall survival, but recovery of renal function is also associated with improved survival. In general, 50% of patients will recover renal function, though in some series renal recovery has been documented in 85% of patients. The only factors predictive of renal recovery are the absence of interstitial fibrosis on renal biopsy, and reduced renal recovery in patients with pure light chain myeloma. There is a suggestion that renal recovery is less likely in patients with more severe renal dysfunction at presentation. For patients with myeloma who remain on dialysis and leave hospital alive, median survival is 20 months, with a significant number of patients (up to 30%) surviving more than 3 years. The median time to renal improvement is 36–70 days. A small number of patients (7% in one series) will recover renal function several months after presentation.

Overall, therefore, the renal failure of myeloma should be treated as a medical emergency, and dialysis should be instituted early. Despite the poor prognosis of myeloma, it is not so poor as to refuse dialysis to patients with reasonable quality of life, and a significant minority of patients will survive several years.

LIGHT AND HEAVY CHAIN DEPOSITION DISEASES, AL AMYLOID AND CRYOGLOBULINAEMIA IN MYELOMA

These are much rarer causes of ARF in myeloma than cast nephropathy, interstitial nephritis, dehydration, hypercalcaemia and urosepsis. Light chain deposition disease (LCDD) presents either with proteinuria (often nephrotic) or with ARF (in 80% of patients). Renal function often deteriorates rapidly. Systemic deposition of light chains can cause hepatomegaly, cardiomegaly and neuropathy. A significant number of patients (up to 30%) do not have detectable monoclonal immunoglobulin in blood or urine. Renal histology shows a characteristic nodular glomerulosclerosis, and deposition of monoclonal light chains in tubular and glomerular basement membranes by immunochemistry. In about 80% of reported cases, κ light chains have been described; the reason for this predominance is unclear. Granular deposits are seen in tubular basement membranes by electron microscopy, and non-fibrillar deposits in the mesangial nodules.

Practice Point. Management of myeloma renal failure

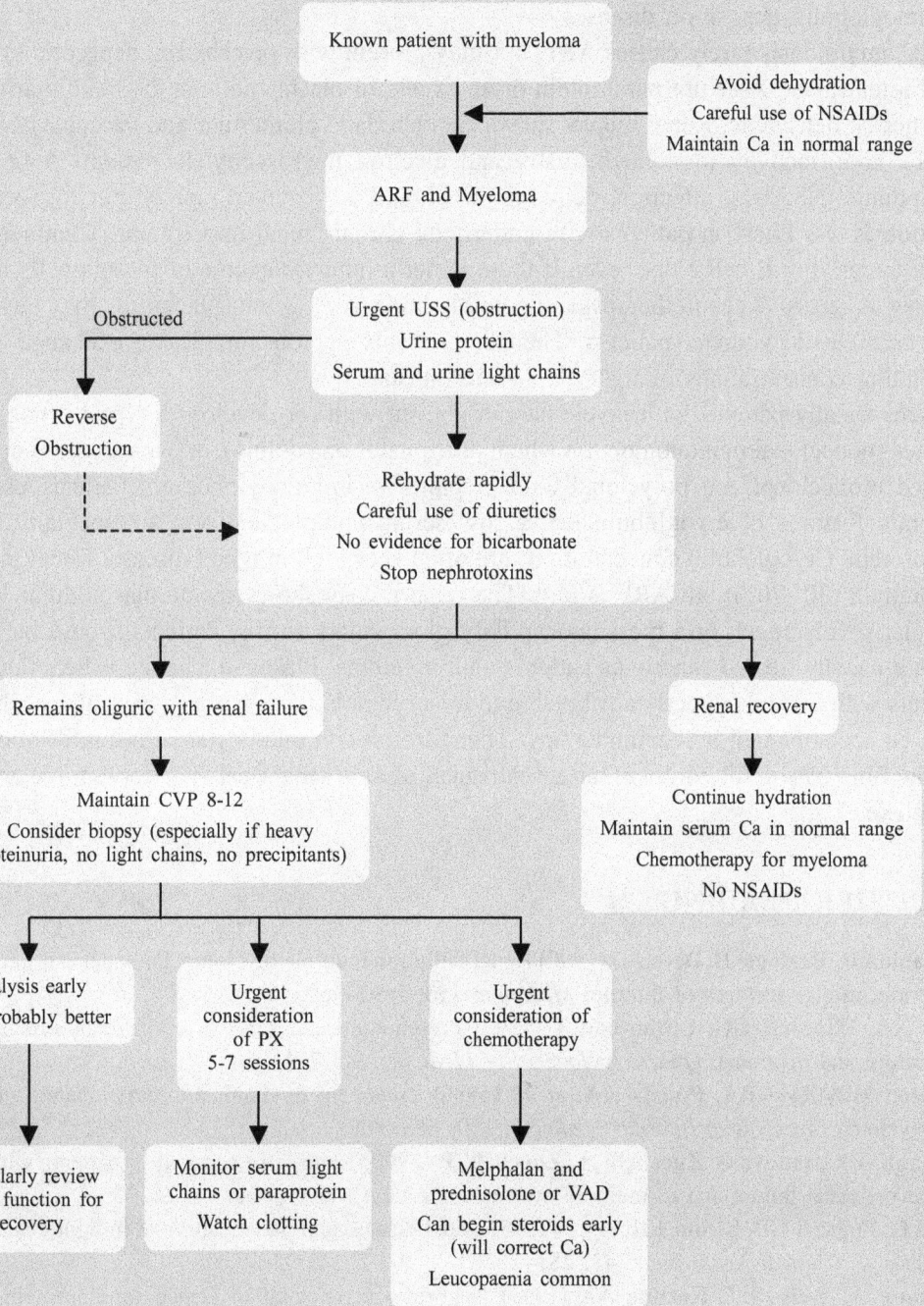

```
                    Known patient with myeloma
                                |
                                |          Avoid dehydration
                                |<———————  Careful use of NSAIDs
                                |          Maintain Ca in normal range
                                v
                         ARF and Myeloma
                                |
                                v
                      Urgent USS (obstruction)
     Obstructed              Urine protein
                       Serum and urine light chains
          |                     |
          v                     |
      Reverse                   |
     Obstruction                v
          |            Rehydrate rapidly
          |            Careful use of diuretics
          — — — — — —> No evidence for bicarbonate
                       Stop nephrotoxins
                                |
              ——————————————————————————————————————
              |                                     |
              v                                     v
   Remains oliguric with renal failure       Renal recovery
              |                                     |
              v                                     v
      Maintain CVP 8-12                     Continue hydration
  Consider biopsy (especially if heavy   Maintain serum Ca in normal range
proteinuria, no light chains, no precipitants)  Chemotherapy for myeloma
              |                                  No NSAIDs
     ————————————————————————
     |           |          |
     v           v          v
Dialysis early  Urgent    Urgent
HD probably   consideration consideration of
  better       of PX      chemotherapy
             5-7 sessions
     |           |          |
     v           v          v
Regularly review  Monitor serum light   Melphalan and
renal function for chains or paraprotein  prednisolone or VAD
  recovery      Watch clotting        Can begin steroids early
                                      (will correct Ca)
                                      Leucopaenia common
```

Tubular casts are not seen. Heavy chain deposition disease is rarer, but has similar features. Survival ranges from 1 month to 10 years, but is usually very poor (median 20 months) even with aggressive treatment. Patients with overt myeloma should receive chemotherapy. Patients without a detectable B cell clone should probably also receive chemotherapy if they have evidence of ongoing end-organ damage. There are no data on the benefits of plasma exchange in monoclonal immunoglobulin deposition diseases.

AL amyloidosis rarely causes ARF, but may present with proteinuria, nephrotic syndrome or renal impairment. A serum paraprotein or an excess of plasma cells in the bone marrow may or may not be detectable. Renal biopsy shows characteristic glomerular and vascular lesions which can be confirmed by immunochemistry and electron microscopy. In patients with ARF, any precipitants (NSAIDs, infection, dehydration) should be reversed rapidly, but recovery of renal function is less likely in patients with underlying chronic renal impairment. Treatment is aimed at the underlying B cell clone, even if there is not a numeric excess of plasma cells in the bone marrow. Aggressive chemotherapy, and possibly bone marrow transplantation, may be appropriate (and curative) in younger patients. There is probably no role for plasma exchange, since high circulating concentrations of light chains are unusual.

Occasionally patients with myeloma can present with (or develop) a type I cryoglobulin (an isolated monoclonal immunoglobulin which precipitates on cooling), or even a type II cryoglobulin (mixed monoclonal and polyclonal cold precipitable immunoglobulins). Patients usually have systemic features of cryoglobulinaemia, low serum complement levels (especially C4) and a paraprotein. Cryoglobulin concentrations are often very high in type I disease. Renal involvement is common (30–70%) but ARF is rare. The renal biopsy shows glomerular nodular lesions and vascular involvement, or a mesangiocapillary glomerulonephritis. Patients should be kept warm and are usually treated exactly as patients with myeloma. Plasma exchange is beneficial in some patients with features directly attributable to the cryoglobulin (especially vascular occlusion), but must be accompanied by chemotherapy. There are no controlled trials. Plasmafiltration (using a hollow fibre plasmafilter rather than a centrifugal plasma separator) may not remove cryoglobulin complexes.

FURTHER READING

Alexanian R, Barlogie B, Dixon D (1990) Renal failure in multiple myeloma. Pathogenesis and prognostic implications. *Archives of Internal Medicine*; 150: 1693–1695

Irish AB, Winearls CG, Littlewood T (1997) Presentation and survival of patients with severe renal failure and myeloma. *Quarterly Journal of Medicine*; 90: 773–780

Johnson WJ, Kyle RA, Pineda AA, et al. (1989) Treatment of renal failure associated with multiple myeloma. *Archives of Internal Medicine*; 150: 863–869

Pasquali S, Casanova S, Zucchelli A, Zucchelli P (1990) Long-term survival in patients with acute and severe renal failure due to multiple myeloma. *Clinical Nephrology*; 34: 247–254

Pozzi C, Fogazzi GB, Strom EH, et al. (1995) Renal disease and patient survival in light chain deposition disease. *Clinical Nephrology*; 43: 281–287

Solomon A, Weiss DT, Kattine AA (1991) Nephrotoxic potential of Bence Jones proteins. *The New England Journal of Medicine*; 324: 1845–1851

Winearls CG (1995) Acute myeloma kidney. *Kidney International*; 48: 1347–1361

Zucchelli P, Pasquali S, Cagnoli L, Ferrari G (1988) Controlled trial of plasma exchange in ARF due to multiple myeloma. *Kidney International*; 33: 1175–1180

Chapter 23

RENAL TRACT OBSTRUCTION & ACUTE RENAL FAILURE
Roger Walker

INTRODUCTION

Renal tract obstruction is an important cause of acute renal failure (ARF). In a community based study, it was responsible for ARF in 36% of patients (Feest *et al*. 1993). In general, ARF secondary to renal tract obstruction is reversible and associated with a favourable renal prognosis.

The urinary tract transports urine unidirectionally at relatively low pressure from the collecting ducts to the exterior. Obstruction to urinary flow leads to increased urinary tract pressure proximal to the obstruction, with the potential to damage those structures subjected to the pressure rise. Urinary tract obstruction may result in a spectrum of renal dysfunction, ranging from minimal renal impairment to established ARF, dependent on a number of factors:

- Is the obstruction unilateral or bilateral?
- How complete is the obstruction?
- Is there obstruction in the presence of superadded infection?
- How long has the obstruction been present?
- Was there pre-existing renal impairment/previously one or two functioning kidneys?

Severe acute renal failure typically occurs as a result of sudden and complete bilateral obstruction, or secondary to unilateral obstruction where the contralateral kidney is either non-functioning or absent.

DEFINITIONS

Obstructive uropathy — the anatomical impedance to the flow of urine anywhere along the urinary tract.

Obstructive nephropathy — the damage to renal parenchyma that results from obstruction to the flow of urine.

Hydronephrosis — a descriptive term referring to renal pelvis and calyceal dilatation; it **may or may not** be due to obstruction.

PATHOPHYSIOLOGY

The pathogenesis of renal dysfunction during obstructive uropathy is poorly understood. Much of what is known comes from work performed in experimental models of acute obstruction. However, these models are often poorly representative of human disease, where obstruction is usually partial and chronic. Tubule obstruction increases the hydrostatic pressure in Bowman's capsule (P_{BC}) leading to a reduction in glomerular filtration rate (GFR) (see **Chapter 1**). In addition, tubule obstruction causes changes in renal blood flow (RBF) that may alter P_{GC} and subsequently GFR (see below). The changes in RBF depend on whether the obstruction is unilateral or bilateral, and on whether it is complete or partial.

Following acute **unilateral** obstruction there is a classical **triphasic response** of the kidney in terms of renal blood flow and ureteric pressure:

Phase 1: 0–90 min: increased renal blood flow (RBF) and increased collecting system pressure.

Phase 2: 90 min–4 h: decline in RBF with the elevated collecting system pressure maintained.

Phase 3: 4–18 h: further decline in RBF and gradual fall in collecting system pressure.

Initially, GFR is maintained despite collecting system pressures rising from a resting level of 6–12 mmHg to as high as 50–70 mmHg. GFR is maintained by:

- Concomitant rises in filtration pressure due to raised blood flow.
- Increased pyelolymphatic flow.
- Increased pyelovenous flow.
- Extravasation into peri-renal spaces.

Preservation of GFR occurs such that even with obstruction over longer periods, a urine flow of ~2 mL/min can still be maintained, with 80–90% of the filtrate being absorbed in the tubules. In complete unilateral obstruction, GFR in the obstructed system falls by 52% at 4 h to 2% at 48 h. In **bilateral ureteric obstruction**, or unilateral obstruction in a solitary functioning kidney, the triphasic response to obstruction does not occur. After 48 h of bilateral ureteric obstruction, GFR falls to 22% of its normal level. Decreased RBF, increased collecting system pressures and falling GFR eventually lead to established intrinsic renal failure.

Histopathology

The renal histopathological changes that occur following urinary tract obstruction include:

- 1–7 days: flattening of renal papillae and dilatation of distal nephron.
- 7–14 days: atrophy and necrosis of collecting tubules.
- 14–28 days: progressive dilatation of distal and collecting tubules.
- >28 days: 50% decrease in medulla, thinning of cortex, proximal tubule atrophy, glomerular changes first noted.

Obstruction damages the polar regions of the kidney initially. In addition, the renal pelvis and ureter show proximal dilatation, muscular hypertrophy and hyperplasia, and increased collagen and elastin deposition. Transforming growth factor beta (TGF-β) plays a major role in the development of fibrosis in the obstructed kidney. TGF-β up-regulation in children 2 weeks following obstruction, and in adults at 4–6 weeks, has led some authors to suggest that obstruction should be relieved within these time frames. Indeed, it is now generally accepted that **obstruction should be relieved within 2–4 weeks**, although recovery can occur after longer periods.

The above discussion refers to obstruction in the **absence** of infection. **Where infection and obstruction coexist**, damage to renal tissue occurs more rapidly and there is a significant risk of developing, life-threatening gram negative sepsis. This occurs as a results of pyelovenous and pyelolymphatic flow in an obstructed system and facilitates direct movement of organisms from the urinary tract to the systemic circulation, leading to systemic sepsis. In this clinical scenario, urgent imaging and decompression with either a percutaneous nephrostomy or JJ stent is mandatory (see below).

AETIOLOGY

The causes of urinary tract obstruction are divided into **congenital** and **acquired** (see **Table 1**) and according to whether it is due to an **intraluminal**, **intramural** or **extraluminal**. Congenital causes such as PUJ obstruction, strictures, reflux and ureteric/urethral valves, are predominantly

Table 1. Acquired causes of urinary tract obstruction

Intraluminal	Intramural	Extraluminal	
Calculus*	Ureteral strictures	Malignancy	Gynaecological
Papillary necrosis*	schistosomiasis	prostate*	fibroids
Blood clot*	tuberculosis	bladder*	endometriosis
Fungus ball	drugs (e.g. NSAIDs)	colorectal*	tubo-ovarian abscess
Stricture	ureteral instrumentation	ovarian	ovarian cyst
Urothelial tumour*	Urethral strictures*	uterine	pregnancy
Intrarenal obstruction	Diseases	cervical*	Male
sulphonamides	(functional obstruction)	Retroperitoneal	bladder outlet obstruction*
aciclovir	diabetes mellitus	lymphoma	Retroperitoneal disease
myeloma	multiple sclerosis	germ cell tumour	retroperitoneal fibrosis
	stroke	sarcoma	tuberculosis
	spinal cord injury	vascular	sarcoidosis
	Parkinson's disease	aortic aneurysm	haemorrhage
		iliac artery aneurysm	urinoma
		Gastrointestinal disease	Iatrogenic*
		pancreatitis	pelvic surgery
		appendicitis	JJ stent
		diverticulitis	
		Crohn's disease	

*Highlights those conditions most commonly seen in clinical practice.

detected in children, although they can occasionally present in adult life. Although these conditions may lead to chronic renal damage, they rarely cause ARF *per se*, and are not discussed further here.

CLINICAL PRESENTATION

Symptoms associated with urinary tract obstruction vary according to:

- the time over which obstruction occurs (acute versus chronic);
- whether obstruction is unilateral or bilateral;
- the aetiology of the obstruction;
- whether the obstruction is complete or partial;
- whether infection coexists;
- the anatomical level/site of obstruction.

Symptoms

Pain is the predominant symptom associated with urinary tract obstruction. This results from raised intra-ureteric and intra-pelvic pressures. Acute obstruction is usually associated with loin pain that may radiate to the groin or testis/labia. It may be colicky (intermittent) or a dull constant ache. Acute bilateral obstruction is associated with the onset of anuria. Bilateral obstruction (or unilateral obstruction with a non-functioning contralateral kidney) can present with all the features of ARF described in **Section 2**.

Fever associated with loin pain suggests that infection coexists with obstruction; this requires urgent investigation and treatment. Obstruction of the lower urinary tract may cause bilateral renal obstruction; in addition to voiding difficulties (e.g. poor stream, complete urinary retention), back pain maybe a feature.

In a previously asymptomatic individual presenting with ARF, the first indication of possible upper urinary tract obstruction may be the presence of **hydronephrosis** on **ultrasound** imaging. An algorithm for the radiological management of this common clinical scenario is given in **Chapter 6**.

Signs

Acute ureteric obstruction is associated with hypertension due to increased renin secretion. Other clinical signs are as for ARF of any cause (see **Chapter 4.1**).

INVESTIGATIONS

1. Urine (see also Chapter 4.2)

- Urine dipstick
  Presence of blood suggests nephrolithiasis, urothelial malignancy or inflammation.

- Urine microscopy

  White cells or organisms suggest infection

  Crystalluria may be seen in nephrolithiasis.

- Urine biochemistry

  Acute obstruction — similar to pre-renal azotaemia (low urinary Na^+, increased osmolality)

  Chronic obstruction — similar to ATN (high urinary Na^+, decreased osmolality, decreased urine: plasma creatinine ratio).

- Urine cytology

  Presence of malignant cells suggests renal tract obstruction is due to transitional cell carcinoma.

2. Biochemistry

- The typical biochemical profile of acute renal failure will be observed in acute, severe bilateral obstruction or unilateral obstruction in a solitary kidney.
- Hypophosphataemia, hypocalcaemia and hypomagnesaemia may be seen in long standing obstruction (secondary to tubule dysfunction and resultant urinary losses).

3. Imaging

Imaging of the renal tract is discussed in detail in **Chapter 6**.

TREATMENT PRINCIPLES

General Principles

The aims of management are:

- to relieve obstruction;
- allow recovery of renal function;
- diagnose the cause of urinary tract obstruction.

Note that under certain circumstances, obstruction may not actually be the cause of ARF, but may coexist with other aetiologies. In this setting, treatment should still include relief of the obstruction, in addition to appropriate management of the coexistent pathology.

Specific Actions

Lower tract drainage

In the case of lower tract obstruction, catheterisation is performed. Catheterisation should also be performed in cases of upper tract obstruction, as lower tract obstruction may coexist and catheterisation facilitates accurate measurement of urinary output. Where upper renal tract obstruction exists, or where upper tract dilatation persists and renal function fails to improve following bladder catheterisation, then upper urinary tract drainage should be performed.

Upper tract drainage

- **Antegrade percutaneous nephrostomy versus cystoscopy and retrograde JJ stent insertion**

Upper urinary tract obstruction can be relieved by nephrostomy or retrograde insertion of a JJ stent. Whilst no differences between the two procedures, in terms of complications and recovery, has been demonstrated in clinical trials, there are several theoretical advantages to the percutaneous approach. Where available, this should be the method of choice for draining the upper urinary tract, particularly in patients with ARF.

The advantages of percutaneous drainage over JJ stent insertion are as follows:

- Percutaneous drainage can be performed without the need for general anaesthesia.
- JJ stents obstruct the ureter and require higher renal pelvic pressures to drain compared to a nephrostomy.
- JJ stents are less effective at draining an obstructed ureter due to extrinsic compression than a nephrostomy.
- JJ stents inhibit normal ureteric peristalsis; peristalsis returns following percutaneous drainage of an obstructed system, and may facilitate spontaneous passage of ureteric calculi.
- Retrograde manipulation of a stone and insertion of a JJ stent in an infected obstructed system raises intrapelvic pressure, and increases pyelovenous and pyelolymphatic flow of infected urine leading to systemic sepsis.
- Antegrade insertion of a JJ stent can be performed via nephrostomy; this is often the easiest insertion route when obstruction has been caused by compression of the ureter by bulky tumour.
- Antegrade ureteropyelography can be performed at a later stage permitting visualisation of the site of obstruction and planning of definitive management.

Cystoscopy and retrograde JJ stent insertion for upper tract obstruction might be preferred where:

- Therapeutic intervention may be possible e.g. stone management, although this is not recommended in the acutely unwell/ARF patient.
- Coagulopathy exists.
- Failed percutaneous drainage.
- Necessary expertise for percutaneous nephrostomy placement is unavailable.
- The situation is less urgent and a planned elective procedure is acceptable.

After drainage of the upper or lower urinary tract has been performed, renal function should be monitored, followed by definitive treatment of the obstruction, if appropriate. If infection and obstruction coexist following percutaneous drainage, antegrade ureteropyelography should be delayed for at least one week to allow full resolution of infection. Definitive treatment depends on the underlying aetiology and whether renal function recovers. If recovery of renal function does not occur following the relief of obstruction, other causes of ARF should be considered.

OUTCOME

The extent of recovery of renal function can be difficult to predict. Anecdotal reports suggest that recovery of renal function can be observed up to 18 months after relief of the obstruction. As discussed earlier, renal tract obstruction is usually partial and chronic, rather than complete which may account for the observed recovery of renal function following extended periods of obstruction. Renal outcome is less favourable with:

- increased duration of obstruction,
- increased severity of obstruction,
- superadded infection,
- pre-existing renal impairment.

Renal recovery is more complete following relief of bilateral obstruction or of unilateral obstruction where the contralateral kidney is absent or non-functioning (the "renal counterbalance" mechanism).

Following relief of obstruction, recovery of renal function occurs in two phases:

Tubule phase: 0–2 weeks

Glomerular phase: 2 weeks–3 months

Plasma creatinine (and creatinine clearance) improves almost immediately, probably due to ↑ tubule secretion of creatinine. Major improvements usually occur by 2 weeks and further small improvements occur up to 3 weeks.

Following relief of obstruction, some patients may experience a **post-obstructive diuresis**. The mechanisms underlying this include:

- Physiological excretion of retained water and salt (solute-obligated diuresis; retained urea also contributes).
- Impaired sensitivity of collecting duct to ADH.
- Inability to maintain a medullary solute concentration gradient due to increased medullary blood flow during obstruction (solute washout).
- Increased atrial natriuretic peptide levels (ANP) resulting in natriuresis and diuresis.

Salt and water loss is maximal over the first 24 h and usually complete by day 3. **Post obstructive diuresis** can occur following relief of bilateral obstruction from any cause, relief of unilateral obstruction of a solitary kidney and relief of urinary retention (see below). Hourly urine output should be carefully monitored; solute and water losses should be appropriately replaced (see **Chapter 8.1**). Predicting which patients will recover is difficult. Following relief of obstruction, tubule recovery occurs in the first 2 weeks, followed by recovery of glomerular function. Therefore, improvements in DTPA MAG3 renography or GFR are not typically seen in the first two weeks, and these investigations are unhelpful within this time frame. In practice, it is often a matter of relieving the obstruction, performing serial creatinine measurements and awaiting recovery of function. Generally, ARF due to obstruction, both in terms of renal recovery and patient mortality, has been shown to have a good prognosis compared to other causes (Feest *et al.* 1993).

SPECIFIC CONDITIONS

Bladder Outlet Obstruction and Acute Renal Failure (see Table 2)

In one community based study of ARF, prostatic disease accounted for 25% of cases of ARF (Feest *et al.* 1993). Indeed, approximately 14% of patients with benign prostatic hyperplasia (BPH), one of the commoner causes of bladder outlet obstruction, have a degree of renal insufficiency. All patients who present with urinary retention should have their serum creatinine measured, since they are at risk of acute renal failure. The term **high-pressure chronic retention** has been coined to describe those patients with urinary retention and associated renal failure. In this group, high bladder storage pressures may occur, resulting in upper tract dilatation and renal dysfunction. Bilateral upper tract dilatation occurs due to thickening of bladder detrusor muscle wall impairing ureteric peristalsis, or to detrusor post-void pressure remaining high within the bladder, thus preventing adequate upper tract drainage. It does not occur due to simple high-pressure reflux up the ureter.

Table 2. Causes of bladder outlet obstruction

Anatomic
Benign prostatic enlargement (BPE: histologically usually benign prostatic hyperplasia)
Prostatic carcinoma
Urethral stricture
Bladder neck contracture
Bladder calculi
Clots (clot retention secondary to haematuria)
Functional
Sphincter dysynergia (striated and smooth)

Clinical presentation

Patients often present with painless urinary retention, and may describe urinary incontinence, frequency due to overflow, or non-specific features including weight gain, ankle swelling and shortness of breath:

- 52% of patients present with elevated blood pressure.
- 38% have peripheral oedema.
- 24% have an elevated jugular venous pressure.

Treatment

Relief of the obstruction is rapidly achieved by urethral catheterisation. Some bleeding from the bladder wall may occur following catheterisation. This is usually self-limiting and rarely requires intervention or a 3-way catheter/irrigation. Urethral catheters should never be clamped following relief of urinary retention.

Jones *et al.* (1991) demonstrated that following relief of the obstruction in patients with chronic retention and renal failure:

- 80% follow a clinically unremarkable recovery.
- 20% have a urine output of >4 L a day.
- 10% develop significant thirst requiring oral fluids.
- 5% require intravenous fluids due to postural hypotension.
- 1% suffer prolonged post-obstructive diuresis/chronic salt loss.

They also suggest that patients at highest risk of ongoing salt and water loss/postural hypotension, are those whose urine output is >200 mL/h for more than 12 hours. With regard to replacing fluid losses, many patients can be managed on oral fluids alone. It is important not to convert a physiological diuresis into an iatrogenic one from over-zealous fluid replacement. Occasionally a paradoxical increase in serum $[K^+]$ can occur following relief of obstruction; this is due to pseudo-hypoaldosteronism caused by defective response of the distal tubule to aldosterone. It is self-limiting and the hyperkalaemia rarely requires treatment. A small percentage of patients ($\leq 1\%$) will have prolonged or irreversible distal tubule damage resulting in an ongoing salt-losing diuresis.

Following treatment of ARF, definitive management of the patient's bladder outlet dysfunction is undertaken (details of this can be found in urological texts). If surgery (TURP) is proposed, it has been suggested this is left until 2 weeks following relief of obstruction to allow significant improvement in renal function to occur, and in particular to allow resolution of uraemic bleeding diathesis.

URINARY STONE DISEASE (UROLITHIASIS) AND ACUTE RENAL FAILURE

Pathophysiology

Urinary lithiasis was the second most common cause of urinary tract obstruction causing ARF (approximately 10% of patients) in the study referred to above (Feest *et al.*). Whilst deleterious effects to one kidney result from an obstructing ureteric calculi, ARF occurs following obstruction of one kidney where the contralateral unit is absent or non-functioning, or where bilateral obstructing ureteric calculi occur simultaneously (rare). Calculi increase the risk of urinary sepsis and thus systemic gram-negative sepsis. Urinary stones form in the collecting ducts and can impact and obstruct anywhere from the infundibulum of the renal calyces to the urethral meatus. The most common site of impaction is the renal pelvis or ureter (specifically below the PUJ, pelvic brim at the level of the internal iliac artery, and vesicoureteric junction).

Clinical Presentation

- *History*

Pain radiating from the loin to groin area (classically colicky).

Ureteric colic and sepsis can present as an acute abdomen.

Asymptomatic obstructive stone disease can occur.

Past history of stone disease.

Predisposing conditions (Type 1 renal tubular acidosis, medullary sponge kidneys, hypercalcaemia, neurogenic bladder, ileostomy, high urinary uric acid [gout and treated myeloproliferative diseases] and cystinuria).

- *Examination*

Pyrexia.

Loin tenderness.

Investigations (refer also to **Section 2** of this volume)

Urine microscopy: haematuria (>85%), crystalluria, white blood cells, organisms.

Urea, electrolytes and creatinine: may show changes of ARF.

KUB radiograph.

IVU (provided normal renal function and no contraindications).

Ultrasound and MAG 3 renogram, if IVU not possible.

Treatment

Dependent on:

- size and site of stone (≤5 mm — spontaneous passage the rule, especially in lower ureter);
- degree of obstruction;
- presence/absence of contralateral kidney;
- presence/absence of infection;
- severity of pain (? requires ongoing opiate analgesia);
- impairment of renal function.

   With obstructing stone disease, as with other causes of obstruction to the urinary tract, controversy exists as to when one should intervene to relieve the obstruction to prevent irreversible renal damage. **The patient who presents with signs of sepsis, ureteric obstruction and ARF clearly needs urgent relief of obstruction.** This is best achieved by percutaneous nephrostomy drainage (see above). If expertise is not available or percutaneous drainage fails, an alternative approach is cystoscopy and retrograde insertion of JJ stent. Signs of sepsis require antibiotic therapy from presentation (see **Chapter 19**). Antimicrobials are also required to cover nephrostomy placement or JJ stent insertion. Following relief of obstruction, a period of time is allowed for renal function to improve and sepsis to settle. A post-obstructive diuresis may occur if the contralateral kidney is non-functioning or absent (which it will be in the case of ARF). A detailed discussion about the definitive treatment of calculi is beyond the scope of this book.

   Patients with obstructing stones should be told to drink normally and not "drink plenty". In acute obstruction, increasing fluid intake is likely to cause further distension of the collecting system, increase pain and possibly cause urinary extravasation from small tears in the calyceal fornix. As obstruction is established, GFR falls and excess fluid is excreted by the contralateral kidney. There is no evidence that excessive increases in fluid intake facilitate stone passage, and indeed recent evidence suggests it may be deleterious. All patients with stone disease should undergo full or limited evaluation for any underlying metabolic or structural abnormality causing their stone episode. This is generally undertaken when they are stone free.

MALIGNANT OBSTRUCTION

Ureteric obstruction from malignant disease arising from the pelvis or retroperitoneum, may occur as a presenting feature of the disease, or as a late development in a patient with known malignancy. Obstruction occurs due to local extension or to extrinsic compression from nodal metastases. Ureteric obstruction is generally a sign of advanced disease and, even if disease is newly diagnosed, the outlook is often poor. The malignancies most commonly causing acute ureteric obstruction and renal failure include cervix, bladder, prostate, gastrointestinal, ovary and breast (see also **Chapter 21**).

In patients with ARF and malignancy, the principles of investigation and management include:

- Identification of the level and degree of obstruction (unilateral or bilateral? — most commonly bilateral).
- Identification of underlying aetiology of obstructing lesion, stage, grade and histological diagnosis.
- Establishing prognosis, given the above information.
- Establishing treatment options (surgery, chemotherapy, radiotherapy) and their relative success rates.
- Establishing patient/relative wishes if this represents progression of a known or untreatable malignancy.
- Deciding if active management to be undertaken to treat ARF.
- Draining the obstructed system — antegrade percutaneous nephrostomy versus JJ stent (see below).
- Undertaking definitive treatment (medical/surgical) or planning palliative care.

If definitive treatment of the underlying condition is to be undertaken, preservation of renal function is very important. Once the decision is made to treat, rapid drainage of the obstructed system should be performed. **Note** that, in patients presenting with suspected malignant obstruction following primary treatment with radiotherapy, there is a 10% chance that the obstruction is due to fibrosis rather than recurrent disease. If the patient was primarily treated with both radiation and surgery, this figure increases to approximately 30%.

In advanced malignancy, the traditional view has been to allow the patient a relatively comfortable death from ARF, rather than prolonging life only to suffer at a later stage from pain/instrumentation, etc. Appropriate provision of good palliative care services is essential.

The principles of establishing urinary drainage, detailed in the treatment section above, also apply in malignant disease, with the following caveats:

- Insertion of JJ stent from below is often difficult with malignant disease in the pelvis.
- Antegrade percutaneous nephrostomy and antegrade insertion of JJ stent is usually more successful and obviates the need for a general anaesthetic.

- Even if passed across the site of extrinsic compression from malignancy, a JJ stent may not relieve obstruction as well as percutaneous nephrostomy drainage.
- The nephrostomy should be clamped for 48 h prior to removal to ensure that there is adequate drainage and no deterioration in renal function.

RENAL ALLOGRAFT OBSTRUCTION

Ureteric obstruction must be excluded as a cause of graft dysfunction in the renal transplant patient (see also **Chapters 6** and **24**). Ureteric obstruction in the transplant patient will result in ARF. The causes of ureteric obstruction in transplant kidneys are shown in **Table 3**.

Table 3. Causes of ureteric obstruction in transplant kidneys
Ischaemic stenosis
Oedema
Blood clot
Calculus
Lymphocoele
Tumour
Fungus ball
Kinked/redundant ureter

In a series of 1,000 transplant recipients, 3.7% patients developed ureteral obstruction (Shoskers *et al.*, 1995). The median time to obstruction was 16 weeks, although ranging from 4 h to 400 weeks. In the majority of cases, obstruction occurred at the ureterovesical junction. The causes of obstruction in this series were presumed ischaemic stricture (56%), lymphocoele (16%), redundant, kinked or twisted ureters (8%), calculus (5%), abscess, obstructing lower pole vessel, PUJ obstruction, double renal pelvis (3% each). Early ureteric obstruction may be associated with a ureteric or bladder leak. Leaks occurred in 2.5% patients in the series reported above. In addition to the causes of upper urinary tract obstruction, lower urinary tract obstruction represented 0.7% cases; this should be managed as described in the section on bladder outlet obstruction.

Clinical Presentation

The transplanted kidney is denervated and patients with ureteric obstruction do not present with typical symptoms of renal colic. Where pain is present it is often non-specific abdominal pain or tenderness over the graft. Pain may be a symptom if associated with urinary leakage or infection. More common presenting features include decreasing urine output, or an acute deterioration in graft function.

Investigations

Following routine biochemical and microbiological assessment, ultrasound examination is required. In addition to the finding of upper tract dilatation the use of doppler ultrasound and resistive index measurement may be of value in obstruction the transplant setting (see **Chapter 6**). Radionuclide scans (e.g. DTPA or MAG3 isotope renogram) also aid diagnosis of allograft obstruction as discussed in **Chapter 6**.

Treatment

If deterioration of renal function is due to suspected intraluminal or intramural obstruction a percutaneous nephrostomy should be placed. Retrograde JJ stenting can be performed as an alternative, but the ureteric opening may be difficult to cannulate and the advantages of the antegrade approach over the retrograde route, discussed above, particularly apply here. In cases of equivocal obstruction a percutaneous nephrostomy can be placed to see if graft function improves.

Following nephrostomy placement, urine output and renal function are monitored and time allowed for infection to resolve, if associated with obstruction. Subsequent antegrade pyelography allows anatomical definition of the site of obstruction and diagnosis of the cause of obstruction. Following percutaneous drainage, spontaneous passage of obstructing calculi or clot may occur or oedema resolve — in this case, no further action need be taken. If antegrade ureteropyelography demonstrates obstruction, non-surgical treatment includes antegrade insertion of a JJ stent. This may allow resolution of oedema or even treat milder forms of obstruction. Balloon dilatation of strictures has been used but the long-term results are poor. If more conservative/endo-urological manoeuvres fail, open surgery will be necessary. This occurred in 73% of cases in the series reported by Shoskes.

Calculi in the transplant kidney and ureter can be treated as for native calculus disease. Extra-corporeal shock wave lithotripsy and percutaneous nephrolithotomy can be safely performed in the transplant kidney. Ureteroscopic management may be more demanding due to retrograde cannulation of the neoureteric orifice, but newer flexible endoscopes and energy sources (YAG laser) make this possible in specialist centres.

If ultrasound scanning reveals obstruction to be due to extrinsic compression (most commonly a **lymphocoele** in the post-transplant period) percutaneous drainage may result in resolution of obstruction. Subsequent lymphocoele recurrence may require open drainage or marsupialisation.

Prevention

Many of the urological complications of transplantation are technical in nature. In most cases, obstruction is due to ureteric stenosis, probably secondary to ischaemic ureteric injury at the time of organ retrieval or preoperative preparation. Technical ability and experience reduce the incidence of ureteric obstruction. At organ retrieval and preparation, the peri-ureteral connective tissue and the triangle of renal hilum, great vessels and medial lower pole should not be dissected. The insertion of a JJ stent at the time of transplantation also appears to have reduced the incidence of complications.

FURTHER READING

Feest TG, Round A, Hamad S (1993) Incidence of severe acute renal failure in adults: Results of a community based study. *British Medical Journal*; 306: 481–483

George NJR, O'Reilly PH, Barnard RJ, Blacklock NJ (1983) High pressure chronic retention. *British Medical Journal*; 286: 1780–1783

Jones DA, George NJR, O'Reilly PH, Barnard RJ (1988) The biphasic nature of renal functional recovery following relief of chronic obstructive uropathy. *British Journal of Urology*; 61: 192–197

Jones DA, Gilpin SA, Holden D, *et al.* (1991) Relationship between bladder morphology and long-term outcome of treatment in patients with high pressure chronic retention of urine. *British Journal of Urology*; 67: 280–285

Shoskes DA, Hanbury D, Cranston D, Morris PJ (1995) Urological complications in 1,000 consecutive renal transplant recipients. *Journal of Urology*; 153: 18–21

Walsh P, Retik A, Vaughan Jr E D, Wein A (1998) Campbells urology. 7th Edition. London: WB Saunders Company

SECTION 4

SPECIALIST SCENARIOS

Chapter 24 _____

THE RENAL TRANSPLANT RECIPIENT
Anthony Warrens

INTRODUCTION

There is no cause of acute renal failure (ARF) that affects an individual's native kidneys which cannot also affect a transplanted kidney (with the obvious exception of most congenital abnormalities). However, the transplanted kidney is subjected to a range of insults almost unknown to the native kidney, including the terminal events of the donor's life, an inevitable period of both warm and cold ischaemia, and vascular and ureteric re-anastomosis. These bring with them increased risks of ARF. In addition, the allograft kidney is continuously exposed to immunosuppressive and other drugs and is at risk of the complications of such therapy. Finally, by definition, allografted kidneys are transplanted into a patient population which has, as its defining characteristic, the fact that each individual has developed renal failure. Thus, a transplanted kidney may develop ARF from the same cause as may have induced it in the recipient's native kidneys. From the above observations, it is unsurprising that the distribution of renal disease in the transplanted population is very different from that of the community at large.

PATHOPHYSIOLOGY

1. Complications of the Process of Transplantation

Ante-mortem damage in the donor

Much of this is discussed elsewhere in this book in the context of very sick patients. ARF is a common problem for the seriously ill, particularly if they have been sick for more than a day or two. Successful cadaveric donation requires a period of planning such that people who are ultimately used as donors often fall into this category. Considering their outcome, they are unequivocally seriously ill in their last few days. Even with the advent of the use of non-heart-beating donors, a patient can only be considered for donation if there is a period of time between realising that he is not going to recover and actual death, in order to plan the harvesting and to gain consent.

Therefore, even although the tests of renal function may suggest the donor's kidneys are functioning normally, it is very common for these kidneys to have sustained some degree of damage even before the harvesting operation begins. The most common problem ante-mortem is hypotension and so, at the time of harvesting, the kidneys may be relatively ischaemic or possibly even in the early stages of acute tubular necrosis (ATN). Alternatively, or in addition, it is common for donors to develop acute bacterial infections, often associated with multiple instrumentations in the intensive care unit. It is well recognised that sepsis is a predisposing factor to ATN in the native kidney. Mechanisms underlying this will be dealt with in detail elsewhere in this book (see **Chapter 19**). However, in brief, it appears that endotoxin binds the surface of cells such as macrophages (via its receptor CD14). This results in the elaboration of cytokines such as interleukin-1 (IL-1) and tumour necrosis factor (TNF). Numerous other potential mediators of tissue damage are generated, including thromboxanes, leukotrienes, nitric oxide, free radicals, platelet activating factor and complement. As a result of this, the endothelial cells of the kidney become activated and demonstrate increased expression of activation markers and a prothrombotic phenotype. Some of these factors represent the final common pathway of tissue injury, as will be discussed below.

Recent work has demonstrated that there are other mechanisms active in the donor which may render their kidneys susceptible to subsequent damage following transplantation. Many organ donors die as a result of intra-cerebral catastrophes. Such events have been shown to be associated with increased expression of several pro-inflammatory cytokines. In addition, MHC class I, class II and the co-stimulatory molecule, B7, are up-regulated in the kidney following cerebral trauma, which would be compatible with increased immunogenicity. The mechanism underlying this effect has not been well characterised. These observations probably explain why donor brain trauma may have a negative effect on allograft survival.

The superiority of using living donors rather than cadavers is well established. A major factor in this is the ability to control the warm and cold ischaemic times. However, it is clear from the above discussion that there are other major advantages in taking an organ from someone who is, by definition, in good health at the time of donation.

Ischaemia-reperfusion injury

Every transplanted kidney will suffer from some degree of ischaemia. In the live donor this will be short, but in the cadaver, particularly one with a prolonged terminal illness, it may be rather long. The period of ischaemia is divided into warm and cold periods. The period of warm ischaemia may, in the context of hypotension of the donor or other factors, begin before harvesting and stops with the perfusion of the harvested kidney with cold preservation solution. This marks the beginning of the cold ischaemic time which continues until the vascular clamps are removed following the anastomosis of the donor renal artery and vein(s) to the recipient.

Warm ischaemia is much more damaging than cold, largely because of the higher demand for energy at higher temperatures. For this reason the tolerance of warm ischaemia is measured in minutes while that of cold ischaemia is in hours.

A significant part of the damage consequent on ischaemia in an allograft results from the fact that the changes in the tissue induced by ischaemia alter the way it interacts with circulating leukocytes, partly by increased expression of endothelial cell adhesion molecules, such as intercellular adhesion molecule-1 (ICAM-1). There is increased adhesion to recently ischaemic tissue and this plays a significant factor in the damage of what is referred to as "ischaemia-reperfusion injury".

Vascular factors

The kidney is usually very good at regulating its own blood flow (see **Chapter 1**). However, following ischaemia, its ability to autoregulate is impaired. In part, this may be due to the swelling of tubular epithelial cells which occlude adjacent capillaries, but it is exacerbated by the seepage of vasoactive mediators through the leaky, ischaemic endothelium. During reperfusion, increased adhesion of leukocytes to endothelium decreases perfusion further. Vasoactive factors involved include nitric oxide, endothelin, thromboxanes and platelet activating factors.

Epithelial cell damage

We have just mentioned the tubular cell swelling associated with ischaemia. At its extreme, this may result in sloughing of the tubular epithelium and subsequent obstruction of the nephron. Various factors have been implicated in this process, including the intracellular accumulation of calcium, the generation of reactive oxygen species, depletion of ATP, and the activation of phospholipases and proteases.

Acidosis

Ischaemia leads to increased anaerobic glycolysis and, with it, an accumulation of acid. At mild levels of acidosis, this may actually be protective of cells from ischaemic damage, but, at lower pH, acidosis may contribute to diminished tissue blood flow and injury.

Leukocytes in ischaemia-reperfusion injury

Leukocytes are present in greater numbers after an ischaemic event and may contribute to tissue damage by potentiating an inflammatory response, as well as by blocking small vessels and impairing local perfusion. Activated leukocytes can release cytokines, proteases, myeloperoxidase, elastases and other enzymes, and reactive oxygen species. All of these can mediate tissue damage. Activated neutrophils have increased adhesiveness and are also intrinsically "stiffer", which causes further physical obstruction to the flow of blood. Some of the products of activated neutrophils are themselves vasoconstricting.

The initial interaction of leukocytes with endothelium involves the binding of selectins to their ligands. Following this initial transient selectin-mediated adhesion, leukocytes are immobilised via the binding of integrins on the leukocytes with members of the immunoglobulin superfamily on the endothelium, such as ICAM-1. One example is the binding of the leukocyte β2 integrins, LFA-1 and/or Mac-1, to ICAM-1 on endothelial cells.

These molecules are affected by the inflammatory process. P-selectin is found to be expressed strongly in transplants demonstrating acute cellular rejection but less strongly in those showing ATN. ICAM-1 expression is increased following ischaemia-reperfusion injury. It has been shown that the inhibition of the interactions of ICAM-1 with either LFA-1 or Mac-1 may have an effect in ameliorating ischaemic injury. *In vitro* data suggest that, while these probably represent the most important molecules, other factors may also be involved.

Much effort has been expended in attempting to reverse the potentially deleterious effects of ischaemia prior to transplantation by altering the constituents of the cold perfusion fluid used to preserve the kidney during its period *ex vivo*. High concentrations of potassium and magnesium are used to mimic intracellular fluid concentrations. In order to prevent consequent cell swelling, other components are used which do not cross the cell membrane. Numerous other additives, some of them designed specifically to reverse the effects of various inflammatory molecules, have been included in various studies. However, none has yet gained widespread popularity.

Surgical complications

At the simplest level, kidney transplantation consists merely of three anastomoses: the artery, the vein and the ureter. Problems at each can result in acute renal failure. Ureteric problems may result in obstruction. This may be associated with an abnormality of the ureteric tissue itself, or blockage of a stent placed in order to protect the anastomosis. Turbulent flow resulting from an imperfect venous anastomosis may result in acute renal vein thrombosis. Acute problems at the arterial anastomosis are a less common cause of ARF, although occasionally acute haemorrhage may induce ATN, or thrombosis may result in acute irreversible renal failure secondary to infarction of the kidney.

2. Drug Complications

For almost two decades, cyclosporin has been the mainstay of immunosuppression in transplantation. It works by inhibiting the calcineurin-mediated transduction of a signal from the cell surface (following appropriate engagement of the T cell receptor) to the nucleus, which would otherwise result in the production of interleukin-2 (IL-2), a potent T cell growth factor. Recently, a second calcineurin inhibitor, tacrolimus (formerly known as FK506) has been introduced. Paradoxically, the major side effect of each is nephrotoxicity. Cyclosporin has an effect on intra-renal blood flow. It is associated with an acute increase in renal vascular resistance, probably as a result of a disproportionate increase in vascular tone of afferent glomerular arterioles. The mechanism underlying this change in vascular resistance is unclear. There are conflicting data about a role for nitric oxide and prostacyclin, but it seems likely that cyclosporin administration increases the production of endothelin. Vasodilatory prostaglandins may partially reverse the vasospasm induced by cyclosporin (which is why non-steroidal anti-inflammatory drugs, which inhibit prostaglandins, may enhance cyclosporin-mediated nephrotoxicity). Cyclosporin also increases the glomerular generation of platelet aggregating factor and initiates vascular smooth muscle contractile responses which may explain the ameliorating effect of calcium channel blockers on cyclosporin nephrotoxicity.

In addition, cyclosporin may have a direct toxic effect on tubular function. Biochemical abnormalities of cyclosporin nephrotoxicity seem to be disproportionate to the reduction in GFR that occurs. Finally, cyclosporin is known to activate endothelial cells and can, in rare cases, precipitate a haemolytic uraemic like-syndrome.

The other immunosuppressive drugs used in renal transplantation do not themselves have direct nephrotoxic effects. However, the allografted kidney may be damaged as a result of infections resulting from over-zealous immunosuppression. Also, certain drugs, particularly antibiotics, which may be associated with nephrotoxicity (either direct or allergic), are commonly required in renal transplant recipients because of the risk of infection.

3. Rejection

Rejection is classified into hyperacute, acute and chronic, based on the underlying pathogenic mechanisms. Hyperacute rejection is caused within minutes to hours of the vascular clamps being removed at operation. It results from pre-existing antibodies binding to the endothelium of the newly transplanted graft, which then activate endothelial cells and the complement and coagulation cascades. It results in early loss of the graft. It should never occur nowadays since the presence of these antibodies should be detected in the obligatory pre-transplant direct crossmatch between recipient serum and donor cells.

Acute rejection results from the stimulation *de novo* of an immune response to the allograft. Either or both of the cell-mediated and humoral arms of the immune response may be important in acute rejection. Cell-mediated responses include tubulitis and interstitial infiltrates. Antibody-mediated acute rejection tends to be associated with vascular lesions and is often more severe. The two frequently coexist.

Chronic rejection is an ill-defined entity, many presumed cases of which are now being reclassified as "chronic allograft nephropathy", since there is no uniform immunological rejection process that underlies it. While it may be triggered by damage mediated by the immune system, which may continue, a large element of the underlying pathophysiology is related to the scarring and remodelling processes. It is a slow, indolent deterioration of renal function and therefore does not present with acute renal failure. However, a patient with impaired function due to chronic allograft nephropathy is at increased risk of ARF.

4. Recurrent Disease

Everyone who needs a renal transplant has lost the use of his or her own kidneys. However, the majority of causes of renal failure are chronic progressive diseases. If these recur in the transplant, which many of them do, they tend to present with chronic renal failure again. Because anyone with chronic renal impairment is much more easily tipped into acute renal failure by precipitants that might leave normal kidneys unscathed, this is a factor that ought to be considered in the pathogenesis of acute renal failure in the transplanted kidney. Some recurrent diseases can cause rapid onset of ARF, however, such as haemolytic uraemic syndrome and anti-glomerular basement membrane disease, and their early recognition is critical if the graft is to be saved.

AETIOLOGY

1. Acute Tubular Necrosis

This is the commonest cause of ARF in the renal transplant unit, occurring in up to half of all transplanted patients in the immediate post-operative period. The term "delayed graft function" is used in most of these cases since very often no biopsy material is available to confirm the diagnosis. The behaviour is typical. Commonly, urine is produced from the ureter following release of the vascular clamps, but some hours after the operation the urine output begins to tail off. During this period, daily creatinines reveal that there is no significant improvement in GFR following transplantation. Since delayed graft function is such a common feature following transplantation and usually resolves, there is no reason to proceed to an early biopsy to confirm the diagnosis. Indeed, in the non-sensitised patient, it takes some days before the kidney is at risk of immunological damage. After a few days, it is no longer possible to be quite so sanguine about the diagnosis since acute rejection may develop against the background of delayed graft function. In such a situation, the normal indicator of developing rejection, serum creatinine, is not informative. It is therefore necessary to investigate more aggressively, in most cases by performing a renal biopsy.

The definition of delayed graft function is not cast in stone. Clearly, as long as the creatinine is falling there is function, although this may take a few days to happen. Operationally, it is useful to consider that delayed graft function (presumed to be due ATN consequent on donor events, the circumstances of the harvesting and transplantation procedures) has occurred if the patient requires dialysis at any stage after the first twenty-four hours of transplantation. The first twenty-four hours are excluded from this definition since it is occasionally necessary to dialyse somebody for post-operative fluid overload or biochemical abnormalities.

In the majority of cases, delayed graft function slowly resolves, as with other causes of ATN. However, in some cases, the patient never regains function of the transplanted kidney. It is almost certain that this kidney will have been biopsied and more information will be available as to why the kidney has not functioned. This situation is best referred to as primary non-function. Unfortunately, this term is often confused with delayed graft function.

It is clear that ATN/delayed graft function has a deleterious effect on long-term outcome. However, this is only true if the period of delayed graft function is prolonged. It seems that if the kidney starts working within seven days, this is not necessarily a poor prognostic factor.

Although the vast majority of episodes of ATN occur as a result of the transplant procedure in the immediate post-operative period, ATN may occur at any stage for any of the reasons that may induce it in a native kidney. As the transplanted kidney often has an element of impaired function, it is more susceptible to the insults that might induce ATN in the native kidney.

2. Rejection

The second commonest cause of ARF in the transplant patient is rejection. As outlined above, this is subclassified into hyperacute, acute and chronic rejection.

Hyperacute rejection should not occur nowadays. When it did, it presented within minutes to a few hours of the clamps being removed from the vascular anastomoses with a painful swollen graft, microscopic haematuria and no function.

Acute rejection is by far the most common form of rejection to cause ARF. It rarely occurs before the end of the first week following transplantation and it is relatively uncommon after the first six months. However, late acute rejection episodes do occur, most often precipitated by an injudicious reduction in immunosuppression. It should always be considered in a patient whose allograft function is deteriorating, even many years after transplantation. Acute rejection usually presents with a rise in creatinine which may be relatively rapid. Formerly, when less aggressive immunosuppression was used, the graft may have swollen and become tender. However, this is relatively uncommon today. It is important to remember that acute rejection may occur in a non-functioning graft. For this reason it is common practice to biopsy the graft displaying delayed graft function on a regular, often weekly, basis.

As stated above, chronic rejection, or chronic allograft nephropathy, does not present with ARF. However, a patient with chronic allograft nephropathy is at an increased risk of ARF, like any other patient with impaired function.

3. Infection

Urinary tract infection (UTI) may also present with an acute rise in creatinine. It is common following transplantation, as in any post-operative period, but particularly since it is the urinary tract on which the procedure has been performed. This is compounded by the presence of prosthetic material if it is the practice of the operating surgeon to protect the ureteric anastomosis by leaving a stent *in situ*. As time passes, urosepsis is made more likely by slow passage of urine in the context of delayed graft function, any abnormality of the vesico-ureteric junction resulting from the surgery, and by immunosuppression.

It is always important to consider this diagnosis before proceeding to biopsy since a biopsy of an infected kidney runs the risk of generating a parenchymal abscess. Urinary tract infection may present with frequency, haematuria and dysuria, as usual. However, it may be surprisingly asymptomatic in transplant recipients. Hence, a low threshold of suspicion is required.

4. Calcineurin-Inhibitor (Cyclosporin/Tacrolimus) Nephrotoxicity

Either cyclosporin or tacrolimus may cause an acute rise in serum creatinine. If caught early, this responds rapidly to a reduction in circulating levels. Many believe that these drugs (and perhaps cyclosporin in particular) may be associated with chronic irreversible changes in renal function, but these are again indolent and slowly progressive, and would only be associated with ARF in the context of another insult.

5. Urinary Tract Obstruction (see also Chapter 23)

Because of the abnormal anatomy of the transplanted ureter, with the possible placement of a stent, urinary obstruction is not uncommon following transplantation. In addition, urine outflow may be obstructed by pressure external to the pelvicalyceal system, such as a collection of lymph (lymphocoele), blood (haematoma) or urine (urinoma). The first two usually resolve spontaneously, but may have to be drained if they are obstructing outflow or if they become infected: the same may be said of a urinoma, but, in that case, the source must be identified and closed.

Obstruction presents usually with no more than a rise in creatinine. It is rarely symptomatic. Occasionally, the patient presents with oligoanuria. For this reason, an ultrasound scan is a necessary investigation when the serum creatinine rises. Interpretation is complicated slightly by the fact that the pelvicalyceal system of the transplanted kidney is often more prominent than that of a native kidney, without necessarily implying the presence of obstruction to urinary outflow.

An alternative investigation would be a nuclear medicine perfusion scan, using DTPA or MAG3 (see **Chapter 6**).

6. Renal Vein Thrombosis

The most common cause of renal vein thrombosis is an abnormality of the venous anastomosis. However, a disproportionate number of patients with renal vein thrombosis are found to have thrombophilia. Renal vein thrombosis presents with acute, sometimes painful, swelling of the kidney associated with acute haematuria. Function deteriorates rapidly.

CLINICAL PRESENTATION

The presence of an acute rise in serum creatinine in a transplant recipient should be regarded as an urgent observation. If associated with oligoanuria, haematuria or pain over the transplant, it is a medical emergency. One approach is summarised in **Practice Point 1**.

Acute Graft Pain

This is most likely due to infection or a vascular accident. Infection may be parenchymal (acute pyelonephritis), urinary (urinary tract infection or, occasionally, pyonephrosis) or perirenal. In the last case, consider infection of a lymphocoele, haematoma or urinoma. If the cause of the pain is vascular it may be due to a haemorrhage (most likely from a hole in the renal artery) or infarction (venous or arterial). Acute rejection is rarely painful with current immunosuppression.

Macroscopic Haematuria

This is most likely a feature of urinary tract infection, but may be due to renal vein thrombosis.

Reduction or Cessation in Urine Output (oligo-anuria)

Obstruction is the most likely cause, although it may occur with any cause of ARF. It is important to remember that total anuria may not occur, even with total obstruction of the transplant kidney, since there may be some residual urine produced by the native kidneys.

Asymptomatic Rise in Creatinine

Any of the causes of ARF may present in this way. A rise in creatinine is, in fact, much the commonest presentation of ARF. It is, of course, much less specific than any of the other three presentations. The following is a stepwise approach to dealing with this (summarised in **Practice Point 2**):

1. Assess the significance of the change. In many patients, serum creatinine values fluctuate rather widely. Sometimes it is appropriate merely to repeat the creatinine.

2. A rise in creatinine accompanied by a disproportionate rise in urea is suggestive of hypovolaemia. In any case, it is important to undertake a fluid assessment on transplant patients, since concentrating defects of the renal tubules are very common.
3. Arrange a renal ultrasound to exclude pelvicalyceal dilatation associated with acute obstruction. Also, if possible, request Doppler studies to check that there is a signal from both artery and vein. The clinical scenario is likely to be much more acute in the context of either renal vein or arterial thrombosis.
4. Arrange urgent urinary microscopy and culture to exclude urosepsis.
5. Check a 12 h trough level of the appropriate calcineurin inhibitor (cyclosporin or tacrolimus).
6. If there is no other explanation, it is appropriate to proceed to percutaneous transplant biopsy. Before doing so, check clotting screen and full blood count.

TREATMENT PRINCIPLES

It may be enough merely to optimise the patient's fluid volume status.

If the levels of calcineurin inhibitor are too high, then it may be appropriate to omit a single dose and restart regular therapy at a lower dose. Some patients are exquisitely sensitive to calcineurin inhibitors and so therapeutic ranges should be treated only as a general guide.

Urinary tract sepsis should obviously be treated with appropriate antibiotics.

Obstruction should be treated urgently. This usually involves the insertion of a percutaneous nephrostomy under ultrasound guidance. If an obvious reversible cause for obstruction, such as a blocked ureteric stent, can be identified, it should be removed.

Treatment of acute rejection is very context-specific. You should take into account the level of immunological risk for a given patient, the immunological track record of this and previous transplants, current medication, and the nature of histological findings. For example, in a high risk patient, known to be sensitised, who has a biopsy showing acute severe vascular rejection (antibody-mediated), it may be appropriate to increase the B lymphocyte component of immunosuppression. Indeed, many would advocate the use of plasma exchange or immunoadsorption in this scenario. At the other end of the spectrum, in an immunologically low risk patient, the most appropriate treatment of a mild first episode of acute rejection would be a course of methylprednisolone. Whatever treatment is given at this stage, attention should be focused on the background immunosuppression to which the patient returns following acute therapy. Immunosuppression is a very contentious and, to some extent, idiosyncratic art. There are no right answers and this area is still subject to multiple clinical trials. In addition, new agents are constantly being introduced. Each transplant unit will have its own policies on immunosuppression.

OUTCOME

A large percentage of patients who receive a renal allograft undergo an episode of ARF. The vast majority of these episodes are reversed and the patient returns to good renal function. Most units expect that 90% of grafts transplanted are still functioning at 1 year and 70–75% are still functioning at 5 years. The unsolved problem in transplantation is the chronic decline in function rather than ARF.

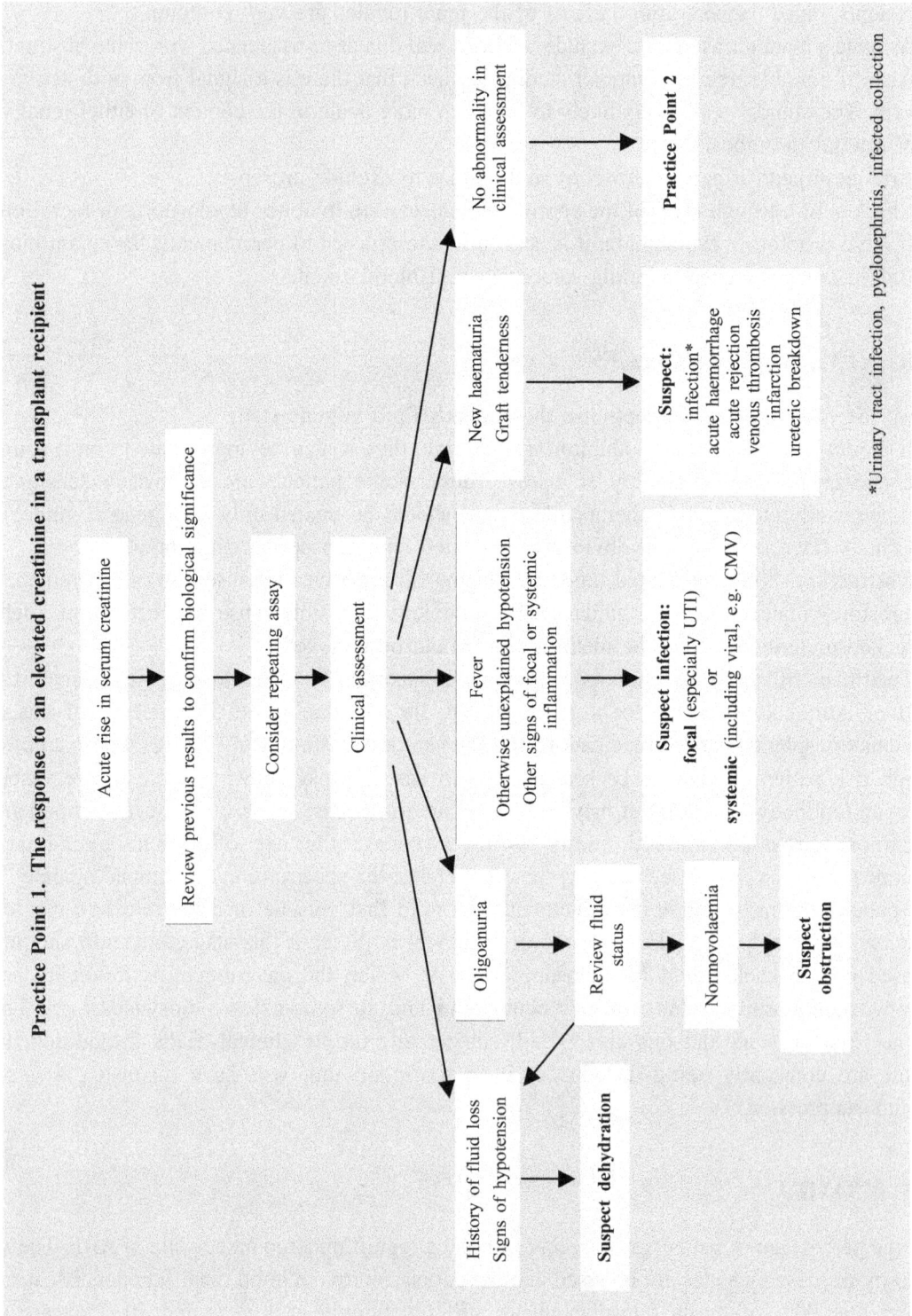

Practice Point 1. The response to an elevated creatinine in a transplant recipient

Acute rise in serum creatinine

↓

Review previous results to confirm biological significance

↓

Consider repeating assay

↓

Clinical assessment

Clinical assessment branches to:

No abnormality in clinical assessment → **Practice Point 2**

New haematuria / Graft tenderness → **Suspect:** infection* / acute haemorrhage / acute rejection / venous thrombosis / infarction / ureteric breakdown

Fever / Otherwise unexplained hypotension / Other signs of focal or systemic inflammation → **Suspect infection: focal** (especially UTI) **or systemic** (including viral, e.g. CMV)

Oligoanuria → Review fluid status → Normovolaemia → **Suspect obstruction**

History of fluid loss / Signs of hypotension → **Suspect dehydration**

*Urinary tract infection, pyelonephritis, infected collection

Practice Point 2. The response to a validated elevated serum creatinine in the absence of abnormal clinical features

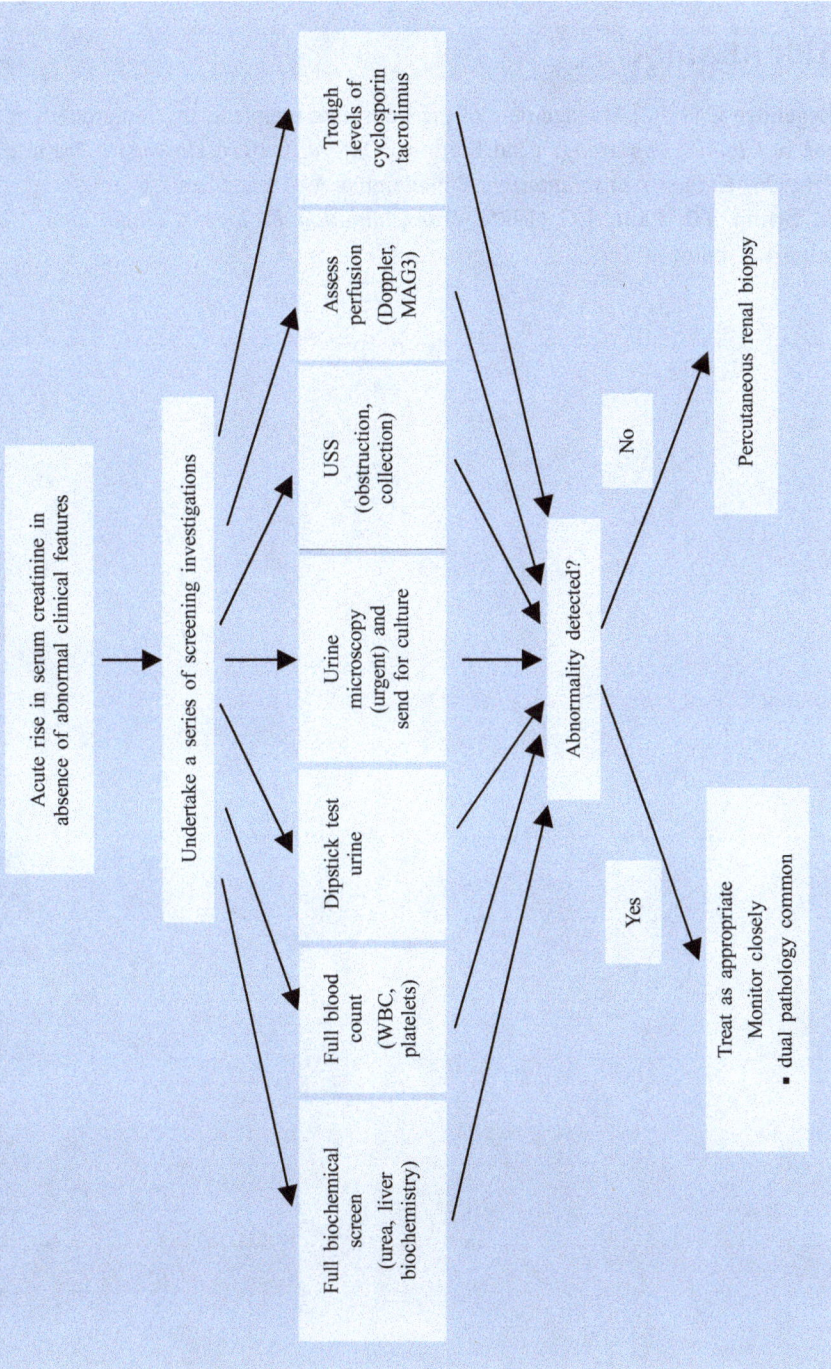

Acute rise in serum creatinine in absence of abnormal clinical features

↓

Undertake a series of screening investigations

- Full biochemical screen (urea, liver biochemistry)
- Full blood count (WBC, platelets)
- Dipstick test urine
- Urine microscopy (urgent) and send for culture
- USS (obstruction, collection)
- Assess perfusion (Doppler, MAG3)
- Trough levels of cyclosporin tacrolimus

↓

Abnormality detected?

No → Percutaneous renal biopsy

Yes → Treat as appropriate
Monitor closely
- dual pathology common

ACKNOWLEDGEMENT

The author would like to thank Mr Finn Morgan for his critical reading of the manuscript.

FURTHER READING

Kreis H, Legendre C (1992) Management of the transplant recipient. In: Cameron JS *et al.* (eds.). *Oxford Textbook of Clinical Nephrology* (2nd Edition). Oxford: Oxford University Press; p. 1520

Morris PJ (1996) *Kidney Transplantation.* Philadelphia: WB Saunders

Tilney NL, Strom TB, Paul, LC (1996) *Transplantation Biology: Cellular and Molecular Aspects.* Philadelphia: Lippincott

Chapter 25 _____

THE LIVER UNIT
Steven Holt

INTRODUCTION

Renal impairment complicates more than 50% of acute liver failure cases, and is often present in association with chronic liver disease. This may be due to liver impairment itself (such as hepatorenal syndrome), its complications, or its treatment. Alternatively, both organs may be affected by systemic conditions such as infection, vasculitis, or hereditary disorders; these are mainly dealt with in other chapters, and only briefly reviewed here.

The first part of this chapter deals with the hepatorenal syndrome and the renal complications of treatment for cirrhosis, a common cause of hospital admission. Thereafter, special situations in which hepatic and renal derangement is seen will be discussed.

THE LIVER

The liver performs a number of important functions directly related to the kidney with metabolic, immunological, hormonal, nutritional and detoxifying roles. It derives around 25% of its oxygen supply from portal vein blood, the hepatic artery supplying the remainder. Hepatocytes make up 25% of the liver substance, the other cells being interstitial (or Ito) cells, tissue macrophages (Kupffer cells) or vascular and biliary structures. As well as hepatic failure causing renal dysfunction, there are subtle changes in hepatic function that are induced by renal failure, including altered carbohydrate, lipid and protein metabolism leading to reduced glycolysis, increased gluconeogenesis and hypertriglyceridaemia.

THE HEPATORENAL SYNDROME

Hepatorenal syndrome (HRS) may be defined as "renal failure in patients with liver disease, in the absence of clinical, laboratory or anatomical evidence of other causes of renal failure". HRS represents one end of the spectrum of multi-organ dysfunction associated with severe liver disease. This continuum can range from minimal systemic upset to profound systemic vasodilatation with activation of all compensatory vasoconstrictor mechanisms. The lack of consensus on the definition of HRS has caused difficulty in the interpretation and comparison of studies in this field. Since HRS is largely a diagnosis of exclusion, previous definitions have relied heavily on urinary findings and, latterly, have been considered somewhat too strict. There are now

Table 1

A. Major diagnostic criteria for hepatorenal syndrome

Acute/chronic liver disease

Creatinine clearance <40 mL/min or serum creatinine >136 μmol/L

No shock, bacterial infection, nephrotoxic drugs, fluid losses

No sustained improvement after volume expansion

Proteinuria <500 mg/day

Normal renal imaging

B. Additional diagnostic criteria (which may be indicative, but are not required for the diagnosis of HRS)

Urine volume <500 mL/day

Urine sodium <10 mmol/L

Urine osmolality >plasma osmolality

Urine microscopy <50 red blood cells per high power field

Serum sodium <130 mmol/L

internationally agreed criteria for the definition of HRS (see **Table 1**). All of the major criteria (**Table 1A**) must be present for the diagnosis of HRS, while additional criteria (**Table 1B**) represent supportive evidence, but are not necessary for the diagnosis.

There has been a move to subdivide HRS into types I and II. Type I represents severe or rapidly progressive renal failure and can be defined as: (i) a two-fold increase in serum creatinine; (ii) an initial creatinine level of >220 μmol/L; or (iii) a reduction of creatinine clearance to <20 mL/min in less than 2 weeks. Type II has a more insidious course. The rationale for this distinction is that it distinguishes patients with rapid renal decline from patients with diuretic resistant ascites, since there is a feeling that the pathogenesis and response to treatment may differ. However, since this is only a relatively recent development there is as yet little evidence that this subdivision is helpful in prognosis or management. There are numerous factors that predict the development of the HRS, essentially relating to the severity of the liver disease. However, notably absent are liver function tests and the aetiology of liver disease.

Pathophysiology of Hepatorenal Syndrome

The kidneys in HRS suffer from a form of "functional" renal failure:

i. There is rapid reversal of renal dysfunction after orthotopic liver transplantation or hepatic recovery.
ii. Kidneys taken from patients with HRS work normally when transplanted into a patient with a normal liver.
iii. There are no characteristic histological findings in the kidney at post mortem in patients dying from HRS.

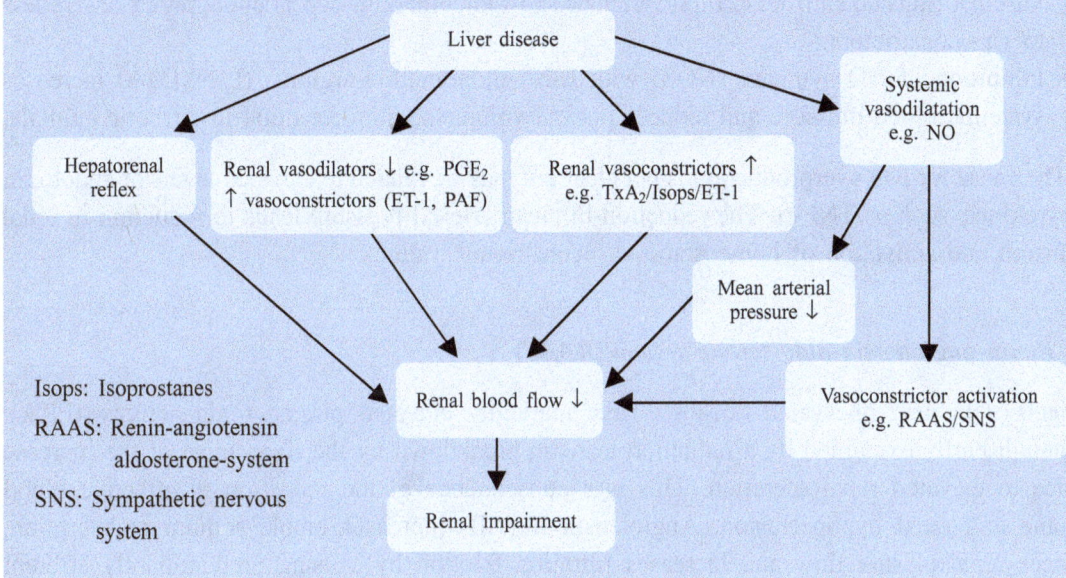

Figure 1. Summary of pathways leading to renal impairment in hepatorenal syndrome

In angiographic studies of patients dying with HRS, a normal angiographic picture may be obtained post mortem, in contrast to the severe peripheral pruning of the angiogram taken before death, suggesting intense renal vasoconstriction.

These clinical observations, in the absence of a well-validated animal model, suggest that HRS is secondary to a dramatic reduction in renal blood flow. Tubule function appears to be intact, at least early in the syndrome, since there is avid sodium retention and oliguria.

There are three components to the reduction in renal blood flow (see **Figure 1**):

i. Development of a hyperdynamic circulation.
ii. Increased levels of endogenous renal vasoconstrictors.
iii. Neurally mediated reflex vasoconstriction.

1. Development of a Hyperdynamic Circulation

In both acute liver failure and cirrhotic liver disease a hyperdynamic circulation develops, manifest by an increased cardiac output, low mean arterial pressure and reduced systemic vascular resistance.

(a) *Endogenous vasodilators*

A number of vasodilatory compounds have been suggested to be important in the reduction in systemic vascular resistance, including adrenomedullin, atrial natriuretic peptide (ANP), calcitonin gene related peptide (CGRP), glucagon, prostacyclin (PGI_2), met-encephalin, nitric oxide (NO), substance P and vasointestinal polypeptide (VIP). Overproduction of the vasodilator NO is likely to be the main cause for the reduction in systemic vascular resistance in liver disease:

(i) Plasma levels of nitrite and nitrate, metabolic products of NO, are elevated in proportion to the degree of liver dysfunction.

(ii) Vascular rings taken from cirrhotic animals show endothelium-dependent hyporesponsiveness to vasoconstrictors.

(iii) Inhibition of NO synthase (NOS) with L-N^G-monomethyl-arginine (L-NMMA) increases systemic blood pressure and reduces plasma volume/sodium retention in cirrhotic animals.

The cause for NO overproduction is not clear but may be related to elevated levels of endotoxin or cytokines, such as TNF-α. The reduction in mean arterial pressure leads to reduction in renal perfusion and activation of homeostatic vasoconstrictor systems.

(b) *Renin-angiotensin-aldosterone system (RAAS)*

Patients with decompensated cirrhosis have markedly elevated plasma renin activity (PRA). Although partly explained by a reduction in renin breakdown by the liver, most of the increase is due to elevated renal secretion. This is a consequence of the reduction in effective blood volume and renal hypoperfusion. Angiotensin II (AII) increases tubule sodium reabsorption, reduces renal plasma flow and increases filtration fraction by causing predominantly efferent renal arteriolar vasoconstriction. The failure of homeostatic mechanisms to increase afferent flow results in detrimental effects of angiotensin.

(c) *Sympathetic nervous system*

Early experiments in patients with HRS focused on the observed enhanced activity in the sympathetic nervous system (SNS). Cirrhotic patients with ascites have high levels of circulating norepinephrine and demonstrate increased renal vascular response to adrenergic stimulation. However, the usual homeostatic renal response to catecholamines involves increases in counter-regulatory vasodilator prostaglandins (e.g. PGE$_2$/PGI$_2$), abrogating the vasoconstrictor effect of alpha adrenoceptor stimulation. This mechanism may be defective in patients with HRS.

2. Increased Formation of Renal Vasoconstrictors

In addition to activation of the SNS and RAAS, other vasoconstrictor systems are activated.

(a) *Prostanoids*

In patients with decompensated cirrhosis without renal impairment there are changes in prostaglandin synthesis and excretion which are complex. Synthesis of the vasodilator PGI$_2$ and vasoconstrictor thromboxane A$_2$ (TxA$_2$) are increased, while the most important renal vasodilator PGE$_2$ is reduced. However, inhibition of TxA$_2$ does not improve renal function, suggesting that this compound may not be an important mediator of renal dysfunction in HRS.

The monocyte and macrophage derived leukotrienes (e.g. LTA$_4$, B$_4$, C$_4$) are renal vasoconstrictors and are also elevated in liver disease. This is due both to reduced hepatic clearance, and also to increased synthesis due to upregulation by pro-inflammatory cytokines. The action of free radicals on arachidonic acid can result in compounds known as the isoprostanes. These have prostaglandin like structures and can act on TxA_2-like receptors resulting in renal vasoconstriction. Synthesis of isoprostanes is upregulated in HRS.

(b) *Endothelin*

The endothelins are a homologous group of vasoconstrictors with additional activities as mitogens and angiogenic factors. Endothelin-1 (ET-1) reduces renal blood flow and glomerular filtration rate, at doses that do not affect systemic blood pressure, by preferential constriction of efferent arteries. ET-1 is synthesised by the vascular endothelium in response to numerous stimuli (injury, ischaemia, endotoxin, inflammatory mediators, thrombin, transforming growth factor β (TGF-β), turbulent flow, stretch, shear). Plasma ET-1 and -3 are increased in hepatic dysfunction, and especially in HRS, although their effects on the kidney are less well characterised.

3. Neurally Mediated Reflex Vasoconstriction

The existence of a neural connection between the liver and the renal circulation has been suspected for some years. The infusion of glutamine into the systemic circulation has no effect on renal function in experimental animals. However, if infused into the portal vein it causes hepatocyte swelling and a reduction in renal blood flow and glomerular filtration rate. Evidence for the existence of a similar pathway in humans comes from a study of renal haemodynamics during transhepatic portosystemic shunt procedures (TIPSS). Inflation of the balloon causes an immediate increase in portal pressure with a simultaneous reduction in renal blood flow. Spinal transection, renal denervation or section of the vagal hepatic nerves abolishes this effect. In humans, lumbar sympathectomy improves renal function in HRS, although this procedure is rarely performed.

TREATMENT PRINCIPLES

Once the diagnosis has been established, treatment is supportive, although the mortality remains high consequent upon the substantial mortality of liver disease. Hepatic recovery or transplantation leads to resolution of HRS but, prior to this, early and aggressive supportive management is vital.

Fluid management

Central venous monitoring is mandatory to ensure an adequate intravascular volume and to assess the response to fluid challenge, since hypovolaemic ARF is a major differential diagnosis. Colloid solutions should be used to replace intravascular volume and, although the use of human albumin solutions has recently been questioned, they remain the treatment of choice. In particular, 20% human albumin solution is often used, as this has a relatively low sodium concentration (≈ 77 mmol/L) and causes less haemodynamic instability in cirrhosis. Urinary catheterisation is sometimes required to assess the urine output and response to therapy. Daily weights are very useful, but often difficult, due to patient immobility (weighable beds or slings can be used).

Treatment of the underlying liver disease

In the context of acute liver failure, intensive care or high dependency bed facilities are required. In acute liver failure some patients will recover spontaneously, as will their ARF. Otherwise liver transplantation, either hetero- or ortho-topic, depending on the aetiology of liver failure, may be required. One of the most common clinical scenarios leading to the development of HRS is acute alcoholic hepatitis, which often occurs on the background of established cirrhosis. In this setting, aggressive treatment with nutrition and steroids (prednisolone 30 mg o.d.) may lead to hepatic recovery (although the latter remains controversial). HRS arising in the context of decompensated cirrhosis, without obvious precipitants, remains the most difficult clinical scenario, with the most ominous prognosis.

Antibiotics

In all cases, it is normal practice to prescribe antibiotics because of the high morbidity and mortality associated with sepsis in liver disease. Prophylactic treatment with broad-spectrum antibiotics is therefore advocated (e.g. **cefotaxime 1 g 12 hourly iv ± metronidazole 400 mg 8 hourly iv or piperacillin/tazobactam 4.5 g 8 hourly iv; see also Appendix A**). The liver failure patient is also susceptible to systemic fungal infection and fungal prophylaxis is often warranted (e.g. **fluconazole 200 mg iv daily**).

Dopamine

Dopamine improves renal blood flow in some situations, but in the small studies in the context of HRS, the results are contradictory. In practice, dopamine (at 2.5 µg/kg/min) is often tried once maximal intravascular filling has been attained. It should be discontinued if no clinical effect is apparent after 24 h (e.g. improved renal function or increased urine output).

Paracentesis

In patients with decompensated liver cirrhosis, ascites is often present and may be exacerbated by aggressive fluid replacement. Very high intra-abdominal pressures secondary to ascites can reduce renal blood flow by increasing renal vein pressure and parenchymal compression; paracentesis may therefore be beneficial.

Trans-jugular intrahepatic porto-systemic shunts (*TIPSS*)

In the context of decompensated chronic liver disease, a TIPSS procedure may improve renal function. Often this occurs after transient deterioration, possibly induced by radiocontrast media used during the procedure. Although no prospective data exist, TIPSS may prove to be a useful stabilising therapy.

Vasopressin analogues

The vasopressin analogues **terlipressin (1–2 mg 4 hourly)** and **ornipressin (6 U/h for 4 h)** with colloid support have both been reported to induce transient regression of HRS in patients with cirrhosis, and may be useful as a therapeutic bridge to transplantation. The mechanism is presumed to be due to peripheral vasoconstriction together with a reduction in sympathetic nervous system activation, and a consequent increase in renal blood flow. Treatment withdrawal is, however, usually followed by relapse.

N-acetylcysteine

N-acetylcysteine is well tolerated and safe. It has theoretical advantages in terms of its action as an antioxidant, and may improve organ function by increasing oxygen extraction. In a pilot study, it has been shown to be useful in improving renal function in early HRS, predominantly in the context of alcoholic hepatitis (**150 mg/kg over 4 h (max 12 g) then 100 mg/kg/day for 5 days**).

Other therapies

Lumbar sympathectomy has been anecdotally reported to reverse the syndrome, but is not routinely performed. Head out of water immersion undoubtedly improves systemic haemodynamics but the practicalities of this therapy mean that it is impossible to use in practice. LeVeen (peritoneovenous) shunting has no effect on renal dysfunction and has been largely discontinued. The renal vasodilator prostanoids and their analogues have been tried in combination with other agents in this condition, but with negligible success. Thromboxane synthase inhibition is equally ineffective, as mentioned above. Blockade of sympathetic nervous system activity and the renin angiotensin system is counterproductive as this causes a further reduction in blood pressure and renal perfusion. Other potential but unproven therapies include thromboxane receptor antagonists, endothelin receptor antagonists and other free radical scavengers.

Orthotopic liver transplantation remains the definitive therapy for HRS when liver dysfunction does not improve quickly. In the context of HRS, this is reserved for patients with acute hepatic failure. If cirrhotic patients develop severe renal dysfunction they are virtually never transplanted. Renal function usually improves within a week of transplantation. Post transplant, patients have a lower glomerular filtration rate compared to those without renal impairment preoperatively, but serum creatinine levels are no different.

Prognosis

Renal impairment in the setting of cirrhosis has a grave prognosis with >95% mortality within 3 weeks and a mean survival of 1.7 weeks. In the largest study of 200 cirrhotic patient with HRS, only 2 spontaneously recovered. Although some studies have estimated that spontaneous recovery rates are higher, these usually follow improvement in hepatic function. It should be noted that uraemia is not usually the immediate cause of death, but patients typically die of sepsis or liver failure.

Renal Replacement Therapy in Hepatorenal Syndrome

The results of renal replacement therapy for HRS have been universally poor, particularly when the underlying condition is cirrhosis. There is little benefit in instituting renal replacement therapy unless there is a realistic hope of hepatic recovery or liver transplantation. However, when an improvement in hepatic function is anticipated, slow continuous haemofiltration is the preferred modality (see below).

Hepatorenal Syndrome Summary

HRS is an ominous development with a mortality in excess of 95%. If hepatic recovery or transplantation is anticipated/possible, aggressive renal support, including renal replacement therapy, is warranted as bridging therapy (see **Practice Point**).

CIRRHOSIS

In the UK, the commonest aetiologies of cirrhosis are alcoholic liver disease, chronic viral hepatitis (hepatitis B and C) and autoimmune conditions like primary biliary cirrhosis (PBC). Whereas each of these conditions can be associated with a variety of renal pathologies, renal impairment usually occurs as a result of treatment for the complications of cirrhosis or the development of HRS in the context of progressive disease.

This section will outline the management of complications of liver disease and more specifically the iatrogenic consequences upon the kidney. Renal disorders associated with the range of cirrhotic diseases will then be discussed.

As described above, cirrhosis leads to the development of a hyperdynamic circulation with some inevitable impairment of renal function (although not necessarily as severe as HRS). The renal impairment of early cirrhosis is rarely reflected in serum urea or creatinine levels. Urea is often lower than expected since its production is impaired by liver dysfunction, and creatinine is lower than expected due to low muscle mass and low meat intake. However, most patients with clinically significant cirrhosis have an impaired creatinine clearance when measured. Renal blood flow and glomerular filtration rate are reduced by ~60% compared to a non-cirrhotic population. The reduction in renal blood flow is roughly proportional to the severity of the hepatic impairment, such that the lowest values are seen in those with most severe liver derangement. Plasma creatinine concentrations that appear to be within the normal range may be associated with glomerular filtration rates of only 20–60 mL/min. Therefore, even minor renal insults can lead to profound functional impairment.

Ascites

One of the most frequent problems encountered in cirrhotic patients is the development and management of ascites. As a consequence of reduced renal blood flow and SNS/RAAS activation, cirrhosis is associated with marked sodium retention and reduced free water clearance. While the development of ascites itself only occasionally leads to renal impairment, in the rare circumstance of compression of the renal vein with tense ascites, inappropriate management is often associated with deterioration in renal function.

Practice Point. Active management of the hepatorenal syndrome

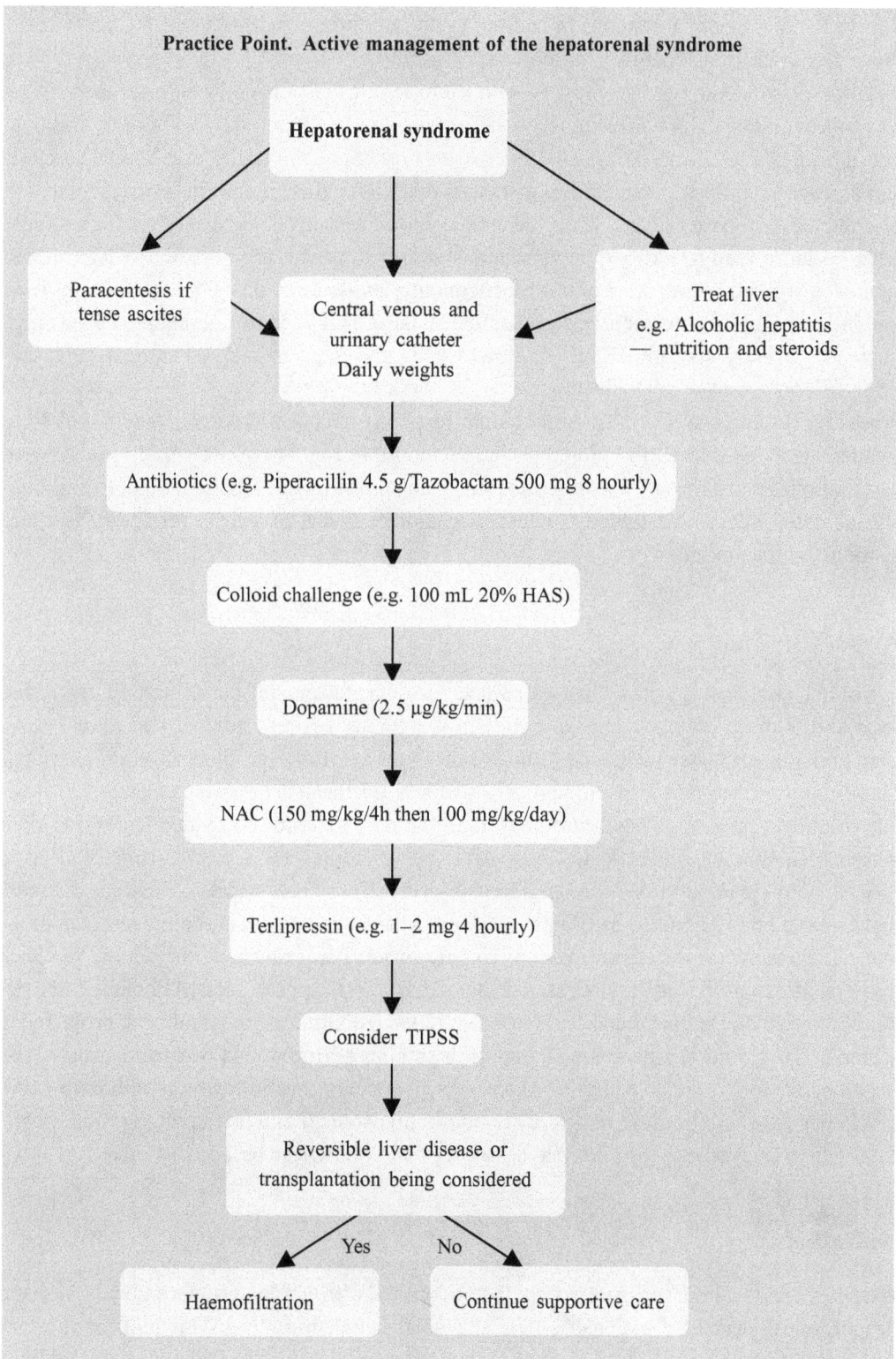

```
                        Hepatorenal syndrome
         ┌──────────────────────┼──────────────────────┐
         ▼                      ▼                      ▼
  Paracentesis if      Central venous and        Treat liver
  tense ascites  ────▶ urinary catheter   ◀───  e.g. Alcoholic hepatitis
                       Daily weights             — nutrition and steroids
                              │
                              ▼
         Antibiotics (e.g. Piperacillin 4.5 g/Tazobactam 500 mg 8 hourly)
                              │
                              ▼
              Colloid challenge (e.g. 100 mL 20% HAS)
                              │
                              ▼
                   Dopamine (2.5 µg/kg/min)
                              │
                              ▼
              NAC (150 mg/kg/4h then 100 mg/kg/day)
                              │
                              ▼
                Terlipressin (e.g. 1–2 mg 4 hourly)
                              │
                              ▼
                       Consider TIPSS
                              │
                              ▼
                Reversible liver disease or
             transplantation being considered
                   │                    │
                 Yes                    No
                   ▼                    ▼
           Haemofiltration      Continue supportive care
```

General therapeutic measures

The simple management approach is of sodium (~ 80 mmol/day) and fluid (~ 1.5 L/day) restriction but these are often inadequate in the control of ascites.

First line pharmacological therapy is with diuretics, initially usually aldosterone antagonists such as spironolactone (50–400 mg/day) or amiloride (5–20 mg/day). There is frequently a delayed natriuresis when initiating this therapy and attempts to rapidly escalate dose should be resisted as excessive dosing can lead to a sudden diuresis and reduction in intravascular volume. In the context of in-patient care, fluid balance is monitored by daily weights which should not decrease by more than 0.5 kg/day. Hyperkalaemia is a frequent complication of spironolactone therapy, even if renal impairment is not biochemically evident. In this situation, simply reducing or stopping the diuretic is effective. Furosemide is used as a second line agent (20–80 mg/day) and increases urinary sodium excretion; however, it may lead to marked intravascular volume depletion and exacerbate renal dysfunction.

Increasing dosage should be titrated against response and, if a dose increase is not followed by enhanced response, no further dose escalation should occur. There is a small group of patients who are completely refractory to diuretics at any dose, and in such patients increasing the dose merely increases the risk of toxicity. Thus, if it is clear that a patient is refractory to diuretics, they should be discontinued.

Paracentesis

Large volume paracentesis has been established as a safe and efficient therapy for ascites in cirrhosis and is more effective than diuretics in improving ascites. It has a less than 1% risk of bleeding and a much lower incidence of bowel perforation. However, this procedure is associated with perturbation of systemic haemodynamics unless performed in associated with intravenous plasma volume expansion. These cardiovascular changes may not be evident by blood pressure measurement alone but are reflected by activation of homeostatic mechanisms leading to an increase in sympathetic and or renin-angiotensin drive. There are studies indicating that subtotal paracentesis can be safely performed without albumin replacement, but complete removal of ascites without replacement causes severe haemodynamic upset. Paracentesis with volume replacement by albumin, dextran-70 and hemaccel, but not dextran-40, appear safe. Although there is still debate about which replacement fluid to use, 20% albumin is the author's preferred fluid replacement. This fluid has been associated with smaller perturbations of cardiovascular indices when compared to synthetic colloids. At present it appears that intravenous albumin (100 mL 20% HAS per 1.5 L ascitic fluid removed) is safe in this context and has advantages on theoretical grounds. Cheaper synthetic colloids have not yet been shown to be equally effective and safe.

Pressure effects

Tense ascites exerts a high pressure within the abdominal cavity. This pressure may be transmitted to retroperitoneal structures increasing IVC and renal venous pressure. This reduces the forward pressure gradient through the kidney. Since blood pressure is often low this pressure gradient can cause a fall in renal blood flow leading to renal failure. In practice, gross haemodynamic upset only occurs when the intra-abdominal pressure is very high (>40 mmHg) and the abdomen is very taut. Treatment is to perform therapeutic paracentesis. If ascites is thought to be the main problem causing renal impairment, then only a small amount of fluid needs to be removed (usually ~200–500 mL), since pressure falls rapidly with relatively little fluid removal.

Drugs Causing Renal Failure in Cirrhosis

Diuretics

Diuretics are frequently and appropriately prescribed to cirrhotic patients in order to mobilise ascites. However, if used excessively, they can lead to intravascular volume depletion and acute tubular necrosis. Because serum urea and creatinine tend to be lower in cirrhotics, due to lower muscle mass and poor protein intake, renal dysfunction may be overlooked unless clearance studies are performed.

Non-steroidal anti-inflammatory agents (NSAIDs)

The reduction in renal perfusion that accompanies liver dysfunction, is counteracted by the effects of locally produced prostaglandins in maintaining renal blood flow. This adaptive response is abrogated by NSAIDs, which cause a profound reduction in renal blood flow, leading to worsening renal function and impaired sodium and free water excretion. **Use of these drugs is absolutely contraindicated in liver disease.**

Angiotensin converting enzyme inhibitors (ACEI)

ACEI are detrimental to renal function in cirrhosis even when blood pressure is not reduced and when basal renin activity is low. There is a fall in urine output and sodium excretion.

Demeclocycline

Demeclocycline antagonises ADH receptors causing nephrogenic diabetes insipidus. Although effective at increasing serum sodium concentrations, it markedly reduces GFR due to a reduction in renal blood flow.

Aminoglycosides

Patients with liver impairment are more sensitive to the nephrotoxic effects of the aminoglycosides and levels need to be carefully monitored (see **Appendix A**).

Variceal Haemorrhage

Chronic liver disease is associated with the development of portal hypertension and varices. These can bleed and lead to hypotensive/hypovolaemic renal impairment. Acutely bleeding patients require rapid resuscitation with blood and clotting factors. If patients are actively bleeding, various medical manoeuvres can be used to stop bleeding by reducing portal pressure — these may be dangerous if renal function is impaired:

- Blood transfusion in the setting of renal impairment can cause hyperkalaemia and fluid overload; thus intravascular volumes need to be carefully and continuously reassessed (see **Chapters 5** and **8**).
- Vasopressin and terlipressin can lead to systemic (including some renal) vasoconstriction, an increase in tubule water permeability (thus reabsorption) and a reduction in urine output.
- GTN can lead to systemic vasodilatation and renal hypoperfusion.
- TIPSS is performed using X-ray screening and intravenous contrast, and can thus lead to contrast nephropathy.

In order to avoid exacerbating uraemia, phosphate enemas should be given to speed the clearance of the "blood meal".

Obstructive Jaundice

Obstructive jaundice occurs when there is an obstruction to the bile flow in the liver, causing accumulation of bilirubin, bile acids (cholic, deoxycholic, chenodeoxycholic) and bile salts (glycine or taurine conjugated acids). Bilirubin concentration rises from ~12 µmol/L (<1 mg/dL) to ~350 µmol/L (30 mg/dL) after uncomplicated complete biliary obstruction, but it may rise as high as ~1200 µmol/L (100 mg/dL) if renal failure occurs. The concentration of bile acids in the systemic circulation is usually negligible (<1 µmol/L), but is higher in the portal circulation because of enterohepatic circulation. Free levels are low (nM) since most bile acids are found bound to albumin and lipoproteins. Following biliary obstruction levels rise up to ~800 µmol/L. Most commonly, this occurs due to biliary stone disease, but it can occur in other situations such as malignancies of the pancreas or biliary system.

Previous studies have noted that ~10% of patients with obstructive jaundice have renal failure. Apart from renal dysfunction, cholaemia *per se* predisposes to sepsis and poor wound healing. The mortality rate for jaundiced patients undergoing biliary surgery is around 16–18% and this rises to 70–80% in patients who develop ARF. This is a huge increase in risk compared to the ~0.1% risk of biliary tract surgery in the non-jaundiced patient.

In a study of patients with cholangiocarcinoma, the renal functional abnormalities were proportional to the degree of jaundice and hepatic dysfunction, and no abnormality of renal function or sodium excretion was observed in patients with mild disease (bilirubin <300 µmol/L). In patients with moderate disease (bilirubin ~300–500 µmol/L), creatinine clearance was decreased but urinary sodium increased, and no reduction in renal blood flow was found. In patients with severe jaundice (bilirubin >500 µmol/L), renal blood flow, GFR, sodium excretion and free water clearance were all impaired.

Mechanisms of renal impairment

In acute biliary obstruction there is a fall in glomerular filtration rate and renal plasma flow, but an increase in urine volume. The consequent intravascular volume depletion and increase in renin angiotensin and sympathetic nervous system activity causes renal vasoconstriction, further decreasing renal blood flow.

The reduction in renal blood flow is mediated by afferent or efferent vasoconstriction and a number of vasoactive mediators have been proposed including TxA_2, AII, endotoxin or sympathetic stimulation. However, denervation of the kidney or inhibition of cyclo-oxygenase with indomethacin does not protect animals from renal impairment, and no change has been reported in PRA. The reduction in glomerular filtration rate seems in part to be mediated by alterations in renal vascular tone, specifically cortical vasoconstriction, and it is likely to be multi-factorial. Micropuncture experiments have demonstrated marked increases in proximal tubule sodium reabsorption as well as increased reabsorption more distally, after biliary obstruction.

Following biliary obstruction circulating levels of endotoxin and TNF-α are found to increase. Endotoxaemia occurs in ~85% of patients with biliary obstruction and is thought to be due to enhanced absorption of gut derived endotoxins secondary to the low intestinal bile acid concentrations and reduced secretion of immunoglobulin A. The clearance of endotoxin may be impaired following obstruction, leading to systemic endotoxaemia, renal vasoconstriction and oxidative stress (**Figure 2**). Lactulose decreases systemic and portal endotoxin levels by speeding bowel content flow, thus reducing bowel flora. *In vitro*, lactulose can directly lower TNF-α production by endotoxin stimulated monocytes. Oral lactulose and bile salts have been shown to

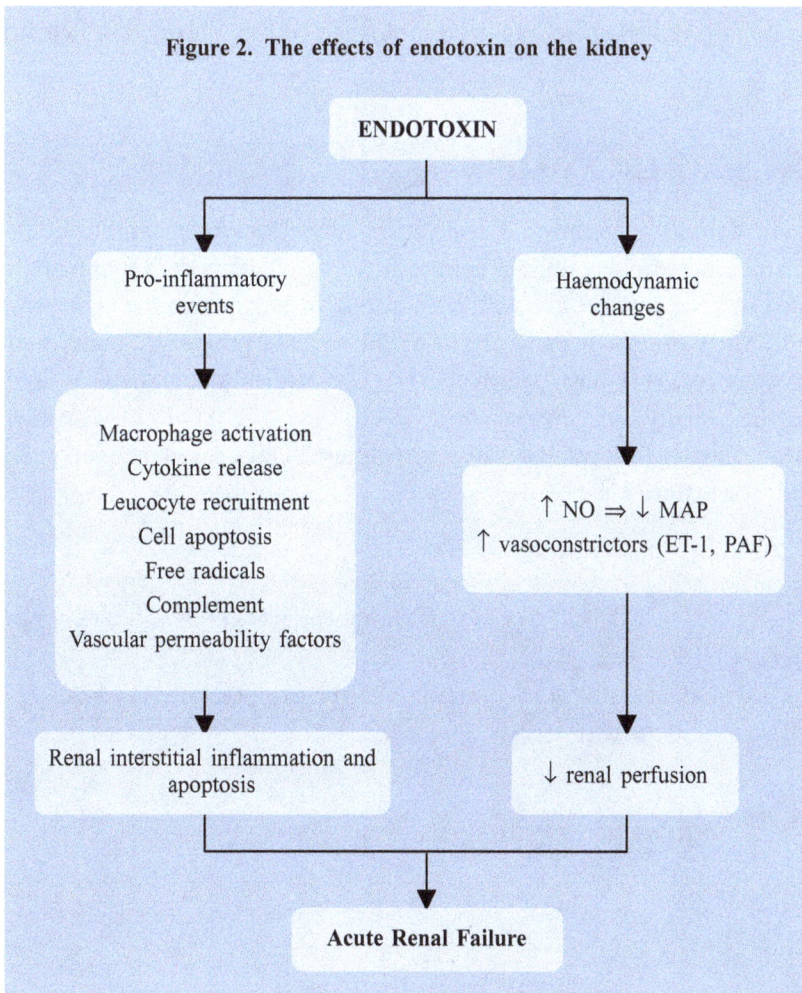

Figure 2. The effects of endotoxin on the kidney

decrease post-operative rates of renal failure and mortality, suggesting a link between endotoxin absorption and/or immune activation and renal impairment during endotoxaemia.

Data from bile infusion experiments suggest that bile salts directly cause diuresis, natriuresis and kaliuresis. Dialysis or cholestyramine treatment of bile, abolishes the diuretic effects of bile infusion. Tubule micro-perfusion experiments suggest that bile salts act directly in PTC to impair fluid reabsorption by up to 30%. At high levels, bile salts inhibit ATPase activity, disrupt lipid membranes and lysosomes. Bilirubin has no direct renal effects when infused alone. However, the infusion of bile salts alone into the dog renal artery is not associated with a reduction in glomerular filtration rate or renal plasma flow. This suggests that while bile acids/salts may be directly responsible for the increase in urine volume, they are not necessarily implicated in the pathogenesis of renal dysfunction, except via induction of hypovolaemia.

Treatment of renal dysfunction associated with biliary obstruction

The most important therapy is to relieve biliary obstruction and to maintain adequate intravascular volumes. Lactulose 10–20 mL 6–8 hourly should be administered. Animal studies suggest that N-acetylcysteine may be beneficial, and anecdotally it appears to improve renal function when used in humans but no controlled studies have been performed. Renal function usually corrects as bilirubin levels fall, unless there has been prolonged biliary obstruction, when improvement takes longer.

FULMINANT HEPATIC FAILURE

Fulminant hepatic failure is defined as encephalopathy developing rapidly after the onset of jaundice in the face of previously normal hepatic function. Patients with fulminant hepatic failure should be treated in specialist centres with access to liver transplantation. The presence of renal failure complicating fulminant hepatic failure is an adverse prognostic sign, predicting higher mortality and slower recovery postoperatively. The cause of fulminant hepatic failure in the UK is usually drugs (especially paracetamol) or viral hepatitis (see **Table 2**). Treatment of ARF in fulminant hepatic failure follows the same principles as discussed above (see **Hepatorenal Syndrome**) and in **Section 2**.

Table 2. Causes of fulminant hepatic failure

Paracetamol and other drugs (halothane, isoniazid, sulphonamides, phenytoin, ketoconazole, NSAIDs)

Viral hepatitis (HBV±δ, HCV, HEV, CMV, EBV, HSV)

Pregnancy

Wilson's disease

Malignancy (especially lymphoma)

Veno-occlusive disease

Reye's syndrome

ELECTROLYTE DISTURBANCES IN LIVER DISEASE

Electrolyte disturbances associated with liver disease, especially that of alcoholic aetiology, include a fall in serum sodium, magnesium, potassium, calcium and phosphate (see **Table 3** and **Chapter 8**).

Electrolyte	Causes	Comments
Hyponatraemia	↑ADH (2° to ↓ systemic vascular resistance) ↓hepatic metabolism of ADH ↑RAAS/SNS activity Altered intra-renal prostaglandin production ↓distal sodium delivery Drugs[2]	May exacerbate encephalopathy
Hypomagnesaemia	Nutritional inadequacy Reduced absorption — diarrhoea — steatorrhoea Renal wasting — diuretics — hypophosphataemia — ethanol directly ↓ PTH secretion from parathyroid gland	Symptomatic hypomagnesaemia is associated with deficit of 0.5–1 mmol/kg Give IV Mg^{2+} (magnesium sulphate) up to 160 mmol Mg^{2+} over 2–5 days Oral Mg^{2+} replacement is not well absorbed and tends to exacerbate diarrhoea, but magnesium glycerophosphate can be used at a dose of 24 mmol Mg^{2+} daily in divided doses
Hypokalaemia	Nutritional inadequacy GI/renal losses	
Hypocalcaemia	Nutritional deficiency Vitamin D deficiency	Ensure Ca^{2+} measurements corrected for albumin are used
Hypophosphataemia	Nutritional inadequacy Vomiting/diarrhoea (2° to alcohol) Antacid use (phosphate binding) Renal tubule losses (direct effect of alcohol) Glucose infusions (cause insulin induced cellular phosphate uptake)	

Table 3. Electrolyte disturbances in liver disease[1]

[1]Calcium, magnesium and phosphate disturbances are discussed in detail in **Chapter 8.5**.

[2]e.g. diuretics, antihistamines, paracetamol, anticholinergics, phenothiazines, tricyclics, biguanides, sulphonylureas, NSAIDs, barbiturates, opiates.

The degree of hyponatraemia roughly parallels the severity of the liver disease, and a serum sodium <125 mmol/L carries a poor prognosis. In addition, hyponatraemia may exacerbate encephalopathy. Mild hyponatraemia (130–135 mmol/L) probably need not be treated but signals caution. In particular, fluid restriction is often difficult since this needs to be in the region of <500 mL/day to be effective. In contrast, sodium restriction may be useful. Diuretics should be stopped if sodium is reducing or is <135 mmol/L. Demeclocycline should not be used. ADH antagonists are currently undergoing trials and may be useful in the future. Occasionally ultrafiltration with a continuous technique has been used, but should not be used for correction of hyponatraemia unless clinically symptomatic.

ACID-BASE CHANGES IN LIVER DISEASE

Many processes that take place in the liver generate acid and some generate alkali. For example, glucose is metabolised to lactate generating protons (acid), while lactate is reconverted to pyruvate using up protons. With a normal Western diet around 1 mEq of acid is generated per kg per day (see **Chapter 8.4**).

Alkalosis

Many patients with moderate to severe liver disease have some component of respiratory alkalosis, manifest by a low P_aCO_2. This may be caused by vascular shunting and hyperventilation, in addition to impaired metabolism leading to high levels of progesterone and ammonia that may cause increased sensitivity of the respiratory centres to carbon dioxide. Occasionally a metabolic alkalosis develops, and this is almost always due to GI loss, e.g. vomiting/nasogastric tube.

Acidosis

A normal anion-gap metabolic acidosis (with low bicarbonate) can occur, which may be a metabolic adaptation to the respiratory alkalosis. However, some patients with liver disease have a distal renal tubular acidosis (e.g. Wilson's, autoimmune hepatitis and primary biliary cirrhosis). In some cases, this is due to drugs (e.g. spironolactone) antagonising distal acidification mechanisms. In advanced liver disease, there is also a reduction in sodium delivery to the distal tubule. Treatment consists of giving sodium bicarbonate orally. This not only neutralises acid but also increases sodium delivery.

Advanced liver disease leads to impaired lactate clearance with an increase in half-life by 10–20% in cirrhotics compared to normals. In addition, there is increased lactate production through impairment in oxygen delivery to tissues. If compensatory mechanisms are adequate to keep the pH normal then treatment should be directed at stabilising haemodynamics; however once pH starts to fall the outlook is usually bleak. Non-lactate buffered replacement fluids and haemofiltration may help in normalising acid base balance in the short term (see **Chapter 9.5**).

GLOMERULONEPHRITIS IN LIVER DISEASE

A number of glomerular abnormalities are associated with liver disease. The most common association is that of a mesangiocapillary glomerulonephritis (MCGN) with hepatitis C. However, there are other associations, such as IgA nephropathy in alcoholic cirrhosis (see **Table 4**).

Table 4. Glomerular disease association with hepatic disorders	
Glomerular abnormality	**Common associations**
MCGN type I	Hepatitis C
Membranous nephropathy	Hepatitis B
Alcoholic liver disease	IgA nephropathy/Proliferative post-infectious GN
ANCA positive crescentic nephritis	Alpha1-antitrypsin deficiency

ISCHAEMIC HEPATITIS

This condition occurs when there is poor perfusion of the liver and usually kidney. It is seen in elderly patients who often present with cardiovascular collapse. In this setting, the liver function tests are almost always highly deranged with AST and ALT >1000. Initially the PT may be normal, but there is frequent hyperkalaemia, hyperphosphataemia, an elevated urate and high lactate dehydrogenase (LDH), suggesting tissue damage. Renal impairment is almost invariable. Treatment is directed to restoring hepatic and renal blood flow after which the liver and kidney often recover. However most patients are hypotensive on arrival and rarely respond to any therapy that does not include increase in renal perfusion. If the systemic haemodynamics can be normalised then prognosis is said to be good. The mortality is ~60%.

INFECTION

Hepatitis B Virus

Hepatitis B virus (HBV) is non-cytopathic to the liver, and it is the immune response to the virus, especially the action of HBV-specific cytotoxic T cells, which is the main mediator of liver injury. The situation is slightly different in the post-liver transplant immunosuppressed state, where there is evidence for direct HBV cytotoxicity. In contrast, most of the renal lesions are seen in the presence of circulating virus, and may result from the deposition of viral components within the kidney (**Table 5**).

In the acute phase, the shedding of e antigens and HBV DNA can lead to deposition of immune complexes in medium sized vessels, causing a syndrome indistinguishable from classical polyarteritis nodosa (PAN). Histologically there is fibrinoid necrosis and fibrin deposition, followed by aneurysm formation. In these lesions, surface antigen can be detected, implicating it in the

Table 5. Renal disease in viral hepatitis	
Hepatitis B infection	**Hepatitis C infection**
Polyarteritis nodosa	Mixed cryoglobulinaemia
Membranous glomerulonephritis	Mesangiocapillary glomerulonephritis
Mesangiocapillary glomerulonephritis	Membranous glomerulonephritis
IgA nephropathy	
Cryoglobulinaemia	

pathogenesis of the inflammation. Downstream dysfunction leads to symptoms of end organ damage. In chronic infection, membranous glomerulonephritis is the most common association with hepatitis B. The membranous changes lead to nephrotic syndrome, with impaired renal function. This may spontaneously remit in children but in adults can progress inexorably towards end stage renal failure.

Treatment

In view of the association between the renal lesion and viraemia, anti-viral agents have been used for the treatment of HBV-associated renal disease. Treatment of HBV-associated PAN differs from that of classical PAN, since the usual therapy of steroids and cyclophosphamide may adversely affect outcome, due to massive increases in viral replication. Thus, in HBV-associated cases, treatment regimens are modified to consist of steroids with the addition of an antiviral agent, such as Lamivudine, a nucleoside analogue. Some also advocate plasma exchange. No randomised trials have been performed, but anecdotal evidence suggests that Lamivudine may also improve membranous GN, when associated with HBV infection. The dose of Lamivudine needs to be titrated against renal function.

Hepatitis C Virus

Infection with the hepatitis C virus leads to an acute hepatitis in less than 5% of patients, and fulminant hepatic failure with consequences on renal function is extremely uncommon. However, approximately 1% of the general population of USA and Europe, and up to 15% in the Middle East, are chronically infected with HCV, which is now recognised as a very important cause of liver disease worldwide.

  HCV infection can result in a number of renal and other extra-hepatic complications, independent of its association with hepatic cirrhosis and hepatocellular carcinoma. In the kidney, it has been shown to cause mesangiocapillary and membranous glomerulonephritis, with or without a cryoglobulinaemic vasculitis. Apart from cryoglobulinaemia, which is present in 15% of patients but is associated with vasculitis in only a small proportion of cases, the factors which predispose to renal lesions are uncertain. Viral load or HCV genotype do not appear to be important factors. It is also of concern that HCV prevalence among the dialysis population is much higher than the general population, with rates of up to 20–50% being reported. Fortunately, the incidence of new diagnosis in this group is declining, perhaps reflecting improved infection control.

Mesangiocapillary glomerulonephritis (MCGN)

The MCGN seen in hepatitis C is usually type I. There is endocapillary proliferation due to monocyte infiltration, with EM deposits in the sub-endothelial, sub-epithelial and mesangial areas. There is granular deposition of C3, and immunostaining is also often positive for IgG and M. Clinically, this may manifest as nephrotic syndrome or, less commonly, asymptomatic haematuria and proteinuria. The presence of a circulating cryoglobulin is such a frequent association with this glomerular lesion in Europe, that the diagnosis should be reviewed if no cryoglobulin can be demonstrated; however such cases are described in the USA and Japan. Rarely, the renal lesion may not be MCGN but segmental mesangial proliferation.

Cryoglobulinaemic vasculitis

The cryoglobulin is always almost a mixed type II cryoglobulin (see **Chapter 4.5**) and complement C4 is usually reduced. It is now thought that three-quarters of "essential" cryoglobulinaemia is due to HCV disease. In patients with MCGN almost all have detectable viral DNA in the cryoprecipitate, but less frequently in the circulation. The virus probably initiates a clonal expansion of B cells. The cryocrit appears to correlate with renal prognosis.

Clinical features

The clinical features of cryoglobulinaemic vasculitis occur in less than one third of patients with cryoglobulins and include a purpuric rash, Raynaud's, arthralgia, peripheral neuropathy and weakness. Renal manifestations include nephrotic syndrome, haematuria, hypertension and ARF.

Treatment

Optimal therapy for chronic HCV infection presently includes the combination of alpha-interferon (3 MU × 3/week sc) and Ribavirin (1–1.2 g/day po), given for 6–12 months. With this therapy, approximately 40% of patients will have a sustained response, defined as HCV RNA negative by PCR six months after completion of treatment course. Worse response rates are seen in patients infected with the common genotype 1, and in those with established cirrhosis.

There is some evidence that this treatment regimen can induce renal remission. Unlike HBV, response is usually maintained during treatment, if it is achieved. Treatment with Ribavirin may need to be modified, since it is largely renally excreted and needs dose reduction in renal impairment.

Prognosis

The most common causes of death are cardiovascular, infection, liver failure and malignancy. The renal prognosis is variable, with approximately one third of patients appearing to have a spontaneous remission from glomerular disease. Nevertheless ~10% develop progressive renal impairment.

Other infections which can cause both ARF and liver dysfunction (e.g. leptospirosis, HIV and malaria) are discussed in **Chapter 20**.

THE KIDNEY IN THE LIVER TRANSPLANT PATIENT

Liver transplantation in adults is indicated for a number of conditions, including primary biliary cirrhosis, sclerosing cholangitis, malignancy, metabolic disorders and acute or chronic liver failure (**Table 6**).

Table 6. Indications for consideration of liver transplantation

Paracetamol induced

PH <7.3

PT >100 seconds and Creatinine >300 μmol/L and grade III/IV encephalopathy

Non-paracetamol induced

PT >100 seconds

Or three of:

    Age <10 or >40 years

    Non A/Non B viral hepatitis, halothane, drugs

    Jaundice >7 days before encephalopathy

    Bilirubin >300 μmol/L

    PT >50

Unlike renal transplantation, liver transplantation can be performed across ABO barriers in super-urgent transplantation, but this results in significantly poorer results with 1 year survival around 40% (cf. 80% in non super-urgent transplants).

Although most patients receive an orthotopic liver transplant, some patients are given heterotopic (or auxiliary) liver transplants in acute hepatic failure, where recovery might be expected. The advantage of the latter is that immunosuppression can be gradually withdrawn when the native liver recovers.

Chronic renal impairment occurs in 90% of patients with liver transplants. Many of these patients have chronic toxicity due to immunophillin binding drugs (Cyclosporin A, Tacrolimus), but focal glomerulosclerosis is the most common finding on renal biopsy. Acute renal dysfunction can also occur in association with hepatic graft dysfunction, either with acute or chronic rejection, seen as an HRS like syndrome or with a cholestasis-like picture.

PARACETAMOL POISONING

Paracetamol overdose is a leading cause of mortality and morbidity from deliberate overdose in the UK, and is associated with ~160 deaths/year. Paracetamol is the major metabolite of phenacetin and may chronically give rise to an analgesic nephropathy, but renal failure is more commonly due to acute poisoning. Paracetamol is usually detoxified in the liver by conjugation with glucuronide and sulphation to inactive metabolites. However, this is a saturable process, and once saturated, paracetamol can be metabolised by the cytochrome p450 system to N-acetyl-p-benzoquinoneimine (NAQI). This toxic compound is inactivated by reduced glutathione and converted to mercaptopuric acid. However, when glutathione stores are exhausted, this highly reactive pro-oxidant is able to cause extensive lipid peroxidation, protein modification, macrophage activation and eventually cell death, in both the liver and kidney. In doses <150 mg/kg, no adverse effects are usually seen, and in the UK a nomogram is often used to predict the likelihood of severe hepatic necrosis from blood levels at a given time after ingestion. However, these levels are only a guide and should be adjusted down in cases of patients on enzyme inducing drugs, anorexics, patients with chronic liver disease or a history of multiple overdoses. It is noteworthy that renal impairment, even severe dialysis-requiring ARF, can be seen in the setting of mild derangement of hepatic function. **Mortality in fulminant hepatic failure in this context is directly related to plasma creatinine:**

Plasma creatinine (μmol/L)	Mortality
>300	77%
100–300	60%
<100	35%

Metabolic abnormalities accompanying paracetamol overdose include compensated and uncompensated metabolic acidosis, hyperlactataemia, hypophosphataemia and phosphaturia.

Treatment

Gastric lavage, administration of 50 g activated charcoal or ipecacuanha emesis should be performed if the patient presents within 6 hours. A safe and effective antidote, N-acetylcysteine (NAC), exists and should be given intravenously as soon as possible after ingestion; it probably has some benefit up to 24 h after ingestion or more. Oral methionine (36 mg/kg 4 hourly × 4 doses) is an alternative that is less well tolerated and less effective than NAC. Although this treatment is effective at reducing or preventing damage to the liver, studies showed a trend for a possible beneficial renal effect of NAC therapy, but this did not reach statistical significance. Current treatment regimens involve therapy for just over 20 h, but evidence is accumulating that NAC should probably be continued longer than this.

RENAL REPLACEMENT THERAPY IN LIVER DISEASE

A major consideration in the liver failure patient is that of renal replacement therapy: not only which modality is indicated, but also the question of who and who does not benefit from such therapy. Traditionally, it has been considered that patients with cirrhosis who have developed renal failure do badly on renal replacement therapy (RRT) with 100% mortality in some studies. Thus, some physicians do not routinely offer RRT to such patients unless there is a realistic hope of hepatic recovery. In the setting of sepsis induced renal failure with cirrhosis, few studies have shown that RRT improves outcome. However, recent data suggest that, although exceptional, some patients do survive such that RRT should be considered in all patients with any hope of hepatic recovery or transplantation.

Patients with fulminant hepatic failure will usually be offered RRT, since some recover spontaneously or are listed for hepatic transplantation. Patients with hepatic and renal impairment due to alcoholic hepatitis pose a difficult problem, since few recover. In this circumstance, many adopt a trial of RRT with defined end points, e.g. a week of haemofiltration during which time patients are given steroids and antibiotics. If hepatic or renal function has not improved, then RRT is withdrawn.

Continuous Renal Replacement Therapy (see also Chapter 9.5)

The use of continuous pumped venovenous haemofiltration is the preferred modality of renal replacement therapy in liver disease. This modality of therapy has the advantage of causing minimal haemodynamic upset, particularly little or no rebound increase in cerebral perfusion pressure. Haemofiltration offers a theoretical advantage over dialysis in terms of middle molecule removal. The type of membrane may be important in view of adsorption of cytokines. Some membranes are effective at trapping cytokines and, at least in the first hour of use, there is some evidence of improvement in endothelial dysfunction. This provides a rationale for frequent membrane changes; however the economics and practicalities of replacing membranes for this indication would require more evidence of benefit. For haemodiafiltration these patients usually require special non-buffered solutions, since standard solutions are generally lactate based and the liver cannot adequately metabolise this to bicarbonate, leading to a worsening lactic acidosis. Thus non-buffered salt solutions are used with the addition of bicarbonate via the return limb or other venous access. These solutions can be made up using standard litre bags of normal saline, dextrose-saline, and 5% dextrose, but this is labour intensive. Alternatively, large volume bags of both standard and bespoke solutions are available (e.g. 5 L bags containing NaCl 110 mmol/L, $MgCl_2$ 1.0 mmol/L, $CaCl_2$ 1.3 mmol/L ± K 4 mmol/L, with addition of 8.4% $NaHCO_3$ at 25 mL/h per litre cycle). However these are expensive and many units opt to measure lactate while starting on lactate containing solutions, only changing to lactate-free solutions if the serum lactate begins to rise.

Peritoneal Dialysis

Peritoneal dialysis is difficult in patients with liver disease. It has theoretical advantages over extracorporeal approaches in that it causes minimal systemic haemodynamic compromise. However, complications include bleeding and infection. Taking this together with issues around portal hypertension and ascites, few units perform PD in patients with significant liver disease.

Haemodialysis

Intermittent haemodialysis (HD) is relatively contraindicated in liver disease. Studies have shown that acute HD leads to severe haemodynamic disturbance in liver patients and to an increase in intra-cerebral pressure. This is thought to be due to haemodynamic upset associated with high blood pump speeds and the loss of cerebral autoregulation in cirrhotic patients. This leads to a reduction in perfusion pressure of the brain. The lower perfusion pressure causes ischaemia and generation of osmoles (e.g. lactate), known as idiogenic osmoles, in the intra- and extra-cellular cerebral fluid. There is also a danger of rapid electrolyte correction, especially sodium, with central pontine myelinolysis reported after rapid correction of hyponatraemia. Intermittent haemodialysis is therefore relatively contraindicated in patients with cirrhosis or hepatic failure.

Dialysis technology has improved since the seminal studies of Davenport *et al.* in this group of patients, suggesting that intermittent haemodialysis could be revisited. To minimise hazards, the dialysis prescription would then include using colloid line priming, biocompatible membranes, dialysate cooling, daily dialysis, very low pump speeds (~100 mL/min), long hours of dialysis (in excess of 6 h) and very low UF rates.

Anticoagulation

Many patients with liver disease do not synthesise clotting factors well and are therefore relatively auto-anticoagulated. Thus, most extracorporeal circuits in these patients do not need routine anticoagulation, especially if predilution is used, e.g. 1–2 L/h. However, in practice, it is often noted that circuits do not last long, and heparin may not be the anticoagulant of choice, since antithrombin III and cofactor II are low in these patients. Prostacyclin is usually effective as an anticoagulant and has the advantage of increasing oxygen extraction by peripheral tissues, which may reflect microcirculatory changes. However, it is a vasodilator and since these patients are often hypotensive this may require addition or increase in inotropic support. If prostacyclin is added prior to the arterial limb, much of it (~50–60%) is removed by the filter. The use of regional citrate anticoagulation can be considered but it is technically difficult to perform and the dose of citrate needs to be low, since generally the liver is incapable of dealing with the citrate load (see **Chapter 9.5**).

Haemoperfusion and Other Experimental Procedures

A number of studies using charcoal or other sorbents in the management of liver failure patients has been published. The rationale for this therapy is the removal of hepatically derived toxins, contributing to the genesis of the cardiovascular and neurological problems. These small studies claim improvement in physiological and neurological indices, but this therapy has yet to gain wide acceptance.

Recently a single case of percutaneous hepatocyte transplantation has been published in abstract form, with collagenase digested hepatocytes infused into the splenic artery causing an increase in urine output soon after transplant, and improved renal function for several weeks. The hepatic assist device has also been promoted as a possible solution. This consists of hepatocytes grown onto a hollow fibre cartridge, similar to a haemodialysis filter, through which blood passes. The idea is that the hepatocytes "process" the blood passing through the filter. The data suggest that this may be useful in short-term supportive treatment.

FURTHER READING

Arroyo V, Gines P, Rodes J, Schrier RW (eds.) (1999) *Ascites and Renal Dysfunction in Liver Disease.* Oxford: Blackwell Science

Davenport A (1999) Is there a role for continuous renal replacement therapies in patients with liver and renal failure? *Kidney International*; 56: suppl 72

Epstein M (ed.) (1996) *The Kidney in Liver Disease* (4th Edition). Philadelphia: Hanley and Belfus

Hawker F (1991) Liver dysfunction in critical illness. *Anaesthesia and Intensive Care*; 19: 165–181

Moore K (1997) The hepatorenal syndrome. *Clinical Science*; 92: 433–443

Chapter 26 _____

THE HAEMATOLOGY UNIT
Jo Thompson

INTRODUCTION

Many haematological diseases or complications of their specific therapy may result in acute renal failure (ARF); they are summarised in **Table 1**. Malignant diseases (including myeloma) account for most cases of ARF encountered on the haematology wards and are discussed in detail in **Chapters 21** and **22**. This chapter concentrates on renal failure secondary to sickle cell disease, and ARF in the context of bone marrow transplantation.

Table 1. Haematological conditions associated with renal failure	
Benign	
• Sickle cell disease (SCD)	this Chapter
• Paroxysmal nocturnal haemoglobinuria (acute haemoglobinuric ARF)	see Chapter 12
• Acute intravascular haemolysis (acute haemoglobinuric ARF)	see Chapter 12
• Microangiopathic haemolytic anaemia (MAHA)	see Chapter 15
Malignant	
• Acute leukaemias	see Chapter 21
• Chronic leukaemias	see Chapter 21
• Lymphoma	see Chapter 21
• Myeloma	see Chapter 22
Complications of therapy	
• Drug toxicity	see Chapter 11
• Sepsis	see Chapter 19
• Tumour lysis syndrome	see Chapter 21
• Bone marrow transplantation	this Chapter

1. SICKLE CELL DISEASE AND ACUTE RENAL FAILURE

DEFINITION

Homozygous sickle cell disease (SS) results from inheritance of a single point mutation in the β-globin gene from both parents. Substitution of valine for glutamic acid at the sixth residue of the β-globin molecule causes a change in the spatial configuration of haemoglobin. This can result in polymerisation of haemoglobin, leading to alteration of red cell shape into a characteristic sickle. The homozygous state (SS) is the most common disorder causing sickled red cells. However, it can also result from the inheritance of one S gene in combination with another abnormal haemoglobin gene, e.g. haemoglobin C (SC disease), or in conjunction with the inheritance of a complete or partial deletion of the β-globin gene from the other parent (S-β thalassaemias). The prevalence of the HbS gene varies geographically. It is most common in areas of West and Central Africa where, in some areas, heterozygotes account for >25% of the population. The gene also originates from Saudi Arabia and East Central India. With migration to the New World and Europe, sickle cell disease is now a worldwide problem.

PATHOPHYSIOLOGY

Decreased red cell survival, haemolysis, vaso-occlusion, sequestration and altered immune status ultimately account for the varied clinical manifestations of this disease. These are summarised in **Table 2** and are of relevance when determining the likely aetiology of ARF.

Pre-existing renal impairment may go unrecognised or be underestimated, as high metabolic demands, poor nutritional status, reduced muscle mass and the haemodilutional effect of anaemia contribute to much lower levels of serum creatinine than in age- and race-matched controls.

With improvements in the prevention and treatment of some early life-threatening complications, the long-term outlook for patients with this condition is improving. The majority of patients now survive into middle age and beyond. End-organ damage to the lungs, heart and kidneys is becoming an increasingly important cause of death in the adult population.

Table 2. Clinical manifestations of sickle cell disease

Vaso-occlusion
  dactylitis
  painful bone crisis
  abdominal painful crisis
  stroke
  priapism
  leg ulceration
  retinopathy
  splenic infarction

Multifactorial
  acute chest syndrome
  peptic ulcer disease
  hypersplenism
  sickle lung disease
  renal manifestations

Chronic haemolytic anaemia
  jaundice
  gallstones
  increased metabolic demand
  altered growth and anthropometry
  aplastic crisis

Sequestration
  acute splenic sequestration
  hepatic sequestration

Altered immune status
  Pneumococcal septicaemia
  Pneumococcal and Haemophilus meningitis
  Salmonella septicaemia and osteomyelitis

PATHOGENESIS OF RENAL INJURY IN SICKLE CELL DISEASE

Renal Medullary Ischaemia

Hypoxaemia, hypertonicity and acidosis predispose to haemoglobin polymerisation and sickle cell formation. This occurs particularly within the renal medulla of patients with SS disease, leading to vaso-occlusive damage to the vasa rectae in early childhood. Loss of the countercurrent exchange mechanism (see **Chapter 2**) causes an inability to concentrate urine (hyposthenuria) — this is an almost universal, irreversible finding.

Ischaemic damage to the renal medulla also stimulates prostaglandin synthesis leading to:

- increased glomerular filtration rate (GFR);
- increased effective renal plasma flow (ERPF) — resulting in increased renal size compared to age- and race-matched controls;
- enhanced proximal tubule function — resulting in enhanced tubule secretion of creatinine.

Medullary ischaemia contributes to many other renal manifestations of the disease. Patients with sickle cell trait alone may have microscopic haematuria. Gross haematuria may occur with SS disease and this can be severe and prolonged. Papillary necrosis may occur and there is an increased incidence of asymptomatic bacteruria and urinary tract infection.

Proteinuria

Proteinuria of all degrees is very common. Microalbuminuria occurs in over 30% of young adults and low molecular weight proteins of tubular origin are found even more commonly (>50%). The extent of proteinuria may be underestimated by dipstick testing alone because of hyposthenuria. Heavy proteinuria is common and may lead to nephrotic syndrome.

Acute Renal Failure

ARF can occur in conjunction with any other complication, most notably sepsis. Prolonged painful crises and acute chest syndromes can also result in rapid hypovolaemia and ATN. Analgesics, particularly NSAIDs, are commonly used in painful crisis and may precipitate or worsen renal impairment. During pregnancy, sickle patients are at greater risk of painful crises, pre-eclampsia, haemorrhage and infection. Malaria, a particular risk to the sickle cell patient, can cause rapid intravascular haemolysis, hypovolaemia and a high incidence of ARF, which contributes to its grave prognosis in sickle cell disease.

Many other renal lesions have been described in sickle cell disease, although they do not usually cause ARF *per se*. Almost all types of glomerular pathology have been described, and indeed some may be chance associations. The most common is focal segmental glomerulosclerosis (FSGS). Mesangial proliferation is also commonly seen. Glomerular hyperfiltration, subsequent glomerular hypertrophy and then sclerosis, is undoubtedly the final common pathway to progressive renal failure in this condition.

Table 3 summarises the renal manifestations of sickle cell disease and their clinical significance.

Table 3. Renal manifestations of sickle cell disease

Renal manifestation	Mechanism	Clinical significance
Acute renal failure	Sepsis ATN Drugs — NSAIDs, antibiotics Papillary necrosis Pregnancy	Patients are prone to severe infective insults
Papillary necrosis	Medullary ischaemia	May be incidental finding Gross painless haematuria Renal colic Ureteric obstruction
Urinary tract infection	Decreased resistance to infection Medullary ischaemia	May precipitate sickle cell crisis
Hyposthenuria (Inability to concentrate urine)	Vaso-occlusive damage to vasa rectae Loss of countercurrent exchange mechanism	Increased tendency to hypovolaemia High obligatory urine volumes May disguise degree of proteinuria on dipstick testing
Increased GFR and ERPF	Anaemia, increased cardiac output Altered prostaglandin synthesis in ischaemic medulla	Contributes to lower levels of serum creatinine in SS disease
Increased renal size	As above	Difficulty interpreting whether renal impairment acute or chronic as "normal" size kidneys may be small for SS patient
Enhanced proximal tubule function	As above	Increased fractional excretion of creatinine Overestimation of GFR by creatinine clearance
Haematuria	Disruption and interruption of arteriolae rectae circulation and vessel wall injury	Microscopic haematuria common in patients who carry the sickle cell gene Gross haematuria does occur and can be severe
Proteinuria	Hyperfiltration, glomerulosclerosis Other glomerular pathology	Microalbuminuria in >30% of adolescents with sickle cell disease

	Table 3 (*Continued*)	
Renal manifestation	**Mechanism**	**Clinical significance**
Nephrotic syndrome	Focal segmental glomerulosclerosis (50%) Mesangioproliferative glomerulonephritis Other glomerular pathology Post streptococcal glomerulonephritis Renal vein thrombosis (rare)	Heavy proteinuria is common
Chronic renal failure	Hyperfiltration injury Progressive glomerulosclerosis Tubular damage Cortical and medullary infarction Infection	May be detected late and under-estimated due to low creatinine First sign may be reduced steady state haemoglobin or hypertension

CLINICAL PRESENTATION AND TREATMENT PRINCIPLES

The most common cause of ARF is infection; patients usually also have other organ involvement. Serious infection can occur at many sites, particularly the chest, gallbladder and urinary tract. Less common sites include bone and joints with Salmonella or Staphylococcal infection, leg ulceration and central nervous system infection. Malaria, Dengue fever or other tropical infection may be pertinent in travellers (see **Chapter 20**).

A painful bone crisis (the commonest sickle-related presentation) does not normally lead to ARF, but its dramatic presentation may result from and mask another underlying pathology such as sepsis or accompanying acute chest syndrome. Patients may have also received NSAIDs or nephrotoxic antibiotics.

Under normal conditions patients adapt to high obligatory urine volumes even in tropical climates. When unwell, the patient is prone to rapid hypovolaemia and will be unable to conserve intravascular volume. **High urine output will persist even in states of severe hypovolaemia and may give a false sense of security to the unwary.** A vicious cycle resulting in hypovolaemia and increased vaso-occlusion can occur rapidly, and patients deteriorate quickly. They are particularly susceptible to acidosis from superimposed respiratory problems and reduced tissue perfusion. They also have a greater tendency to hyperkalaemia and may require early intervention with renal replacement therapy.

Established ARF is managed as described in **Section 2**. Other management points relevant to patients with SS disease are discussed in the **Practice Point 1**.

Outcome

Prognosis is good if the underlying cause is treated and the renal impairment really is acute. ARF in sickle cell disease unfortunately often occurs on a background of renal impairment, when the prognosis will clearly be poor. Following ATN, if renal recovery does not take place in the

Practice Point 1. Management of acute renal failure in patients with sickle cell disease

- Prompt treatment of underlying cause, adequate hydration and oxygenation may prevent established ARF (see **Chapter 8**)
- Ensure adequate pain relief, usually with opiate analgesia
- Ensure adequate volume replacement with CVP and blood pressure monitoring
- Give blood to maintain haemoglobin >10 g/dL
- Monitor trends in gas exchange with pulse oximetry and blood gases (see **Chapters 5** and **8.4**)
- Pulmonary infiltration on chest X-ray, cerebrovascular events or prolonged painful crises are indications for exchange transfusion
- Give peptic ulcer prophylaxis (e.g. ranitidine 150 mg b.d.); stress ulceration is common
- Clinical uraemia may occur with surprisingly low levels of urea and creatinine
- Renal replacement therapy can be with CVVHD, IHD or acute PD as appropriate (see **Chapter 9**)

expected manner (**Chapter 3**), a renal biopsy is indicated. This may reveal previously unsuspected chronic glomerular obsolescence and interstitial scarring from ischaemic sickle cell nephropathy.

2. BONE MARROW TRANSPLANTATION

ARF is one of the most frequent complications of bone marrow transplantation (BMT) and adversely affects patient prognosis. Gruss *et al.* (1995) reported a total incidence of 26%, with a higher prevalence in allogeneic than in autologous BMT. In a series of BMT recipients reported by Zager *et al.* (1989), 24% developed ARF, and only 16% of these patients survived. Most cases of ARF occur within the first month after transplantation. The aetiologies of ARF in bone marrow transplant recipients are summarised in **Table 4**. Many of these occur during the conditioning phase of the treatment regimen, when patients are exposed to toxic chemotherapeutic agents, total body irradiation, cyclosporin, and prophylactic antiviral, antimicrobial and antifungal agents.

Table 4. Causes of ARF in bone marrow transplantation

Sepsis	see **Chapter 19**	Haemolytic uraemic syndrome	see **Chapter 15**
Hypovolaemia	see **Chapters 8**	Cyclosporin nephrotoxicity	see **Chapters 11**
• radiation induced diarrhoea	and **10**		and **24**
• graft versus host disease (gut and tissue fluid losses)		Marrow infusion toxicity*	
		Hepatic veno-occlusive disease*	
Nephrotoxic drugs	see **Chapter 11**	BMT associated nephropathy*	
Obstructive uropathy (tumour infiltration, calculi)	see **Chapter 23**	(radiation nephritis-like syndrome)	
Tumour lysis syndrome	see **Chapter 21**		

*Several specific renal syndromes occur uniquely or with disproportionate frequency in bone marrow transplant recipients:

Marrow infusion toxicity

ARF has been described immediately post re-infusion of cryopreserved marrow, possibly predisposed to by pre-existing sepsis. Gross haemoglobinuria may occur post infusion and increases the risk of ARF. The renal tubules become markedly dilated and filled with haemoglobin casts.

Veno-occlusive disease of the liver (VOD)

Veno-occlusive disease of the liver is a common complication in patients undergoing high dose chemotherapy and BMT, and usually occurs within one month of transplantation. The aetiology of VOD is complex and poorly understood. The development of a hypercoagulable state, secondary to low protein C and antithrombin III levels, probably plays a major role in the pathogenesis of VOD. VOD is characterised by jaundice, ascites and hepatic failure. ARF secondary to VOD is similar in its pathogenesis and presentation to the hepatorenal syndrome (see **Chapter 25**).

Haemolytic uraemic syndrome

Haemolytic uraemic syndrome (HUS) tends to occur several months after high dose chemotherapeutic regimens. The clinical features and pathophysiology are described in **Chapter 15**. Treatment strategies include plasma exchange, fresh frozen plasma, immunoglobulin, vincristine, and discontinuation of Cyclosporin A. Despite these therapies, HUS following BMT carries a poor prognosis.

Bone marrow transplant associated nephropathy

Late-onset renal insufficiency occurs between six and twelve months post BMT. It is characterised by azotaemia, hypertension and disproportionate anaemia. This usually presents as a progressive decline in renal function but sometimes presents with a rapid decline in renal function, often associated with ongoing haemolysis. This syndrome is histologically similar to acute radiation nephritis, characterised by endothelial cell dropout and widening of capillary loops. Its incidence has fallen with the use of protective renal shielding during total body irradiation.

Practice Point 2. Management of ARF in the bone marrow transplant recipient

There is rarely any **specific** therapy available for the treatment of ARF in BMT patients.

Detailed assessment of renal function by isotopic GFR should be undertaken to plan dosing schedules of chemotherapy prior to treatment. If renal impairment becomes evident at this stage modification of treatment protocols to reduce toxicity may be necessary.

Prophylaxis for tumour lysis syndrome and marrow infusion toxicity involves hydration and alkaline diuresis (see **Chapter 21**), avoiding nephrotoxic agents where possible, early recognition and treatment of infection and correction of volume depletion.

Careful management of fluid balance and adjustment of dosing schedules for degree of renal impairment are critical in prevention of established renal failure.

Provision of renal support during this critical phase of the treatment may become necessary.

Renal biopsy to obtain a precise diagnosis is usually not possible due to abnormal bleeding tendencies and thrombocytopaenia.

Dialysis requiring patients have a very high mortality and escalation of supportive measures to include ventilation is rarely successful.

FURTHER READING

Davison AM, Cameron JS, Grunfeld J-P, *et al.* (1998) *Oxford Textbook of Clinical Nephrology* (2nd Edition). Oxford: Oxford University Press

Gruss E, Bernis C, Tomas JF, *et al.* (1995) Acute renal failure in patients following bone marrow transplantation: Prevalence, risk factors and outcome. *American Journal of Nephrology*; 15: 473–479

Zager RA, O'Quigley J, Zager BK, *et al.* (1989) Acute renal failure following bone marrow transplantation: A retrospective study of 272 patients. *American Journal of Kidney Disease*; 13: 210–216

Chapter 27 _____

THE OBSTETRIC UNIT
Lucy Smyth and Liz Lightstone

NORMAL PREGNANCY AND THE KIDNEY

Renal Changes in Pregnancy

During a normal pregnancy there are many changes to renal physiology, which must be remembered when interpreting the functional data concerning a pregnant woman's renal function. The typical consequences of a normal pregnancy are discussed below.

Haemodynamic Changes

During pregnancy, renal plasma flow (RPF) increases by 70%. Glomerular filtration rate (GFR) begins to rise as early as 6 weeks after conception, reaching a maximum increase of about 50% towards the end of the second trimester before falling slightly in the third. Vasodilatory agents such as prostaglandins, oestrogens and nitric oxide cause a fall in systemic vascular resistance, and plasma volume increases by 40%. Total body water increases by 6–8 litres, and 900 mmol sodium are retained, at least in part due to the activity of the renin-angiotensin-aldosterone axis. Blood pressure falls by an average of 10 mmHg during the first trimester, rising again slightly in the third.

Anatomical Changes

The kidneys are enlarged due to increased interstitial water and vasodilatation, increasing in length by about 1 cm. Marked dilatation of the collecting system occurs especially in the third trimester, and is usually most dramatic on the right. It is unclear whether this is mainly due to hormonal changes or to compression of the ureters at the pelvic brim by the gravid uterus. Dilatation may persist for up to 6 weeks post-partum.

Biochemical Changes

There is a reduction in measured plasma sodium and osmolality, possibly due to a resetting of the osmotic threshold for ADH release and thirst. Glomerular hyperfiltration produces a fall in urea and creatinine, reducing upper limits of the normal range. A mild respiratory alkalosis results from a fall in pCO_2, induced centrally by progesterone. To partially compensate, urinary bicarbonate excretion increases and plasma bicarbonate levels fall.

ACUTE RENAL FAILURE IN PREGNANCY

Renal symptoms may be related to the pregnancy, may be associated with pre-existing renal disease, or may be a combination of the two. **Patients with pre-existing renal disease are at higher risk of developing pregnancy-associated renal problems.** Whilst certain conditions are particularly associated with the pregnant state, any cause of ARF may be encountered.

AETIOLOGY

Table 1. Aetiology of ARF associated with pregnancy

Aetiology	Examples	
1. Hypovolaemia	Pre-renal failure Acute tubular necrosis Acute cortical necrosis	due to: hyperemesis gravidarum haemorrhage abruption sepsis pre-eclampsia (PET)
2. Infection	Pyelonephritis Septic abortion Puerperal sepsis	
3. Obstruction	Gravid uterus Stones	
4. Endothelial dysfunction	PET Thrombotic thrombocytopaenic purpura (TTP) Acute fatty liver of pregnancy (AFLP)	
5. Underlying renal disease	Exacerbation Predisposition to PET	

PATHOPHYSIOLOGY

Many of the physiological and anatomical changes that occur normally in pregnancy, as well as the development of obstetric complications, can have a bearing on the development of renal failure.

1. Hypovolaemia

The reduction in systemic vascular resistance, and corresponding fall in blood pressure, seen in pregnancy increase the risk of hypovolaemic renal injury.

Hypovolaemia is probably the most common precipitant of renal failure in pregnancy. It is implicated in pre-renal failure, acute tubular necrosis and cortical necrosis. Early in pregnancy, hyperemesis gravidarum is the most common cause, whereas later ante-partum or post-partum haemorrhage are the most frequent culprits. Patients with PET are already volume deplete and hence particularly vulnerable to hypovolaemic damage if subjected to further fluid loss.

Pre-renal failure simply reflects reduced renal perfusion without tubular damage, but unless treated promptly can progress to intrinsic renal dysfunction.

Acute tubular necrosis is the most common cause of ARF in pregnancy and, following supportive treatment, is almost always associated with complete recovery of renal function.

Bilateral renal cortical necrosis characteristically occurs as a result of catastrophic hypotensive obstetric events, such as abruptio placentae, placenta praevia, sepsis, post-partum haemorrhage, amniotic fluid embolism or prolonged intra-uterine death, and is often associated with coagulopathy. It is most likely to affect multiparas early in the third trimester. Typically it presents with acute oliguria or anuria lasting more than 15–20 days, and may be associated with gross haematuria and loin pain. Cortical damage may be patchy or diffuse, and is thought to result from endothelial dysfunction and thrombus formation secondary to severe ischaemic injury.

2. Infection

Dilatation of the renal tract increases the risk of urinary stasis and thus infection, particularly pyelonephritis. Up to 10% of pregnant women have asymptomatic bacteriuria, and if left untreated 40% of these will go on to develop a symptomatic UTI, compared to 1.5% of those with a negative urine culture.

Acute pyelonephritis occurs in 1–2%. In the majority of cases, the organism is *Escherichia coli*. Pyelonephritis causes renal impairment more frequently in pregnancy, particularly if associated with hypovolaemia, and septic shock can ensue.

Septic abortion and *puerperal sepsis*, as with any cause of a sepsis syndrome, can lead to ARF in the context of multi-organ dysfunction.

3. Obstruction

The gravid uterus may contribute to the renal tract dilatation seen in most women, but in some it can cause overt ureteric obstruction. This is more common if the pregnancy is multiple, or if polyhydramnios is present. The obstruction can result in renal impairment, infection and hypertension, and can precipitate preterm labour. Obstruction rather than simple dilatation is more likely to be present if nausea, fevers, oliguria or renal impairment are present. Stones are no more common during pregnancy, but may become dislodged leading to symptoms.

4. Endothelial Dysfunction

Endothelial changes in pregnancy are thought to contribute to a number of renal-associated conditions. **Pre-eclampsia** and the **HELLP syndrome** will be discussed in detail in the next section.

Pregnancy appears to be a predisposing factor for the **haemolytic uraemic syndrome (HUS)** and **thrombotic thrombocytopaenic purpura (TTP)**. Both encompass microangiopathic haemolytic anaemia, thrombocytopaenia, renal dysfunction and fever, with neurological involvement in TTP. Renal dysfunction in HUS tends to be much more severe, often leading to anuria, and almost always occurs post-partum (2 days to 10 weeks). TTP presents ante-partum, usually in the first or second trimester, with only mild haematuria and proteinuria. The pathological findings are similar in both conditions, with widespread thrombotic occlusion of capillaries and arterioles by hyaline platelet thrombi. The presence of high molecular weight multimers of factor VIII-related von Willebrand factor has been found in these conditions, with a reduction in levels during relapse, suggesting their involvement in thrombus formation. Levels of vWF are known to increase in pregnancy, possibly increasing predisposition to the syndrome (see also **Chapter 15**).

5. Underlying Renal Disease

The outcome of pregnancy, both foetal and maternal, in patients with renal failure depends on baseline function (see **Table 2**). Renal impairment pre-conception is associated with risk of renal decline, superimposed PET, intra-uterine growth retardation, preterm delivery and perinatal mortality. The outcome is more likely to be complicated if hypertension is present.

Table 2. Obstetric and renal outcome in patients with pre-existing renal impairment			
	Creatinine <130 μmol/L	Creatinine 130–250 μmol/L	Creatinine >250 μmol/L
Pregnancy complications	25%	50%	85%
Successful obstetric outcome	96%	90%	47%
Permanent decline renal function	<10%	25%	55%

In general, the type of underlying renal disease does not appear to affect outcome. **Systemic lupus erythematosus**, however, is associated with foetal loss, PET and IUGR even if apparently inactive. Severe renal flares can occur in pregnancy, although it is unclear if they are more common. The presence of anti-cardiolipin antibodies, either alone or as part of SLE, has a particularly high association with early and late foetal loss and IUGR. Patients with **scleroderma** and renal involvement are at particularly high risk of malignant hypertension and rapid renal deterioration during pregnancy.

Renal Transplant Recipients

Pregnancy in renal transplant recipients has a successful obstetric outcome in 90%, but IUGR and preterm delivery occur in about 50%. Renal function should not be affected by the pregnancy in those with good graft function (creatinine <130 µmol/L), and no hypertension. Proteinuria occurs in up to 40%, but is not significant in the absence of hypertension, and usually regresses post-partum. However PET has been reported in up to 30% of women. Acute graft rejection appears to be no higher than in the non-pregnant population, but it is recommended that patients wait 1–2 years post-transplantation before conceiving, when the risk of acute rejection is lower, and the level of immunosuppression has been reduced. Experience suggests that the standard immunosuppressive agents used, cyclosporin, azathioprine and lower dose steroids are safe in pregnancy. The pelvic graft does not interfere with normal delivery, and Caesarean section is only required for obstetric reasons.

CLINICAL PRESENTATION

Due to the diverse nature of renal problems that can occur, clinical presentation can be varied and non-specific. However, in some cases the presentation may give clues to the underlying cause, as described in **Table 3**.

Table 3. Clinical and laboratory features associated with ARF in pregnancy

Feature	Possible cause
Loin pain	Pyelonephritis, obstruction
Oedema	PET, underlying renal disease
Hypertension	PET, underlying renal disease
Proteinuria	PET,UTI, glomerulonephritis, SLE
Haematuria	UTI, glomerulonephritis, SLE, stones
Renal impairment	Pre-renal failure, ATN, cortical necrosis, obstruction, glomerulonephritis, SLE, pyelo-nephritis, underlying renal disease
Coagulopathy	PET, HELLP
Thrombocytopaenia	HELLP, HUS, TTP

Particular points should be noted in the history and examination:

History

- Timing in relation to pregnancy (which trimester?).
- Risk of PET.
- History of hypertension on oral contraceptive pill.
- Previous foetal loss, premature labour, IUGR, proteinuria.

Previous medical history (symptoms or diagnosis)

- Underlying renal disease.
- Hypertension.

- Diabetes.
- SLE.

Family history

- Renal disease.
- PET.

Examination

Maternal assessment

- Blood pressure (lying and standing).
- Volume status (**note**: patient may be intravascularly volume deplete despite oedema).
- Loin tenderness.
- Stigmata of systemic disease.

Foetal assessment

- Gestation.
- Movement.
- Foetal ultrasound scan: growth, liquor volume, uterine artery dopplers.
- Cardiotocograph.

INVESTIGATIONS

Table 4. Clinical investigation of ARF in pregnancy	
Investigation	**Comments**
Urine	
Dipstick for protein and blood	Initial screening investigation
Microscopy for red cells & casts	To investigate for underlying glomerulonephritis or SLE
Culture	To investigate for underlying UTI or pyelonephritis
24 h urinary protein excretion	To quantify extent of urinary protein leak
Creatinine clearance	To measure GFR
Blood	
Full blood count	Anaemia and thrombocytopaenia may be present in HUS
Blood film/haptoglobins/reticulocytes	To investigate for underlying haemolysis, e.g. in HELLP or HUS
Urea, creatinine and electrolytes	To estimate renal function
Liver function tests	To investigate for underlying HELLP
Urate	Elevated in PET
dsDNA, ACA, ANA, complement levels	To investigate for underlying SLE/anti-phospholipid syndrome

Table 4 (*Continued*)	
Investigation	**Comments**
Renal ultrasound scan	Increased echogenicity in renal parenchymal disease
	Small size may indicate underlying renal disease
	Obstruction can be difficult to distinguish from dilatation
	Doppler studies can show renal vein thrombosis associated with nephrotic syndrome
Liver ultrasound scan	To look for liver haematoma in HELLP
Nuclear medicine renogram	Can be used to help confirm obstruction
	(A limited one-shot renogram has a radiation dose of <1 cGy)
Renal biopsy	Considered safe throughout pregnancy, although after 32 weeks it is usual to expedite delivery and then biopsy
	Performed with patient in sitting position if heavily pregnant
	Contra-indicated if coagulation impaired, or thrombocytopaenic

TREATMENT PRINCIPLES

General Measures

Joint renal/obstetric care

Patients should always be under the care of an obstetrician and a renal physician experienced in the management of pregnancy-related disease.

Preventative measures

- *Aspirin*

Trials of low-dose aspirin have been carried out with respect to the risk of PET and will be discussed in the next section. However, it is also generally recommended, at 75 mg daily, to those with pre-existing renal impairment, proteinuria, hypertension, diabetes, anti-cardiolipin antibodies or a history of PET.

- *Low molecular weight heparin*

This is generally given in a prophylactic dose (e.g. enoxaparin 40 mg daily) to patients with nephrotic range proteinuria, and combined with aspirin for those patients with anti-cardiolipin antibodies who have a history of previous foetal loss or thrombosis. Patients who are severely nephrotic, or who have proven thrombosis, may need full anticoagulation (e.g. enoxaparin 1 mg/kg every 12 h), which can be monitored by measuring factor Xa levels.

Acute renal failure

The management of ARF with or without oliguria is the same in pregnancy as in any other patient. The emphasis has to be on optimising fluid balance, and requires the use of central venous pressure monitoring together with accurate fluid balance recording.

Practice Point 1

- CVP monitoring must be used if there is ARF
- Aggressive rehydration is often required, but must be according to CVP
- Fluid overload must be avoided in patients with PET who are particularly at risk of pulmonary oedema
- Diuretics should not be used until volume losses have been replaced
- Pre-renal failure will be reversed by the above management, but renal causes such as ATN may require a period of supportive management, possibly including dialysis

---

Hypertension

The management of hypertension in pregnancy is discussed in the next section on pre-eclampsia. Although PET is the most frequent cause of raised blood pressure in pregnancy, other renal problems may also be responsible.

Dialysis

- *Acute renal failure*

If possible, delivery should be carried out. If dialysis has to be started then daily haemodialysis is usually the preferred option, but there is a risk to the foetus from changes in maternal volume status and anticoagulation.

- *Chronic renal failure*

Dialysis has been instituted and continued in pregnancy in patients with chronic renal failure, but the risk of a poor pregnancy outcome (IUGR, prematurity, foetal loss) is high. Peritoneal dialysis is favoured in some centres, with the aim being to maintain urea <15 mmol/L.

Delivery

Delivery is the cure for PET and HELLP, and facilitates easier maternal management of most other renal conditions. The foetus is at risk of impaired growth. Most obstetricians are happy to deliver a baby after 30–32 weeks gestation if the condition of either the mother or baby warrants it. The best management of mother and baby relies on close and constant collaboration between the obstetric and renal teams. If possible foetal lung maturity should be optimised with steroids for 48 h before delivery. It is usually considered wise to aim for delivery in all patients with renal impairment by 39 weeks. Delivery should be carried out in a unit with appropriate neonatal ICU facilities.

Specific Measures

Infection

Pyelonephritis should be treated in a hospital setting, with appropriate antibiotics, initially intravenously. Intravenous rehydration may be required. A MSU should be taken to confirm effective treatment, and repeated at regular intervals throughout the pregnancy to pick up re-infection. Urinary tract infections (UTI) are associated with pre-term labour. Prophylactic antibiotics should be used in patients with recurrent UTI, or with a history of pyelonephritis in pregnancy.

Obstruction

Obstruction may sometimes be relieved by lying the patient in the left lateral position. However, in most cases a decision has to be made between delivery of the baby or continuing the pregnancy and relieving the obstruction. Percutaneous insertion of nephrostomies under US guidance is generally felt to be the most straightforward solution. Retrograde stenting is more anatomically difficult due to the gravid uterus, but is recommended by some and may carry less risk of being dislodged. Long-term antibiotic cover is required whilst either stents or nephrostomies are in place.

HUS/TTP

Pregnancy-associated HUS is almost always post-partum, and is treated as for all HUS, as discussed in **Chapter 15**. TTP is rarely associated with renal impairment that requires specific intervention; however treatment with plasma exchange may be indicated for neurological indications, and can be safely carried out in pregnancy provided that precise fluid balance is maintained.

OUTCOME

Prompt treatment of obstruction should result in no long-term sequelae, as is the case for pyelonephritis if further bacteruria is eradicated. Pre-renal failure should resolve with adequate rehydration, but ATN may lead to prolonged recovery times and residual renal dysfunction. The prognosis is particularly bad in cortical necrosis, where renal recovery may be incomplete, and often deteriorates over a period of years.

The risks to those with chronic renal impairment will depend on the level of function as previously discussed.

Measures which should be discussed with the patient and undertaken in subsequent pregnancies include:

- Aspirin.
- Treatment of hypertension.
- Delaying pregnancy until underlying condition is treated and quiescent.
- Intensive ante-natal monitoring (placental blood flow, regular foetal growth scans).
- Early delivery (39 weeks routinely, earlier if indicated).

PRE-ECLAMPSIA AND ACUTE RENAL FAILURE

DEFINITION

Pre-eclampsia (pre-eclamptic toxaemia, PET) is a disorder of the vascular endothelium that presents in pregnancy with multi-system maternal and placental involvement. It affects 10% of first pregnancies, with severe symptoms occurring in 1%. Eclampsia describes a grand-mal seizure in association with pre-eclampsia, and occurs in 0.05% of pregnancies.

HELLP syndrome is a severe variant of PET in which there is **h**aemolysis, **e**levated **l**iver enzymes and **l**ow **p**latelets.

PATHOPHYSIOLOGY

In PET, there is early failure of trophoblastic invasion of the maternal endometrial spiral arteries resulting in the formation of a high resistance arterial bed. The endothelium plays an important part in the maintenance of vascular tone and in haemostasis. There is evidence that the endothelium is particularly vulnerable to injury in pregnancy and this can lead to vasoconstriction, platelet activation and increased intravascular coagulation. In PET, a relative excess of circulating vasoconstrictor thromboxane A2 (TxA2) over the vasodilators prostaglandin I2 (PGI2) and nitric oxide, favours vasoconstriction. Evidence of endothelial activation in this condition includes raised levels of circulating endothelin, fibronectin and TxA2, reduced PGI2 levels, activation of the coagulation cascade and increased vascular responsiveness to the pressor angiotensin II. The characteristic renal histological lesion in PET is glomerular capillary endothelial cell swelling (glomerular endotheliosis), with subendothelial deposits of fibrin.

CLINICAL PRESENTATION

The classical presentation of PET comprises:

- Hypertension.
- Oedema.
- Proteinuria.

  However other symptoms include:

- Headache and visual disturbance.
- Epigastric or RUQ pain.
- Nausea and vomiting.

Practice Point 2

Hypertension does not have to be present

Diagnosis can be difficult if there is pre-existing hypertension and/or proteinuria

Patients can be frankly nephrotic

INVESTIGATIONS

- Proteinuria (>300 mg/24 h).
- ↑ urea, creatinine.
- ↑ serum urate.
- ↑ liver transaminases.
- ↑ haematocrit.
- ↓ platelets.
- prolonged clotting times.

TREATMENT PRINCIPLES

The management of PET relies on close monitoring of the mother and foetus in hospital. Blood pressure, proteinuria, renal function, liver function, urate, full blood count and coagulation should all be regularly measured. The foetus should have regular ultrasound assessment for the signs of IUGR.

Aspirin

The largest trial of low dose aspirin as prophylaxis against pre-eclampsia, the MRC CLASP trial, showed only a non-significant 12% reduction in the overall incidence of PET, although it did show a reduction in PET requiring delivery before 32 weeks. It is generally felt that aspirin should therefore be given to women particularly at risk of early-onset PET, such as those with renal disease, hypertension, diabetes, anti-phospholipid syndrome or a history of previous severe PET.

Hypertension

The management of hypertension in pregnancy is essentially the same whatever the underlying cause.

- *Mild/moderate*

Hypertension is usually treated if blood pressure is consistently over 140/90 mmHg. If PET is suspected then admission and bed rest are initially required. If therapy is needed, the first line agent is generally methyldopa. There is also widespread experience of using labetalol, nifedipine and oral hydralazine, which may be added in or used if methyldopa is not tolerated (see **Table 4**). Pure β-blockers should be avoided as they may impair placental flow, and ACE inhibitors should not be used, particularly in the 2nd and 3rd trimesters, because of the risk of foetopathy.

Blood pressure should not be lowered too drastically or the utero-placental circulation may be compromised, but the target mean arterial pressure should be less than 125 mmHg (i.e. 150/100).

Table 4. Anti-hypertensive treatments in PET		
Drug	**Route of administration**	**Dose**
Methyldopa	Oral	250–500 mg 2–3 times daily
Labetalol	Oral	Initially 100 mg twice daily
		Increase if necessary by 100 mg twice daily
		In 2nd and 3rd trimesters, severe hypertension may need t.d.s. regimen
		Total range 100–400 mg t.d.s. (Maximum 2400 mg daily)
Labetalol	IV	20 mg/h, doubled every 30 min; maximum 160 mg/h
Nifedipine (modified release)	Oral	10–20 mg twice daily
Hydralazine	Oral	25–50 mg twice daily
		For GFR <50 mL/min give 8 hourly
Hydralazine	IV	Initially 200–300 µg/min
		Maintenance 50–150 µg/min

- *Acute hypertensive crisis*

Oral calcium channel blockers are the first choice, followed by intravenous hydralazine if required. The patient must be optimally hydrated, using CVP monitoring, before treatment is started to avoid catastrophic hypotension. Intra-arterial blood pressure monitoring is advised.

Magnesium sulphate is used to treat seizures, and is often commenced as prophylaxis against eclampsia, particularly if there are signs of cerebral irritation.

Dose: initially 2 g over 5 min (iv), then 4 g over 15 min, with maintenance of 1–2 g/h for 24–48 h

If there is significant renal failure, then magnesium levels should be monitored.

HELLP Syndrome

ARF should be managed as previously discussed. Severe haemolysis and coagulopathy may require the use of blood and blood products. Patients are at risk of haemorrhage, and liver haematomas in particular are seen. Such patients are at high risk of multi-organ failure, and delivery is imperative.

Delivery

The only cure for PET is delivery, and a continuous assessment must be made as to the relative risks of conservative treatment and delivery to the mother and baby. Renal impairment is almost always an indication to deliver regardless of foetal maturity. If delivery is required before 34 weeks gestation, steroids should be given to aid foetal lung maturity. Epidural analgesia is often used as it helps to lower and maintain a stable blood pressure, although a coagulopathy may preclude this.

Post-Partum

Blood pressure may continue to rise, and seizures may still occur, post-partum. Therefore intensive monitoring of blood pressure, fluid balance, biochemistry, clotting and full blood count should be continued for several days.

Anti-hypertensive medication can usually be stopped within 6 weeks. Methyldopa is generally avoided in the post-partum period due to the side-effect of depression. β-blockers, calcium antagonists or ACE inhibitors can all be safely used when breast-feeding.

Proteinuria resolves within about 3 months of delivery. If it persists, the patient should be investigated for underlying renal disease.

Risk of Recurrence

The risk of a recurrence of PET in a subsequent pregnancy is about 10%. The risk of PET is increased if there is underlying renal impairment. Twenty percent of patients who have had HELLP will develop PET in a subsequent pregnancy, but only a minority will develop HELLP again.

FURTHER READING

Lindheimer MD, Davison JM (eds.) (1994) Balliere's Clinical Obstetrics and Gynaecology: Renal Disease in Pregnancy. 8: 2

Nelson-Piercy C (1997) *Handbook of Obstetric Medicine*. Isis Medical

Sibai BM, Kustermann L, Velasco J (1994) Current understanding of severe pre-eclampsia, pregnancy-associated HUS, TTP, HELLP syndrome and post-partum acute renal failure: Different clinical syndromes or just different names? *Current Opinions in Nephrology and Hypertension*; 3: 436–445

Chapter 28 _____

THE INTENSIVE CARE UNIT
Jeremy Cordingley and Stephen Brett

EPIDEMIOLOGY

The incidence of ARF in intensive care units varies widely depending on the case mix of the particular unit and the definition used, and in some units ARF may occur in as many as 30% of patients. The vast majority of ARF in critically ill patients is secondary to acute tubular necrosis, is multifactorial in origin and commonly associated with the failure of other organ systems. Most studies of associated factors have been small and used varying definitions. Factors linked to ARF in published regression analyses include increasing age, volume depletion, hypotension, bleeding and sepsis. Diagnostic categories associated with an increased incidence of ARF include pancreatitis, liver disease, chronic renal disease, aortic or cardiac surgery and burns. Iatrogenic factors include administration of contrast media and aminoglycoside antibiotics.

The mortality in critically ill patients with ARF is high (50–80%) and is primarily dependent on the cause and co-existing diseases. Mortality has not changed from rates published 20 years ago, despite improvements in supportive care and increased use of continuous renal replacement techniques. Patients are now older, have more comorbid conditions, and ARF is more likely to occur in the setting of multiple organ failure rather than as an isolated event. Mortality is higher in older patients. Toxic nephropathies (e.g. contrast or myoglobin) are associated with a better outcome. Oliguric patients have a higher mortality than non-oliguric. Factors linked to a worse prognosis include the requirement for prolonged inotropic support, mechanical ventilation, heart failure, sepsis, coma and malignancy.

The independent effect of ARF on mortality is difficult to determine because of the many other factors involved. In a study of contrast media nephropathy, controlled for co-morbidities, ARF had an odds ratio for mortality of 5.5, strongly suggesting that the complications of ARF add significantly to mortality (Levy *et al.* 1996). Renal function recovers in most patients with acute tubular necrosis who survive critical illness and, perhaps surprisingly, only a small proportion (<5%) requires long-term renal replacement therapy.

PATHOPHYSIOLOGY

Most critically ill patients with ARF have acute tubular necrosis (ATN) secondary to a combination of circulatory failure and sepsis. The pathophysiology of ATN is incompletely understood but experimental models suggest that tubular ischaemia and/or direct cellular toxicity are important (**Table 1**). For a fuller discussion please refer to **Chapter 8.1**.

Table 1. Pathophysiology of ARF	
Decreased renal blood flow	• hypovolaemia • decreased cardiac output • low or high systemic vascular resistance • elevated intra-abdominal pressure
Intrarenal vasoconstriction	• endotoxin • inflammatory mediators — PAF, IL-1, TNF • endothelin
Medullary capillary obstruction	• activated neutrophils, platelets, red blood cells
Direct cellular toxicity	• e.g. drugs, myoglobin
These factors reduce GFR by:	• cell swelling and shedding • tubular obstruction • back-leak of glomerular filtrate • decreased glomerular permeability

INVESTIGATIONS

The diagnosis of ATN is usually clinically obvious and the degree of investigation will depend on the level of suspicion of an alternative or additional renal diagnosis. Causes of ARF are listed in **Table 2**.

Appropriate oliguria secondary to poor renal perfusion can be confirmed by the finding of low urinary sodium (<20 mmol/L) and high urine osmolality (>500 mOsm/L). These tests are impossible to interpret if the patient has received diuretics, natriuretics (e.g. dopamine), or osmotically active agents such as contrast media.

Creatinine clearance can be measured in catheterised patients with a short (2 or 4 h) urine collection, providing that the bladder is emptied at the start of the collection period and there is accurate timing and urine volume measurement.

The time course of renal failure should be established by reference to previous biochemical tests of renal function. An onset longer than a few days should prompt further investigation. Ultrasound of the urinary tract will exclude obstruction and allow measurement of renal size. Urine microscopy is essential to exclude an inflammatory renal disease. Red cell casts and fragmented red blood cells in the urinary sediment are found in glomerulonephritis, vasculitis and interstitial nephritis. Eosinophils in the urine suggest drug induced interstitial nephritis. Urine and blood cultures are mandatory to exclude infection. If the urinary sediment is not suggestive of an active renal disease, obstruction has been excluded, renal function was previously normal, and there are adequate clinical reasons for ATN to have occurred, then further investigations for the cause of ARF are unnecessary. The presence of red cell casts or clinical features suggestive of an alternative renal diagnosis should prompt referral to a nephrologist.

Renal biopsy is usually reserved for patients who do not have an obvious aetiology for ARF, those with a history or examination suggesting another renal disease, or those in whom renal

Table 2. Causes of ARF in the ICU	
Pre-renal	Hypovolaemia
	Low cardiac output
	Hypotension
	Elevated intra-abdominal pressure
	Renal artery/renal vein thrombosis
Renal	Acute tubular necrosis
	Acute cortical necrosis
	Nephrotoxins
	Glomerulonephritis
	Vasculitis
	Interstitial nephritis
	Hepato-renal syndrome
	Thrombotic microangiopathies — HUS, TTP
	Severe pyelonephritis
	Cryoglobulinaemia
	Malignant hypertension
	Myeloma
Post-renal	Intrinsic renal obstruction
	Ureteric obstruction
	Urethral obstruction

function does not recover when expected (usually about 6 weeks). Renal biopsy in the critically ill patient with ARF carries a significant risk of haemorrhage. Coagulation tests including bleeding time should be checked and deficiencies corrected. Desmopressin (DDAVP) at a dose of 0.3 µg/kg may be given to increase endogenous levels of von Willebrand factor.

PREVENTION OF ACUTE RENAL FAILURE

Avoidance of Risk Factors

1. *Nephrotoxic drugs*

Avoidance of nephrotoxic drugs in the critically ill is particularly important, as there are frequently already many other factors likely to cause deterioration in renal function. In some circumstances, it may be difficult to avoid using a potentially nephrotoxic drug. It may be possible to use a less toxic formulation such as liposomal amphotericin, or a different dosing regimen such as once daily aminoglycosides. Where drug monitoring is possible, levels should be measured frequently and doses adjusted accordingly.

2. *Iatrogenic haemodynamic instability*

ARF is associated with impairment of autoregulation of renal blood flow. It is therefore important to prevent avoidable recurrent reductions in blood pressure that can occur in the intensive care unit as a result of, for example, excessive administration of sedative or anaesthetic agents, or changing or kinking of inotrope infusion lines. Administration of excessive anaesthetic induction agent for endotracheal intubation to a hypovolaemic patient with high sympathetic tone can lead to a severe fall in blood pressure. Careful medical and nursing care should allow these events to be anticipated and avoided.

3. *Elevated intra-abdominal pressure*

Increased intra-abdominal pressure can lead to the abdominal compartment syndrome characterised by cardiovascular, respiratory and renal dysfunction. Causes of acute elevated intra-abdominal pressure are listed in **Table 3**.

Table 3. Causes of acute elevated intra-abdominal pressure	
Cause	**Example**
Haemorrhage	post-operative
Fluid	ascites
Tissue oedema	sepsis, ischaemia, prolonged surgery
Gas	visceral distension, pneumoperitoneum
Tumour	gastro-intestinal, gynaecological
Others	abdominal packs, diaphragmatic hernia reduction

Deterioration in renal function because of elevated intra-abdominal pressure occurs as a result of several factors. Renal blood flow falls secondary to a reduction in cardiac output (CO) and increased renal venous pressure. In addition, there is direct compression of the renal parenchyma, reducing filtration and activating homeostatic mechanisms directed at sodium and water retention. With increasing pressure, oliguria and anuria eventually occur. Intra-abdominal hypertension is usually clinically obvious from examination of the abdomen. A measurement of intra-abdominal pressure is useful and can be obtained by instilling 100 mL of sterile water into the bladder via a urinary catheter. The drainage bag tubing is clamped and a needle connected to a pressure transducer is inserted proximal to the clamp through the rubber bung in the catheter usually used to obtain microbiological specimens. Alternatively, the catheter can be connected to sterile tubing which is held up as a manometer and the height of fluid measured with a tape measure using the symphysis pubis as zero. A similar method can be applied using the nasogastric tube. Normal intra-abdominal pressure is less than 5 mmHg. Clinical problems occur at pressures greater than 15–25 mmHg. Acute elevated intra-abdominal pressure is a medical emergency; surgical decompression is the only useful treatment and may involve leaving the abdominal cavity open. Fluid loading will help to stabilise the situation in the short-term. Renal function normally recovers after abdominal decompression.

Haemodynamic Management

• *Intravascular volume*

Optimisation of intravascular volume is the first stage in improving CO and renal blood flow. Using central venous pressure monitoring, 200 mL fluid boluses should be given until there is a sustained rise in venous pressure (see **Practice Point** later in chapter). If there is a clinical suspicion that CO is still low it should be measured (pulmonary artery catheter or oesophageal Doppler monitoring). Fluid boluses should then be administered until stroke volume reaches a plateau. Further fluid will be required to maintain intravascular pressures as peripheral rewarming occurs. There are few data as to whether crystalloid or colloid solutions are superior for volume resuscitation. Colloids are favoured in the UK and Europe and crystalloids in the USA. Much larger volumes of crystalloids are required to achieve the same haemodynamic end-points because of rapid redistribution throughout the extracellular space. Critically ill patients do not have intact endothelial systems and thus colloid solutions leak into tissues with a resultant shorter plasma half-life than in healthy subjects. This has two consequences: firstly, they are less impressive volume expanders than might be anticipated; and secondly, the colloid present in tissues is osmotically active and thus contributes to increased tissue oedema.

Positive pressure ventilation and positive end-expiratory pressure (PEEP) result in increased intrathoracic pressure. Venous return and stroke volume fall with a resultant reduction in CO and renal blood flow. Fluid loading will somewhat reverse these effects. However, patients with poor lung compliance may require very high intrathoracic pressures to maintain alveolar recruitment and oxygenation. In addition, the pulmonary capillary endothelium may be leaky in patients with ARDS. In these circumstances further fluid loading may result in increased pulmonary interstitial oedema and a further deterioration in lung compliance, requiring even higher airway pressures to maintain gas exchange. Thus a judgement about fluid loading must be made for individual patients to provide a suitable balance between optimising renal blood flow and maintenance of gas exchange.

The role of the pulmonary artery catheter in the management of critically ill patients is controversial (see **Chapter 5**). Some authors have suggested that the use of a pulmonary artery catheter is associated with increased mortality even after adjusting for variations in illness severity. No prospective randomised studies to address this issue have been carried out. In general, a pulmonary artery catheter is not indicated unless there are concerns about low CO.

• *Cardiac output*

If CO remains low (cardiac index (CI) <2.8 L/min/m^2) after fluid resuscitation, with continued evidence of impaired tissue perfusion (oliguria, hypotension), an inotrope should be added. Choice of inotrope depends on the clinical circumstances. In the presence of high vascular resistance, dobutamine or a phosphodiesterase inhibitor would be appropriate. In patients with low vascular resistance, epinephrine, or addition of norepinephrine to dobutamine or a phosphodiesterase inhibitor, would be indicated. It must be emphasised that the effects of these agents in individual patients may be unpredictable.

How far should CO be increased? In many patients with a CI <2.8 L/min/m^2 after fluid resuscitation it will be difficult to increase CO substantially because of severity of illness or pre-existing myocardial disease. In such circumstances, excessive doses of inotropes may cause dangerous tachyarrhythmias. Over the last 20 years there has been interest in using supranormal levels of CI (>4.5 L/min/m^2) and oxygen delivery and consumption as therapeutic targets in critically ill patients. This was based on the observation that survivors of high-risk surgery had higher levels of these indices. However, randomised studies of this approach in critically ill patients have not shown an improved outcome, although it may have a role in the prevention of multi-organ failure in high-risk surgical patients.

- *Blood pressure*

If oliguria persists after achievement of an adequate CO, and mean arterial pressure (MAP) is still low (<70 mmHg), a vasoconstrictor should be added. Norepinephrine is the agent of choice and has been shown to increase urine output and GFR in patients with hyperdynamic septic shock. Norepinephrine should be used cautiously in patients with low CO or if requiring another inotrope to maintain CO. Blood pressure should not be increased further if stroke volume starts to fall. Most patients will pass urine with a MAP of 70 mmHg, but some patients with pre-existing hypertension may require MAP up to 80–90 mmHg.

- *End-points of resuscitation*

There is no single marker or measurement that provides assurance that cardiovascular resuscitation is complete. Indices used to assess resuscitation are listed in **Table 4** and include measures of global and regional perfusion. Intramucosal gastric pH is a marker of regional perfusion that has been correlated with patient outcome, but there are few data on its use as a target for resuscitation. Normal practice is to optimise intravascular volume. If clinical improvement does not occur, CO monitoring is instituted and inotropic drugs added as necessary.

Table 4. Assessment of resuscitation

	Clinical	Invasive
Global	Heart rate	Stroke volume and CO
	Blood pressure	Mixed venous O$_2$ saturation
		Oxygen delivery and consumption
		Base deficit
		Lactate
Regional	Core-peripheral temp gradient	Intramucosal gastric pH
	Urine output	Hepatic venous O$_2$ saturation
	Conscious level	

Diuretics

• *Furosemide*

Furosemide inhibits the Na-K-2Cl symport in the thick ascending limb of the loop of Henle. It is highly protein bound, limiting its filtration, and reaches the tubular lumen by secretion into the proximal tubule. Furosemide causes diuresis and natriuresis but does not alter GFR. In addition, furosemide induces renovascular and systemic venous dilatation, probably mediated by prostaglandins. Infusion of furosemide has a greater diuretic effect than bolus dosing. Furosemide causes hypokalaemia and hypomagnesaemia that may aggravate tachyarrhythmias which are common in critically ill patients. Urinary calcium and phosphate losses are also increased. Ototoxicity occurs at high doses and is more likely with concomitant administration of aminoglycosides.

Interest in the use of furosemide in critically ill patients has been stimulated by experimental work, which has shown a potential reno-protective mechanism. The renal medulla is an area where oxygen tension is low because of the countercurrent arrangement of the blood supply. This is also an area of high metabolic activity because of active transport mechanisms involved in the uptake of chloride and sodium in the thick ascending limb of the loop of Henle. Oxygen supply is therefore only just sufficient to meet demand under normal circumstances. Isolated perfused kidney experiments have demonstrated that the thick ascending limb is very susceptible to hypoxic injury, but that this can be ameliorated by agents that inhibit metabolic activity such as digoxin and furosemide.

Prospective randomised controlled studies of large bolus doses of furosemide in patients with ARF have failed to show any clinical benefit. More recent studies of furosemide infusion in patients with ARF have also not demonstrated any benefit. No longer-term studies of prophylaxis in the critically ill have been reported. Thus the *clinical* evidence for a reno-protective effect of furosemide is lacking. Use of furosemide in intensive care however remains common, and frequently used indications are oliguria and adjustment of fluid balance. Bumetanide is an alternative loop diuretic. There are few data concerning the use of bumetanide in ARF.

Dose of furosemide:

- **Infusion: 1 to 40 mg/h according to response.**
- **Bolus: start with 10–20 mg. Increase according to response. Maximum dose 1 g/24 h.**
- **Doses should be administered at a rate not exceeding 4 mg/min.**

The use of thiazide diuretics has not been investigated specifically in critically ill patients and they are not available for intravenous administration.

• *Mannitol*

Mannitol is an osmotic diuretic that acts primarily by increasing sodium and water loss from the proximal tubule and loop of Henle. GFR is unchanged. Other effects that make mannitol potentially helpful in the prevention of ARF include a reduction in tubular cell swelling, relief of tubular obstruction, renal vasodilatation and free-radical scavenging (although good evidence for this is lacking). Extracellular volume expansion can precipitate pulmonary oedema in susceptible patients, and very high doses of mannitol have been reported to cause ARF.

Case reports from the 1960s popularised the use of mannitol in patients with obstructive jaundice; however subsequent small randomised trials failed to show any benefit. There have been no large randomised trials of mannitol in critically ill patients. Perioperative studies conducted mainly in patients having vascular surgery or surgery for obstructive jaundice have been too small to demonstrate any effect. Published clinical case series have promoted a role for mannitol in the prevention of renal failure following rhabdomyolysis (see **Chapter 12**).

The dose of an intravenous mannitol bolus to induce diuresis is 0.5 to 2 g/kg.

In summary, there is no evidence from clinical trials that diuretics prevent or alter the course of ARF. An increase in urine output following administration of diuretics is evidence of a milder degree of renal injury. However, the use of diuretics is widespread and may be helpful in allowing less fluid restriction. Before administering any diuretic it is important to ensure that intravascular volume is adequate, as use of diuretics in a hypovolaemic patient will further reduce renal perfusion and may lead to a deterioration of renal function.

Inotropes

The effects of inotropes on regional perfusion in critically ill patients is not always what might be predicted from the results of animal or normal volunteer studies. This is because of the complex interactions between blood volume, vascular tone and myocardial function that are different in critically ill patients, due to factors such as alterations in autonomic function and the presence of an inflammatory state. There are few published data on the potential reno-protective effects of inotropic agents in critically ill patients because of the difficulties of studying such a multifactorial problem over a long time course. Commonly used dilutions for infusion and dose ranges are listed in **Table 5**.

Table 5. Dilutions and dose ranges of inotropes		
Inotrope	**Dilution**	**Dose range**
Dopamine	200 mg in 50 mL 5% dextrose	2–20 µg/kg/min
Dopexamine	50 mg in 50 mL 5% dextrose	0.5–6 µg/kg/min
Dobutamine	250 mg in 50 mL 5% dextrose	1–20 µg/kg/min
Norepinephrine	4 mg in 50 mL 5% dextrose	start at 0.02 µg/kg/min
Epinephrine	4 mg in 50 mL 5% dextrose	start at 0.02 µg/kg/min
Milrinone	20 mg in 50 mL 5% dextrose	0.1–0.75 µg/kg/min

- *Dopamine*

Dopamine is a naturally occurring catecholamine with effects varying according to dose. At an infusion rate of up to 2 µg/kg/min effects are mainly via dopaminergic receptors. At higher doses of 2–10 µg/kg/min β-adrenergic effects are dominant, with increasing α-adrenergic stimulation above 10 µg/kg/min.

Dopamine has been used for many years, both as prophylaxis against ARF and for treatment of oliguria in critically ill patients. Dopamine has several effects that might be beneficial in this setting. As an inotrope, dopamine increases CO even at so-called low "renal dose" (up to 3 µg/kg/min) which results in increased renal blood flow. It causes renovascular dilatation and is a proximal tubular diuretic, inhibiting sodium reabsorption in the proximal tubule. In the clinical setting, it has been difficult to demonstrate increased renal blood flow secondary to specific renal vasodilatation over and above effects attributable to increased CO.

A number of clinical studies have demonstrated increased GFR and urine output with low-dose dopamine, but no large studies have specifically used ARF or patient outcome as end-points. Despite this, low-dose dopamine is in common use. Generally dopamine is started at 2–5 µg/kg/min and, if blood pressure is low, it can be increased up to 10 µg/kg/min to take advantage of further beta and alpha-adrenergic activity. Higher infusion rates can result in marked vasoconstriction. Normal doses of metoclopramide do not antagonise the renal effects of a low-dose dopamine infusion. Patients with septic shock receiving other catecholamines show a reduced renal and haemodynamic response to low-dose dopamine. Dopamine clearance varies widely between critically ill patients resulting in a large range of blood levels with similar dosage. Adverse effects include tachyarrhythmias and increased alveolar-arterial oxygen gradient because of worse ventilation-perfusion matching. Even low-dose dopamine infusion has a marked inhibitory effect on anterior pituitary function, leading to decreased prolactin, thyrotrophin, luteinising hormone and growth hormone levels. In addition dopamine has an immunosuppressive effect primarily via inhibition of T cell function. Of concern are theoretical arguments that dopamine may increase oxygen demand in the juxtacortical medulla, which has a precarious oxygen balance at the best of times.

In summary, despite potential favourable short-term effects on renal function, which have led to the widespread adoption of low-dose dopamine as a standard therapy, there are no definitive outcome data (renal or survival) to show any advantage of using dopamine. In addition, the pituitary and immunosupressant effects are potentially harmful to the critically ill patient.

- *Dopexamine*

Dopexamine is a synthetic dopamine analogue that is a dopamine-1 and less potent dopamine-2 receptor agonist. It is also a beta agonist, primarily at β-2 adrenoreceptors and inhibits neuronal reuptake of norepinephrine. Dopexamine is thus an inodilator and infusion results in increased CO and decreased peripheral resistance with increased renal and splanchnic blood flow. Renal effects of dopexamine in human volunteers include increased GFR, diuresis and natriuresis. Studies in intensive care patients have suggested that dopexamine may improve splanchnic flow assessed by plasma disappearance rate of indocyanine green dye and lidocaine metabolism.

Dopexamine is usually started at dose of 0.05 µg/kg/min and increased according to response. Tachycardia is common and may require reduction in infusion rate. Hypokalaemia and hyperglycaemia may occur because of β-2 effects. As with all vasodilators, it is necessary to maintain adequate intravascular filling pressures to prevent falls in stroke volume and blood pressure.

There have been no long-term studies in critically ill patients to assess the role of dopexamine in prophylaxis of ARF. Several small perioperative studies of patients undergoing cardiac or vascular surgery have reported inconsistent results. Dopexamine has also been used as part of treatment directed at increasing perioperative oxygen delivery in patients undergoing major surgery. Two small prospective randomised studies have demonstrated a reduction in postoperative morbidity and mortality in this setting.

In summary, dopexamine has potentially attractive effects for maintaining renal perfusion but clinically important results have yet to be demonstrated.

• *Dobutamine*

Dobutamine is a synthetic β-adrenergic agonist which increases heart rate and CO. Blood pressure may rise in patients with low CO and high systemic vascular resistance, but may fall, particularly in the presence of hypovolaemia or low vascular tone. The effects of dobutamine on renal blood flow are dependent on changes in CO. As well as increasing heart rate, large doses of dobutamine can induce tachyarrhythmias, particularly in combination with other beta agonists. In practice, dobutamine is best suited for patients with low CO and elevated systemic vascular resistance. There is rarely any additional benefit from increasing the dose above 10 μg/kg/min.

• *Norepinephrine*

Norepinephrine is a potent α- and β-adrenoreceptor agonist. The effects of norepinephrine on the kidney in normal awake man are to reduce renal blood flow with increased filtration fraction and unchanged GFR. After the introduction of norepinephrine into clinical practice in the 1950s, it was used widely for the management of different types of shock. Unfortunately, there were many reports of tissue ischaemia related to its use, including induction of ARF. Indeed norepinephrine is infused intra-arterially to induce animal models of ischaemic renal failure. During the 1980s, there were a number of case series reporting that norepinephrine improved urine output and GFR in volume resuscitated patients with hyperdynamic septic shock, typically with mean arterial blood pressures of about 50 mmHg. Other groups have reported increased GFR in volume resuscitated haemodynamically stable patients using low doses of norepinephrine.

These data have led to a resurgence in the use of norepinephrine, particularly in patients with hyperdynamic septic shock, when it is clearly superior to dopamine. Caution should be used in patients who are hypovolaemic or with low CO as the primary reason for oliguria, as norepinephrine can cause reduced renal and splanchnic perfusion in these circumstances. Hypovolaemia must be corrected before starting norepinephrine. In patients with severe sepsis, escalating doses of norepinephrine may be required to maintain systemic vascular resistance. In these circumstances, it may be necessary to change to an alternative vasoconstrictor such as angiotensin or vasopressin.

• *Epinephrine*

Epinephrine is a potent α- and β-adrenergic agonist with alpha effects predominating at higher doses. Renal effects in normal volunteers are reduced renal blood flow, increased filtration fraction and unchanged GFR. Adverse effects include tachycardia, tachyarrhythmias, excessive vasoconstriction and elevated blood glucose and lactate. Metabolic rate and oxygen consumption are increased. The renal effects of epinephrine in critically ill patients have not been investigated but are likely to vary according to clinical circumstances, as is the case with norepinephrine. In hypovolaemic patients, epinephrine is likely to cause further renal vasoconstriction and a fall in GFR. Following fluid resuscitation epinephrine may improve renal function in patients with low CO. In hyperdynamic, hypotensive patients epinephrine may improve GFR by increasing arterial pressure but norepinephrine is preferred in this situation.

- *Phosphodiesterase inhibitors*

Milrinone and enoximone are phosphodiesterase (isoenzyme III) inhibitors. Administration results in decreased systemic vascular resistance, positive inotropy and lusitropy (improved ventricular relaxation). In practice milrinone is preferred to enoximone because of its shorter half-life and lower incidence of adverse effects. Milrinone is renally excreted and a reduced dose is necessary in patients with renal impairment. Adverse effects include tachycardia and hypotension, particularly in hypovolaemic patients.

Milrinone is started by administering a slow loading dose of 50 µg/kg followed by a continuous infusion of up to 0.75 µg/kg/h. Milrinone is useful for patients with a low CO and high systemic vascular resistance. Patients with poorly compliant left ventricular function (i.e. diastolic dysfunction) often benefit. Such patients include those with ischaemic cardiac damage, those with chronic hypertension and those recovering from surgery for aortic valve stenosis. If blood pressure falls norepinephrine can be added to maintain blood pressure. In summary, milrinone may be useful for improving renal perfusion because of increased CO but blood pressure should not be allowed to fall too low.

Theophylline and other methylxanthines are non-selective phosphodiesterase inhibitors and adenosine antagonists, and alter intracellular calcium concentration by direct and indirect actions. Cardiovascular effects include positive inotropy, chronotropy and systemic vasodilatation. In the kidney, methylxanthines are diuretic and natriuretic agents. In addition, adenosine antagonism is theoretically beneficial in preventing reductions in GFR from inhibition of tubulo-glomerular feedback. Although theopyllines have been beneficial in animal models of ARF there are few data concerning clinical use. A small study has showed a protective effect in radiocontrast nephropathy.

Dose of intravenous aminophylline: up to 500 µg/kg/h by infusion adjusted according to response and plasma theophylline levels which should not exceed 20 mg/L.

- *Other agents*

Atrial natriuretic peptide (ANP) increases GFR by afferent arteriolar dilatation, efferent arteriolar constriction and an increase in glomerular permeability. A large prospective randomised study using an ANP analogue in patients with ARF failed to show an improvement in mortality and it is unclear whether specific subgroups of patients would benefit from this drug.

Urodilatin is a natriuretic peptide found in the kidney that has less systemic hypotensive effects. Its use has been reported in small case series of transplant patients with encouraging results but no large randomised studies have been published.

Practice Point. Practical management of oliguria

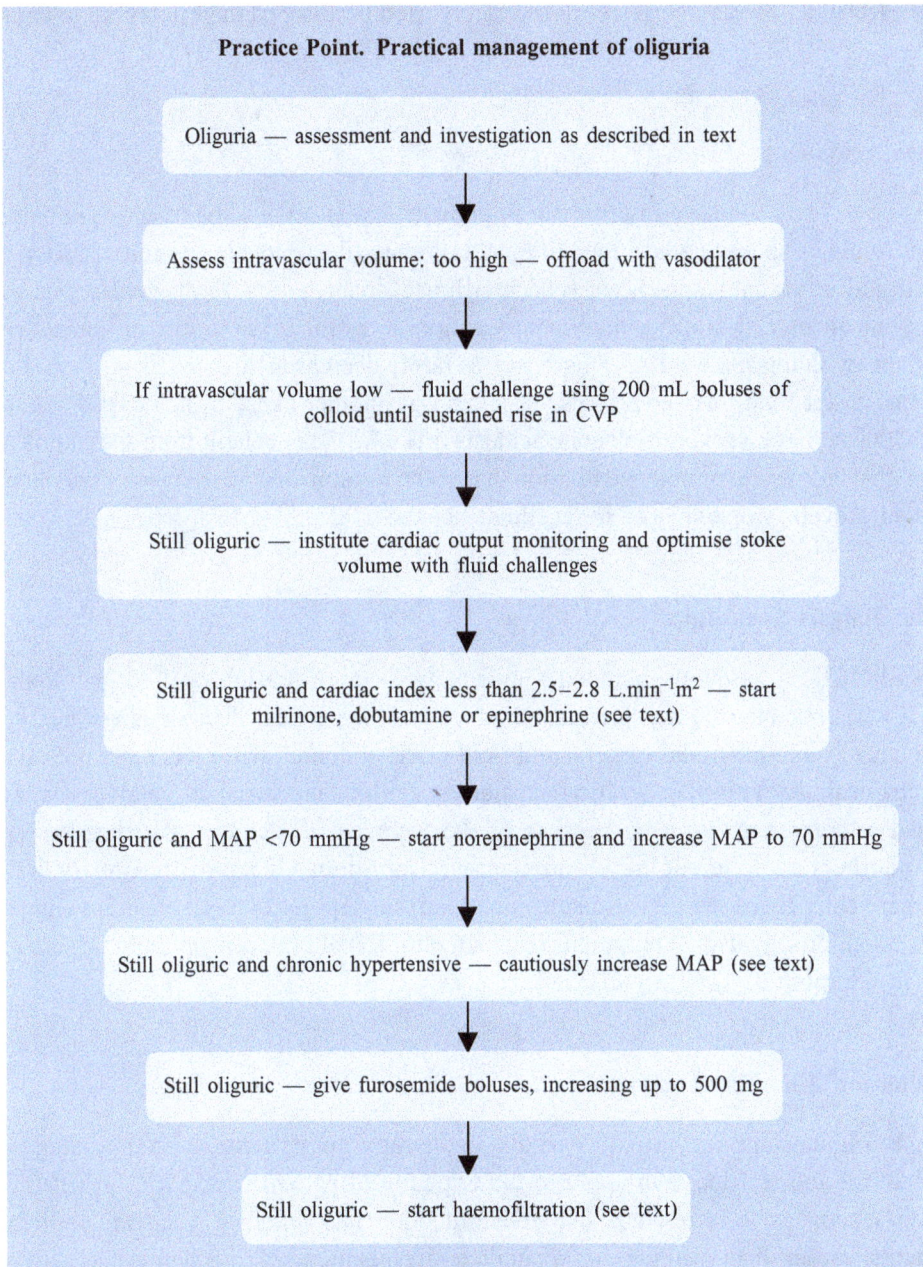

Oliguria — assessment and investigation as described in text

$\downarrow$

Assess intravascular volume: too high — offload with vasodilator

$\downarrow$

If intravascular volume low — fluid challenge using 200 mL boluses of colloid until sustained rise in CVP

$\downarrow$

Still oliguric — institute cardiac output monitoring and optimise stoke volume with fluid challenges

$\downarrow$

Still oliguric and cardiac index less than 2.5–2.8 L.min^{-1}m^2 — start milrinone, dobutamine or epinephrine (see text)

$\downarrow$

Still oliguric and MAP <70 mmHg — start norepinephrine and increase MAP to 70 mmHg

$\downarrow$

Still oliguric and chronic hypertensive — cautiously increase MAP (see text)

$\downarrow$

Still oliguric — give furosemide boluses, increasing up to 500 mg

$\downarrow$

Still oliguric — start haemofiltration (see text)

MANAGEMENT OF ESTABLISHED ARF

The management of metabolic emergencies resulting from ARF is described in **Chapter 8**.

Hyperkalaemia

Hyperkalaemia is usually managed with insulin and dextrose infusions until haemofiltration can be started. Severe hyperkalaemia with ECG changes is managed with calcium gluconate and sodium bicarbonate. Ion exchange resins are rarely used because of their potential to cause faecal impaction.

Metabolic Acidosis

Metabolic acidosis is common in critically ill patients and is usually the result of impaired tissue perfusion. Acidosis should not ascribed to renal failure until cardiovascular resuscitation has been completed and other causes such as ischaemic bowel, pancreatitis and severe sepsis excluded. Measurement of arterial blood lactate concentration is useful in these circumstances.

In patients with unsupported ARF base excess rarely decreases by more than 2 mmol/day. Any fall at a rate faster than this should raise suspicion of another cause of acidosis. Patients with a very low CO who have a severe metabolic acidosis (pH <7.2) may benefit from sodium bicarbonate, providing that adequate minute ventilation has been established to remove generated carbon dioxide and prevent worsening of intracellular acidosis.

Filtration/Dialysis Techniques

In the adult ICU, continuous pumped venovenous haemofiltration with or without dialysis (CVVHDF) has become the accepted standard of care. Peritoneal dialysis is frequently contra-indicated because of abdominal surgery, and fluid in the abdomen will hinder attempts at weaning from mechanical ventilation. In addition, clearances are low and variable. Venovenous access has superceded arteriovenous systems because of the technical difficulties associated with arterial access and the development of blood pumps. Continuous haemofiltration (±dialysis) is haemodynamically more stable than intermittent dialysis, and retrospective studies suggest lower morbidity and mortality using continuous renal support. Renal replacement therapies are discussed in detail in **Chapter 9**.

Indications for Filtration/Dialysis

Traditional indications for initiating dialysis therapy in patients with end-stage chronic renal failure are too restrictive to apply to the critically ill patient with ARF. In general therapy is started as soon as it is obvious that renal function has failed to keep up with metabolic requirements, rather than waiting for a marked derangement of biochemistry to develop. In addition, early haemofiltration allows a normal feeding regimen to be continued. The usual indications are listed below, but in practice haemofiltration is often started before these indices are reached:

- uncontrolled hyperkalaemia;
- metabolic acidosis persisting after fluid and cardiovascular resuscitation, BE < −10 mmol/L;
- oligo/anuria despite circulatory resuscitation;
- fluid overload;
- urea >30 mmol/L, creatinine >500 μmol/L;
- uraemic complications (pericarditis, encephalopathy or neuropathy).

Vascular Access

Access for veno-venous techniques is via a specific double lumen catheter that is sited via either subclavian, internal jugular or femoral vein. An appropriate length catheter should be used to ensure the tip is not sited in the right atrium (see **Chapter 9.6**). Femoral catheters are associated with more recirculation but this is not usually clinically significant if using a continuous filtration/dialysis technique . All intravascular access lines are a potential source of infection and should be inserted aseptically and inspected regularly for evidence of infection. Catheter changes are usually carried out for suspected or proven infection, rather than on a routine basis. A line infection is suggested by inflammation around the skin puncture site, pyrexia, or an increase in white cell count or CRP without other explanation. A new puncture site is preferred to re-wiring of an old line because of reduced infective complications but re-wiring may be indicated in the presence of coagulopathy or restricted venous access sites. Lines are normally filled with heparin when not in use to prevent thrombosis. Flow can sometimes be improved by swapping the venous and arterial lumens but this practice increases recirculation.

Anticoagulation

Many different methods have been used to anticoagulate the extracorporeal circuit. The most frequent is to use unfractionated heparin. The circuit is primed with heparin, the patient is given a bolus dose of heparin as the system is connected and heparin is infused at 100–1000 i.u./h into the circuit prior to the filter. The patient's APPT should be monitored and should not exceed twice control. It is often possible to have lower or normal APPT levels without the filter clotting. Activated clotting time (ACT) is an insensitive test for the dose range of heparin used for haemofiltration. Adding protamine to the returning blood (for example by adding to the replacement fluid) has been used to achieve regional anticoagulation of the extracorporeal circuit.

Epoprostanol (Flolan®) is an alternative to heparin. It is a reversible platelet inhibitor with a short half-life (3 min). It is therefore useful for patients who may be at risk of bleeding or if heparin is contra-indicated, for example because of heparin-induced thrombocytopaenia. The dose of epoprostanol prostacyclin is 5–20 ng/kg/min (see **Table 21, Chapter 9.5**). As epoprostanol is a vasodilator, blood pressure may fall particularly with higher infusion rates. Epoprostanol is expensive.

Alternative anticoagulants used in intensive care include low molecular weight heparin and, recently described, infusion of citrate pre-filter together with calcium infusion post-filter. Other measures which will help to reduce clotting in the extracorporeal circuit include using high flow rates (200 mL/min) and pre-dilution. Pre-dilution is the addition of fluid prior to the filter in the extracorporeal circuit (see **Chapter 9.5**).

Bleeding is one of the commonest complications associated with blood filtration techniques. This may be secondary to agents used to anticoagulate the extracorporeal circuit, or to coagulopathy associated with renal failure, sepsis or the patient's primary illness. In addition, platelet function deteriorates with time during extracorporeal circulation, a fact which may not be apparent from monitoring platelet count alone. (Bleeding time is the only common clinically available test that includes platelet function). It is therefore appropriate to err on the side of under-anticoagulating the circuit, as clotting of the filter is preferable to a potentially catastrophic haemorrhage. For patients with active bleeding it may be preferable to use no anticoagulant.

Types of Dialysis/Replacement Fluid

Dialysis and replacement fluids commonly contain physiological concentrations of sodium, chloride calcium and magnesium. Lactate is included as a buffer because bicarbonate is unstable in solution. Concentration of potassium varies and choice depends on whether it is necessary to reduce serum potassium quickly. Extra potassium chloride can be added to bags if necessary.

Administered lactate is normally converted to bicarbonate in the liver to replace bicarbonate that is filtered. However, in some circumstances such as severe sepsis, liver dysfunction or low CO, the production of bicarbonate is inadequate and patients will develop a progressive metabolic acidosis despite treatment with haemofiltration/dialysis. Note that although the metabolic acidosis may already be partly due to lactic acid this is not the result of administered lactate.

Treatment of progressive acidosis in this situation is firstly to ensure that the circulation has been optimised. Secondly, sodium bicarbonate should be administered either by using bicarbonate replacement fluid or by direct intravenous infusion. If given intravenously, 100–200 mmol sodium bicarbonate per hour may be necessary to control metabolic acidosis. This situation is often accompanied by hypoglycaemia, which is a very poor prognostic sign. Magnesium and calcium levels may fall as a result of bicarbonate infusion.

Lactate-free replacement fluids are available and do not contain any buffer. Therefore use of lactate free fluid will result in a metabolic acidosis if bicarbonate is not administered simultaneously. In addition, lactate-free fluids contain a low sodium concentration (110 mmol/L) and will cause severe hyponatraemia if not used in conjunction with sodium bicarbonate. Dialysis and replacement fluids do not contain phosphate. Although phosphate concentrations usually rise in ARF, levels will fall after several days of haemofiltration and replacement will be required.

Haemofiltration alone will usually be sufficient for metabolic control in elderly patients. Patients who are catabolic, in particular young men, will frequently require the higher clearances obtained by haemodiafiltration. Dialysis fluid is run at either 1 or 2 L/h countercurrent to blood flow in the filter (see **Chapter 9.5**).

General Supportive Management

Ventilation

As discussed in the fluid management section, positive pressure ventilation and positive end-expiratory pressure (PEEP) can have important deleterious effects on renal function. Normal ventilatory strategy is to adjust tidal volume to 6–8 mL/kg with a respiratory rate that obtains a minute volume to maintain $PaCO_2$ in the normal range. Inspired oxygen concentration (FiO_2) and PEEP are set to maintain arterial oxygen saturations (SaO_2) above 90%. In patients with poor lung compliance an inverse ratio (inspiration: expiration 2:1) and higher levels of PEEP are used to increase mean intrathoracic pressure and improve alveolar recruitment and oxygenation. Peak airway pressure is usually limited to 35–40 cm H_2O to reduce barotrauma. Prone positioning or administration of inhaled nitric oxide may be used to improve oxygenation, although these manoeuvres remain under investigation. As lung function improves the ventilator is set to modes allowing patient triggering and support is gradually reduced. Tracheostomy is often performed to reduce laryngeal trauma and improve patient comfort during weaning.

Red cell transfusion

Until recently it was common practice to transfuse all critically ill patients to a haemoglobin concentration of 10 g/dL in order to maximise oxygen delivery. Recent evidence suggests that liberal transfusion of red cells is detrimental and for most patients it is preferable to limit red cell transfusion to a target of 7–9 g/dL. The reasons for an adverse effect of red cell transfusion in critically ill patients are unclear but may be related to the immunosuppressive effects of neutrophils in donor blood (an effect utilised in the past to suppress renal transplant rejection). For patients with ischaemic heart disease a higher target haemoglobin is indicated (10 g/dL).

Nutrition

Early feeding of critically ill patients is associated with improved outcome. High calorie feeding during the catabolic phase of critical illness helps to limit, but does not prevent, endogenous protein breakdown. Total daily caloric intake should be about 30–35 kcal/kg and may be calculated using the Harris-Benedict equation and an appropriate stress factor. ARF in itself does not add much to energy requirements but the underlying condition such as sepsis may add significantly. With the advent of readily available renal replacement techniques it is not necessary to restrict protein administration, which should be 1.5–2.0 g/kg per day. Amino acid losses from continuous filtration/dialysis techniques can be as high as 15 g/day. Non-protein calories are usually provided as one third fat and two thirds carbohydrate. Excessive calorie load, as carbohydrate, increases carbon dioxide production and can slow weaning from mechanical ventilation.

Electrolyte content of feed can be varied according to clinical requirements although in practice patients receiving continuous filtration/dialysis therapies rarely require restricted potassium diets. Phosphate losses can be high and require replacement. Vitamin and trace element requirements are higher in the critically ill. In particular, the water soluble folinic acid, B vitamins and vitamin C should be supplemented during haemofiltration. The non-essential amino acid glutamine is an important substrate for intestinal mucosal metabolism. Glutamine supplementation improves intestinal mucosal integrity in critically ill patients and is commonly practised. Fluid requirements are assessed daily but use of continuous filtration/dialysis techniques means that volume of feed is not a factor in limiting intake.

Enteral feeding is generally accepted as the preferred route in critically ill patients and is associated with improved gastrointestinal mucosal function. Absence of bowel sounds is not a contra-indication to starting enteral feeding. Feeding is initiated via nasogastric tube by slowly increasing the rate of feeding. Return of large gastric aspirates is usually managed by administration of prokinetic agents. If aspirates remain large it is necessary to consider placement of a nasojejunal feeding tube either by administration of prokinetic agents or by an endoscopic technique. An alternative is feeding via a jejunostomy formed at the time of surgery. Parenteral nutrition should be considered only if enteral feeding has failed or is contra-indicated. Particular attention should be paid to reserving one intravenous line exclusively for feed to reduce infective complications.

Stress ulcer prophylaxis

Significant bleeding from the upper-gastro-intestinal tract from stress ulceration is rare and has been associated with mechanical ventilation, coagulopathy and reduced mucosal perfusion. Agents used as prophylaxis include antacids, sucralfate and H2 receptor antagonists. A recent large prospective randomised trial (Canadian Critical Care Trials Group) of sucralfate versus ranitidine in mechanically ventilated patients showed a significantly reduced incidence of clinically important haemorrhage in patients treated with ranitidine. However, there was no difference in length of intensive care stay or mortality. Common practice is to administer sucralfate or an H2 receptor antagonist until enteral feeding is established. Use of sucralfate in patients with severe renal impairment is contra-indicated because of aluminium absorption. The dose of ranitidine should be reduced for patients with renal failure.

Infection

Treatment of infection is discussed in detail in **Chapter 19**. Broad-spectrum antibiotics are usually administered until definitive microbiological results are available, with doses adjusted to the level of renal and hepatic function and mode of renal support. In the absence of obvious infection a high index of suspicion should be maintained and regular specimens taken for investigation. Prevention of infection is important as all critically ill patients are functionally immunosuppressed. All tubes running into the patient are potential routes of infection. The urinary catheter can be removed in the presence of anuria. Intravascular catheters should only be sited if they can be justified and be removed as soon as possible. When possible, non-invasive respiratory support is preferred as endotracheal intubation is associated with a high incidence of nosocomial pneumonia. Connecting tubes (e.g. transducer lines, ventilator tubing) are changed regularly. Cross infection between patients is nearly always the result of transfer by medical and nursing staff and is reduced by meticulous hand washing.

Specific Problems

Postoperative patients

Management of postoperative patients should follow the general principles outlined above. In addition, the following can be postoperative causes of oliguria:

- Bleeding is common in postoperative patients and is either due to coagulopathy or inadequate haemostasis. Bleeding is often obvious and visible (drains or wound sites) but occasionally is only suspected from haemodynamic alterations or fluid requirements. Coagulopathy should be corrected and surgeons contacted early as re-exploration is often required.
- Intra-abdominal hypertension — elevated intra-abdominal pressure may occur after emergency abdominal surgery and should be treated urgently (see earlier section).
- Aortic surgery — renal dysfunction is common after aortic surgery, particularly after emergency aneurysm repair, but no drugs have been demonstrated to be useful for prophylaxis. Cholesterol embolism occurs often after aortic or angiographic procedures but rarely results in ARF.
- Cardiac surgery — postoperative cardiac tamponade may present as oliguria. A high index of suspicion is necessary as the usual clinical signs are not always present. An intra-aortic balloon pump can obstruct the renal arteries if positioned too distally in the aorta.

Rhabdomyolysis

Please refer to **Chapter 12**.

Contrast media nephropathy

Few patients are admitted to the intensive care unit as a result of contrast media associated ARF. A more common problem is the use of radiocontrast agents in critically-ill patients who already have a degree of renal dysfunction. Risk factors include concurrent renal dysfunction, diabetes, myeloma, hypovolaemia, and type and dose of contrast agent. No agents have been reliably demonstrated to reduce the incidence of contrast nephropathy and the best prophylaxis is adequate fluid loading.

Elevated intracranial pressure

For patients with renal failure and raised intracranial pressure a continuous renal replacement technique is mandatory to prevent surges in intracranial pressure. A sudden rise in intracranial pressure is caused by rapid solute removal during intermittent dialysis and may be fatal.

FURTHER READING

Allgren RL, Marbury TC, Rahman SN, *et al*. (1997) Anaritide in acute tubular necrosis. Auriculin Anaritide ARF Study Group. *The New England Journal of Medicine*; 336: 828–834

Bellomo R, Ronco C (eds.) (1995) *ARF in the Critically Ill. Update in Intensive Care and Emergency Medicine 20.* Berlin. Springer-Verlag

Boyd O, Grounds RM, Bennett ED (1993) A randomized clinical trial of the effect of deliberate perioperative increase of oxygen delivery on mortality in high-risk surgical patients. *Journal of the American Medical Association*; 270: 2699–2707

Brezis M, Rosen S (1995) Hypoxia of the renal medulla — its implications for disease. *The New England Journal of Medicine*; 332: 647–655

Bumaschny E (1998) The abdominal compartment syndrome. *Current Opinions in Critical Care*; 4: 236–244

Cook D, Juyatt J, Marshall J, *et al*. (1998) A comparison of sucralfate and ranitidine for the prevention of upper gastrointestinal bleeding in patients requiring mechanical ventilation. Canadian Critical Care Trials Group. *The New England Journal of Medicine*; 338: 791–797

Gattinoni L, Brazzi L, Pelosi P, *et al*. (1995) A trial of goal-orientated haemodynamic therapy in critically ill patients. SvO2 Collaborative Group. *The New England Journal of Medicine*; 333: 1025–1032

Hebert PC, Wells G, Blajchman MA, *et al*. (1999) A multicenter, randomized controlled clinical trial of transfusion requirements in critical care. Transfusion Requirements in Critical Care Investigators, Canadian Critical Care Trials Group. *The New England Journal of Medicine*; 340: 409–417

Levy EM, Viscoli CM, Horwitz RI, *et al*. (1996) The effect of ARF on mortality. *Journal of the American Medical Association*; 275: 1489–1494

Martin C, Papazian L, Perrin G, *et al*. (1993) Norepinephrine or dopamine for the treatment of hyperdynamic septic shock? *Chest*; 103: 1826–1831

Shilliday IR, Quinn KJ, Allison EM (1997) Loop diuretics in the management of ARF: A prospective, double-blind, placebo-controlled, randomized study. *Nephrology Dialysis and Transplantation*; 12: 2592–2596

Webb AR, Shapiro MJ, Singer M, Suter P (eds.) (1998) *Oxford Textbook of Critical Care*. Oxford: Oxford University Press

Appendix A _____

DRUG PRESCRIBING IN ACUTE RENAL FAILURE
Katy Glynne

PRINCIPLES OF DRUG PRESCRIBING IN ARF: A STEPWISE APPROACH

1. Assess the Severity of Renal Failure

Creatinine clearance (CrCl) is often used as a measure of glomerular filtration rate (GFR). CrCl is measured from either a 24 h urine collection or derived from equations, e.g. Cockcroft-Gault equation:

$$\textbf{Male patients}: \text{CrCl (mL/min)} = \frac{1.23\,(140 - \text{age in years})\,\text{weight in kg*}}{\text{serum creatinine (µmol/L)}}$$

$$\textbf{Female patients}: \text{CrCl (mL/min)} = \frac{1.04\,(140 - \text{age in years})\,\text{weight in kg*}}{\text{serum creatinine (µmol/L)}}$$

*For obese patients use Ideal Body Weight (IBW), for other patients use Actual Body Weight if <IBW

IBW calculation: Males   = 50 kg + (2.3 × number inches >5 ft)
Females = 45.5 kg + (2.3 × number inches >5 ft)**

**For patients <5 ft tall, subtract 2.3 kg × number of inches <5 ft.

The assessment of CrCl using Cockcroft-Gault needs to be interpreted with caution in patients with ARF, where two serum creatinine levels measured in 24 h vary by more than 20 µmol/L. This may represent non-steady state serum [creatinine] — therefore one may underestimate the degree of renal impairment.

2. Determine the Need for Dose Adjustments

The following types of drugs need major dose adjustments in ARF:

- Drugs that are normally excreted via the kidneys.
- Drugs that are metabolised to pharmacologically active metabolites, requiring intact renal excretory function for their elimination (see **Table 1**).

Table 1. Common parent drugs with metabolites dependent on renal excretion

Allopurinol	Diazepam	Propanolol
Azathioprine	Primidone	Sulphonamides
Cephalosporins	Pethidine	
Chlordiazepoxide	Morphine	

3. Determine the Requirement for a Loading Dose (LD)

- LD aims rapidly to achieve therapeutic plasma concentrations.
- If no LD is given, it will take 4½ drug half-lives ($t^{½}$) to reach steady state plasma levels.
- Always consider a LD when ARF results in a significantly prolonged drug $t^{½}$, or when rapid attainment of therapeutic plasma levels is critical.
- It is generally recommended that a standard LD is administered to patients on continuous renal replacement therapy (CRRT, see also **Chapter 9.5**).

4. Calculate Maintenance Doses (MD)

- Maintenance doses for varying degrees of renal failure are given in the tables below, and are adjusted as follows:
  - Lengthening dosing interval, corresponding to the degree of delayed drug excretion or metabolism (most practical for drugs with a long half-life).
  - Reducing the amount of drug administered in proportion to the degree of ARF, leaving the dosing interval unchanged. This usually leads to more steady blood concentrations.

- In CRRT, the dose chosen is based on an estimation of CrCl achieved by the extracorporeal system used (see also **Chapter 9.5**). For haemofiltration, the volume of ultrafiltrate collected each hour can be used to represent the CrCl:
  - When the ultrafiltration rate is >15 mL/min, the dose selected should reflect that administered to patients with moderate renal failure (see below).
  - When the ultrafiltration rate is <15 mL/min, the dose should follow that recommended for patients with severe renal failure (see below).

5. Therapeutic Drug Monitoring

- Close monitoring of the plasma concentration of drugs is advised where the margin between therapeutic and toxic levels is small.
- **Peak levels** reflect the highest concentration after the rapid distribution phase of the drug, before substantial elimination has started.
- **Trough levels** are the lowest levels observed, as they are obtained prior to administration of the next dose. The trough level is closely related to the total body (systemic) clearance of the drug.

Table 2. Drugs not significantly excreted via the kidneys

Alfentanil	Hydrocortisone acetate/sodium succinate
Aminophylline (Increased incidence of gastrointestinal & neurological side-effects in renal impairment at plasma levels above optimum range. Monitor levels, adjust according to response)	Isoniazid — 300 mg/day maximum. Inactivated hepatically. HD removes drug; give dose after dialysis
Amiodarone	Isosorbide Mononitrate
Amlodipine	
Budesonide	Labetalol
	Lorazepam
Calcium acetate/carbonate/gluconate/resonium	Methylprednisolone
Carbamazepine	Naloxone
Ceftriaxone (No adjustment needed unless renal & hepatic impairment coexist, in which case the maximum dose is 2 g/day)	Nifedipine
Chloramphenicol	Norepinephrine
Chlormethiazole	Octreotide
Chlorpromazine	Omeprazole
Clindamycin (no supplemental dose needed in HD & PD. Sometimes interval is lengthened in severe renal & hepatic impairment)	Ondansetron
Cyclizine	Phenytoin ($\downarrow$ protein binding & volume of distribution in ARF. Request free phenytoin levels if possible. Otherwise, total phenytoin levels should be adjusted for albumin levels & uraemia)
Cyclosporin (renal excretion of drug is a minor pathway, but monitor for nephrotoxicity. Pharmaco-kinetics affected by hepatic disease, monitor serum drug levels. No supplement required after dialysis)	Phytomenadione (vitamin K)
Dalteparin	Propofol
Dexamethasone	Pyrazinamide
Diltiazem	
Dobutamine	Rifampicin (600 mg/day maximum. No significant removal by dialysis. Caution in hepatorenal syndrome)
Dopamine	Salbutamol
Dopexamine	Sodium valproate
Doxazosin	Tacrolimus
Enoxaparin	

Table 2 (*Continued*)	
Epinephrine	Thyroxine
Epoietin alpha/beta	
Epoprostenol (prostacyclin)	Verapamil
	Warfarin
Fusidic acid (sodium fusidate)	

DRUG DOSAGES IN ACUTE RENAL FAILURE AND RRT

Dosage recommendations in ARF often use data extrapolated from studies of the drugs in patients with chronic renal failure (CRF) who have a CrCl <10 mL/min. This is important, as pharmacokinetic profiles of drugs used in ARF may differ from those measured in patients with CRF. Specifically, extra-renal drug excretion progressively decreases, the longer the duration of renal failure. The preservation of non-renal clearance observed early in the course of ARF suggests that dosing schemes extrapolated from patients with stable chronic renal failure could possibly result in ineffectively low drug concentrations. Individualized pharmacokinetic dosing for patients with ARF is therefore essential early in the course of the patient's therapy.

Note that many drugs are not significantly renally cleared, and dose adjustments are **NOT** necessary for patients with ARF and/or receiving RRT. These are listed in **Table 2**.

The following information serves as a guide for prescribing some of the more commonly used drugs that are renally excreted and/or nephrotoxic in adult patients (antineoplastic agents are discussed in **Chapters 11** and **21**). For patients undergoing intermittent haemodialysis, if a supplemental dose is required, it may be simplest to schedule drug administration times so that they follow dialysis. *To the best of the editors' knowledge, at the time of going to press, all drug doses listed are accurate and as recommended in the relevant Data Sheet Compendia. However, owing to intermittent changes in dosing recommendations, the reader is advised to check all drug doses in the* **current** *British National Formulary and/or Data Sheet Compendia.*

ANTIMICROBIAL AGENTS

Aminoglycosides

In ARF (CrCl <20 mL/min) use the following prescribing principles (**NOT** once-daily dosing):

- Need **standard LD** in ARF.
- Subsequent dose adjustment by dose reduction and/or interval extension, depending on serum levels.
- Serum levels must be measured for efficacy and toxicity.
- In patients on renal replacement therapy, measure post-dialysis drug levels.
- For obese patients (>20% ideal body weight) use dosing weight (DW),

$$DW = IBW + 0.4(\text{actual body weight} - IBW).$$

- Dose administered over 30 minutes

Take *trough level within 1 h of the next dose. If trough elevated, extend dosing interval to 12, 24, 36 or 48 h as appropriate. Take **peak level 30 mins after the end of the infusion. If peak level low, increase dose and dosing interval.

Gentamicin

Normal dose	GFR 30–70 mL/min	GFR 10–30 mL/min	GFR 5–10 mL/min	HD Dose	CVVHD Dose
LD = 1–2 mg/kg					
MD = 1.7 mg/kg 8 hourly	MD = 80 mg 12 hourly (60 mg if <60 kg)	MD = 80 mg daily (60 mg if <60 kg)	MD = 80 mg every 48 h (60 mg if <60 kg)	MD = 80 mg post HD (60 mg if <60 kg)	MD = 80 mg daily (60 mg if <60 kg)

*Peak serum concentration should not be >10 mg/L; **Trough serum concentration should be <2 mg/L; concurrent penicillin Rx may result in sub-therapeutic levels.

Penicillins

Drug Normal dose	GFR 20–50 mL/min	GFR 10–20 mL/min	GFR <10 mL/min	HD Dose	CVVHD Dose	Comments
Ampicillin IV/IM 0.5–2 g 6 hourly Oral: 0.25–1 g 6 hourly	Unchanged	250–500 mg 6 hourly	250 mg 6 hourly	250 mg 6 hourly after HD	250–500 mg 6 hourly	Do not mix with aminoglycosides Sodium content of injection 2.7 mmol/g
Benzylpenicillin IV/IM: 0.6–14.4 g daily in 2–6 divided doses 1 MU = 600 mg Meningitis: up to 14.4 g daily Endocarditis: 4.8 g daily	Unchanged	75% of normal dose	20–50% of normal dose	As for GFR <10 mL/min after HD	75% of normal dose	Maximum dose in severe ARF: 4–6 MU daily 1 MU contains 1.68 mmol Na^+ and 1.7 mmol K^+ Increased incidence of seizures in ARF
Co-amoxiclav (amoxycillin/clavulanic acid) IV: 1.2 g 8 hourly (increasing to 6 hourly in severe infection) Oral: 375 mg 8 hourly Maximum 625 mg 8 hourly	Unchanged	IV: 1.2 g stat, then 600 mg IV 8–12 hourly Oral: 375 mg or 625 mg 12 hourly	IV: 1.2 g stat, then 600 mg IV daily Oral: 375 mg 8–12 hourly	As in GFR <10 mL/min	As in GFR 10–20 mL/min	CSM advice: cholestatic jaundice may occur if treatment >14 d or up to 6 weeks after R_x stopped Each 1.2 g vial contains: Na^+ 3.1 mmol, K^+ 1 mmol

Penicillins (Continued)

Drug Normal dose	GFR 20–50 mL/min	GFR 10–20 mL/min	GFR <10 mL/min	HD Dose	CVVHD Dose	Comments
Piperacillin IM/IV: Serious infection: 4 g 6–8 hourly; Mild infection: 2 g 6–8 hourly or 4 g 12 hourly	4 g 8 hourly	4 g 8–12 hourly	4 g 12 hourly	2 g 8 hourly after HD; HD removes 30–50% in 4 h	4 g 8–12 hourly	Each 1 g of Pipril contains 1.85 mmol Na$^+$
Piperacillin/tazobactam IV: 4.5 g 8 hourly	4.5 g 8 hourly	4.5 g 12 hourly	4.5 g 12 hourly	4.5 g 12 hourly	4.5 g 12 hourly	Each vial contains 9.37 mmol Na$^+$

Carbapenems

Drug Normal dose	GFR 20–50 mL/min	GFR 10–20 mL/min	GFR <10 mL/min	HD Dose	CVVHD Dose	Comments
Imipenem + cilastatin IV: 500 mg 6–8 hourly (up to 1 g 6–8 hourly)	0.5–1 g 8 hourly	0.5–1 g 12 hourly	250 mg 12 hourly or 3.5 mg/kg 12 hourly whichever is lowest	250 mg 12 hourly dose after HD	250–500 mg 12 hourly or 3.5 mg/kg 12 hourly whichever is lowest	Risk of seizures; Cilastatin prevents renal metabolism of imipenem by dihydropeptidase-1 (DHP-1)
Meropenem IV: 0.5–2 g 8 hourly	1–2 g 12 hourly	1 g 12 hourly	up to 1 g daily	500 mg–1 g daily dose after HD	1 g 12 hourly	Stable to DHP-1, therefore does not require addition of DHP-1 inhibitor

Cephalosporins

May be nephrotoxic in combination with aminoglycoside antibiotics, diuretics, and volume depletion. Rarely allergic interstitial nephritis

Drug Normal dose	GFR 20–50 mL/min	GFR 10–20 mL/min	GFR <10 mL/min	HD Dose	CVVHD Dose	Comments
Cefuroxime IV/IM: 0.75–1.5 g 6–8 hourly	0.75–1.5 g 8 hourly	0.75–1.5 g 8–12 hourly	750 mg 12 hourly	As per GFR <10 mL/min Dose after HD	750 mg 12 hourly	
Cefotaxime IV: up to 2 g 8 hourly	Unchanged	Unchanged	0.5–1 g 8–12 hourly	As per GFR < 10 mL/min Dose after HD	1 g 12 hourly	↓ dose further for hepatic & renal failure
Ceftazidime IV: 1–2 g 8–12 hourly	GFR 31–50 mL/min 1 g 12 hourly	GFR 16–30 mL/min 1 g daily	GFR <15 mL/min 0.5–1 g every 24–48 h	0.5–1 g every 24–48 h Dose after HD	0.5–1g 12 hourly	Volume of distribution increases with infection

Macrolide antibiotics

Drug Normal dose	GFR 20–50 mL/min	GFR 10–20 mL/min	GFR <10 mL/min	HD Dose	CVVHD Dose	Comments
Clarithromycin IV: 500 mg 12 hourly infusion over 60 min Oral: 250–500 mg 12 hourly	Unchanged	250–500 mg 12 hourly	250 mg 12 hourly	As per GFR <10 mL/min	As per GFR 10–20 mL/min	Doses given for renal impairment are for IV and oral routes
Erythromycin IV: 0.25–1 g 6 hourly Oral: 0.25–0.5 g 6 hourly	Unchanged	Unchanged	50–75% of normal dose Maximum 1.5 g daily	As per GFR <10 mL/min	Unchanged (unknown dialysability)	Ototoxicity with high doses in ESRD Volume of distribution increases in ESRD

Fluoroquinolone antibiotics

Drug Normal dose	GFR 20–50 mL/min	GFR 10–20 mL/min	GFR <10 mL/min	HD Dose	CVVHD Dose	Comments
Ciprofloxacin IV: 100–400 mg 12 hourly PO: 0.25–0.75 g 12 hourly	Unchanged	50% normal dose	50% normal dose	IV: 200 mg 12 hourly PO: 0.25–0.5 g 12 hourly	IV: 200 mg 12 hourly PO: 0.5–0.75 g 12 hourly	

Miscellaneous antibiotics

Drug Normal dose	GFR 20–50 mL/min	GFR 10–20 mL/min	GFR <10 mL/min	HD Dose	CVVHD Dose	Comments
Co-trimoxazole (trimethoprim + sulfamethoxazole) Treatment of PCP IV: 60 mg/kg 12 hourly	Unchanged	60 mg/kg 12 hourly for 3 days, then 60 mg/kg daily	60 mg/kg daily	As per GFR <10 mL/min Dose after HD	As per GFR 10–20 mL/min	In ARF only give if HD facilities available
Linezolid IV/oral: 600 mg 12 hourly	Unchanged	Unchanged	Unchanged	Unchanged Dose after HD	No data	Manufacturer advises metabolites may accumulate if Cr Cl <30 mL/min
Metronidazole IV: 500 mg 8 hourly	Unchanged	Unchanged	Unchanged	Unchanged Dose after HD	Unchanged	500 mg/100 mL infusion provides 14 mmol Na^+
Teicoplanin IV/IM: **Severe infection** LD = 3 × 400 mg doses 12 hourly MD = 400 mg daily	Day 1–3 standard dose. From day 4 give 50% normal dose daily, or 100% every 48 h	Day 1–3 standard dose. From day 4 give 33% normal dose daily, or 100% every 72 h	Day 1–3 standard dose. From day 4 give 33% normal dose daily, or 100% every 72 h	As per GFR <10 mL/min	As per GFR 10–20 mL/min	**For patients with renal impairment, a reduction in dose is not required until day 4 of therapy**

Miscellaneous antibiotics (Continued)

Drug Normal dose	GFR 20–50 mL/min	GFR 10–20 mL/min	GFR <10 mL/min	HD Dose	CVVHD Dose	Comments
Vancomycin IV 0.5 g 6 hourly or 1 g 12 hourly Measure serum levels at 3rd or 4th dose. Draw **trough** within 60 mins before dose Trough: 5–10 μg/mL	Give 15 mg/kg, or 1 g stat, starting dose, with subsequent doses based on renal function and serum concentrations of drug measured at 24 h intervals. Take trough level before next dose. Aim for trough <10 μg/mL	As per GFR 20–50 mL/min	As per GFR 20–50 mL/min	1 g once or twice weekly Not removed, no supplement needed	As per GFR <10 mL/min	Infusion rate NOT faster than 10 mg/min For dialysis patients, measure random level on days 4–5 of Rx. Repeat dose when random level <10 μg/mL

Antifungal antibiotics

Drug Normal dose	GFR 20–50 mL/min	GFR 10–20 mL/min	GFR <10 mL/min	HD Dose	CVVHD Dose	Comments
Amphotericin IV: 0.5–1.5 mg/kg/day infused over 6 h Liposomal products: 1–5 mg/kg/day infused over 1 h See individual product sheets	Unchanged	Unchanged	Normal dose every 24–36 h	As per GFR <10 mL/min Not removed by HD	Unchanged Liposomal preparations should be infused into venous return line	Highly nephrotoxic; can cause distal RTA, ↓K⁺, ↓Mg⁺, nephrogenic DI. Only 3–5% of drug is renally excreted, but nephrotoxicity occurs in >80% patients. Toxicity *amplified* by concomitant cyclosporin A, aminoglycosides or Pentamidine; *lessened* by saline loading

Antifungal antibiotics (Continued)

Drug Normal dose	GFR 20–50 mL/min	GFR 10–20 mL/min	GFR <10 mL/min	HD Dose	CVVHD Dose	Comments
Fluconazole IV/Oral: 200–400 mg daily, depending on indication	Unchanged	Unchanged	50% normal dose	Standard dose on dialysis days only post HD	Unchanged	No adjustment needed for single dose therapy
Itraconazole IV/Oral: 100–200 mg 1–2 times daily	Unchanged	Unchanged	50% normal dose	100 mg 12–24 hourly	100 mg 12–24 hourly	Manufacturer recommends avoidance of IV product if CrCl <30 ml/min

Antiparasitic antibiotics

Drug Normal dose	GFR 20–50 mL/min	GFR 10–20 mL/min	GFR <10 mL/min	HD Dose	CVVHD Dose	Comments
Chloroquine Oral, IV: consult data sheet	Unchanged	Unchanged	50% normal treatment dose	As in GFR <10 mL/min	Unchanged	Chloroquine sulphate injection 5.45% w/v (equivalent to 40 mg chloroquine base/ mL) is available
Quinine Dihydrochloride LD = 20 mg/kg to a maximum of 1.4 g, then after 8–12 h: MD = 10 mg/kg (up to 700 mg) 8–12 hourly	5–10 mg/kg 8 hourly	5–10 mg/kg 8–12 hourly	5–10 mg/kg daily	As per GFR <10 mL/min Dose after HD	As per GFR 10–20 mL/min	Marked tissue accumulation Monitor for signs of cardiotoxicity

Antiparasitic antibiotics *(Continued)*

Drug Normal dose	GFR 20–50 mL/min	GFR 10–20 mL/min	GFR <10 mL/min	HD Dose	CVVHD Dose	Comments
Quinine Dihydrochloride Reduce to 5–7 mg/kg if parenteral therapy needed for >48 h						In ESRD: reduce dose after 2 day to prevent toxic accumulation

Antiviral agents

Drug Normal dose	GFR 20–50 mL/min	GFR 10–20 mL/min	GFR <10 mL/min	HD Dose	CVVHD Dose	Comments
Aciclovir **IV**: 5–10 mg/kg 8 hourly, depending on indication. Consult data sheet. Infuse over at least 1 h	5–10 mg/kg 12 hourly	5–10 mg/kg daily (some units use 3.5–7 mg/kg daily)	2.5–5 mg/kg daily	As per GFR <10 mL/min Dose after HD	As per GFR 10–20 mL/min	Rapid infusion can worsen renal impairment Adequate hydration of the patient should be maintained Reports of neurological toxicity at maximum recommended doses
Oral: Simplex treatment: 200–400 mg 5 times daily for 5 days Zoster treatment: 800 mg 5 times daily for 7 days	Unchanged	Simplex: Unchanged Zoster: 800 mg 8 hourly	Simplex: 200 mg 12 hourly Zoster: 800 mg 12 hourly	As per GFR <10 mL/min Dose after HD	As per GFR 10–20 mL/min	Consider IV R_x for Zoster infection if patient severely immunocompromised

Antiviral agents (Continued)

Drug / Normal dose	GFR 20–50 mL/min	GFR 10–20 mL/min	GFR <10 mL/min	HD Dose	CVVHD Dose	Comments
Ganciclovir IV Treatment: LD: 5 mg/kg 12 hourly for 14–21 days; MD: 5 mg/kg daily IV Prevention: as for treatment, except induction length is 7–14 days	2.5 mg/kg 12 hourly	2.5 mg/kg daily	1.25 mg/kg daily	1.25 mg/kg daily post HD on dialysis days only, maximum 3 times weekly	2.5 mg/kg daily	Frequent granulocytopaenia & thrombocytopaenia

Sedatives

Drug / Normal dose	GFR 20–50 mL/min	GFR 10–20 mL/min	GFR <10 mL/min	HD Dose	CVVHD Dose	Comments
Diamorphine IV: 2.5–5 mg 4 hourly (halve dose in elderly) SC/IM: 5–10 mg 4 hourly, ↑ing dose as necessary	Unchanged	Use small doses e.g. 2.5 mg 6 hourly SC/IM and titrate to response	Use small doses e.g. 2.5 mg 8-hourly SC/IM and titrate to response	As per GFR <10 mL/min	As per GFR 10–20 mL/min	**Caution with regular dosing.** May lead to accumulation of active metabolites. ↑cerebral sensitivity in ARF can lead to excess sedation and serious respiratory depression
Fentanyl IV/IM: consult data sheet	Unchanged Titrate to response	75% normal dose	50% normal dose	As per GFR <10 mL/min Not removed by HD	As per GFR 10–20 mL/min	For intractable pain in renal patients, try Fentanyl patches

Sedatives (Continued)

Drug Normal dose	GFR 20–50 mL/min	GFR 10–20 mL/min	GFR <10 mL/min	HD Dose	CVVHD Dose	Comments
Morphine IV/SC/IM: 5–20 mg 4 hourly (higher in severe pain or terminal illness)	75% normal dose Adjust to response	2.5–5 mg 4 hourly	1.25–2.5 mg 4 hourly	As in GFR <10 mL/min 75% morphine & metabolites removed during HD	As in GFR 10–20 mL/min Active metabolites removed	Potential accumulation of morphine-6-glucuronide, an active renally excreted metabolite, more potent than morphine. Its half-life is increased from 3–5 h in normal renal function, to 50 h in ESRD Reduced plasma protein binding causes increase in sensitivity to drug effects
Midazolam Sedation: IV over 30 sec, 2 mg followed after 2 min by increments of 0.5–1 mg if sedation not adequate; usual range 2.5–7.5 mg. Elderly 1–2 mg	Unchanged	Unchanged	50% normal dose	As in GFR <10 mL/min	Unchanged	Hepatic elimination ↑sensitivity in ARF

Acid suppressants

Drug Normal dose	GFR 20–50 mL/min	GFR 10–20 mL/min	GFR <10 mL/min	HD Dose	CVVHD Dose	Comments
Cimetidine IV/IM: See data sheet. Dosage regime depends on prophylaxis versus active bleed	Unchanged	50% normal dose	25–50% normal dose	As for GFR <10 mL/min Dose after HD & every 12–24 h, between HD sessions	As for GFR 10–20 mL/min	↑serum creatinine (competes for tubule creatinine secretion). May cause confusion in renal or hepatic disease. ARF reported
Ranitidine IM/slow IV: 50 mg 6–8 hourly	Unchanged	Unchanged	50 mg IV 12 hourly	As per GFR <10 mL/min Dose after HD	As per GFR 10–20 mL/min	Preferred to cimetidine
Sucralfate Stress ulcer prophylaxis 1 g 6 times daily oral	4 g daily	2–4 g daily	2–4 g daily	As for GFR <10 mL/min	As for GFR 10–20 mL/min	Only use with caution in dialysis and ARF. Only use for short periods. Aluminium may accumulate

CARDIOVASCULAR AND ANTIHYPERTENSIVE AGENTS

ACE inhibitors (ACEIs, see also **Chapters 11 and 13**)

Drug Normal dose	GFR 20–50 mL/min	GFR 10–20 mL/min	GFR <10 mL/min	HD Dose	CVVHD Dose	Comments
Captopril Oral: 6.25–50 mg, 1–3 times daily	Start low & adjust according to response	As for GFR 20–50 mL/min	As for GFR 20–50 mL/min	As for GFR <10 mL/min	As for GFR 10–20 mL/min	Once daily dosing in severe renal impairment is effective
Enalapril Oral: 2.5–40 mg daily	Unchanged	Start with 2.5 mg daily then dose according to response	As for GFR 10–20 mL/min	As for GFR <10 mL/min	As for GFR 10–20 mL/min	Enalapril maleate is a pro-drug that needs hepatic conversion to enalaprilat, with a long half-life. It is thus not suitable as an ACE inhibitor test-dose drug
Fosinopril Oral: 10–40 mg once daily	Unchanged	Unchanged, start with low dose	Unchanged, start with low dose	As for GFR <10 mL/min	As for GFR 10–20 mL/min	
Lisinopril Oral: Initially 2.5 mg daily; maximum 40 mg daily	50–75% normal dose Titrate according to response	50–75% normal dose Titrate according to response	25–50% normal dose Titrate according to response	As for GFR <10 mL/min	As for GFR 10–20 mL/min	
Perindopril Oral: 2–8 mg daily	GFR 30–60 mL/min 2 mg daily	GFR 15–30 mL/min 2 mg alternate days	GFR <15 mL/min 2 mg alternate days, adjust according to BP	As for GFR <15 mL/min	As for GFR <15 mL/min	

Beta-blockers

Drug Normal dose	GFR 20–50 mL/min	GFR 10–20 mL/min	GFR <10 mL/min	HD Dose	CVVHD Dose	Comments
Atenolol Oral: 50–100 mg daily	Unchanged	Unchanged	50 mg once daily	As for GFR <10 mL/min	Unchanged	Significant accumulation in ARF
Bisoprolol Oral: 5–10 mg daily (max. 20 mg daily)	5–20 mg daily	5–20 mg daily	5–10 mg daily	As for GFR <10 mL/min	As for GFR 10–20 mL/min	
Metoprolol Oral: 50–100 mg 2–3 times daily IV: 5–15 mg	Unchanged	Start with small doses/normal interval	Start with small doses/normal interval	Dialysed. Start with small doses	Probably dialysed. Start with small doses and titrate in accordance with response	Can cause hypoglycaemia in dialysis patients
Sotalol Oral: 80–640 mg daily in single or divided doses IV: 0.5–1.5 mg/kg 6 hourly	50% normal dose	25% normal dose	Avoid or use with caution	Unknown dialysability Dose as per GFR <10mL/min Use lowest dose possible	Unknown dialysability Dose as in GFR 10–20 mL/min	↑QT interval predisposing to Torsades de pointes

Vasodilators

Drug Normal dose	GFR 20–50 mL/min	GFR 10–20 mL/min	GFR <10 mL/min	HD Dose	CVVHD Dose	Comments
Hydralazine Oral: 25–50 mg twice daily IV infusion: 200–300 μg/min initially decreasing to 50–150 μg/min	Start with small dose and adjust according to response	Start with small dose and adjust according to response	Start with small dose and adjust according to response	As per GFR <10 mL/min	As per GFR 10–20 mL/min	Avoid long-term use due to accumulation of metabolites in severe renal insufficiency and dialysis patients
Sodium Nitroprusside IV: 0.3–8.0 μg/kg/min Range: 10–400 μg/min	Unchanged	Unchanged Avoid prolonged use	Unchanged Avoid prolonged use	As per GFR <10 mL/min	As per GFR 10–20 mL/min	Rapidly metabolized to cyanogen which is converted to thiocyanate (toxic) Avoid prolonged use in ARF. Accumulation of thiocyanate-dialysable

Cardiac glycosides

Drug Normal dose	GFR 20–50 mL/min	GFR 10–20 mL/min	GFR <10 mL/min	HD Dose	CVVHD Dose	Comments
Digoxin Digitalisation: 1–1.5 mg in divided doses over 24 h followed by 62.5–500 μg daily adjusted according to response	Digitalisation — see comments 125–250 μg daily	As per GFR 20–50 mL/min Monitor levels	Digitalisation — see comments 62.5 μg 3 times a week after HD, or 62.5 μg daily Monitor levels	As per GFR <10 mL/min	As per GFR 10–20 mL/min	Digitalisation in renal impairment: 750 μg–1 mg. Interval between normal or reduced doses may need to be lengthened Steady state plasma monitoring advised. Normal range: 0.8–2 ng/mL. Draw serum no sooner than 12 h after a dose in ESRD (6–8 h after a dose with normal renal function)

Appendix B _____

NUTRITION IN ACUTE RENAL FAILURE
Marie Kelly

Patients with ARF are at increased risk of developing malnutrition secondary to:

- pre-existing nutritional deficits;
- disease-related nutritional deficits;
- prolonged hospitalization.

Prompt assessment of patient's nutritional requirements and the implementation of a tailored nutritional prescription may help to reduce morbidity associated with ARF. Patients should always be referred for nutritional assessment to identify those at risk of developing malnutrition (**Table 1**).

Table 1. Nutritional assessment tests	
Measurement/Tests	**Examples**
Anthropometric	Body mass index (BMI); % body weight loss Triceps skinfold thickness (TST)
Biochemical parameters	Albumin, pre-albumin
Urea kinetics/Nitrogen requirements	Urea appearance rate (UAR) Protein catabolic rate (PCR)
Energy requirements	Indirect calorimetry/predictive equations
Subjective scores	Subjective global assessment (SGA)
Dietary assessment	Food records

NUTRITIONAL REQUIREMENTS

The optimum nutritional prescription should take into account:

- the patient's nutritional status;
- the degree of catabolism associated with the underlying disease;
- dialysis requirements.

Energy Requirements

- Recent studies have shown that the energy requirements for ARF patients are no higher than for patients with normal renal function.
- In sepsis, energy requirements can be increased by as much as 25% — these increased requirements reflect the degree of catabolism only and not the ARF *per se.*
- Energy requirements can be measured by indirect calorimetry, although it is more common in clinical practice to use predictive equations to calculate the Basal Metabolic Rate (BMR; see **Table 2**).

Addition of an appropriate stress factor (**Figure 1**) and activity factor to the BMR will provide an estimate of the Total Energy Expenditure (TEE):

$$\textbf{BMR + Stress \% + Activity Factor \% = TEE.}$$

The activity factor for bedbound immobile patients is 10%, for bedbound mobile/sitting patients is 15–20% and for mobile patients is 25%.

Table 2. Calculating energy requirements[1]		
Age (yrs)	Men	Women
10–17	BMR = 0.074 × wt + 2.754	BMR = 0.056 × wt + 2.898
18–29	BMR = 0.063 × wt + 2.896	BMR = 0.062 × wt + 2.036
30–59	BMR = 0.048 × wt + 3.653	BMR = 0.034 × wt + 3.538
60–74	BMR = 0.0499 × wt + 2.930 (n = 189)	BMR = 0.0386 × wt + 2.875 (n = 109)
75+	BMR = 0.0350 × wt + 3.434 (n = 112)	BMR = 0.0410 × wt + 2.610 (n = 96)

[1]This table allows estimation of basal metabolic rate (BMR) in megajoules (MJ). To convert MJ to kcal multiply by 238. Need to allow for true weights for those patients who have had amputations [taken from Schofield WN (1985). Predicting basal metabolic rate, new standards and review of previous work. *Hum Nutr Clin Nutr*; 39 Suppl 1: 5–41].

Protein Requirements

The classification of catabolic patients is given in **Table 3**. Protein requirements for both normocatabolic and catabolic patients can be estimated using **Table 4** (Elia, 1990).

Normocatabolic/non-dialysis dependent patients

The practice of using low protein diets to manage impaired renal function in non-dialysis patients with ARF is no longer encouraged. Studies that have examined optimal protein intake in ARF now suggest using between 0.8–1.0 g/kg/day for non-dialysis dependent patients.

Figure 1. "Stress factor" nomogram

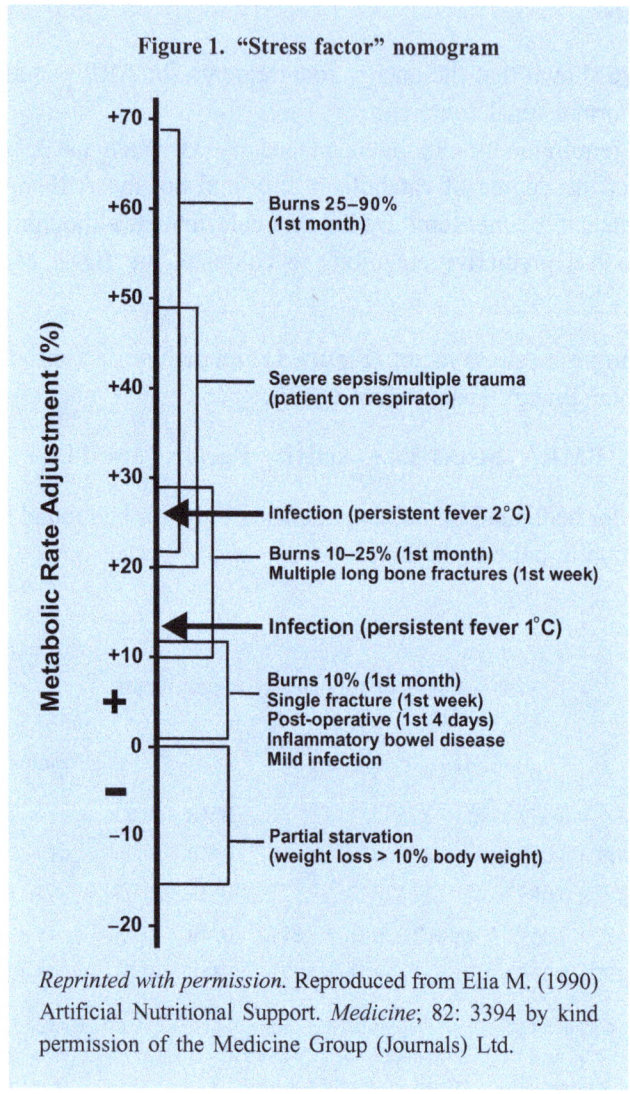

Reprinted with permission. Reproduced from Elia M. (1990) Artificial Nutritional Support. *Medicine*; 82: 3394 by kind permission of the Medicine Group (Journals) Ltd.

Table 3. Classification of catabolic patients

Urea Nitrogen Appearance (UNA) > Daily N intake	Catabolism
<6 g	Normocatabolic
6–12 g	Moderate
>12 g	Severe

Urea nitrogen appearance equals the sum of daily losses of urea nitrogen plus the change in body urea nitrogen.

Moderately/severely catabolic patients

The availability of dialysis, i.e. HD/CRRT, has allowed protein intakes of >1 g/kg/day in these patients. Catabolic patients dialyzed by CRRT can now tolerate relatively large protein intakes, i.e. 1.3–1.5 g/kg/day.

Table 4. Estimation of nitrogen requirements

Need to use the same % stress factor as that used to calculate energy requirements (Elia, 1990)

	Nitrogen (g/kg/day) mean (range)	Protein (g/kg/day) mean (range)
Normal	0.17 (0.14–0.20)	1.06 (0.88–1.25)
Hypermetabolic (% change for nomogram)		
5–25%	0.20 (0.17–0.25)	1.25 (1.06–1.56)
25–50%	0.25 (0.20–0.30)	1.56 (1.25–1.88)
>50%	0.30 (0.25–0.35)	1.88 (1.56–2.19)
Depleted	0.30 (0.20–0.40)	1.88 (1.25–2.50)

For obese individuals with a BMI of >30 kg/m^2 use approximately 75% of the value estimated from body weight. For those with a BMI >50 kg/m^2 use approximately 65% of value estimated from weight.

Dialytic losses

In addition to protein requirements, patients on dialysis require an additional nitrogen/protein allowance to compensate for losses occurring during dialysis. As a general guide, additional losses of amino acids/protein during dialysis are given in **Table 5**.

Table 5. Additional losses of amino acids/protein during dialysis

Type of dialysis	Estimated average losses
Intermittent Haemodialysis (HD)	1–1.5 g N/dialysis session; 6–9 g protein/session
Continuous Renal Replacement (CRRT)	1.5–2.0 g N/day; 9–12.5 g protein/day

N.B. The provision of adequate non-protein calories is essential to prevent the process of gluconeogenesis and the associated rise in blood urea nitrogen (BUN) due to the breakdown of both endogenous (muscle tissue) and exogenous (nitrogen provided) proteins to meet energy requirements.

ELECTROLYTES AND MINERALS

Potassium

Normocatabolic/non-dialysis dependent patients

A restriction of dietary potassium intake of 0.8 mmol/kg/day is usually required to treat an elevated serum potassium in the ARF patient not on dialysis. Since most foods, particularly fruit and vegetables, contain potassium, management of hyperkalaemia is aimed at avoiding the high potassium foods and restricting the amounts of fruit and vegetable consumed. A list of high potassium foods to avoid is summarized in **Table 6**.

Table 6. High potassium foods to avoid	
Fruit	**Vegetables**
Apricots (fresh or tinned)	Spinach
Bananas	Mushrooms
Dried fruits, e.g. currants, dates, raisins, prunes, sultanas	Potatoes — baked/roasted/chipped (unless par-boiled)
Rhubarb	Oven ready chips
Avocado pears	Instant mashed potato
Oranges	Soya products
Kiwi fruit	Crisps
Drinks	**Miscellaneous**
Fruit juice, e.g. orange, apple, tomato, pineapple	Salt substitutes, e.g. Ruthmol or Selora
Fruit squash is suitable	Marmite, Oxo, Bovril
Ribena or blackcurrant drinks	Liquorice, chocolate, fruit gums, fudge
Lucozade (canned)	Chocolate biscuits and cakes
Coffee	Rich fruit cakes
Drinking chocolate	**LIMIT:**
Ovaltine	Milk — allow ½ pint/day
Evaporated and condensed milk, milkshakes	Milk product, i.e. custard, milk puddings, yoghurts, cheese
Coffeemate	

In addition, the avoidance of excessive amounts of milk and milk products, i.e. yoghurt, milk puddings and cheese, which are high in potassium, will have the added effect of reducing phosphate intake. For practical purposes, a system using 4 mmol K$^+$ fruit and vegetable exchanges is frequently used to control the potassium intake from these sources. A brief list of these exchanges is summarized in (**Table 7**).

Table 7. Sample list of 4 mmol K⁺ fruit exchanges
Each fruit portion contains equivalent amounts of potassium
1 apple/plum/small pear
5–6 cherries
½ orange/grapefruit/kiwi/peach
10 grapes
4 oz tinned fruit (not apricots)

N.B: Fruit exchanges such as oranges may be included in a K⁺ lowering diet, providing they are used as part of the exchange system and that the total intake does not exceed the total K⁺ allowance.

Moderately/severely catabolic patients

Since potassium is lost during intermittent dialysis, patients can tolerate slightly higher intakes of potassium of 1 mmol/kg/day. This may mean the difference of 1–2 extra fruit or vegetable portions per day. Very catabolic patients requiring CRRT are frequently unable to take food orally and rely totally on nutritional intervention, i.e. enteral/parenteral feeding. Since potassium intake can be controlled and potassium losses are increased by CRRT, it is much more common to see hypokalaemia in this group of patients and additional supplementation is required.

Sodium

ARF patients who are oedematous and/or require intermittent HD are usually required to follow a fluid restriction i.e. 500 mL for insensible losses plus the equivalent of the previous days urinary output. Patients following such a restriction and who are managing to select an oral diet should avoid foods with a high salt content, which will exacerbate their thirst. An intake of 80–100 mmol Na⁺ (no added salt diet) is usually recommended to help achieve fluid balance in these patients. A list of high salt foods to avoid is summarized in **Table 8**.

Patients who are dialyzed by CRRT can usually tolerate considerably greater sodium intakes to replace dialytic losses, i.e. 100–200 mmol Na⁺/day. Since most of these patients are receiving

Table 8. High salt foods to avoid	
Meat	Processed, e.g. ham, bacon, tongue, sausages, meat pasties, meat pies
Fish	Smoked and tinned fish. Shellfish and fish paste, fish fingers and fish cakes
Dairy products	Cheese
Vegetables	Tinned, e.g. baked beans, peas, instant potatoes
Snacks	Crisps and other snacks, salted nuts
Miscellaneous	All soups, yeast extracts, gravies and stock cubes

intensive nutritional support, i.e. enteral/parenteral nutrition, their sodium intakes can be easily tailored to meet their requirement.

Phosphate, Calcium and Magnesium

Requirements for minerals in ARF are not well documented. Serum levels should be monitored regularly to assess requirements and the need for supplementation.

Normocatabolic/non-dialysis dependent patients

Hyperphosphataemic patients requiring dialysis therapy for an extended period of time, and who are consuming excessive amounts of high phosphate foods (see **Table 9**), may be asked to reduce their intake of these foods temporarily. This strategy does not apply to patients who are consuming a poor intake and whose intake may be supplemented with additional high energy milk products.

Table 9. High phosphate foods to avoid	
Dairy Products	Milk (allow ½ pint daily). Cheese, yoghurt, milk puddings
Meat	Veal, liver
Fish	Containing edible bones, e.g. sardines, pilchards
Beverages	Ovaltine, Horlicks
Snacks	Nuts

Moderately/severely catabolic patients

During the early stages of presentation, dialytic and nutritional therapies are aimed at reducing hyperphosphataemia and hypermagnesaemia and normalizing serum calcium levels. Enteral and parenteral feeding regimens are subsequently modified to meet these demands. Since feeding is frequently associated with intracellular shifts in serum mineral levels, it is important that serum levels are monitored regularly. Serum levels of K^+, Mg^{2+} and PO_4^{2-} may decrease rapidly following feeding and require immediate supplementation to facilitate the on-going anabolic processes. Hypophosphataemia may be further exacerbated when the CRRT dialytic fluid is phosphate free but has a high glucose concentration, i.e. 2.5%.

Micronutrients[2]

Water soluble vitamins — are recommended daily to supplement reduced vitamin intakes in these patients due to poor nutritional intakes, potassium lowering cooking methods, restrictive fruit and vegetable intakes, and to replace dialytic losses.

---

[2]*NB:* Very little information is documented about vitamin and trace element requirements in ARF; most of the recommendations are derived from studies carried out on healthy populations and from patients with chronic renal failure.

Fat soluble vitamins (A, D, E, and K) — are not routinely prescribed for renal patients in the short-term. However, since it has been documented that Vitamins A, D and E are reduced in ARF, while Vitamin K is normal/elevated, a preparation containing Vitamins A, D (1,25 dihydroxycholecalciferol) and E should be considered in the long term management of these patients.

Trace elements

The high protein binding properties of trace elements and their decreased renal and gastrointestinal excretion increases the risk of toxicity in parenterally fed patients. Patients fed on oral and enteral feeds are not at risk since excess can be excreted via the gut.

NUTRITIONAL THERAPY

A large number of patients with ARF present with anorexia and weight loss. Nutritional management is aimed at developing a strategy which may include the hospital diet only and/or the addition of sip-feeds, or more intensive therapy such as enteral or parenteral nutrition.

Table 10. Sip-feeds, composition/100 mL

Name (Manufacturer)	Presentation (mL)	Energy (kcal)	Protein (g)	Na$^+$ (mmol)	K$^+$ (mmol)	Phosphorus (mg)	Indication
Ensure Plus (Abbott)	200 mL carton	150	6.25	5.2	5.13	92	1.5 kcal/mL milk type, high protein
Enlive (Abbott)	240 mL carton	125	4	0.87	0.33	9	1.25 kcal/mL juice type, low electrolyte
Fortifresh (Nutricia)	200 mL carton	155	6.5	1.87	3.85	97	1.55 kcal/mL yoghurt tasting
Provide Xtra (Fresenius)	200 mL carton	125	3.8	1.2	1.2	40	1 Kcal/mL juice type, fat free
Protein Plus (Fresenius)	200 mL carton	125	10	3.9	3.8	100	1 kcal/mL milk type, high protein
Fresubin (Fresenius)	200 mL carton	100	3.4	3.3	3.2	47	1 kcal/mL milk type
Fortisip (Nutricia)	200 mL carton	150	5	3.5–7.1	3.75	80	1.5 kcal/mL milk type
Fortimel (Nutricia)	200 mL carton	100	9.7	2.17	5.13	202	1 kcal/mL milk type, high protein

Oral Diet

Hyperkalaemic patients will require a renal diet (low potassium). Patients managing only part of the hospital food will require additional foods or sip-feeds to meet their energy and protein requirements. The most appropriate sip-feeds for patients on fluid restrictions are those which are energy dense. Alternative sip-feeds may be selected for their low electrolyte or high protein content. Patients should be encouraged to taste the product before it is prescribed. A brief list of sip-feeds is summarized in **Table 10**.

Patients who are at risk of becoming nutritionally compromised, and who are unable to achieve an adequate intake from a combination of sip-feeds and oral diet, should be considered for additional nutritional intervention i.e. nasogastric feeding.

ENTERAL FEEDING

Indications

Enteral feeding is strongly recommended in patients with a functioning gastrointestinal tract.

Choice of Feed

Commercially there are a large number of feeds available which may be administered nasogastrically or nasoduodenally (**Table 11**). Haemodialysis patients and/or fluid restricted patients will benefit

Table 11. Tube feeds, composition/100 mL							
Name (Manufacturer)	Presentation (mL)	Energy (kcal)	Protein (g)	Na^+ (mmol)	K^+ (mmol)	PO_4^{2-} (mmol)	Indication
Specialized Feeds							
Nepro (Abbott)	237 mL can	200	7	3.48	2.7	70	2 kcal/mL; low electrolyte
Two Cal HN (Abbott)	237 mL can	202	8.4	6.5	6.3	106	2 kcal/mL; high protein, high electrolyte
Suplena (Abbott)	237 mL can	201	3	3.5	2.9	79	Protein, electrolyte and fluid restricted
Standard Feeds (isotonic)							
Osmolite (Abbott)	500 mL RTH 1000 RTH	100	4	3.97	3.79	72	1 kcal/mL
Jevity (Abbott)	500 mL RTH 1000 mL RTH	100	4	3.91	3.79	72	1.4 g fibre/100 mL
Clinifeed ISO (Nestle)	375 mL can	100	2.8	1.5	3.79	45	low protein

from the use of a concentrated, high energy, low electrolyte feed. All feeds listed meet either the recommended daily allowances for vitamins, or are specially adapted for vitamin requirements in chronic renal failure. Patients dialyzing by CRRT can usually be managed on less concentrated feeds, i.e. 1 kcal/mL. Increased flexibility can be achieved by mixing feeds or adding high-energy supplements to produce a feeding regimen tailored to the patient's requirements.

Total Parenteral Nutrition (TPN)

Energy/protein requirements

The nutritional requirements for patients on parenteral nutrition are also estimated using predictive equations, as described above. Exceeding energy requirements may be harmful. Glucose-containing

Table 12. Vitamin and trace element preparations, composition/vial or ampule

Preparation (Kabi Pharmacia)	Content		Dosage
Solvito N (vial)	Vitamin B1	3.2 mg	
	Vitamin B2	3.6 mg	
	Nicotinamide	40 mg	1/day
	Vitamin B6	4.0 mg	
	Pantothenic acid	15.0 mg	
	Biotin	60 µg	
	Folic acid	0.4 mg	
	Vitamin B12	5.0 µg	
	Vitamin C	100 mg	
Vitlipid N Adult (ampule)	Retinol palmitate corresponding to retinol (A)	990 µg (3,300 iu)	1/day
	Ergocalciferol (D)	5 µg (200 iu)	
	Alpha-tocopherol (E)	9.1 mg (10 iu)	
	Phytomenadione (K)	150 µg	
Additrace (ampule)	Fe	20 µmol	2/week
	Zn	100 µmol	
	Mn	5 µmol	
	Cu	20 µmol	
	Cr	0.2 µmol	
	Se	0.4 µmol	
	Mo	0.2 µmol	
	F	50 µmol	
	I	1 µmol	

dialysis fluids used in some CRRT systems can result in excessive glucose intake, which when combined with a parenteral source may induce severe metabolic disturbances.

$$\text{A glucose intake} > \frac{4\,\text{mg CHO} \times \text{wt (kg)} \times 60\,\text{min} \times \text{number of hours patient fed}}{1000} = \text{g CHO/day}$$

is associated with excessive CO_2 production and lipogenesis. A combination of glucose and lipid as an energy source will minimize these effects. Due to decreased lipoprotein lipase activity, the amount of lipid prescribed may need adjusting if the patient becomes lipaemic. Usually, 1 g/kg/day will not exacerbate the problem.

Patients routinely receive both glucose and lipids, and a combination of essential amino acids and non-essential amino acids, in standard solutions. Since glutamine has been reported to enhance immunological function and maintain gut integrity, it is seen as an essential component of the nutritional regimen in certain centres. Patients managed on parenteral nutrition also require simultaneous feeding with token amounts of enteral feed to maintain normal intestinal structure and function.

Electrolytes

Requirements vary greatly from day to day and between patients. Daily monitoring is essential to ensure the regimen prescribed meets the patient's requirements and avoids metabolic complications.

Vitamins/trace elements

ARF patients requiring long standing nutritional support are usually prescribed standardized doses of vitamins and trace elements that contain adequate amounts of soluble vitamins and trace elements. Examples of available preparations are given in **Table 12**.

FURTHER READING

Bellomo R, Martin H, Parkin J, *et al.* (1991) Continuous arteriovenous haemodiafiltration in the critically ill; influence in major nutrient balances. *Intensive Care Medicine*; 17: 399–402

Druml W (1993) Nutritional support in acute renal failure. *Clinical Nutrition*; 12: 196–207

Elia M (1982) The effect of nitrogen and energy intake on metabolism of normal, depleted and injured man. *Clinical Nutrition*; 1: 173–192

Elia M (1990) Artificial nutritional support. *Medicine International*; 82: 3392–3396

Macfie J, Yule AG, Hill GL, *et al.* (1981) Glucose or fat as a non-protein energy source: A controlled clinical trial in gastroenteral patients requiring intravenous nutrition. *Gastroenterology*; 8: 103–107

Monson P, Mehta RL (1994) Nutrition in acute renal failure: A reappraisal for the 1990s. *Journal of Renal Nutrition*; 4: 58–77

Vitamin & essential trace elements (1986). Recommendations during intravenous nutrition theory and practice. *Proceedings of the Nutrition Society*; 45: 383–390

Appendix C

BIOCHEMISTRY

These normal values were compiled by Dr Mandy Donaldson, Mr John Meek and Miss Oonagh Prendiville, Department of Clinical Chemistry, Hammersmith Hospitals NHS Trust. Note that values vary from one laboratory to another. Please check with your own laboratory.

Blood

Analyte	Reference Ranges	Units
Alanine aminotransferase (ALT)	Female <31 Male <37	IU/L
Albumin	33–47	g/L
Alcohol	N/A	mg/100 mL
Alkaline Phosphatase	9 years–18 years 50–500 Adult 30–130	IU/L IU/L
Aluminium	<0.3	umol/L
Ammonia	<40	umol/L
Amylase	0–90	IU/L
Angiotensin converting enzyme	10–70	IU/L
Aspartate aminotransferase (AST)	Female <31 Male <37	IU/L IU/L
Beta-2- Microglobulin	1.2–2.4	mg/L
Bicarbonate	24–30 Pregnancy 18–22	mmol/L
Bilirubin (total)	2–17	umol/L
Bilirubin (conjugated)	<50	umol/L
Blood gases (arterial)		
pH	7.36–7.44	
pO2	11.7–15.3	kPa
pCO2	4.5–6.0	kPa
BE	−3 to +3	mmol/L
SB	23–28	mmol/L

Analyte	Reference Ranges	Units
C reactive protein (CRP)	<10	mg/L
Calcium	2.15–2.65	mmol/L
Chloride	95–108	mmo/L
Cholesterol	Female 3.5–6.0	mmol/L
	Male 3.5–6.5	mmol/L
Copper	12–20	umol/L
Creatine Kinase (CK)	Female <170	IU/L
	Male <200	IU/L
Creatine Kinase MB fraction (CKMB)	<6	ng/ml
Creatinine	Adult Female 55–110	umol/L
	Adult Male 60–125	umol/L
Digoxin (therapeutic)	1.0–3.0	nmol/L
Ferritin	Female 20–50 years 10–120	ug/L
	Female >50 years 20–300	ug/L
	Adult Male 20–300	ug/L
Gamma-glutamyl transferase (GGT)	Female <30	IU/L
	Male <50	IU/L
Glucose (plasma)	Fasting 3.0–6.0	mmol/L
	Non fasting 3.0–7.8	mmol/L
Glycated Haemoglobin (HbA1c)	4.3–5.5	% of total
HDL-Cholesterol (HDL)	Female 1.00–2.20	mmol/L
	Male 1.00–1.90	mmol/L
Immunoglobulin A (IgA)*	0.8–2.8	g/L
Immunoglobulin G (IgG)*	5–16	g/L
Immunoglobulin M (IgM)*	0.50–1.90	g/L
Immunoglobulin E (IgE)*	3–150	IU/ml
Iron	Female 7–27	umol/L
	Male 9–29	umol/L
Lactate	0.6–1.8	mmol/L
Lactate dehydrogenase (LDH)	120–500	IU/L
LDL- cholesterol	2.0–5.0	mmol/L
Lead (whole blood)	<0.6	umol/L
Lithium (therapeutic)	0.5–1.0	mmol/L
Magnesium	0.7–1.0	mmol/L
Osmolality	285–295	mmol/Kg
Oxalate	1.0–3.0	umol/L
Paracetamol (toxic)	>1.5	mmol/L
Parathyroid hormone (PTH)	1.1–6.8	pmol/L
Phosphate (inorganic)	0.8–1.40	mmol/L
Potassium	3.8–5.5	mmol/L
Salicylate (toxic)	>2.5	mmol/L

Analyte	Reference Ranges	Units
Sodium	135–145	mmol/L
Total cholesterol:HDL ratio	Ideal <5	g/L
Total Protein	64–83	g/L
Transferrin	1.5–3.0	g/L
Transferrin saturation index (TFI)	20–45	%
Triglycerides	Female <1.8	mmol/L
	Male <2.20	mmol/L
TSH	0.3–3.8	mU/L
Urea	Female 2.5–7.0	mmol/L
	Male 3.0–8.0	mmol/l
Uric acid	Female 0.14–0.37	mmol/L
	Male 0.18–0.44	mmol/l
Vitamin D (25-Hydroxycholecalciferol)	7–50	mg/mL
Zinc	11–18	umol/L

Urine

Analyte	Reference Ranges	Units
Albumin/creatinine ratio	0–3.0	mg/mmol creat
Calcium	Male 2.5–10	mmol/24 h
	Female 2.5–9.0	mmol/24 h
Calcium/creatinine ratio	0.10–0.32	mmol/mmol creat
Citrate	<0.5	mmol/24 h
Copper	<1	umol/24 h
Creatinine	11.5–13.5	mmol/24 h
Creatinine clearance	80–140	mL/min
	Pregnancy 120–160	
Cystine	<0.13	mmol/24 h
Magnesium	6–10	mmol/24 h
Microalbumin	0–30	mg/L
Oxalate/Glycollate	0.1–0.46	mmol/24 h
Phosphate	16–32	mmol/24 h
Potassium	60–80	mmol/24 h
Sodium	150–250	mmol/24 h
Total Protein	<0.2	g/24 h
	pregnancy <0.3	
Urea	350–450	mmol/24 h
Uric Acid	<2.4	mmol/24 h

Miscellaneous

Analyte	Reference Ranges	Units
Cerebrospinal fluid		
Glucose	Approximately 60% blood level	mmol/L
IgG	<40	mg/L
Protein	0.15–0.45	g/L
Lactate	1.2–2.1	mmol/L
Angiotensin Converting Enzyme	0.1–0.4	IU/L
Pleural fluid		
Protein	Exudate >30	g/L
	Transudate <30	g/L

HAEMATOLOGY

Analyte	Reference Ranges	Units
Haemoglobin	Male 13.0–16.8	g/dL
	Female 11.5–14.9	g/dL
Red blood cell	$4.3–5.7 \times 10^{12}$	
Haematocrit	0.391–0.502	ratio
Mean corpuscular volume	82.0–98.0	fL
Mean corpuscular haemoglobin	26.7–33.0	pg
RDW	38.1–58.3	fL
Platelets	120–400	$\times 10^9$/L
White blood cells	3.20–11.0	$\times 10^9$/L
Neutrophil number	1.90–7.7	$\times 10^9$/L
Lymphocyte number	0.30–2.80	$\times 10^9$/L
Monocyte number	0.10–0.90	$\times 10^9$/L
Eosinophil number	0–0.4	$\times 10^9$/L
Basophil number	0–0.1	$\times 10^9$/L
ESR	<20	mm/h
Serum B12	200–900	pg/mL
Serum folate	1.8–14.0	ng/mL
Red cell folate	110–700	ng/mL
Coagulation		
Reticulocyte %	0.79–1.81	%
Absolute Reticulocyte count	20–85	$\times 10^9$/L
High fluorescence reticulocyte %	0.0–2.5	%
Prothrombin time	9.6–11.6	seconds

Analyte	Reference Ranges	Units
Activated partial thromboplastin time	24–32	seconds
Thrombin time	15–19	seconds
International normalized ratio	2.0–6.0	
Fibrinogen	1.8–3.6	g/L
Factor VIII	0.45–1.58	u/mL
Von Willebrand Factor	0.5–2	u/mL
Antithrombin III	0.75–1.25	u/mL
Protein C	0.7–1.4	u/mL
Protein S function	0.6–1.35	u/mL
Activated protein C resistance	2–4	ratio
Russell viper venom time	35–50	seconds
Haptoglobin	52–224	mg/dL

HAEMODYNAMIC VALUES AND DERIVED VARIABLES

Normal Values

Mean arterial pressure (MAP)	70–105 (1/3 systolic BP + 2/3 diastolic BP)	mmHg
Stroke volume (SV)	70–100	mL
Cardiac output (CO)	4–6	L/min
Right atrial pressure	0–5	mmHg
Right ventricular pressure	20–25/0–5	mmHg
Pulmonary artery pressure	20–25/10–15	mmHg
Pulmonary artery wedge pressure	6–12	mmHg
Mixed venous oxygen saturation (SvO_2)	70–75	%

Derived Variables

Variable	Calculation	Normal Range
Cardiac index (CI)	$\dfrac{CO}{\text{Body surface area}}$	2.5–3.5 L/min/m^2
Stroke index (SI)	$\dfrac{SV}{\text{Body surface area}}$	40–60 mL/ m^2
Systemic vascular resistance (SVR)	$\dfrac{MAP - RAP \times 79.9}{CO}$	960–1400 dyn.sec/cm^5
Pulmonary vascular resistance (PVR)	$\dfrac{MPAP - PAWP \times 79.9}{CO}$	25–125 dyn.sec/cm^5

Variable	Calculation	Normal Range
Oxygen delivery (DO_2)	$0.134 \times CO \times Hb_a \times SaO_2$	950–1300 mL/min
Oxygen consumption (VO_2)	$0.134 \times CO \times (Hb_a \times SaO_2 - Hb_v \times SvO_2)$	180–320 mL/min
Oxygen extraction ratio	$1 - \dfrac{SaO_2 - SvO_2}{SaO_2}$	0.25–0.3

INDEX

www.ingramcontent.com/pod-product-compliance
Lightning Source LLC
Chambersburg PA
CBHW081214220326
41598CB00037B/6772